STERN'S GUIDE TO THE CRUISE VACATION

2000 EDITION

STERN'S

GUIDE TO THE

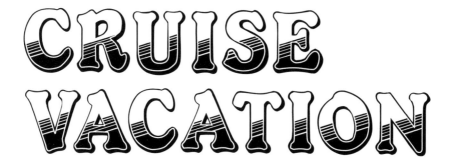

CRUISE
VACATION

Steven B. Stern

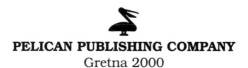

PELICAN PUBLISHING COMPANY

Gretna 2000

First edition, 1974
Second edition, 1984
First Pelican edition, 1988
Fourth edition, 1991
Fifth edition, 1994
Sixth edition, 1995
Seventh edition, 1997
Eighth edition, 1998
Ninth edition, 1999
Tenth edition, 1999

Library of Congress Cataloging-in-Publication Data

Stern, Steven B.
    [Guide to the cruise vacation]
    Stern's guide to the cruise vacation / Steven B. Stern—10th ed., [2000 ed.]
        p. cm.
    Includes index.
    ISBN 1-56554-681-4 (pbk. : alk. paper)
    1. Ocean travel Guidebooks. I. Title. II. Title: Guide to the cruise vacation
G153.4.S75 1999b
910'.2'02—dc21   99-32984
                                                                        CIP

Manufactured in the United States of America
Published by Pelican Publishing Company, Inc.
1000 Burmaster Street, Gretna, Louisiana 70053

Contents

Preface

Over the past thirty-five years, I have had the pleasure of experiencing some marvelous vacations and unforgettable moments aboard cruise ships. I have seen the cruise industry grow from a formal haven for the very rich to a fun-filled, exciting, bargain holiday for a broad cross section of our population. Every year greater numbers of travelers are wisely spending their vacation dollars on a cruise. It has been estimated that the cruise passenger market has increased from a half-million to close to eight million people during the last twenty-five years, and is predicted to rise to ten million with the turn of the century.

This guide has been written to familiarize those who have never encountered the delights of the open sea with what they can expect from a cruise vacation, as well as to assist seasoned sailors in making intelligent selections for their next ship and cruise grounds. Chapter 11 offers a detailed description of each major cruise line and the vessels of its fleet. Included are overall ratings for each ship (Ribbon Awards) as well as a description of medical facilities, photographs, sample menus, and daily programs for each cruise line. Chapter 14 summarizes the overall ratings (Ribbon Awards) and goes on to rate ships from each major cruise line in eleven specific categories.

The book also includes a description of the various cruise grounds and ports of call, setting forth points of interest, restaurants, beaches, sports facilities, and what you can cover with only limited time ashore. In Chapter 10 the airlines and various classes of travel are evaluated with helpful hints on saving money and selecting the best flight. Chapter 12 describes the most expensive, top-luxury suites on vessels that offer such accommodations, and chapter 13 is devoted to the emerging, popular concept of alternative dining venues aboard ship.

Author's Note

Over the past decade numerous ships have been removed from service or purchased by other cruise lines, and several cruise lines have merged, been acquired by competitors, or ceased operations. This trend should continue into the new millennium, and some of the ships and cruise lines listed in this edition may be acquired by other cruise lines, sold, receive new names, or cease operations before next year. Therefore, we have provided a history of each cruise ship in Chapter 11 so that our readers can keep track of and evaluate the genealogy of each vessel.

New Ships Coming on Line

With the ever-increasing growth of the cruise industry, the major cruise lines are continuously building new vessels both to expand their fleets and to replace older ships. During the period extending from summer 1999 to the end of 2000, the following new vessels are scheduled to enter service:

Carnival Cruise Line
   102,383-ton *Carnival Triumph*—July 1999
   102,383-ton *Carnival Victory*—August 2000

Costa Cruises:
   82,000-ton *Costa Atlantica*—2000

Celebrity Cruises:
   85,000-ton *Millennium 1*—June 2000

Disney Cruise Line:
   83,338-ton *Disney Wonder*—1999

Hapag-Lloyd:
   28,000-ton *Europa*—August 1999

Holland America:
   63,000-ton *Volendam*—August 1999
   63,000-ton *Zaandam*—November 1999

Norwegian Cruise Line:
   78,000-ton *Norwegian Sky*—August 1999

P & O
   76,000-ton *Aurora*—May 2000

Princess Cruises:
   77,000-ton *Ocean Princess*—December 1999

Radisson Seven Seas Cruises:
   30,000-ton *Navigator*—August 1999

Renaissance Cruises:
   30,200-ton *R-3*—June 1999
   30,200-ton *R-4*—October 1999

Royal Caribbean International:
- 136,000-ton *Voyager of the Seas*—November 1999
- 136,000-ton *Explorer of the Seas*—November 2000

Silversea Cruises
- 25,000-ton *TBN*—July 2000

Star Cruises
- 76,800-ton *Superstar Virgo*—July 1999

Star Clippers
- 5,000-ton *Royal Clipper*—November 1999

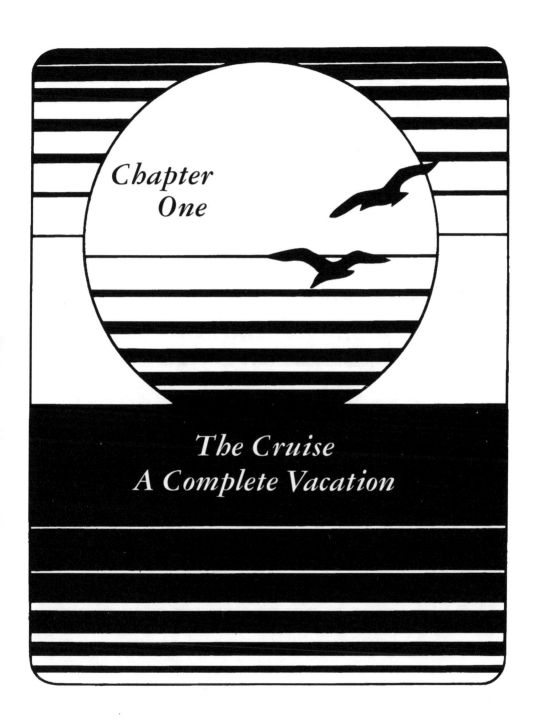

Chapter One

*The Cruise
A Complete Vacation*

An Introduction to Cruising (with four case studies)

Lively and exciting, yet serene and relaxing; romantic and glamorous, yet interesting and broadening; elegant and luxurious, yet casual and economical; gregarious and convivial, yet intimate and private. All of these descriptions, although antithetical at first glance, in fact apply to the cruise vacation. A cruise is a truly unique travel experience—the ultimate escape from reality that does not lend itself to a simple definition.

Taking a cruise vacation is partaking in a varied program of exciting activities with interesting and congenial fellow passengers from diverse walks of life. It may be indulging in the finest gourmet cuisine prepared by Continental chefs and impeccably served by an experienced crew who cater to your every whim. It is unwinding and relaxing in comfortable, posh surroundings with an impressive variety of facilities and modern conveniences. It is traveling to exotic ports of call, viewing breathtaking scenery, and exploring historic points of interest. It is a cool dip in the pool, breakfast in bed, a relaxing sauna and massage, moonlit walks on deck, costume balls, movies, bridge tournaments, games, entertainment, cocktail parties, shopping, sunning, dancing, romance, companionship, enlightenment—and, best of all, this can be yours for less than you would spend on any comparable vacation.

Although the price of any cruise will vary on the basis of your accommodations, economy-conscious travelers who book minimum cabins can obtain the best possible buy for their vacation dollar. If you reside in the Southeast, for example, you can take a seven-day cruise from Miami stopping at four Caribbean ports for as little as $950. If you live in the Midwest, you can purchase an "air-sea package" (offered by numerous cruise lines), fly to Puerto Rico, and cruise to South America plus five additional Caribbean islands in a seven-day period for as little as $1,200, including your room, all meals and entertainment, round-trip air fare, and transfers to and from the airport and ship. To duplicate these trips—flying from place to place by plane and frequenting restaurants and hotels with food and accommodations comparable to those found on the ship—would easily cost twice as much.

On a land vacation, you will have a greater opportunity for in-depth sightseeing and pursuing more time-consuming activities, such as golf and fishing. However, to visit as many varied places and to engage in activities similar to those offered on a cruise would require you to be constantly on the move. One of the most unique characteristics of the cruise vacation is that everything is conveniently located aboard ship. You need not run around seeking out restaurants, nightclubs, hairdressers, laundries, or companionship—it is all right there. Additionally, you are afforded the opportunity to visit many glamorous and diverse foreign countries without the necessity of lugging around heavy baggage, waiting in line at several airports, and constantly changing hotels. After you have spent a busy day in port sightseeing, swimming, and shopping, you can return to your friendly, familiar floating hotel to dine, drink, dance, and be entertained before you finally retire to awake the following morning already delivered to your next exciting port of call.

Cruising has grown impressively in popularity over the past few decades. New modern luxury liners are being built, and older vessels are being remodeled to meet the ever-increasing lure of travelers to the high seas. This demand can be attributed, perhaps, to the fact that today's cruise offers something for just about everyone—young and old, singles and couples, adults and children, gourmets and gourmands, the gregarious and the inhibited, sun-worshippers and those who prefer indoor relaxation. The rich can reserve the most expensive suite aboard and ensconce themselves in the lap of luxury, and the not-so-rich often can enjoy the same food, entertainment, and public facilities while booking a less expensive cabin. Those who desire recreation can participate in a diverse range of events and activities around the clock, while those who wish to relax can sit back and let the experienced staff and crew serve and entertain them. The athletic types can join the exercise class, work out in the gym, jog around the deck, and on shore can swim, play tennis, or catch a fast eighteen holes of golf; while the spectator types can watch a movie, attend a lecture, or view the nightly entertainment. The working person can find a cruise that coincides with his or her one-, two-, or three-week vacation, while retired persons can opt to cruise for three or four months around the world.

Four Case Studies

John and Martha

John, a bookkeeper from Omaha, Nebraska, and his wife, Martha, who have just seen the last of their three children graduate from college, are looking forward to letting loose and having the time of their lives on a very special cruise. They get up early the first morning at sea to watch the sunrise while enjoying some coffee, juice, and rolls on deck. After a few deep knee bends and stretches at the exercise class, they are ready for a hearty breakfast in the dining room with fresh pineapple and melon, smoked salmon, a cheese omelet, sausages, fried potatoes, toast, and pastries.

Following breakfast, they participate in a Ping-Pong tournament and deck games at the pool, followed by some trap shooting and a free salsa lesson. After a cool dip in the pool, they are ready for an elegant lunch in the dining room with an opportunity to try some exotic foreign dishes. Sunning and swimming fill up the early hours of the afternoon, still leaving time for the duplicate bridge tournament. A little workout on the exercycle at the gym, followed by a sauna and massage, helps John work off a few of those piña coladas he was sipping all afternoon. He then showers and shaves while Martha is having her hair set at the beauty shop.

John and Martha don their fancy clothes in time to attend the captain's cocktail party and practice the new dance steps they learned earlier. Then comes the "welcome aboard" dinner in the dining room, complete from caviar to crêpes suzette. Martha wants to play a few games of bingo before the evening variety show, and John tries his luck at blackjack and roulette in the casino.

After the evening's entertainment in the main lounge, a few cold cuts, cheeses, and desserts at the midnight buffet just hit the spot; and then it is time to go up to the discotheque to swing with the night owls into the wee hours. Following a leisurely stroll around the deck, our active couple is ready for bed. It was never like this in Omaha!

Michael and Vivian

Michael, an overworked New York attorney, and his wife, Vivian, a harassed primary-school teacher, never had a chance to take a trip when they got married last June. This cruise represents a long-overdue honeymoon. They start their first day at sea by enjoying a leisurely breakfast in bed, followed by some quiet hours soaking up the sun on deck. One shuffleboard game, a short swim in the pool, and a stroll up to the bridge are just enough excitement to help them work up an appetite for a delicious buffet lunch served on deck by the pool.

A little more sun, a few chapters of a good book, a first-run movie in the theater, some tea and cakes on the promenade deck, and our honeymooners are ready for rest and relaxation in their cabin before dressing for the evening. They elect to drink the bottle of champagne their travel agent sent them while enjoying some hot hors d'oeuvres in the lounge; then it's off to the dining room for an eight-course gourmet meal. After the evening entertainment, Michael and Vivian have the first opportunity since their wedding to dance to a romantic orchestra. A chance to gaze at the stars on deck caps off the night. What new marriage couldn't use a day like this?

Joan and Ron

Joan, who works in a Miami insurance office, wants to make the most out of her one remaining week of vacation time. She wants to relax and visit some new places, and she wouldn't object to meeting a tall, dark, handsome stranger if he came along. On the first day at sea, she misses breakfast in the dining room but enjoys some juice, croissants, and coffee served on the deck for the late sleepers. Off comes the cover-up, revealing her new bikini. She takes a stroll around the pool to let all those who are interested know she is aboard.

The eleven o'clock dance class is a must, since it affords her a controlled atmosphere for meeting other passengers. At the class she meets two women from California, and they decide to sit at the same table for lunch. The understanding maître d' arranges a large table for singles, where Joan and her two new friends are joined by another woman traveling alone and four eligible bachelors. The group decides to spend the afternoon at the pool swimming and playing backgammon. Several of the other singles come over to watch, and by the afternoon "singles-only" cocktail party, Joan has already met most of the other single passengers aboard ship.

Ron, one of the eligible bachelors at Joan's table, is an advertising executive from Boston who is recently divorced and in search of some feminine companionship. He initially decides that he and Joan are basically looking for different things; however, her popularity with other single female passengers indicates that she is a good mixer and a potential source of introductions. By participating in the deck games and making frequent trips to the numerous bars, Ron manages to meet a few more women, and those he missed show up at the "singles-only" cocktail party. By dinnertime, he has three or four interesting prospects for the evening. He decides to have a drink with Joan and her friends before dinner; however, he passes up the planned evening entertainment and goes straight to the discotheque where he can dance with all of the other young women he has met.

After dinner, Joan prefers to see the variety show, browse through the shops, and try the "one-arm bandits" before joining the other singles at the discotheque at midnight. By the time she arrives, Ron has already run through a half-dozen possibilities and decided that he really can't relate to any of them. Ron asks Joan to dance, and both feel a strange new chemistry that wasn't evident earlier that evening. Joan and Ron won't give permission to print the rest of the story; therefore, you can select your own ending.

Scotty and Jamie

Scotty, age eight, and his big sister Jamie, age fourteen, could hardly sleep the night before their mom and dad took them on their first seven-day Caribbean cruise. By sharing a four-berth cabin with their parents, it only cost an extra $375 apiece to bring them along.

The first afternoon aboard ship was exciting. The band was playing, passengers were partying and throwing colorful streamers overboard, and crew members were passing out drinks and sandwiches. Upon arriving at their cabin, Scotty was delighted to find that he had been assigned an upper berth, but Jamie pouted when her dad told her that the other top bunk was hers.

After the ship set sail, Scotty migrated to the electronic game room, where he met numerous other youngsters around his age. After a while, he and a new friend went up on deck to play Ping-Pong and shuffleboard by the pool. At five o'clock, there was a get-together at the disco for teens, which Jamie anxiously attended. A member of the ship's social staff outlined the special events and programs that would be offered throughout the cruise for the teenage set. At the same time, there was a similar meeting for the pre-teens at the ice-cream emporium. Here Scotty learned about the daily movies, bingo, deck sports, pool games, scavenger hunts, masquerade balls, talent shows, and "Coke-tail" parties that would dominate his days aboard ship.

After dinner, Scotty and his new friend went to the movies, followed by pizza and a soda in the special pizzeria restaurant. Jamie attended the first-night-aboard party in the show lounge, where she was introduced to the cruise staff and took part in the audience participation games. After the party, she went to the disco, which was already packed to the rafters with enthusiastic young passengers getting to know each other.

Days ashore were especially enjoyable. The varied ports of call offered pristine white-sand beaches, water sports, horseback riding, tennis, historic sights, cute souvenir shops, and scenic drives. Mealtimes were also great fun. Each evening, the dining room was decorated in a different ethnic theme and the attentive waiters were dressed to blend in. Scotty was able to order hamburgers and hot dogs for lunch and a big, fat steak and fries for dinner. Jamie, an aspiring gourmet, elected to sample the more esoteric offerings.

On the last evening aboard, the lights were turned down and all the waiters paraded around the dining room carrying baked Alaskas with sparklers while the passengers sang "Auld Lang Syne." The seven days had passed too quickly and our two young sailors were very sad the morning the ship sailed back into its homeport. They had visited exciting and different islands, made many new friends, and participated in numerous good times. As for Mom and Dad . . . they showed up at dinner, bedtime, and when the youngsters needed quarters for the game machines. When Scotty and Jamie were asked how they liked the cruise, their joint answer was, "Awesome!"

The remaining chapters of this book are designed to familiarize you with the different aspects of the cruise vacation. Chapter 2, entitled "Getting Ready for the Cruise," starts by detailing how to go about planning and booking a cruise and proceeds to set forth objective standards for selecting a ship. The chapter goes on to delineate the factors that will determine the cost of your cabin and list the items you will want to be certain to bring along. Chapter 3 describes your day at sea, depicting the customary facilities found aboard ship as well as the typical program of round-the-clock activities. The dining experience is then portrayed with descriptions of the numerous meals and varieties of cuisine as well as some suggestions relating to multiple sittings and tipping. Chapter 4 analyzes the pros and cons of cruising for singles. The desirability and cost of bringing along your children are explored in chapter 5, together with a description of the events and facilities aboard ships that are designed specifically for their interests. In chapter 6, you will find a summary of the various cruise areas and highlights of the most popular cruise stops, with suggestions on what you can see and do during your day in port. Chapters 7, 8, and 9, respectively, describe where to go in each port to swim, play tennis, and jog.

Chapter 10 evaluates the major airlines, the equipment, and differences in the various classes of travel and goes on to make suggestions on obtaining the cheapest air fares. Chapter 11 includes a description of every major cruise line and cruise ship, including my overall ratings (in the form of Ribbon Awards), photographs, sample menus, and daily programs. Chapter 12 describes the most expensive, top-luxury suites on vessels that offer such accommodations, and chapter 13 describes alternative dining specialty restaurants that recently have been added to many ships. Chapter 14 summarizes my Ribbon Awards and goes on to evaluate sample ships of each line in eleven specific categories.

The growing concern of prospective cruisers as to available medical facilities on the various ships is covered in this edition. An analysis of medical care at sea is discussed in chapter two, and the facilities, equipment, and personnel available aboard each ship (as represented by the cruise lines) is included in chapter 11.

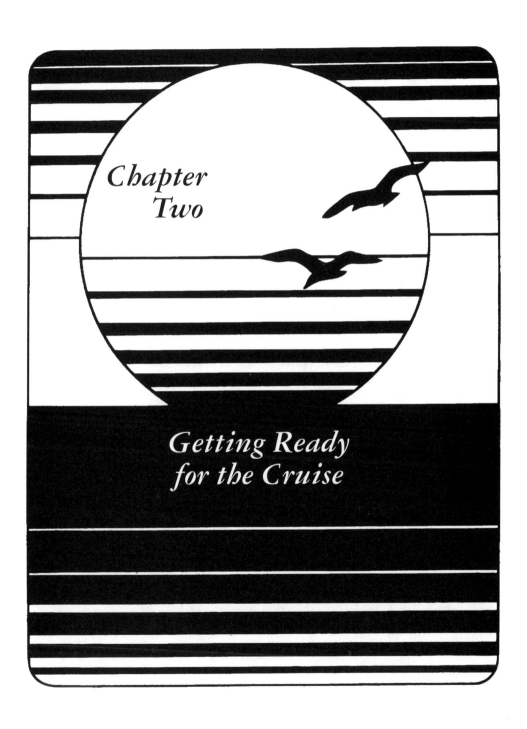

Chapter
Two

Getting Ready
for the Cruise

Planning and Booking a Cruise

When planning a cruise, you must consider a number of factors. First of all, you must decide at what time of year you will be taking your cruise vacation. If you choose to travel in the late fall or winter, you may prefer cruising in the warmer climate and calmer waters of the Caribbean, South Pacific, Indian Ocean, or Far East. Transatlantic crossings at this time of year can be a bit rough for all but the hardiest seadogs.

On the other hand, a late spring, summer, or early fall cruise in the Mediterranean to the Greek Islands, Turkish Coast, and Middle East or in the Baltic, North Sea, or up to the fjords, can afford a very interesting opportunity to mingle with passengers from other countries. Transatlantic crossings at these times of year are not necessarily rough, but they are not recommended for your first exploration of the sea. Be aware that ships crossing the Atlantic by the southern route will encounter better weather, permitting more days on deck than those ships taking the northern route.

After you have decided upon the time of the year to go and the general geographic area to see, the next step is to find out which ships will be cruising in that area on the dates you have available. (If you are set on cruising on a specific ship, then you will be sailing at any given time to any given place, I recommend that you consult a copy of the *Official Steamship Guide International.* This magazine is subscribed to by most travel agencies, is updated seasonally, and contains a complete list of prospective cruises for all ships for the upcoming twelve-month period as soon as the line makes the dates public. *Ocean Cruise News, Portholes, Cruise Business News,* and *Cruise Travel* magazines are periodicals that list prospective cruises and include articles describing ships, ports of call, and updates on what is going on in the cruise industry.

Of course, you can check with your travel agent. In the seventies and early eighties, I found that many of the employees at travel agencies had rarely, if ever, sailed on a ship and did not specialize in cruise vacations; therefore, they could not do much more than furnish you with a few brochures that they may have had on hand. Fortunately, with the growing popularity of cruises, this situation has changed, and most of the better agencies today are staffed with employees who have expertise in this area. They may also participate in familiarization trips offered by the cruise lines. However, be sure that the advice you are getting is firsthand. The fact that one of the agent's other customers had a ball on a banana freighter that hit some out-of-the-way ports in the South Pacific does not mean that you will also enjoy this type of cruise.

Over the past few years, numerous travel agencies that specialize in cruising have sprung up. Frequently they can offer deep-discount tickets due to prior arrangements with some of the cruise lines. You will want to check the cruise/discount-fare advertisements in the travel section of your Sunday newspaper, as well as the various cruise periodicals. Once you have cruised on a particular line, you will be placed on its mailing list and be provided from time to time with brochures offering special discounted sailings.

When consulting the available guides, you will also have to consider the length of time you have for your vacation. If you have only a week or ten days, seek out a ship with a correspondingly shorter itinerary. However, if you have two weeks or more, you can also consider the longer cruises.

Now that you have traced the ships that are sailing in the geographic area of your choice during the period you have scheduled for your vacation, you will want to study the credentials and offerings of each of these vessels. Do you prefer French food, Italian service, Scandinavian *joie de vivre,* Dutch hospitality, or British efficiency? Do you wish to storm seven ports in seven days, or do you prefer spending three or four relaxing days at sea? Do you desire the intimacy of a small ship, or is a large superliner your cup of tea? These are the questions that you must ask, and the following section of this chapter, as well as chapters 11 and 14, are devoted to helping you arrive at your decision.

After you have finally selected a vessel, it is desirable to include a second and even a third choice, for now you must determine whether space on the ship you desire is still available. A later section of this chapter on "Costs and Your Cabin" will point out the factors to be considered in choosing accommodations.

When booking reservations for a cabin, you can either go to your travel agent or directly to the cruise line office in your locality. Booking through a travel agent generally has the advantage of having someone else obtain your tickets, make all arrangements, provide you with necessary instructions, and maybe even throw in a bottle of the bubbly when you arrive on ship. However, if your agent tells you that the space you desire is not available, do not give up. Either call another agent or contact the line directly, request that you be wait-listed, and explain how you are dying to cruise on their ships but can go only at a certain time and for a certain price. Call them up every week or so to check on whether there has been a cancellation. Persistence may pay off because vacationers often change their minds, and there are usually a great number of last-minute cancellations.

To play it safe, you can accept a more expensive room, for example, and ask to be wait-listed for the first cheaper one that becomes available. I do not know for a fact what procedures the various lines follow; however, it is possible that some cruise lines will sell a room that becomes available to a new customer rather than to one who has already accepted another room and has been wait-listed. Therefore, if you are set on obtaining specific accommodations, you may have a better chance if you do not accept a substitute; however, you may also be left behind. Here again it will pay off to contact the numerous travel agencies that specialize in cruising since they may have an inventory of pre-purchased accommodations or a little extra clout with the cruise line.

As you would expect, it is more difficult to book cruises for holidays such as Christmas, New Year's, Easter, Thanksgiving, Memorial Day, the Fourth of July, and Labor Day. Everyone wants to go away at these times, and you must book far in advance (as much as six months to a year for a Christmas or New Year's cruise on some ships).

Selecting a Ship

What kind of ship you select will depend upon your feelings about people, food, relaxation, activity, aesthetics, and so on. Whereas one reader may be delighted by a ship that offers a diverse Continental menu of gourmet delights, another may feel dissatisfied because the kitchen staff cannot prepare a thick, juicy sirloin steak. One couple may fall in love with a cruise ship because of the super time they had dancing to good music every evening and taking part in a masquerade ball, but another couple may feel that the same ship was not a good buy because it offered no "big-name" entertainment. The fact that any particular ship may appeal to one does not mean it will appeal to another. Also, the food and service on any given ship can vary from time to time, just as it does in a restaurant or hotel. A change in chefs, for example, can make a big difference.

How, then, can you compare ships and make a selection? To a certain extent, you will rely on the opinions of others. You are encouraged to discuss this with your travel agent as well as with friends (holding similar interests and tastes) who have cruised on the ships you are considering. Acquire all the brochures and other promotional matter printed by the cruise lines. These pamphlets usually contain pictures of the public rooms and cabins, prices, enumeration of facilities, description of ports of call, and a deck plan. If your travel agent does not have the relevant brochure for the ship in which you are interested, you can write directly to the line. Do not hesitate to contact the line about any specific bit of information you may wish to obtain.

To assist you further with your selection, detailed descriptions, per diem fares, and ratings for most cruise ships, as well as photos, sample menus, and activity programs, appear in chapters 11 and 14 of this book.

The following is an analysis of many of the factors that I recommend you consider in comparing potential cruises:

Ports of Call

Check to see at which ports the ship will be calling and then review what each of those ports has to offer (see analysis of ports in chapter 6). Do you prefer spending your days ashore shopping, sunning at a beautiful beach, exploring archeological ruins, hiking through natural scenery, or visiting historic museums? Be certain that the ship stops at a port that will afford you an opportunity to pursue the activities you enjoy.

When sailing the Caribbean, St. Thomas, St. Croix, and Curaçao are considered to have the most diversified shopping, with the best bargains in French perfume being found in Martinique, Guadeloupe, and St. Martin. The finest beaches for swimming and sunning are found in the Grand Caymans, Bermuda, St. Thomas, St. Croix, St. John, Virgin Gorda, Aruba, Barbados, Antigua, Anguilla, St. Martin, Grenada, the Bahamas, and Cozumel. Archeology buffs will want to visit Guatemala and the ports of the Yucatán. Those wishing to tour historical points of interest, museums, and monuments will find the best offerings in Caracas, Puerto Rico, and Martinique.

Although the beaches of the Mediterranean, Baltic, and North Sea don't compare with those of the Caribbean, the offering of historic points of interest, art, museums, and shopping is far superior in the Mediterranean and Northern European ports. Today it is possible to cruise almost anywhere in the world, including such faraway areas as the South Seas, the Far East, Australia, Africa, the Indian Ocean, and even Antarctica.

As mentioned earlier, you will want to determine how many ports are on the itinerary of the cruises you may be considering. For example, some ships visit as many as five ports on a seven-day cruise, whereas others stop at only one or two. Do you prefer a busy itinerary where you are in port almost every day, or do you prefer spending the majority of your days on the open sea?

Next, you should check out the period of time the ship is docked at each port. Too often a ship may be in port for so short a period that there is not time to visit the places you have mapped out. For example, several ships stop in Montego Bay for only five hours, not leaving sufficient time to drive to Dunn's Falls or take the jungle river raft ride down the Martha Brae. Other ships dock at San Juan only in the later afternoon and evening to permit passengers to gamble, while leaving insufficient time to explore the island. There are still other ships that include in their brochures "ports of call" where the vessels dock for merely an hour to pick up passengers. Certain Mediterranean cruises drop anchor at Gibraltar, Cannes, Genoa, and Naples to receive embarking passengers but don't stop long enough to permit any exploration. You should carefully analyze the itinerary of each ship you are considering.

Dining

As pointed out in detail in the next chapter, the dining experience aboard ship is one of the highlights of the cruise. Therefore, a good deal of consideration should be given to the fare offered by the different lines. Although many ships rate far above the average restaurant in this department, the types and varieties of victuals do vary from ship to ship.

Most of the lunch and dinner menus offer an interesting assortment of foods with an emphasis on ethnic dishes that are representative of the nationality of the dining room staff and chef. Thus, French cuisine will be most prevalent on the French Cruise Lines (riverboats) and *Club Med II;* Italian dishes on Costa and Princess lines; Greek specialties on Royal Olympic Cruises; German offerings on the Euro-Lloyd/Hapag-Lloyd, Deutsche Seereederei, and K D River Cruises of Europe lines; Japanese food on Crystal Cruises; and a mixed Continental menu on most of the other lines. If you require kosher food, baby food, or have any special dietary restrictions, you should check with the ship line in advance to determine whether the required foods will be available. An emerging concept is the inclusion of an alternative specialty restaurant in addition to the main dining room, which affords passengers an opportunity to break up the nightly routine and opt for a more intimate dining experience. *Radisson Diamond* features an indoor/outdoor Italian restaurant atop ship with strolling musicians; and ships of Crystal Cruises offer both Italian and Asian specialty restaurants. The *Vistafjord, Disney Magic, Song of Flower, Grand Princess, Silverwind, Silver Cloud, R-1, R-2,* and the *Rotterdam* VI have added Italian specialty restaurants, and many ships, including those of the Costa and Princess lines, have separate pizza parlors as well. Casual, alternative-dining restaurants are featured on all of the newer Princess, Carnival, Renaissance, RCI vessels, and the *Marco Polo.* Wine, caviar, and espresso bars are rapidly being added to many of the newer vessels.

In chapter 11, you will find sample menus from ships representing the various lines. Because the menus tend to be similar for ships of the same line, these samples should give you some idea of what to expect. (*Caution:* You will see steak and lobster offered on almost all of the menus, but the quality may vary radically. Beef shipped from the United States and lobster caught off the coast of Maine may be quite a bit more tender than beef picked up in Mexico or lobsters caught in the Caribbean.) In addition, food and dining room service often will be superior on the flagship of each line. Generally, the chefs and waiters earn the privilege of serving on the flagship by working their way up the ladder on the other vessels. The ratings for dining quality found in chapter 14 may assist you in comparing the ships of the various cruise lines.

Service

The quality of service rendered by the dining room staff, the cabin stewards, and social staff can significantly affect your enjoyment of the cruise. A pleasant, efficient waiter can perk up a mediocre meal; an understanding and helpful cabin steward can minimize the inconvenience of a small or otherwise inadequate cabin; and a tactful, perceptive social director can bring together people of common interests and add an additional dimension to your vacation.

Naturally, the quality of service varies from line to line and even among ships of the same line. I have found that ships with Italian dining room and cabin staffs offer the best all-around service. These waiters and stewards seem to have received the best training, maintain the best attitudes, and are the most anxious to please. I found the mixed European crew on Crystal, Radisson Seven Seas, Silversea, Celebrity Cruises, Princess, Renaissance, Seabourn, Costa, and the *Seabourn Goddesses, Vistafjord,* and *Seabourn Sun* to be superior in these areas. The Greek ships tend to economize and overwork their crews, with the obvious results. Some of the English and French crews often seem disenchanted with their lot; however, this is usually the exception and not the rule. Those ships using mixed service crews from the Caribbean islands, South America, India, Asia, and Mexico do so as an economy factor. Unfortunately, these people do not have the training or "know-how" of most of the European crews. The Holland America and other lines' use of Indonesian and Filipino waiters and room stewards has proved to be somewhat of a mixed bag— some cruisers find them charming and attentive, while others have found the service mediocre because of the serious language problem and lack of experience. The all-American crews with American Hawaii Cruises and The Delta Queen Steamboat Company were often inexperienced. The nationality of the dining room and cabin crews is indicated in chapter 11.

Service may vary from one year to the next on the same ship, especially when a line is striving to improve this area. Therefore, obtain knowledgeable opinions on the standard of service for any ships you are considering.

Medical Care at Sea

Considering the millions of people of all ages and levels of health who cruise each year to exotic and remote areas where access to state-of-the-art hospitals and well-trained physicians may be limited, one must conclude that the availability and quality of medical facilities and personnel aboard ship should be a major consideration when selecting a particular vessel.

Certainly, a significant segment of the cruising population that opts for longer cruises to more out-of-the-way destinations is retired and getting on in years. Although when encountering an emergency at home, these senior citizens can call 911 and be rushed to a modern hospital, when they find themselves in the middle of the Pacific or docked at a primitive port in New Guinea, the best they can hope for is a decent medical facility and physician aboard ship. Many younger passengers have infirmities that could require special medical attention, while others may suffer accidental injuries either on the ship or during port explorations. Here again, the only available emergency equipment and supplies may be at the ship's medical facility.

Therefore, the experience and specialties of a ship's physician and nurses, the technological equipment and pharmaceuticals available, as well as the x-ray, operating, and emergency facilities should receive as much consideration by older cruisers and those with pre-existing medical problems as the level of dining, activities, and shore excursions.

Generally, the larger vessels carry more medical staff and are equipped with expanded facilities in anticipation of a greater demand by both passengers and crew members. Many smaller ships have also made ample provision for medical emergencies. However, over the years I have found that ships unwisely economize in this department. Ships sometimes carry too small a medical staff to cope with the passenger/crew load, hire physicians for short durations or who are not trained to deal with multiple emergencies, have limited equipment and supplies available, and tend to downplay their responsibility for passenger health needs.

The American College of Emergency Physicians has published *Guidelines of Care for Cruise Ship Medical Facilities.* Among the numerous recommendations are the following:

1. A medical staff, available around the clock, board-certified in emergency medicine, family practice, and internal medicine, with two to three years of clinical experience, emergency/critical care experience, advanced trauma and cardiac life-support skills, minor surgical skills, and fluency in the major language of passengers and crew.

2. Emergency medical equipment and medications including primary and backup cardiac monitors, primary and backup portable defibrillators, electrocardiograph, wheelchairs, refrigerator/freezer, extrication device, C-collar immobilization capability, trauma cart supplies, airway equipment, volume pumps, ventilators, pulse oximeter, external pacer capability, portable oxygen sufficient until patient can disembark ship, and medications comparable to those required to run two emergency department code carts including advanced cardiac support drugs.

3. Basic laboratory capabilities including x-ray unit, capability to perform hemoglobin, urinalysis, pregnancy, and glucose tolerance tests, a microscope, and a universal crew-blood-donor list.

4. A passenger information program regarding on-board health and safety, a pre-assessment of passengers' medical needs, and a program to meet Physical Disabilities Act standards.

5. A crew screening program covering all communicable diseases and certain other conditions, as well as a crew safety program.

6. Examination and treatment areas and an in-patient holding unit adequate for the size of the ship.

Dr. Deryck Gowland heads up the hospital staff on *Grand Princess,* one of the largest and most impressively equipped medical facilities at sea. He suggests that ship doctors be trained in advanced trauma and life support, have broad experience in family and emergency medicine, and be backed up by sufficient registered nurses with similar practical experience to formulate an efficient emergency-response team to deal with cardiac arrest and other serious medical traumas. He advises that when the combined passenger/crew population exceeds 1,000, a second physician is advisable, as well as an expanded nursing staff. Facilities should include a well-stocked computer-controlled pharmacy, a satisfactory range of x-ray facilities, a fully equipped operating theater, biochemistry and full-blood-count equipment, at least one or two intensive care wards which include a cardiac monitor, EKG machine, and pulse oximetry, and, if possible, a tele-medical facility enabling the shipboard doctor to consult with and obtain advice from hospitals and specialists ashore while giving advice or performing procedures with which he may not be familiar at sea.

My personal medical-cruise guru, Dr. Joseph Daddino, Director of Medical Education at Resurrection Medical Center in Chicago, Illinois, and a frequent cruiser, suggests that ships need one physician and two nurses per 1,000 (or less) passenger/crew population.

We have attempted to elicit information as to the experience of the medical personnel and the extent of the medical facilities, equipment, and systems aboard each cruise ship. However, it would be naive to believe that one could obtain totally honest responses when surveying the various cruise lines as to the quality of the facilities, equipment, and staff aboard their ships. No cruise line would admit to be remiss in any of these areas, although my personal observation leads me to suspect some are inadequately staffed or equipped to handle the passenger and crew load they carry.

Any potential cruiser with a medical problem, in a high-risk group, or with general concerns as to medical facilities aboard a particular ship would be well advised to contact the medical director of the cruise line in advance of booking the trip to determine if the caliber of medical support and facilities he or she may require will be available. Probably, it would be prudent to make a written inquiry and request a written reply so that the party responding is careful to research the matter before making any representations. Similar investigation can be made into the ship's ability to satisfy special dietary needs, as well as possible inoculations that may be advisable. When in doubt, an ounce of prevention is worth a pound of cure, or some such euphemism.

Note: After the short summaries of each ship listed in Chapter 11, we have added a code designating the medical personnel, facilities, and equipment that the cruise line has represented is available aboard the vessel. Where the cruise line has not responded to our inquiries, the failure to respond is indicated. I must emphasize that this information was given by an employee of the cruise line, has not been verified by the author or publisher, and may have changed by the time you read this information. A written inquiry made directly to the medical director of the cruise line is your most prudent course.

CODE DESIGNATING MEDICAL PERSONNEL,
FACILITIES, AND EQUIPMENT

C   Number of wheelchair-accessible cabins.

P   Number of physicians.

EM   Certified in emergency medicine.
CLS   Certified in advanced trauma and cardiac life support.
MS   Ability to perform minor surgical procedures.

N   Number of Nurses Experienced in Emergency Medicine or Critical Care.

Emergency medical equipment, lab equipment, and facilities.

CM   Primary and backup cardiac monitors.
PD   Primary and backup portable defibrillators.
BC   Equipment for biochemistry, full blood count, and urinalysis.
EKG Electrocardiograph machine.
TC   Trauma cart supplies.
PO   Pulse oximeter.
EPC External pacer capability.
OX   Portable oxygen
WC   At least one wheelchair for 300 passengers and crew
OR   Operating room sufficient for minor surgery. (If this is important, you need to obtain details from the cruise line.)
ICU Intensive care unit
X   X-ray unit
M   Microscope
CCP Computer-controlled pharmacy
D   Dialysis equipment
TM   Tele-medical capability
LJ   Life jackets located at Muster Stations (as well as in cabins) sufficient for all passengers. This is not required by SOLA; some cruise lines have a limited number at the Muster Stations. Where "LJ" is included, it indicates that the cruise line has represented to me that it has life jackets sufficient to accommodate all passengers at Muster Stations, in addition to those in the cabins.

Facilities for Physically Challenged

The cruise lines and ships that have provided the most facilities and accommodations for the physically challenged are Celebrity, Crystal, Disney, Princess, Royal Caribbean, the *Seabourn Sun, SuperStar Leo* and *Virgo, Carnival Destiny* and *Triumph,* and P & O's *Arcadia* and *Oriana.*

Other Facilities

The facilities will vary from ship to ship, with the most facilities being found on the larger craft. The megaships (more than 70,000 gross registered tons) of Royal Caribbean, Princess, Celebrity, Disney, Holland America, Costa, and Carnival cruise lines, as well as the *Queen Elizabeth 2 (QE2)*, and *Norway,* for example, have just about every facility found in a large resort hotel, and then some. However, even the mid-size and smaller vessels make clever use of the area they have, offering passengers almost the same facilities as the larger ships but on a smaller scale. The age of the ship may be a factor here, and if you are considering an older ship, it is important to find out if it has been recently remodeled.

Consider and compare the public rooms, swimming pools (number and size), deck areas, restaurant facilities, gymnasium, sauna, deck sports, library, elevators, movie theater, chapel, dance bands, bars, game rooms, hospital, cabins, bathrooms, and so on. Some of the more common facilities are included in the descriptions of the various ships in chapter 11. A better description and pictures of these facilities can be found in the ship's promotional brochures. Be careful! These brochures are like most advertising material; they have a tendency to portray the ship as larger and more beautiful than it may appear on actual inspection.

Activities

Although almost all ships offer a wide range of varied activities, not all ships subscribe to the same program. Golf addicts will want to consider those ships that offer golf clinics, joggers should check out which ships afford jogging decks, and amateur chefs may wish to select a ship with gourmet cooking lessons. The vast range of daily activities is more thoroughly described in the next chapter, and chapter 11 contains sample daily programs from ships of most of the major cruise lines.

In general, I have found that the ships offering regular cruises from Florida, California, and New York have the most activities per day at sea, with the Royal Caribbean, Holland America, Celebrity, Norwegian, Carnival, Costa, and Princess lines leading in this department. Ships sailing the Mediterranean and Northern Europe seem to offer the least activities (probably because they spend the majority of days in port). Several of the lines offer "once-a-year, special activity" cruises featuring classical or jazz music festivals, gourmet-cooking classes, wine seminars, or Broadway theater.

If you are cruising with children, be sure to note those vessels that offer a special children's program. I was particularly impressed with the children's programs on Princess and Premier cruise lines ("The Big Red Boats"), which include special counselors, children's activities, special discos, electronic game rooms, and ice-cream and pizza parlors. Most of the larger ships also have good facilities and programs for children. With Disney's entrance into the cruise market in 1998, the other lines will have to increase their programs to provide for cruising families if they want to remain competitive.

Many of the vessels built in the nineties have special areas and facilities for business meetings and seminars, as well as public computer rooms with instructional classes.

Accommodations

As previously explained, each ship prints an attractive brochure that includes a deck plan describing the size of each room, number of closets, dresser space, bathroom facilities, type of beds (single, double, or bunk), and general layouts. Thus, it is possible for you to review these facts before booking your cabin. Generally, you will pay more for added space, with the deluxe suites going for two to three times the price of the average cabin. There is often a difference between similarly priced accommodations on different ships. If living quarters are one of your major concerns, then this comparison of rooms will be an important factor in your selection of vessels.

You may find that a few of the older ships offer larger rooms and greater closet space, but check to see how recently they have been remodeled. If it has been more than ten years, some of the rooms can get a trifle seedy. Some of the rooms on the ships making regular short cruises out of Miami and Athens have suffered a great deal of wear and tear and could stand to be rejuvenated.

I have been especially impressed with the accommodations in the average room on the vessels of Silversea, Windstar Sail Cruises, Holland America, Celebrity, Carnival (post-1980 ships), Renaissance, Seabourn, Disney, and Crystal, as well as on the *QE2, Vistafjord, Radisson Diamond, Paul Gauguin, Mozart, Seabourn Goddesses*, and the newer ships of Princess Cruises, which also include many rooms with outdoor balconies for those who enjoy sitting out on their own private patio overlooking the sea.

Ships built during the past ten years have put a greater emphasis on providing balconies. Prime examples are the Princess and Silversea cruise lines, the newest ships of Celebrity Cruises, Renaissance, Disney, and Holland America Line, and the *Radisson Diamond* and *Paul Gauguin*. Although cabins with balconies fetch a higher price, many cruisers after experiencing the joys of a "balcony at sea" find this luxury well worth the extra tariff. Balconies attached to suites tend to be larger and more utilitarian than those adjoining standard cabins, and on a few ships they include an outdoor Jacuzzi tub.

Price

What do you get for your money? The answer may depend upon whether you are looking for quality or quantity, although it is not necessary to sacrifice either. If you divide the price of the cruise by the number of nights afloat, you will arrive at the average cost per day, which can serve as one standard of comparison. Do not use days afloat because this may be deceptive. A ship that leaves at 7:00 P.M. on a Sunday and returns at 8:00 A.M. on Saturday may be advertised as a "seven-day cruise," when in fact you are spending only six nights and five days aboard.

After you arrive at your average daily cost, then determine what kind of cabin this amount of money will purchase on comparable ships. Also compare the miles traveled and the number of ports of call. The existence of the "air-sea package," mentioned earlier and described later, will significantly affect your calculations. If you are comparing two ships and one offers an air-sea package, you must add in the cost of air transportation before making your comparison.

The price of cruising has escalated over the past decade, reflecting the increased demand by travelers as well as the increased cost of food, fuel, and labor. A number of the great "luxury" vessels of the sixties such as the *France,* the *Michaelangelo,* and the *Raffaello* were retired because the French and Italian lines could not afford to keep up the high standard of food and service without losing millions of dollars each year. However, the cruise vacation still represents one of the best bargains around for travelers.

You will find that cruises on the ships of Silversea Cruises, Crystal Cruises, Radisson Seven Seas Cruises, and the *QE2, Seabourn Goddesses, Legend, Pride, Spirit, Sun* and *Vistafjord* are the most expensive. However, these vessels offer a certain elegance and such a high standard of service that many travelers are willing to pay a little extra. The tariff for the choice cabins on the *QE2* and on the ships of the Princess, Holland America, Celebrity, Windstar, Disney, and Royal Caribbean lines will run almost as high. A luxury suite on almost any fine cruise ship will cost the most. Price comparisons for many of the ships can be found in chapter 11.

Beware of some of the "super-low" rates. When a ship offers a cruise for 50 percent less than another, something has to go (and it usually isn't the ship owner's profits). This does not mean that they will not offer many of the same amenities of the more expensive cruises; however, the food, service, and accommodations will not be of the same quality. One exception would be "loss leaders" offered by lines attempting to open up a new cruise market or attempting to fill their ships to capacity during the off-season. These can be real bargains. Many of the lines offer significant discounts on selected sailings or for customers who pay their fare well in advance. You will want to check this out with your travel agent or the ship lines you are considering. In addition, numerous travel agencies purchase blocks of space on ships and offer them to their customers at discount rates. These discount agencies generally advertise in travel sections of newspapers and cruise periodicals.

In recent years, almost all of the cruise lines have adopted varying discount policies. For selected sailings at different times of the year, you will find discounts ranging from 10 to 50 percent. Some of these discounted fares are advertised and available to everyone, while others are only offered through discount travel agents, tour operators, wholesale travel agents, private clubs, travel newsletters, and business organizations. In fact, the majority of cruisers today probably are not paying the fares published in the brochures. This is a disturbing trend because you do not know whether you have received the best reduction until you are aboard ship comparing prices with fellow passengers. However, for better or worse, the practice exists, and those of you wishing to obtain the best bargain have to do your homework.

Age of Ship

Unlike a fine wine, ships do not necessarily improve with age. Unless a ship is well maintained and frequently refurbished, it will soon show signs of wear. Fortunately, most lines frequently rebuild and refurbish their crafts so as to prevent deterioration. Chapter 11 indicates the age of the ships as well as the last date they were significantly refurbished. These dates will be of interest to you in comparing the various vessels.

The most exquisite public areas with bright modern decor can be found on the new Silversea, Crystal, Celebrity, Royal Caribbean, Princess, Carnival, and Holland America ships, as well as on the *QE2, Seabourn Sun, Radisson Diamond,* and on the yacht-like vessels of Seabourn, Renaissance, Windstar, and Cunard's *Seabourn Goddesses.* For a more traditional decor and elegance, you may prefer the public areas of some of the vintage ships; however, do not expect to find the quaint, stately elegance of the old *Queen Mary, Queen Elizabeth,* or *Isle de France.* Sadly, it no longer exists.

By October 1, 1997, all ships were required to meet the standards of "Safety at Sea" (SOLA), an international treaty that addresses the safe operation of ships and has been signed by all seafaring nations who are members of the International Maritime Organization. Most of the standards deal with fire safety and involve refitting cabins with sprinkler systems and smoke detectors. For economic reasons, many of the cruise lines have taken their older ships out of service because of the potential cost to meet these standards. Cunard's *Sagafjord* and Holland America's *Rotterdam* were two of the earlier victims; however, both were acquired by other ship lines, renamed, and recycled. Many of the ships built by the major cruise lines in the sixties and seventies have also been sold to smaller cruise lines servicing the economy and foreign markets.

People

People who like people will love cruising. There is no other vacation that affords you as great an opportunity to meet people from all over the world and from all walks of life. This does not mean that you will like everyone you meet any more than you like all of your neighbors or relatives. However, the camaraderie of a cruise offers an ideal climate to make new friends and strike up conversations with people from many different places.

What kind of people will be your fellow passengers? Although there is always a cross section of varied backgrounds, the majority of passengers will be indigenous to the area surrounding the port of embarkation. Passengers from New York and the East Coast will predominate on a cruise emanating from New York. If the cruise departs from California, you can expect a majority of travelers to be from the West Coast and states of the Southwest. Midwesterners tend to leave from Miami, Fort Lauderdale, and the Caribbean; however, today you will find many Easterners and Californians on these cruises. The development of the air-sea package has changed this lineup somewhat, and cruise lines are flying passengers from all over the country to meet their ships.

Cruises commencing in Mediterranean or Northern European ports will have many Europeans, with the majority being of the same nationality as the vessel. Again, this is changing because more and more people from the United States and Canada are taking these cruises as part of a European vacation. In fact, on one of my most recent North Sea-Baltic cruises, 90 percent of the passengers were from the United States. Cunard's ships tend to attract more British, Germans, and Northern Europeans. Club Med appeals to Northern Europeans as well as to the French. Holland America also can boast a partial European clientele. Costa's ships, when cruising the Mediterranean, are booked mostly by Italians, and when cruising South America, mostly by South Americans.

Entertainment

As mentioned previously, the opportunity to witness big-name performers is important to many travelers, while others are just as content to dance to good music and make their own fun. The quality of entertainment has vastly improved over the past few years, and many stars and talented artists are now performing on ships. When ships offer big-name entertainers, they will advertise the event. Generally, the cruises on the larger ships leaving from New York or Florida offer the best talent because many of these performers actually rotate ships, staying on the Caribbean circuit. I have found less in the way of talent during European and Pacific cruises. The *Norway* and *QE2* have a policy of carrying well-known entertainers on every cruise, as does Holland America on its annual world cruise and the *Seabourn Sun* on its longer cruises.

Some of the best entertainment on ships is of a more informal variety, with emphasis on audience-participation events such as adult games for prizes, dancing, costume balls, gambling, talent shows, and so on. Most ships also offer a wide selection of first-run movies. Many of the more recently built vessels offer closed-circuit TV movies or videos in your cabin. The newest Celebrity ships feature interactive televisions on which you can select your own videos. If the caliber of entertainment and entertainers is an important consideration, be certain to check out what will be offered on the cruise you are investigating.

Size of Ship

In chapter 11, I have set forth the size of the major cruise ships, including tonnage, length, width, number of decks, passenger capacity, and number of cabins. Thus, you will be able to easily compare the relative sizes of each vessel. The larger ships of the Carnival, Royal Caribbean, Star, Princess, Celebrity, Costa, and Holland America lines and the *QE2* and *Norway* tend to offer more facilities, entertainment, dining options, and activities for all age groups, while the smaller vessels are more intimate, friendlier, easier to negotiate, less congested, and can dock at a greater number of ports. Most ships built during the seventies were in the medium-size category, ranging from 16,000 to 23,000 tons. However, during the eighties and nineties the cruise lines introduced many new ships in the 45,000- to 85,000-ton and up range, as well as an assortment of small yacht-like vessels. During the late nineties and into the next century, vessels weighing in over 100,000 G.R.T. have become the fad. Although these behemoths may offer endless options not available on other vessels, passengers must be willing to accept long lines, long waits, and long walks.

For those who can afford the high tariffs, the highest standard of food and service and the most comfortable accommodations are found on the *Seabourn Sun* (formerly *Royal Viking Sun*), Crystal Cruises' ships, first class on the *QE2,* on the suite decks of Celebrity and Holland America, on the new "R-Class" ships of Renaissance, and on the smaller vessels of the Cunard Line's Seabourn Brand, Radisson Seven Seas, and Silversea. Young children and teens will be better accommodated on the larger ships, where there are more activities and special programs designed to entertain them.

Nationality of Crew

Chapter 11 also covers the nationality of the service crew for each ship. The nationality of the crew often sets the tone for the cruise, and on European and Mediterranean cruises it may determine the official language spoken. The difference in the nationality of the crew and what it may mean is discussed in this chapter under "Service."

The only major ships with a totally U.S. crew in service today are the *Independence,* which cruises the Hawaiian islands, and ships of the Alaska Sightseeing Tours, American Canadian, The Delta Queen Steamboat Company, and Clipper Cruise lines. Therefore, chances are that you will take a ship with a foreign crew, and it will be quite like spending time in the country the ship represents. You may find that this makes cruising all the more interesting and educational. You will most likely want to try ships of different nationalities each time you take a cruise vacation. Unfortunately, almost all of the lines have switched to crews of mixed nationalities for economic reasons. This move has destroyed much of the old-country charm and flavor and has created some language barriers

OUTSTANDING DINING, SERVICE, AND LUXURY

For those who can afford the steep tariffs, the highest standard of food and service and the most comfortable accommodations will be found on the following ships. **Large vessels** (over 20,000 G.R.T.): *Seabourn Sun, Crystal Harmony,* and *Symphony,* Celebrity's *Century, Galaxy, Mercury, Horizon,* and *Zenith, R-1* and *R-2* of Renaissance Cruises, and "grill class" on the *QE2.* **Medium-size vessels:** *Radisson Diamond, Paul Gauguin, Silver Cloud,* and *Silver Wind.* **Small vessels:** *Seabourn Goddess I* and

II, Seabourn Pride, Legend, and *Spirit, Song of Flower,* and *Renaissance VII-VIII.* The *Song of Flower* and *Renaissance* ships are the best bargains; and on the larger vessels you must opt for a suite or deluxe cabin to enjoy the best experiences.

Costs and Your Cabin

Given a comparable cabin on a comparable deck during the same season for cruises of similar duration, your tariff on most ships in the same category (see chapter 14) should not vary more than 10 to 20 percent.

The rates will be higher for single rooms than for rooms shared by two people. Adding a third or fourth person to the room will bring the tariff down even more. Children under twelve sharing a cabin with two full-fare adults will generally pay only half of the minimum fare (the price charged for the least expensive accommodations on the ship).

The more expensive rooms are usually located on a higher deck and are often a little larger. Outside staterooms with balconies, windows, or portholes go for a higher price than inside ones without a view to the sea. This price differential may range from $200 to $1,000 per person on a seven-day cruise.

Whether or not an outside cabin is worth the extra cost is a matter of personal priorities. You cannot see nearly as much out of a small porthole as you can on deck, and often it is difficult to close the porthole tight enough to keep out the early morning sun. Most of the newer vessels offer full windows or balconies in the more expensive cabins and suites. Should you purchase an outside cabin on the promenade deck, you will be annoyed by the noise of passengers strolling by early in the morning or late at night. However, outside cabins are brighter and generally larger, and most cruisers prefer to have a view of the sea.

Cabins with a double or two lower beds will go for more than those with a lower and an upper bunk. The same room on the same ship will cost more "in season" (mid-December to mid-April in the Caribbean and Pacific; June through September in Europe, with variations) than it will off-season. On transatlantic crossings, you will want to carefully investigate the varying prices for "peak season," "intermediate season," and "low season." You may be able to save as much as 30 percent by sailing eastward in late May rather than mid-June, or by returning westward in early June rather than late July. If your travel agent cannot obtain a discounted rate, he or she may still be able to obtain a cabin upgrade for you if he or she is persistent.

Of course, the longer the duration of the cruise, the more you will pay. This is possibly the only variation that makes real sense. Your per-person cost for a "minimum" room on an average seven-day cruise may range from $850 to $1,750. For ten-day cruises, your average minimum cost may vary from $1,100 to $2,100, and for fourteen-day cruises from $1,750 to $3,500. Do not be misled by newspaper advertisements publicizing rooms starting at $100 per day, per person. Often there are only a handful of rooms at this modest cost, and they are only available to those who book many months in advance. The average-priced room will be at least 50 percent higher than the minimum-priced one. If your decision as to whether or not to take a cruise is dependent upon the minimum offering, you should start making plans nine months to a year in advance.

The higher the deck, the more you will pay. Possibly the greatest differential on any given cruise is based upon which deck your cabin is located. Contrary to popular belief, the least motion will be felt in the interior of the lower decks. You do not have to be a student of science to comprehend this principle if you can just imagine a tree blowing in the wind.

The difference in cost between the most expensive and the least expensive cabin on the same ship can vary from 100 percent to 250 percent on the average ship, and to 500 percent on the super-luxury liners. Although there will exist a difference in area, closet and dresser space, and general accommodations between rooms, all passengers on a cruise enjoy the use of all public facilities, participate in the same activities, and eat the same food. Only your immediate neighbors will know which cabin you occupy, and only snobs will care, so if economy is a major consideration, book the most inexpensive cabin available. However, if you tend toward claustrophobia or feel that lounging around a comfortable room is a prerequisite to enjoying your vacation, then you will have to pay for expensive quarters. On many of the smaller luxury vessels, all accommodations are junior suites and all go for about the same fare, with a small variance based on which deck you are located.

The price structure on the QE2 when making transatlantic crossings is somewhat different from other cruises. Passengers booking the more expensive suites and cabins will eat better food served by more experienced waiters and will enjoy larger public rooms generally located on a higher deck.

Before leaving the subject of cost, a final word on port charges and the air-sea package is in order. A universally practiced deception is the tacking on of port charges after quoting the cruise fare. These can run from $60 up to several hundred dollars on longer cruises. Since the cruise line brochures generally quote cabin prices with an asterisk (*) to the effect that port charges will be added, potential customers are often misled as to the total fare. On a more positive note, many of the cruise lines have made arrangements with the private and regularly scheduled air carriers to obtain special package rates for parties who are flying directly to the port of embarkation on the day of the cruise and flying home the day the ship returns to its home port. It works like this: you check in your luggage upon arriving at your home airport; upon landing, you are transported by bus to the dock and your luggage is taken separately from the airport and brought right to your cabin. The airfare is often as low as one-half or even one-quarter of the normal economy rate. In addition, you are saving on taxi fares and tips to porters. The value of the air-sea package may vary from season to season on the same ship, and on some cruise lines it is only available to passengers purchasing medium- and higher-priced cabins. Therefore, when considering different cruises, you must carefully check to see the extent to which the air-sea package is available to you for the particular sailing you contemplate taking.

In recent years, the pricing policy of many of the cruise lines has become confusing at best, and possibly deceptive. Many of the companies will offer a few minimum cabins several hundred dollars lower than the other less expensive cabins. This is done in order to advertise the cruise as starting at a price lower than their competitors. In addition, air-sea packages have become complicated in that some lines offer free air, or air with a slight add-on (under $100), whereas others merely offer airfares that are only slightly reduced from normal coach fares.

To make matters worse, many of the lines offer an assortment of discounts for early bookings. Others discount cabins to tour operators and travel agents guaranteeing to sell a number of cruises. Therefore, you will often find that the couple in the adjoining stateroom with identical accommodations is paying a much different price from what you are paying. For those wishing to obtain discounted rates, it would be desirable to check with your travel agent or an agency that specializes in cruises as to which lines are offering early booking discounts as well as last-minute discounts. You may be able to save 25 to 50 percent by booking six months in advance or just a few days before a cruise. Generally, a cruise line with available cabins a few days prior to sailing will offer substantial cabin upgrades at minimum fares in order to fill up its berths.

Because pricing has become so illusory, my division of ships into four price/market categories (in chapters 11 and 14) is not based upon published fares alone. I also take into consideration the cost of items while on the ship (drinks, tours, tipping, etc.) as well as the passenger market the cruise line seeks to attract and actually does attract. Therefore, you may find certain ships placed in categories that do not always correlate with the prices advertised in periodicals and brochures.

What to Bring Along

Although U.S. citizens no longer need a passport to visit most of the islands of the Caribbean, a valid U.S. passport is a prerequisite when you are traveling in most other parts of the world. To obtain this document, you must apply in person to the Passport Division or passport agencies of the State Department. In some cities this function is handled by the clerk of the federal court or by the federal post office. When making application, you must present a birth certificate or proof that you were either born in the United States or became a naturalized citizen as well as two identical photographs signed by you, together with other identification. Your passport will be good for ten years from the date issued.

This is an indispensable document abroad and should be diligently guarded. Should you lose it or have it stolen, head for the nearest U.S. Embassy or Consulate to report the loss. For this reason, you would be wise to keep a separate record of your passport number, date, and place of issuance. Even though the document may not be required for many trips, it is your best means of identification in any foreign land when cashing traveler's checks or otherwise establishing credit.

Some countries that do not require a passport still require proof of U.S. citizenship, such as a voter registration card. It is also wise to bring along your driver's license and a charge card as additional identification.

Certain foreign countries also require visas and/or vaccination certificates. It is best to check with your travel agent or with the cruise line before each trip to determine which, if any, of these documents you may need.

You will want to bring along money, of course, and the best way to carry money when traveling is in traveler's checks. Do not forget to keep a record of the check numbers in a separate place from the checks so that you are in a position to report a loss. Your charge cards and personal checks might help in an emergency, but do not count on many places honoring them. Most ships will not cash personal checks, much to the dismay and displeasure of the unwary traveler. You will receive information on ship as to how to change your dollars to local currency upon arriving in a foreign port.

The amount of money you will bring along depends upon the length of the cruise as well as your personal spending habits. Generally, on ship, you will need money for tobacco, cocktails, wine, miscellaneous medicines and sundry items, photographs, stamps, laundry, cleaning, games of chance, and tips. On some ships you pay as you go, while on most there is a compulsory "charge it" system in which you are presented with an itemized invoice of your shipboard charges at the close of the cruise. When in port, you will need money for cab fares, restaurants, shopping, and any other activity you plan to pursue. It would be wise to sit down before you leave and analyze how much the foregoing expenditures may run—then add 30 to 40 percent to be safe.

While on the subject of money and shopping, remember that as a U.S. citizen, you will be permitted to bring back duty-free up to $400 of goods purchased abroad ($800 from most Caribbean islands), including up to one quart of liquor or wine. Should your ship stop in any of the U.S. Virgin Islands (most Caribbean cruises do), Guam, or American Samoa, you can increase your purchase limit to $1,200 per person and include one gallon of wine or spirits (provided your purchases in excess of $400 and one quart of liquor or wine are made on one of these islands). Meats, fruits, vegetables, plants, and plant products will be impounded by U.S. Customs unless they are accompanied by an import license from a U.S. government agency. Americans abroad can also mail home gifts of no more than $10 in value ($20 from the U.S. possessions in the Caribbean and Pacific) to friends and family that are free of duty or tax if the recipient does not receive more than one package a day. These gifts do not have to be declared by the sender. Liquor and tobacco products may not be mailed, however.

When getting ready to pack, be certain that you have sturdy, substantial luggage. Should you rise early on the morning your ship pulls into the port of final disembarkation, you may be shocked to see your favorite Gucci bag being tossed from man to man like a football as it makes its way to the dock. Luggage is frequently damaged while being transported on to and off of the ship, so valuable or fragile pieces should probably be left at home. Be sure to bring along a small traveling bag (about 1 foot by 2 feet). These are handy for carrying bathing suits, towels, a change of clothes, suntan lotion, and so on when spending a day ashore.

Your selection of clothes depends to a great extent upon the climate, length of the cruise, and your personal habits. Some travelers prefer to travel light with a few drip-dry garments, while others are not content to wear the same outfit twice. However, on a cruise you are not bothered with having to frequently pack and unpack, and in view of this you may wish to take advantage of the opportunity to display many of your fineries that do not normally make it on your vacations.

On a short cruise (seven days, for example), there are usually only two formal nights, while there are more on the longer cruises. You will find a greater percentage of men wearing a tuxedo on the *QE2, Vistafjord, Seabourn Goddesses, Legend, Pride, Spirit,* and *Sun,* and the ships of the Radisson Seven Seas, Crystal, Silversea, Celebrity, Holland America, and Princess cruise lines, because these ships tend to attract a wealthier, older, and more formal clientele. Although there are always a respectable number of male passengers in plain business suits, this can vary among ships, and to be safe, check with the line before leaving.

For the nonformal evenings, the men will wear suits and sport jackets, except for the "casual" evenings in port when no jacket or tie is required. White slacks and white dress shoes are always very "in," and it would be advisable to bring several nice sport shirts to wear with the white slacks. A robe for the shower, sauna, and pool is advisable, although robes are provided on some of the luxury cruise ships. A comfortable pair of deck shoes will get you through the day, and at night you will need dress shoes to coordinate with your suits and jackets. It is generally helpful to stay with one color when possible so you will not need as many different accessories. And don't forget socks, underwear, pajamas, bathing suits, sports shirts, dress shirts, ties, shorts, slacks, a sweater, and a raincoat. The same items you need aboard ship will generally work out for your shore excursions, so a separate wardrobe is unnecessary.

For the women, several of the chic numbers you have been reluctant to wear at home will be right in order. The number of dresses you pack will depend upon how often you wish to change. Again, it will be helpful to coordinate your choices with the same purse, dress shoes, and other accessories so as to cut down on the bulk of items that must be included in your wardrobe. As a rule of thumb, for every seven nights afloat, you can count on needing a dress outfit for two nights, a casual outfit for two nights, and something in between for the other evenings.

During the day, you will need swimming attire, a cover-up, sandals, shorts, skirts, blouses, slacks, a sweater, raincoat, and undergarments. Round this off with your favorite negligée, and you are ready to sail.

Most ships have laundry and cleaning services that vary from quite cheap to moderately expensive. Many vessels have self-service laundromats so you can feel like you have never left home.

Whether to bring along expensive jewelry is a difficult question. Opportunities for theft exist on a ship, and all jewelry and valuables should be kept locked in the vault when not in use. Most of the newer vessels provide a private wall safe in your cabin.

You may wish to personally carry aboard your jewelry, cosmetics, and medicines and the clothes you plan to wear the first evening at sea. All too often your luggage will not find its way to your room until several hours after the ship sails. You may feel more comfortable and less panicky if you follow this suggestion.

Some of the miscellaneous items you will not want to forget are sunglasses, suntan lotion, prescription drugs (as well as your prescription for an emergency), a traveling alarm clock, and last, but not least, your camera (don't worry about film— all but the most uncommon brands are obtainable). Although most of the ships have their own photographer who will be happy to record your every movement, these pictures can become expensive ($6 each, and up), and they often do not capture you at your best angle. On a cruise, you will experience many beautiful and memorable moments, and you will meet many interesting and often unforgettable people. Don't miss recording them for posterity.

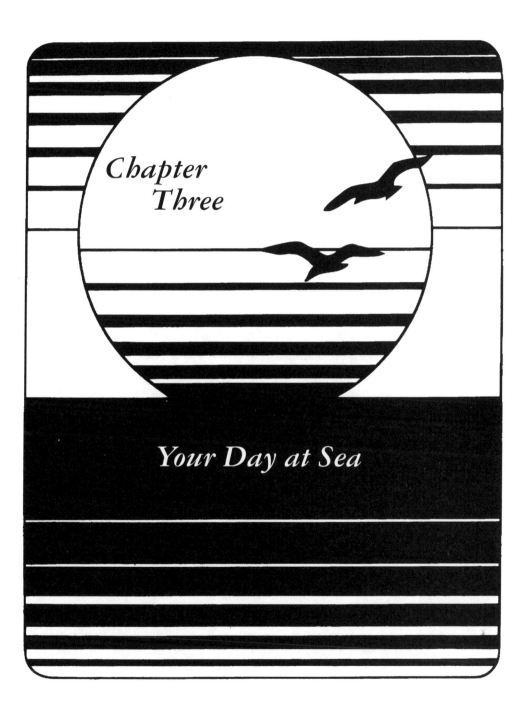

Chapter Three

Your Day at Sea

Although your selection of a cabin will help determine cost, and although the ports of call will elicit "oohs" and "ahs" from your neighbors back home when you exhibit your slides, your daily activities aboard ship as well as your dining experiences will be the decisive factor in forming your overall opinion of the vacation.

Most cruise ships make only brief stops in port, permitting just a superficial exploration of the environs—a preview, if you will, for later in-depth visits. Therefore, it is your day at sea that must be given top priority in selecting a cruise.

Facilities and Activities

The facilities and public rooms found on different ships will vary somewhat with the size of the craft and the duration of the cruise. All of the major cruise lines print elaborate color brochures, which you can obtain from travel agents or by writing to the line directly. These brochures will describe and often illustrate the numerous facilities found aboard.

Almost every cruise ship afloat today is fully air conditioned and equipped with the necessary stabilizers to keep the roll and pitch at a minimum. Most ships have radio rooms, providing the opportunity to place calls and fax messages home. Many have direct-dial telephones in the private cabins. A well-stocked library and cardroom are standard, and you will usually find a ship's hospital and pharmacy with at least one qualified doctor. Hairdresser salons are also available, but make your beauty shop appointments early on formal nights. Most women aboard who have their hair done will want an appointment the day of the captain's dinner.

You will find at least one and as many as four swimming pools. Because of the limited space, however, most pools offer an opportunity, at best, for only a dunk and five or six good strokes. Many ships have gymnasiums, and attached to the gym you will often find Jacuzzis, sauna, and massage rooms. In fact, on many of the larger new ships, there are fully equipped health spas. The ships that have devoted the most area and provide the best facilities are the larger Carnival, RCI, Princess, and Celebrity ships; the Crystal ships; and the *QE2, Radisson Diamond, Disney Magic,* and *Norway.*

The shops aboard ship will offer clothes, jewelry, and trinkets from numerous foreign ports at bargain prices. The larger ships generally have a variety of shops, while the smaller vessels only have one or two. Liquor, cigarettes, and perfume are generally the best buys. However, if your ship is stopping at a "free port," such as St. Thomas, you may wish to wait and compare prices ashore. Almost all ships provide laundry and cleaning facilities, and many have a self-service laundromat.

For those inclined to try their hand at Lady Luck, most cruise ships have slot machines aboard as well as fully stocked casinos, complete with craps tables, roulette, and blackjack. Again, the larger vessels tend to have the more complete casinos—some of the smaller ships only offer slot machines and one or two blackjack tables.

The usual public rooms consist of two or more grand ballrooms, one or more dining rooms, several smaller lounges, show-lounges, cardrooms, a library, a game room, numerous bars, a movie theater, a discotheque, and a buffet restaurant near the pool. Many of the ships built in the nineties have included conference facilities; wine, specialty coffee, and caviar-and-champagne bars; elaborate Broadway-caliber show-lounges; alternate specialty restaurants; computer centers; inventive children and teen areas; and a bevy of high-tech accouterments.

Upon rising each morning, you will find a schedule of the day's activities pushed under the door of your cabin. This very important document will indicate what is going on every minute of the day, which movies will be shown in the theater, and the dress for dinner. You will most certainly want to study this publication carefully so you will not miss any activity or happening in which you may wish to participate (see sample programs in chapter 11).

Your ship will have a cruise director and social staff who are there to organize activities, bring the passengers together (especially the singles), give orientation lectures on ports of call, sell shore excursion tickets, and generally act as mentors to the passengers. Some are excellent and can contribute to making your trip a delight. Others vary from indifferent to detrimental, giving wrong information about places of interest in ports or even bum steers to tourist traps (where they may have a little something going on the side). Be careful to check out the recommendations they may offer on shops and restaurants. It may be advisable to consult your guidebook or one of the tourist magazines that are printed by the tourist boards of the various ports and distributed on ship.

The adventures of John, Martha, Michael, Vivian, Joan, Ron, Scotty, and Jamie described in chapter 1 are just a few examples of the various ways you may elect to spend your days at sea. For those who do not wish just to relax, a cruise also offers a vast range of activities around the clock designed to appeal to every taste. There is probably no resort on earth that offers as much as often.

For the early risers, there are the morning exercise and aerobics classes, walking, jogging, shuffleboard, Ping-Pong, and deck tennis. Many of the larger ships carry a full-time golf pro and offer a morning golf clinic. In addition to the group lessons aboard ship, the golf pro will arrange tours to the local golf courses when ashore. Several lines have occasionally offered a tennis clinic program on some of their cruises that includes daily lessons on the ship and organized games in port. You may wish to attend morning lectures on forthcoming ports of call, especially if you have not been to that port previously. Foreign-language classes in the native tongue of the crew—such as French, Italian, or Greek—are common, as are lessons in bridge, backgammon, and chess. A number of the ships offer investment and estate planning seminars, while others offer cooking and needlepoint lessons, wine tastings, musical concerts, trap-shooting, bingo, and deck horse races. Most cruise ships carry a professional dance team that gives complimentary dance lessons each morning.

After lunch there are duplicate bridge, backgammon, and gin rummy tournaments, as well as first-run movies. For the children and ambitious adults, there are swimming games at the pool and deck sport tournaments. In addition to the usual deck sports, a few ships have miniature golf courses, and many vessels of the Carnival, Celebrity, Costa, Disney, Princess, and Royal Caribbean lines and the *Norway* have basketball courts. At some point in each cruise you are given an opportunity to visit the bridge or tour the kitchen. Late in the afternoon, many passengers squeeze in the hairdresser or a sauna and massage. Many of you will find that just lying out in the deck chair by the pool and soaking up the sun can be one of the nicest experiences during the day. Add music from the ship's calypso band and a rum punch, and it is just like being at a pool on one of the Caribbean islands.

Evenings are usually the most exciting part of the cruise. Even on cruises that hit numerous ports, the majority of evenings are spent at sea. You will probably start out in the cocktail lounges before dinner, where you can sample some hors d'oeuvres, music, and exotic drinks. The captain's welcome-aboard cocktail party is held before dinner, usually on the second night at sea. On this occasion, each passenger is introduced personally to the captain, treated to free drinks, and has an opportunity to meet the other passengers aboard. After dinner each evening, there are parlor games such as bingo and cinema racing (betting on taped horse races). The casinos also are active at this time.

During the majority of evenings at sea, most ships offer a variety show. Several of the lines have a policy of offering two completely different shows each evening, one in the main lounge and one later at night in the cabaret or discotheque. These shows feature singers, comedians, magicians, dancers, puppeteers, and more singers. As pointed out in an earlier chapter, the quality of the entertainment has improved in recent years, with the best entertainers being found on those ships departing from New York, Florida, and California.

One night during each cruise, many of the ships hold a passenger talent show and, on another night, a passenger costume party. These affairs often afford more laughs than many of the second-rate comedians, magicians, and singers who get paid to perform. Once you get into the spirit of things, you may find that the audience-participation events will leave you with more memorable experiences than the average, run-of-the-mill variety show. For those who prefer something different, most ships offer a first-run movie each evening in the theater. The movies are varied throughout the cruise and generally repeated at least once so you can choose which afternoon or evening you wish to give up some other activity. Closed-circuit TV movies or VCRs in your cabin have been introduced on many of the newer vessels. On some ships, these have replaced the movie theater.

Around midnight, almost every cruise ship offers the midnight buffet. Also, later in the evening, things start to swing in the late-night spots, where couples and singles can indulge in some romantic dancing before the traditional stroll on deck. No matter how involved you become in activities, and no matter how tired you may be, you should save a few minutes each night to walk out on deck under the stars and watch the black sea splash against the hull of the ship. Looking out across the sea at such a moment offers a unique opportunity for reflection.

From the foregoing description, it is obvious that there is something for everyone aboard a cruise ship. After a day or two, you should be able to adapt to your own pace and intensity and alternate between playing and relaxing with your usual agility. Chapter 11 includes a sample of daily program schedules for many of the ships.

Dining

Some of your most memorable experiences aboard ships will be your adventures in dining. Over the years, many of the great ships offered some of the finest restaurants to be found anywhere in the world. Dining on many of the vessels with both European kitchen and dining room staffs is comparable to feasting at the best establishments on the Continent.

Can you imagine starting your evening repast with gobs of Beluga caviar, imported gravlax, a dozen escargots, or perhaps a slice of quiche Lorraine, followed by some onion soup with freshly grated gruyère and Parmesan cheeses too thick to cut with a knife? Next comes your fish course of poached salmon or turbot with hollandaise sauce, dover sole amandine, lobster thermidor, or possibly some trout stuffed with crabmeat.

For your entree, you may decide upon roast duckling à l'orange, steak au poivre, rack of lamb, or Chateaubriand with Béarnaise sauce. The entree may be complemented with some sautéed champignons or truffles. For dessert, why not try a Napoleon slice or other French pastry? Many of the ships have the headwaiters going from table to table each evening, preparing bananas flambé, cherries jubilee, or crêpes suzette. To round things off, you may try an assortment of cheeses from Switzerland, Holland, France, and Italy, followed by some after-dinner mints. Naturally, each course should be accompanied by the proper wine, unless you prefer a shot of vodka with your caviar and Cognac with your coffee.

Although this meal could easily cost $80 to $150 per person in a good French restaurant in Paris or New York, most of these goodies are featured for dinner aboard the vessels of many of the cruise lines at least once or twice during each sailing and nightly on the deluxe vessels. However, many of the ships have been cutting back on the more expensive offerings in recent years.

There no longer exists a purely French vessel, other than the riverboats of French Cruise Lines and Club Med II. Seasoned cruisers will always miss the incomparable dining room of the *France*, which was taken out of service in 1974. Alas, the days of unlimited champagne and caviar may be gone forever—ship lines are no longer willing to lose millions of dollars each year just to maintain an image of excellence. However, notable exceptions are the *Seabourn Goddesses, Legend, Pride, Spirit*, and *Sun*, and the other ships of the Silversea, Crystal, Celebrity, and Radisson Seven Seas cruise lines.

There are several ships with Italian kitchens and dining room staffs that offer a wide selection of Italian dishes, including a different variety of pasta with each lunch and dinner. Before the cruise comes to an end, you will have been exposed to spaghetti, macaroni, mostaccioli, rigatoni, cannelloni, lasagna, manicotti, pizza, gnocchi, and a dozen other lesser-known varieties. Among the more popular ships with Italian kitchens sailing from U.S. ports are the vessels of Costa Cruise Lines and most of the ships of Princess Cruises. There are exceptional Italian specialty restaurants on the *Radisson Diamond, R-1* and *R-2, Song of Flower, Rotterdam VI*, and on the two Crystal and Disney ships (see chapter 13).

Many recent cruisers have expressed the opinion that today the *Seabourn Goddesses, Legend, Pride, Spirit*, and *Sun*, the *Song of Flower*, and the other vessels of the Crystal, Silversea, and Celebrity Cruises lines have the finest kitchens afloat. The food on these ships is Continental, with the European chefs creating an amazingly diverse range of culinary delights. The dining room staffs are mixed European. I have found the overall dining experience on these ships to be superior to most ships currently sailing, but still not up to the excellence of the *France* (now defunct). Among the most elegant dining rooms afloat with the most lavish gourmet cuisine are the Queen's Grill and the two Princess Grills of the *QE2*. Unfortunately, these dining rooms are open only to those passengers booking the most expensive suites and rooms. Each of the "R-class" Renaissance ships features two of the most exquisitely furnished alternative restaurants at sea, simply designated "The Grill" and "The Italian Restaurant."

A variety of Continental, ethnic, and American dishes are offered on the ships of most cruise lines. Although the quantity and quality of the food on ships is generally satisfactory, service often suffers from the use of mixed crews, including less experienced waiters and stewards from the Caribbean, Central America, and the Far East. Some of the less widely publicized ships and some of the bargain cruises do not offer the same high quality and vast quantity of food that has come to be associated with cruising.

If you wish to have special dishes that do not appear on the menu, you must make arrangements with the maître d' at least a day in advance. Generally, he will be anxious to accommodate you, and, of course, you are expected to reciprocate at the end of the cruise with a suitable gratuity. Don't hesitate to ask for any dish that may tickle your palate. A cruise is an excellent opportunity to sample all those special preparations for which you never wanted to splurge in an expensive restaurant. Unfortunately, most ships today are discouraging this practice, and the opportunity to order special gourmet dishes has been completely eliminated on most cruises. The corporate policy of most lines to make larger and larger profits has ruled out much of the elegance and special pampering that has long been associated with cruising.

The wine selection aboard many of the ships is perhaps too limited for the tastes of a discerning connoisseur. The prices of wines have escalated in recent years, and the cost of wine on ships is almost as expensive today as the cost in restaurants. Italian and Greek wines are generally the best bargains. On the majority of ships, some of the sommeliers have had too little training, lack the necessary familiarity with and knowledge of wine, and are too harassed to serve it properly. With the ever-growing popularity of wine drinking, one can only hope that the cruise industry will catch up and bring this department up to the level of the remainder of the dining experience. It should be noted that the ships of the Silversea, Radisson Seven Seas, and Seabourn lines give their passengers free wine with lunch and dinner each day.

Because dining is such an important part of the cruise, you should book your table and choose your sitting carefully. The experienced cruiser will go to the dining steward immediately upon boarding ship to make these arrangements.

Many cruises have both a first and second sitting, which results in two entirely different daily schedules. Should you be traveling with friends, be sure that you all take the same sitting. If your friends take the first sitting and you the second, you may never see them. While you are enjoying cocktails, they may be eating dinner, and while you are having dinner, they may be seeing the first show. While you are watching the second show, they may be dancing, and so on. Ships that provide two sittings also provide two schedules for activities, so all passengers have an opportunity to take part in the various events offered.

When deciding upon whether to take the first or second sitting, you must consider your usual eating habits as well as your dining preferences while on a vacation. If you are an early riser, prefer dinner around six-thirty or seven-thirty, and wish to conclude your evening's entertainment to be in bed by eleven or twelve o'clock, you will prefer the first sitting. If, however, you wish to sleep late, partake in cocktail hour, and not eat until eight-thirty or nine o'clock, then the second sitting is for you.

Most ships have tables for parties of two, four, six, eight, and ten. If you are honeymooners or second-honeymooners and want to be alone, you will prefer a table for two. However, if you have a fight, you're out of luck because it may be difficult to switch tables later. If you feel you will prefer other company, ask the dining room maître d' to make the arrangements. The larger the table, the more people you will get to know, and should one or two at your table not be congenial, there certainly will be others who are. Recently, such luxury vessels as the *Vistafjord* and the ships of Silversea, Renaissance, Radisson Seven Seas, Seabourn, and Windstar Sail Cruises have adopted an open-seating policy with no prearranged dining assignments. Thus, passengers can change table companions as often as they wish. Several of the newer ships coming on line offer a special gourmet dining room where a limited number of passengers can enjoy a more intimate upscale dinner on certain evenings. For example, the *Crystal Harmony* and *Crystal Symphony* offer Oriental and Italian restaurants in addition to the main dining rooms, *R-1* and *R-2* feature an English-style grill and a gourmet Italian restaurant, and the *Seabourn Sun*, Vistafjord, Paul Gauguin, Disney Ships, Rotterdam VI, and *Radisson Diamond* also have special (advanced reservation) Italian restaurants; and ships of the Princess, Carnival, Costa, and several other lines have added pizza parlors (see chapter 13 for listings of alternative dining specialty restaurants).

As mentioned earlier, on the *QE2* the dining rooms are divided into four classifications, and there is a difference in food and service between the Queen's Grill and two Princess Grills (for those booking the most expensive cabins), the Caronia (for those booking the middle-priced cabins), and the Mauretania (for those booking the least expensive cabins). On other cruise lines everyone is considered to be in one class, and therefore, whether you pay $1,000 per week or $10,000 per week for your room, you will eat the same food in the same dining room.

All of the cruise ships have adopted the custom of offering numerous feedings in order to give you the impression that you are getting a lot for your money. As a matter of fact, you are, but quite candidly, few of you will be able to attend each gastronomical offering and do it justice.

The first culinary event is the "early bird breakfast," which consists of coffee, tea, rolls, and juice, starting at six or six-thirty in the morning. Regular breakfast in the dining room commences sometime between seven-thirty and eight-thirty and on many ships is available in your cabin at any time. Traditionally, you could ring for a cabin steward who would bring you a hot breakfast from the regular kitchen or a Continental breakfast from his service kitchen. Many of the ships have eliminated this possibility or varied the routine, requiring passengers who wish breakfast in their cabins to fill out and turn in an order form before going to bed. This has the obvious disadvantage of forcing you to decide in advance what time you want to get up and have breakfast.

Breakfast will generally consist of the usual offerings, such as various fruits, juices, cereals, eggs, breakfast meats, rolls, pancakes, and so on. However, the food is usually typical of the nationality of the crew, and pancakes and waffles may appear a little strange on the French and Italian ships. Therefore, on such ships you will normally be better off to stay with an omelet, croissants, and rolls.

Breakfasts are more nearly akin to the North American tastes on the U.S., British, Scandinavian, and most foreign Florida-based ships, where you can have your bacon, eggs, hot toast, griddle cakes, and lox and bagels just like your mother used to make (maybe a little better).

Most ships have an alternate indoor/outdoor breakfast buffet for the late risers. Having your morning coffee while sitting out in the fresh salt-sea air during a morning at sea is especially delightful.

For those who cannot hold out until lunch, there is a late-morning tea and cakes at about eleven o'clock. Of course, by this time many of your fellow passengers may already be working on their second Bloody Mary or screwdriver. Lunch is generally served in the dining room from twelve to two, depending on your sitting. An indoor/outdoor buffet for those passengers who do not wish to dress to go to the dining room for lunch is generally offered. Buffets on ships are usually quite elaborate and include exotic assortments of cold meats (roast beef, duck, ham, chicken, and venison) attractively displayed with numerous salads, cheeses, several hot dishes, and yummy desserts. The most varied and elaborate lunch buffets are served on the *Seabourn Sun*. When in port, you may find it inconvenient to return to the ship at noon. Some of the ships will furnish you with a box lunch to take with you; otherwise, you may wish to utilize the opportunity to sample some of the local restaurants.

About four or four-thirty in the afternoon, tea and cake are served. You then can partake of cocktails and hors d'oeuvres from six-thirty to eight. After cocktails comes the pièce de résistance of your gastronomical day—dinner. The variety of ethnic cuisine was discussed earlier. To break up the monotony, many ships adopt a different theme for each dinner meal. There may be Italian night, French night, or Caribbean night, where the cuisine will be indigenous to the country or area that is being featured. Most ships offer numerous courses, and you are encouraged to sample as many dishes as you wish. The appetizers usually include juices, a fruit cup, some form of seafood cocktail, relishes, smoked salmon, and perhaps caviar on special evenings. The next course is soups and pastas. As a rule of thumb, you are best advised to choose a dish from the same country of origin as the chef; that is, the pastas are better on Italian ships, moussaka is best on Greek vessels, and quiche should be prepared by a French chef. The rolls and breads on the Italian and French ships are usually superb and irresistible.

The entrees are generally divided between fish and seafood offerings and meat and fowl preparations. Most ships permit you to order one of each. Even if you cannot consume all of this food, you may wish to order a course and share it just to have an opportunity to sample something unusual. Most of the better ships offer a standby such as steak or roast beef every evening for those who are not so adventurous. In the event you do not care for anything on the menu, many of the upscale ships will whip up a steak to accommodate you. For those who enjoy wine with the meal, you are best advised to make a selection at lunch or during the prior evening. This will enable the wine steward to have the bottle waiting for you and properly aired. Otherwise, if he is very busy, your wine may not arrive until your dessert. If you do not finish the entire bottle, request that the wine steward store it for you until the following evening.

The desserts are varied, ranging from assorted ice creams and ices to fancy cakes, pastries, and cheeses. As mentioned earlier, many ships have their headwaiters wandering around each night making crêpes suzette and cherries jubilee so that each table receives these desserts at least once during the cruise. Traditionally, flaming baked Alaska is served on almost every ship on the night of the captain's dinner. This affair generally takes place toward the end of the cruise. Staff and crew alike make every human effort to surpass and outdo all that has preceded the event. The food is the best; the service is even better; there are special decorations; and generally a jovial, festive atmosphere prevails.

Last, but not least, is the midnight buffet. This is the gourmand's delight, where everything that has not been consumed previously on the cruise is refurbished and attractively displayed on a buffet table that often covers the width of the dining room. Many ships go further and prepare some special dishes and fancy desserts for the occasion.

On the Princess, Costa, and the newest Celebrity ships there are pizza parlors open in the afternoon and evening and on Carnival's latest ships they are open around the clock. Many other ships offer special ice-cream shops, caviar-champagne bars, and wine and coffee bistros.

Many of the ships built in the nineties are offering a casual dining policy under which all meals are alternatively offered in the buffet restaurant for passengers not wishing to eat in the dining rooms.

The dress for dinner varies from evening to evening, from casual (no tie or coat required) for evenings in port, to formal attire, which is suggested for the captain's cocktail party, the captain's dinner, and other special occasions. It is, of course, permissible for men to wear a plain business suit and tie on formal evenings; and on the less expensive ships and shorter cruises, most of the male passengers do not bother to bring along a tux. The women, however, generally dress to the hilt, as there is no better place to show off a wardrobe. This does not mean that you will have to run out and spend hundreds or thousands of dollars on clothes in order to enjoy a cruise. Few people do. However, you will want to bring along a variety of your special fineries, depending upon the length of the cruise.

The waiters in the dining room will be especially determined to satisfy your every whim because they are hoping to receive a token of your gratitude by way of a tip. You do not tip them at every meal, but wait until the end of the cruise and then place your gratuity in an envelope with a little thank-you note. Most of the ships will indicate the recommended tipping procedures in a bulletin to passengers; on others, you are left on your own. On the Holland America, Silversea, and Seabourn lines, and on the various Russian cruise lines, tipping is not required. On a recent cruise on Holland America I was left with the impression that the waiters and stewards expect to be tipped as on any other ship, while the staff on the *Silversea* and *Seabourn Pride* absolutely refused to accept any gratuity.

If in doubt, the chief purser is a reliable source from whom to obtain an explanation of the usual procedures. Although many people adhere to the usual 10 to 15 percent of the passage divided between waiters, cabin stewards, and others who have performed a special service on their behalf, this is not always suitable. Whether your ticket costs $850 or $2,000, you require the same service, and there is a big difference between spreading around $85 and spreading around $200. You will probably be about average if you tip $3.50 to $4.50 per day per person to your waiter, and a similar amount to your cabin steward. (Some ships recommend that the busboy be tipped a specified amount in addition to the tip you give the waiter. Normally, the waiter shares his tip with the busboy.)

If you are particularly pleased with the service, you may want to tip more, and if the service is unsatisfactory, you should notify the maître d' or the hotel manager early in the voyage so that your trip is not ruined. Don't forget to tip the wine steward, the maître d', the waiters in the bar, and anyone else whom you may call upon for a special service. Their tips will be about the same as you would normally give at home. However, on many ships a 15 percent service charge already has been added to drinks and wine orders.

Dining is most certainly one of the biggest highlights of the cruise, and must therefore be given its due importance when selecting a ship. You will find sample menus from many of the cruise ships in chapter 11. Because the quality of food and service varies from year to year on ships as it does in restaurants, you will want to solicit the opinion of your travel agent and anyone you may find who has recently cruised on the ship that you are considering. My ratings for food and service can be found in chapter 14. These are based upon my most recent cruise on each ship and may vary from year to year, depending upon the kitchen and dining room staffs.

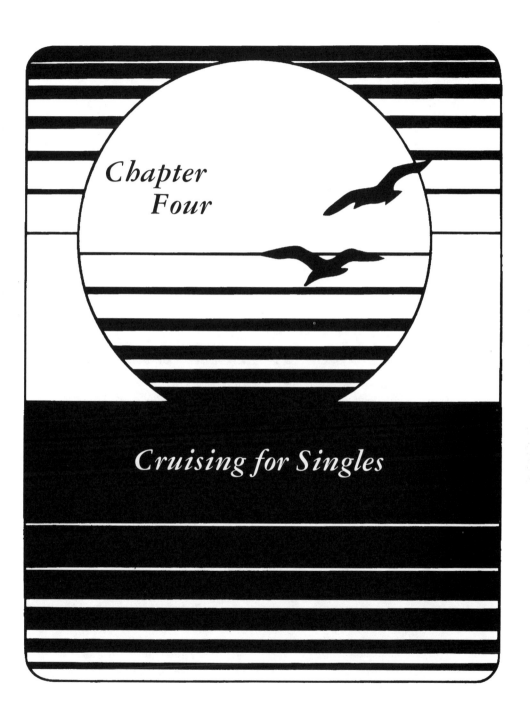

Chapter
Four

Cruising for Singles

With the growing popularity of the cruise vacation and the onslaught of vigorous advertising, more and more singles are being attracted to the high seas. The image of the elderly passenger propped up in a deck chair, covered with blankets, and sipping tea has given way to the younger, sophisticated single of the modern era.

There is no question that the thought of a cruise should conjure up some romantic visions in the mind of the average single. Imagine watching the sun set over the mountains on a balmy, tropical evening as your ship slowly pulls out of port, or dancing to the melodious tunes of a romantic Italian band until the early hours of the morning, followed by a hand-in-hand stroll on deck to view the moon and stars on a clear Caribbean evening.

Of course, cruising has a great deal more than romance to offer the single. In addition to the numerous activities, exciting ports, and fine cuisine (discussed earlier), the cruise offers the single traveler a planned, organized vacation where most major arrangements have already been taken care of. Who could fail to appreciate not having to constantly tote heavy luggage, tip porters, wave down taxis, arrange itineraries, determine a respectable night spot, or suffer the empty feeling of being alone in a strange land?

What kind of companionship can a single person traveling alone expect to find aboard ship? Generally, it takes a day or so to become familiar with the new surroundings and lose your normal inhibitions. By the second evening at sea, all but the most pretentious bores will have warmed up and gotten into the swing of things. Your fellow passengers may smile and nod as you pass them in corridors, the passengers in the adjoining deck chairs may initiate a conversation, and the couple sitting at the next table in the lounge may invite you to join them. The intimate, often cozy atmosphere of the ship, together with the realization that you are all at the mercy of the high seas and that no one is getting off, stimulates a feeling of togetherness and cordiality.

However, the cruise staff of the ship will not leave you to your own devices to find companionship. The entertainment director and social hostess will stimulate co-mingling through singles' cocktail parties, group games, dancing classes, bridge tournaments, and similar get-together functions. Of course, no pressure is ever placed upon anyone to attend these activities, and you are free to just relax, cuddle up with a good book, and do your own thing.

Many of the married couples on ship will be very friendly. The unescorted single may find it quite advantageous to strike up a social relationship with several amenable couples so as not to limit her companionship just to the other singles aboard. A well-traveled couple may prove to be far more interesting company on a shore excursion than some other single who may not share your tastes or interests. In addition, it is often desirable to have an assortment of other people to join in the ship's public rooms when you are avoiding some other single or do not wish to sit alone.

Often your married companions will insist upon buying you a drink; however, you will want to reciprocate at the earliest possible opportunity so as not to give the impression that you are tagging along for a free ride. When sharing taxis or eating at a restaurant in port, etiquette and common sense dictate that you insist upon paying your own share. Your newfound friends will soon abandon you if it turns out that you have become an expense they didn't include in their vacation budget. The women will be well advised to follow the same principle with regard to any male escort who becomes a semi-regular. He may have bargained on paying for a few drinks and an occasional meal, but he probably did not bring along enough cash to take you on as a dependent.

Having touched upon the existence of the feeling of general camaraderie on the cruise and the desirability of not neglecting married couples as potential shipboard pals, we will now explore the question of what kind of companionship the single can expect from singles of the opposite sex. First of all, it is no secret that singles will be in the minority, as they are at most vacation spots. Most newspaper advertisements for "single cruises" are misleading. A travel agency or tour operator will pre-book a number of cabins on a regular cruise and attempt to attract a number of single customers through advertising. Second, single females will generally outnumber single males by two to one.

The greatest number of single females under thirty-five are on shorter cruises, or travel in the summer, or possibly at Christmas or Easter vacation. Single women over thirty-five also tend to travel more during the summer months because this is the season during which most working women take their vacations.

It is difficult to predict during which months you will find the most single male passengers. Single male passengers under thirty-five aboard a Caribbean cruise are somewhat of a rare commodity. Actually, this has been changing, and I have seen a number of younger males on recent cruises of shorter duration, as well as on the seven-day economy ships and the ships of the Carnival line. Should any of my readers be single, male, under thirty-five, and contemplating a cruise, I would advise plenty of rest before the vacation.

But don't despair, women; there is always the crew. At about nine-thirty each evening dozens of young, handsome officers come out of the woodwork in full naval attire and are available for dancing and other forms of socializing until the wee hours of the morning. The policy of most of the lines is to permit the officers to date the single women aboard. They are generally very polite and make excellent shore companions because they are familiar with all of the interesting out-of-the-way spots that the tourists seldom find.

During around-the-world and longer cruises, several of the cruise lines feature "gentlemen hosts" who generally are mature gentlemen (ages 55-70) who receive a free cruise in return for acting as dance and bridge partners for women traveling solo. For many years this program has been available on the *QE2,* and *Vistafjord,* and on the Holland America, Seabourn, Crystal, and Silversea cruise lines. The program was best satirized in the Jack Lemon-Walter Matthau movie Out to Sea.

What, then, is the best cruise for the single? Obviously, you should first select a ship by utilizing the same standards that a couple would consider; that is, food, service, program, ports of call, and so forth. You are still spending your vacation time and hard-earned money, and there is no reason why you should not make your decision with objectivity and discrimination.

However, assuming all else to be equal, the larger the ship, the greater number of singles to choose from as prospective acquaintances and companions. On the other hand, on a very large ship you will find it difficult to become exposed to all of the other passengers early in the trip. It is entirely possible to spend seven days on such a ship without once crossing the path of a fellow passenger who has been on the same ship with you all week. A smaller ship is more intimate, and people warm up more rapidly, but there are fewer people to choose from. You may wish to compare this situation to a small and a large hotel. If you were going to a Caribbean island, would you prefer to stay at a large resort or a smaller, more intimate hotel, assuming similar quality and facilities? The greatest number of younger singles will be found on the three- and four-day cruises, on the ships of the Carnival line, or on less expensive cruises. Most younger singles on more expensive cruises are traveling with their families.

Longer cruises (fifteen to ninety days or more) would not be advisable for the single who feels he or she needs good and exciting companionship to make the trip a success. Although you may get lucky and find "Mr. Right" or "Miss Right" and have the most heavenly time of your life, if you don't you are going to be unhappy for an awfully long time.

When traveling alone, the cabin price is usually higher and there will be a significant savings if you are able to travel with a friend or share a cabin for two. Some of the lines will pair up singles (of the same sex), and others will not. You will have to check with each line in order to determine their current policy. Cabin space in an economy room is limited, and sharing small closets, dressers, and a washroom with even a close friend is often difficult and with a stranger almost impossible. However, if economy is a prime consideration, privacy and comfort may have to be sacrificed. Fortunately, some of the newer ships are being built with a greater number of single occupancy staterooms at rates closer to those charged for each person sharing a double room.

Let me again emphasize that your enjoyment of the cruise vacation does not depend necessarily upon your making friends, finding escorts, or experiencing eternal romance. However, those of you who may be interested in any of these pursuits should consider the following tips:

Let your hair down immediately and freely respond to the fellow passenger's friendly nod or glance. If you insist upon being coy, proper, or aloof, valuable days of the cruise will flee by before you get into the swing of things.

While waiting in the terminal to board ship, survey the prospective group and do not hesitate to introduce yourself to someone who interests you. Inasmuch as you will have to select a table in the dining room as soon as you come on board, this may be as good a time as any to start looking for interesting prospects. (*Note:* Everyone looks a bit dull and seedy when waiting in line to come aboard. Don't worry, they will all look better by tomorrow in different surroundings.)

Upon boarding ship, go right to the dining room steward and sign up for the late dinner sitting at as large a table as possible. The late sitting gives you time to attend cocktail hour each night, and a large table affords you a greater opportunity to meet a variety of other passengers. Even if some of the people at the table turn out to be bores, you should find at least a few that you will relate to. Seating arrangements may be difficult to change after the cruise starts; therefore, it is best to stack your table with as many desirable companions as possible in the very beginning.

Force yourself (if necessary) to make friends with whomever you meet when you first board ship. This can best be accomplished in the bars, in the public rooms, or just walking around the decks—everyone is touring the ship at this point. Each person you meet will introduce you to someone else whom he or she has met, all of which has a pyramid effect, exposing you to the greatest number of people possible in the shortest period of time. Once you have been introduced to the eligible singles on the ship, you can start to become selective. However, if you start out being selective, you may never meet enough other singles to permit you to make a selection.

Make friends with married couples because they often are the best matchmakers around.

During the cruise, singles tend to gravitate to the many bars, lounges, and discotheques, and therefore these are often the best locations to meet other singles (who are looking to meet other singles).

Don't miss the singles' get-together cocktail party, which is usually held the first or second day at sea. No matter how "corny" it may seem to attend this event, the singles' party offers a good opportunity to meet the other singles and to make introductions.

During the first few days, try to attend the card tournaments, dancing classes, deck games, religious services, and other organized events. These social gatherings tend to help break the ice and serve to get the passengers together on a more personal basis.

Stay up for the late, late dancing after midnight. By this time, those not so staunch of heart or steadfast of foot will have retired, the field will be narrowed, and whatever is left is all yours!

Avoid pairing off with one person during the first few days unless you have found a "good one." If you panic and grab the first available, the others will think you are taken and you may blow an opportunity to meet all the other singles. On the other hand, if you really have found a "good one," hold tight, because you are going to have some stiff competition.

Ladies should not depend too heavily on the crew for companionship. Many are married, some are gay, and 99 percent of the balance aren't very sincere and are interested only in lassoing you and bedding you for the duration of the cruise. This obviously won't do much for your opportunity to meet other interesting passengers.

Fellows—move faster than the crew. Your toughest competition will be the ship's officers and waiters. Although they may not beat out the town idiot ashore, while on ship they appear to be Greek gods. Because they are away from their families for long periods of time, they have become quite adroit at the "quick romance." In fact, acquiring the affections of the more select ladies for the duration of the cruise has become the biggest game in town among the younger members of the crew. All is not lost. You have the advantage. You will have the first opportunity to romance the ladies because the crews are usually busy working until the second evening at sea. Stake your claims early. In addition, the ladies will soon realize that the members of the crew are only available at limited times and generally are only interested in one thing. On the other hand, you are available all day and can offer them a little more well-rounded experience.

Pace yourself. Don't wait too long to make your move, or the cruise will be over. On the other hand, the object of your affection may get turned off by someone who is obviously a jerk. On a seven- to ten-day cruise, you can count on the majority of shipboard romances dying midway through the journey. This is because the couples were not well matched and would have broken up after a few dates no matter where they met. Therefore, an attractive candidate who appears to be taken the first day may become very available a little later on.

Don't burn yourself out. Too much sun, food, drink, late hours, and whatever can make you ill and spoil the cruise. You will often stay up until two or three o'clock and still want to get up early because the ship is scheduled to arrive in port later that morning. You will find that a few hours' nap late in the afternoon is revitalizing under such combat conditions.

Those who do find the ultimate mate aboard ship may be interested to know that many of the major cruise lines can arrange weddings when the ship is docked in certain ports; and most of the lines offer special honeymoon packages.

Although the cruising single might not find the same variety of available mates as he or she would at the local singles bar, and although the chance for a lasting romance may be slim, the cruise vacation does offer the single an opportunity to spend a fun and even relaxing vacation, with plenty of companionship while visiting several interesting and exciting foreign ports. (See chapter 14 for how well each ship rates for singles.)

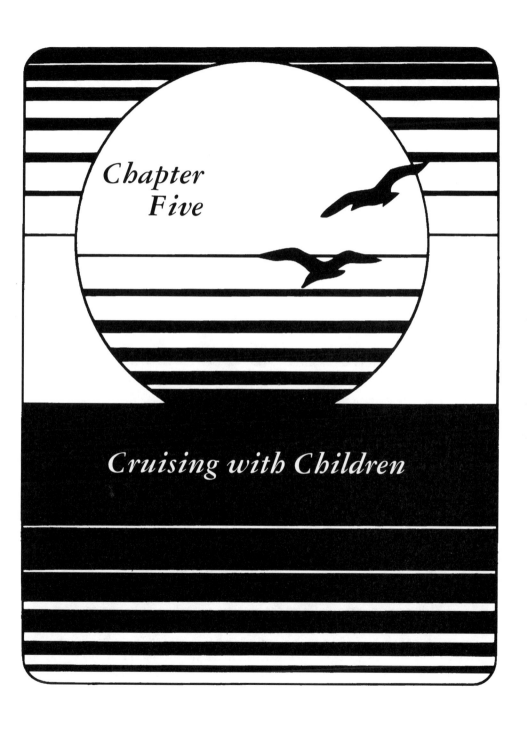

Chapter
Five

Cruising with Children

Prior to considering the pros and cons of cruising with children, you must decide whether to take them along on the vacation in the first place. For those of you who embrace the philosophy that a vacation is an opportunity for a second honeymoon—an escape from dishes, housecleaning, commuter trains, and alarm clocks—there exists no argument that could persuade you to embark upon a family sojourn. Certainly, there is no doubt that travel with children requires a degree of sacrifice on the part of the parent.

However, for those of you who feel that "vacation time" is "family time" and an opportunity to share some pleasant experiences with your children, consideration of a family cruise should be given top priority on your list of possible holidays.

Although children's requirements and interests vary with age, by and large the pre-teen crowd is happy swimming, playing, eating hamburgers, and staying up late. Your first reaction may be to take them for a dip in the neighborhood pool, followed by dinner at McDonald's and the late-night horror show. Upon longer reflection, you may conclude that the purpose of traveling with children is not only to show them a good time, but for you to have a good time with them while broadening their intellectual and cultural horizons. Disney World or a family camping trip may prove to be an excellent first endeavor, but the frequent and seasoned traveler will certainly want to move on to more worldly pursuits.

My personal experience would indicate that there exists no more perfect family vacation than a cruise. Where but on a cruise can you find a sufficient variety of delectable foods, entertainment, activities, and events to meet the personal preferences of parent and child alike? Where but on a cruise can your children be royally entertained from morning until night while you just relax?

One of the truly rewarding pluses for a parent is having to unpack the luggage only on one occasion while still being able to see a variety of exotic places. Many an adventurous family has been discouraged from taking in several European countries or Caribbean islands because of the hassle of dragging children and baggage from airport to airport and from hotel to hotel. On a cruise, you and the children have the unique opportunity of exploring as many different ports as your time may allow while your hotel floats along with you. On those cruises that offer an air-sea package, you part with your bags upon entering your hometown airport, and then do not see them again until they are brought to your private cabin on the ship.

During the day, a cruise offers a great variety of activities for children. In addition to the standard swimming pools, shuffleboard, deck tennis, Ping-Pong, an electronic game room, and gymnasium, which are open continuously, many cruise ships doing the Caribbean provide counselors and a special program for younger children, including scavenger hunts, arts and crafts, and a costume ball. In fact, several of the lines have programs in which the children are picked up after breakfast, entertained and fed all day, and not returned until after they have had their evening meal. In addition to the specially designed activities, the children will usually wish to participate in many of the adult-oriented events. During a typical day at sea, most cruises offer such activities as first-run movies, games around the pool, dancing classes, trap shooting, exercise groups, golf instruction, bingo, horse racing, and other parlor games. Don't be surprised if your children have a great deal of difficulty making their selections from the bulletin of the next day's activities that is pushed under your door every morning. Deciding between a bingo game and a Walt Disney movie can be somewhat difficult for a nine-year-old.

Dining on a ship with children is infinitely simpler and vastly more enjoyable than dragging them around from one restaurant to another in hopes of finding a mutually acceptable establishment. Since you have an assigned table with the same waiter for most of your meals, the waiter will soon learn your children's special needs and be able to efficiently accommodate them. Whether it is a booster chair, chocolate milk, or catsup for the *pommes frites,* you need only ask once and it should be there the remainder of the trip. The waiters are there to please you, and they have been trained to service your entire family in grand style. Although your children will certainly want to sample the numerous international and gourmet offerings, it is possible to arrange for them to have hamburgers, steaks, French fries, or similar "American pie" items at every meal. However, you may be in store for a big surprise when your finicky offspring, who at home insists on having his orange juice strained and the last drop of gravy removed from his meat, orders eggplant Parmesan, Tournedos Rossini, or crêpes suzette.

There is usually no babysitting problem on a ship. During the day and early evening, your cabin steward, whose galley is located only a few steps from your cabin, will be more than happy to look in on your children while they are napping or playing. Late in the evening, you can hire one of the maids to sit with your children for a reasonable price. If your children are not of too tender an age, you may elect to leave them alone in the room. On a ship, you are only moments away from your cabin, and it is convenient to check up on the youngsters frequently without detracting from your own evening. To be safe, it is always advisable to check out the babysitting situation with the cruise line prior to booking your cruise.

In case of an emergency, it is comforting to know that most ships have a hospital, pharmacy, and sailing physician. Contrary to some popularly expressed opinions, ships are as safe a place for children as almost anywhere else. Young children must be cautioned and watched so they do not lean over an open rail or run down wet steps. However, this is certainly no different from preventing them from leaning over an open balcony in a hotel or running around a slippery pool.

It is unlikely that children will be bored. Even before they have an opportunity to search out the many corners of the ship, they will find themselves in port. On most cruises, you will be visiting a different place during a majority of the days afloat. This affords the children an opportunity to stretch their legs and partake in the same activities they would have pursued had you flown to the port rather than sailed. Most ships give lectures and provide you with magazines describing the places of interest in each port prior to your arrival. Thus, there exists ample time and facility to carefully plan your tour of the port so as to include items of interest to the children.

This should not suggest that you must give up your own sightseeing or shopping plans. It is entirely possible in the popular port of St. Thomas to divide your day between shopping for bargains in the wide selection of international stores and then having a leisurely lunch and swim at one of the seaside hotels or magnificent white-sand beaches. Should your ship dock at Montego Bay, your family could raft down an authentic tropical jungle river, climb from the sea up a natural waterfall, ride donkeys through a lush plantation, swim at a clear, palm-laden beach, and take in a native limbo show, all within six to eight hours.

Although almost every cruise will offer most of the activities and programs described above, the best ships for children are probably the larger vessels (over 30,000 tons), because they usually have more facilities, more extensive programs, and more space to move around. The QE2, Norway, "The Big Red Boat," Celebrity, and Princess cruise lines have excellent facilities for preschool children. Through the years, Princess Cruises has had the best programs for pre-teens and teens. Royal Caribbean, Costa, and Carnival have also emphasized children's facilities and activities in recent years. The two new 83,000-ton, 2,400-passenger Disney ships debuting in 1998 and 1999, the Disney Magic and Disney Wonder, are totally geared and designed for families cruising with youngsters. Ships of most of the lines have special programs for children during the summer and on holiday cruises. Most of the larger ships also offer special events for teenagers. When selecting an itinerary, you may be well-advised to concentrate on the shorter cruises (three to seven days) that travel in calm sunny climes, and to avoid cruises where the waters could be choppy and the weather inclement. Those Caribbean cruises embarking from Florida, Puerto Rico, and other islands may be an ideal first venture.

If your children are seven years or older, I would especially recommend taking them on a Mediterranean cruise that visits such historic civilizations as Italy, Turkey, Greece, or Israel, or on a Northern European cruise that may dock at such cities as Southampton (Port of London), Le Havre (Port of Paris), Amsterdam, Hamburg, Copenhagen, Oslo, Stockholm, Helsinki, and St. Petersburg. Such Mediterranean and Northern European cruises are marvelous, painless ways to expand your children's education and exposure to foreign lands and cultures. An adult might prefer visiting a different country each year in order to slowly assimilate the culture rather than barnstorming many countries at one time; however, for a child, it is easier to comprehend, remember, and compare the differences when viewed in close proximity—an experience more akin to reading about different countries in a textbook at school.

Probably the greatest argument for cruising with children is the moderate cost. Almost every ship's schedule of fares provides that a child under a certain age (generally twelve) sharing a room with two adults need pay only one-half or less of the minimum fare (the fare charged for the least expensive accommodations aboard). Thus, on a cruise where the fares range from $1,000 to $2,000 per person, it is possible to book a minimum quad (a room accommodating four persons) and pay $1,000 for each adult and $500 for each child. Travelers who desire more sumptuous accommodations can take a room at the more expensive rate and still only pay $500 for any child who may share that room. Should the ship not be completely filled, you may be able to obtain two adjoining double rooms for the same price as sharing a minimum quad. In any event, it never hurts to check with the chief purser or hotel manager upon getting on the ship to see if such an arrangement is available.

The following cruise lines advertise special programs for young children, pre-teens, and teens: American Hawaii Cruises, Carnival Cruise Lines, Celebrity Cruises, Costa Cruise Lines, Crystal Cruises, Cunard Line (on *QE2* and *Royal Viking Sun*), Disney Cruise Line, Holland America Line, Norwegian Cruise Line, Premier Cruises, Princess Cruises (on most ships), and Royal Caribbean International. All of these lines have special children's facilities, children's menus, reduced rates in a shared cabin, cribs for the cabins, and children's counselors with special programs. Some of them provide private baby-sitters in the evenings.

Of course, every parent knows his or her own children and whether or not they would adjust to the cruise vacation. However, many a parent has been pleasantly surprised at how well-behaved and well-adjusted his children have been on a cruise as compared to their normal behavior at home. Parents often fail to give their children sufficient credit for acquiring maturity. On a cruise, a child for the first time may experience such hedonistic delights as being pampered and waited upon by foreign strangers, tasting the finest culinary creations offered anywhere in the world, witnessing the breathtaking beauty of exotic ports, being lavishly entertained from morning 'til night, and last, but not least, being treated like an adult. Children will more often than not rise to the occasion. Who wouldn't? (See chapter 14 for how well each ship rates for children.)

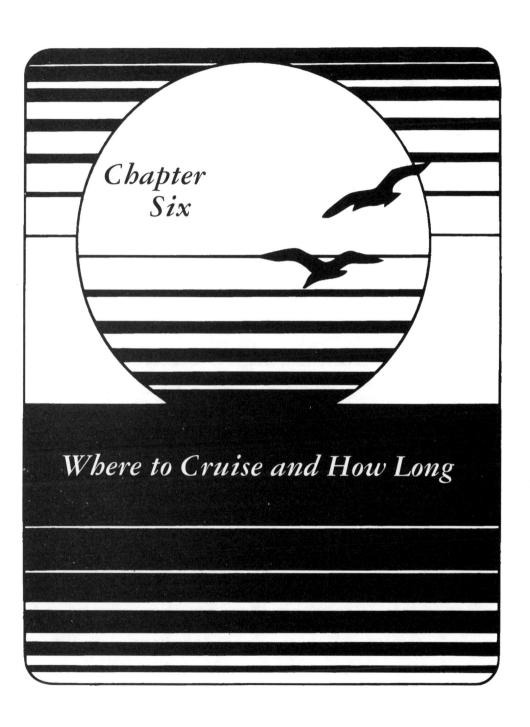

Chapter
Six

Where to Cruise and How Long

Cruise grounds; ports of call; points of interest; and what to do with limited hours in port

Cruising the Seven Seas

Length of Cruise

The possibilities for places to cruise are as infinite as the coastal cities found on a map of the world. Today it is feasible to sail about almost anywhere in the seven seas provided you are endowed with the time, finances, and inclination.

You can board ship at Fort Lauderdale or Miami and sail to Bermuda, the Bahamas, or to any of the tropical islands in the Caribbean. A number of vessels provide embarkations for such Caribbean cruises from Palm Beach, Tampa, Port Canaveral, New Orleans, New York, cities along the Eastern seaboard, and even Puerto Rico, while others include stops in Central and South America.

Should you live near the West Coast, there are numerous cruises leaving from Los Angeles, and San Francisco sailing to Mexico, Central America, South America, Hawaii, Alaska, the South Sea Islands, Australia, and the Orient.

If you are traveling in Europe, you can board ship at LeHavre, Southampton, Bremerhaven, Copenhagen, or Amsterdam for cruises traversing the fjords of Norway or visiting ports in the Baltic, Northern Europe, and even Russia. Perhaps you would prefer a ship leaving Cannes, Monte Carlo, Athens, Venice, Naples, or Genoa, visiting Southern Spain, Northern Africa, Sicily, the Greek islands, the Turkish Coast, or the Middle East. Dozens of ships based in Pireaus (Port of

Athens) offer regular cruises to the myriad of lovely Greek islands as well as to ports in Turkey, Israel, Egypt, and on the Black Sea, and to other Middle Eastern coastal cities. During the spring and summer months, numerous riverboats and barges cruise down the rivers of France, as well as down the Elbe, Rhine, and Moselle Rivers in Germany, the Danube in Austria, the Nile in Egypt, and the waterways of Holland.

Several vessels offer "around the world" cruises extending from forty to ninety days and calling at sample ports in Europe, Africa, Asia, Australia, South America, and various islands along the way. If you do not have time for such a long vacation, it is possible on some of these ships to board and disembark at certain points midway into the cruise. It would be somewhat beyond the scope of this book to cover every conceivable port and every possible itinerary. However, the following sections on "Ports of Call" describe almost all of the popular stops in the more widely traversed cruise areas. The description of each port is not intended to be exhaustive, but is designed to suggest points of interest, scenic places to visit, shopping, beaches, and restaurants for passengers of cruise ships who have from six to twelve hours to spend in port. Current itineraries for the various ships can be found in *Official Steamship Guide International.*

Ports of Call

> Bermuda, the Bahamas, the Caribbean, and South America
> The Mediterranean, Greek Islands,
>   Middle East, and Environs
> Northern Europe, the Baltic, the North Sea,
>   and the Fjords
> Cruises from the West Coast, Mexico,
>   the South Seas, Hawaii, and the Far East
> East Africa and Indian Ocean Cruises
> Transatlantic Crossings

Bermuda, the Bahamas, the Caribbean, and South America

The lush, blue Caribbean is one of the most desirable areas for the cruise vacation because the waters are calm and the variety of islands is endless. Until the seventies, the major cruise ships embarked from New York, resulting in several days at the beginning and end of each cruise being spent in the rougher waters of the Atlantic. During the late fall, winter, and early spring, the weather in the Atlantic is often inclement and the ocean is choppy, making it impossible for you to sit out on deck until your ship is well past Cape Hatteras.

Today, most ships depart from Port Everglades (Port of Fort Lauderdale), Dodge Island (Port of Miami), Tampa, Port Canaveral (Port of Orlando), New Orleans, Palm Beach, or Puerto Rico. These cruises offer the traveler instant sun and the time to visit a greater number of islands because the traveling distance has been reduced. Some of the seven-day cruises from these southern ports make as many as six stops, and the fourteen-day cruises may call on five to twelve different ports.

The islands in the Caribbean area are varied, each with its own individual flavor. The natives of Bermuda, Barbados, Grenada, Jamaica, and the Bahamas still speak with a British accent. French is the official language of Martinique, Guadeloupe, St. Barts, and part of St. Martin. The little towns and brightly painted buildings in Aruba, Bonaire, Curaçao, and the other part of Saint Maarten (St. Martin) are reminiscent of Holland, as are the language and restaurants. Spanish is the native tongue in Puerto Rico, Santo Domingo, and Caracas. Although the United States bought St. Thomas, St. John, and St. Croix (the U.S. Virgin Islands) from Denmark in 1917, the Danes left their mark. Some of the streets still bear names similar to the streets of Copenhagen, and Danish smörbrod and beer can still be purchased in a few local restaurants.

Which islands you will enjoy most depends upon your personal tastes and interests. Many of the ships make a point of stopping at least at one island where there is gambling, one island where there is shopping, and one where there is swimming. Most of the islands offer duty-free shopping bargains of one kind or another, and most have beautiful beaches. Rather than running off to a public beach with limited facilities, consider going to a large hotel or resort where you can make a quick change and enjoy the comforts of the hotel's beach, pool, restaurants, and other facilities. The following are the highlights of some of the more popular ports in this area:

ANGUILLA

The most northerly of the Leeward Islands in the eastern Caribbean lies 5 miles north of St. Martin. Once a part of a federation with St. Kitts and Nevis, Anguilla gained its independence from that association in 1980 and has since been a self-governed British possession. Only 16 miles in length, the island is easily traversed by rental car or taxi.

Anguilla boasts two of the finest resorts in the Caribbean. Malliouhana at Meads Bay is perhaps the most perfect property in the Caribbean, and a marvelous place to spend your day. The beach is among the best on the island, and the incredibly charming indoor/outdoor restaurant perched on a cliff overlooking the sea is not only romantic, but features the imaginative French cuisine of the Rostang family. Whether you opt for lunch or dinner, it is one of those uniquely perfect dining experiences that we constantly seek but rarely find.

Cap Juluca at Maundays Bay is a unique Moorish-style retreat spread along a lovely strand of white-sand beach featuring Eclipse, yet another outstanding restaurant. If time permits, you will want to visit both of these fabulous properties.

The best public beaches are at Shoal Bay and Sandy Ground, where there are some colorful restaurants and small shops. A top choice for a day trip would be a snorkeling expedition to either Sandy Island or Little Cay Bay. Sandy Island, accessible by ferry or motor boat from Sandy Ground, is a tiny islet with a few palm trees surrounded by powder-fine sand and good reefs for snorkeling. The open-air restaurant features barbecued ribs, chicken, and lobster, accompanied by cold beer or rum punch. Little Cay Bay is a picturesque secluded cove accessible only by boat. Here you will find a tiny, white-sand beach with turquoise, azure, and verdant green waters—a romantic spot for a private picnic with good snorkeling possibilities. Other splendid restaurants on the island include Koal Keal and Blanchards.

ANTIGUA

Antigua is a 108-square-mile Caribbean island located about midway between Martinique and St. Thomas and noted most for its numerous white-sand beaches. The travel brochures tout this "Island Paradise" as having 365 beaches—one for each day of the year. The climate is mild, with temperatures varying between the mid-seventies and mid-eighties.

Your ship will dock at Heritage Quay or at Deep Water Harbor near **St. Johns,** the capital. A small shopping center is located near both piers, with several shops featuring local handicrafts, souvenirs, T-shirts, and a few imported items. Points of interest include English Harbour and Nelson's Dockyard, an eighteenth-century naval base, St. John's Cathedral, Clarence House, Fig Tree Hill Drive, Devil's Bridge, and Fort Berkeley. There is an 18-hole golf course at Cedar Valley, and 9-hole courses at Antigua Beach Hotel and Half Moon Bay. Casinos are located at the St. James's Club, the Flamingo Antigua Hotel in St. John, Halcyon Cove Beach Resort at Dickinson Bay, and at the Heritage Quay. The most popular restaurants on the island include Admiral's Inn (seafood), Lobster Pot (Caribbean dishes and seafood), Julian's (Continental), and Alberto's (Italian).

With only six to ten hours in port, I would recommend spending your day at the St. James's Club, Hawksbill Beach Hotel, or at the Rex Halcyon Cove Beach Resort. These resorts are located on lovely strands of white-sand beach with warm, clear waters. They feature adequate swimming pools, numerous shops, water sports (water-skiing, snorkeling, scuba, and sailing), decent tennis courts, a casino, and picturesque restaurants.

THE BAHAMAS

The Bahamas consist of a stretch of hundreds of islands extending off the coast of Florida down to Haiti. Cruise ships generally stop at **Nassau** or **Freeport,** Grand Bahama, which are the most populous and developed of the Bahamian islands.

Several of the cruise lines have purchased and developed pristine "out-islands" in the Bahamas, where their ships stop for a beach party and snorkeling.

Although the Bahamas have gained complete independence from the motherland, you are constantly reminded of the British influence. In Nassau, you can shop in the native straw market adjacent to the docks at Rawson Square, sample some Bahamian conch chowder at a quaint seaside restaurant, take a horse-and-buggy ride through the streets of town, play tennis at any of the large hotels, swim in the absolutely still-clear waters of the beautiful beaches of Paradise Island, or visit the casino and elegant restaurants. The Cafe Martinique (French), the Villa d'Este (Italian), the Buena Vista (Continental), and the Graycliff (Continental) are perhaps some of the best (if not the most expensive) restaurants to be found in the Bahamas.

A short excursion to Coral World on Coral Island is worthwhile. Here you can view sea life and fish indigenous to this part of the world, including sharks, stingrays, and giant turtles. Also located here are an open-air restaurant and a snorkeling trail.

Many passengers enjoy spending their day exploring Paradise Island, which is accessible for a $2 charge by motor launches that depart right at the pier between the cruise ships and town. Until recently this was a beautiful pristine island where visitors could walk along miles of white-sand beach and paths running through pine forests past azure lagoons. Unfortunately, the group owning the Atlantis Hotel Complex purchased the majority of the island, knocked down most of the forests, eliminated the lagoons, and constructed glitzy mega-hotels. The golf course remains on the far side of the island, and the Atlantis Hotels have a large casino, a unique aquarium, and an imaginative pool complex. The beaches at Cable Beach Hotel and the Radisson on Nassau are also excellent for sunning, swimming, and water sports, and are accessible by a 10-minute bus ride.

When shopping at Grand Bahama, you will not want to miss the variety of imported merchandise in the colorful international bazaar, where you can stroll down cobbled streets into shops with imports from Scandinavia, Great Britain, Hong Kong, Japan, India, Spain, and France. You also will want to taste some delectable conch fritters and sausages with ale at one of the atmospheric British pubs, try your luck at El Casino adjoining the bazaar, or swim at one of the white-sand beaches in the fashionable Lucaya area. The best sports facilities on the island are at the Bahama Princess Hotel and the Holiday Inn.

BARBADOS

Barbados is 21 miles long and 14 miles wide with 260,000 inhabitants who are independent members of the British Commonwealth. They enjoy a dry, sunny climate with temperatures varying from seventy to eighty degrees. The island's British heritage is most evident in the capital, **Bridgetown,** with its quaint houses and its statue of Lord Nelson in Trafalgar Square. Taste the local rum that is reputed to be the best in the world; shop at the Terminal at Bridgeport Harbour or in the Broad Street area for duty-free British woolens, Irish linens, English bone china, French perfumes, Japanese cameras, local black-coral jewelry, and Swiss watches; browse through the local arts and crafts offered for sale at Pelican Village off the Princess Alice Highway; see sugar refined at a local factory; or play tennis, sunbathe, and swim in crystal-clear waters on one of the long stretches of fine sand beach or at one of the large, luxury hotels, such as the Sandy Lane, Glitter Bay, Royal Pavillion, and the Coral Reef Club, all of which are located on the west coast, where the waters are extremely calm. There are tennis courts, a golf course, and a beautiful beach at Sandy Lane. Hotels on the Atlantic, east coast, enjoy panoramic vistas; however, the sea is frequently not safe for swimming. All of the resorts offer a variety of dining opportunities. The most popular local restaurants outside the resorts include Bagutelle Great House (Continental), Carambola (Thai and Continental), Sandy Bay (Continental), Ile de France (French), Pisces (seafood), and Josef's (Scandinavian).

Other points of interests include Barbados Museum; Flower Forest, an eight-acre floral park; Harrison's Cave, which you tour by electric tram; Barbados Wildlife Reserve; and the oldest synagogue in the Western Hemisphere, dating back to 1654.

BERMUDA

Bermuda is a self-governing member of the British Commonwealth. It covers 21 square miles and has an English-speaking population of 55,000. The people are very British, and the island boasts a mild climate with lovely scenery, pastel houses, and coral-pink beaches. Temperatures vary from fifty-eight to seventy-six degrees from November through April, and from sixty-five to eighty-six degrees from May through October. You can shop for bargains in friendly shops that feature English bone china and woolens, French perfumes, Danish silver, and Swiss watches; visit the botanical gardens, government house, historical society museum, and the completely restored nineteenth-century fortification at Fort St. Catherine; explore the Crystal Cave, a natural cavern that ranks as Bermuda's most beautiful attraction; play tennis or golf at one of the island's luxury hotels; rent a motorcycle and take a ride across the island; or just swim in the calm, blue waters of a quiet cove along a soft, pink-sand beach. There are some excellent tennis courts at the Southampton Princess and the Sonesta Beach hotels. To the left of the Southampton Princess Hotel is one of the most beautiful stretches of pink-sand beach, inlets, and coves to be found anywhere in the world. You may wish to have your waiter on the ship pack a box lunch with a bottle of wine so you can picnic on this lovely public beach. The Southampton Princess also offers numerous gourmet restaurants, as well as those specializing in seafood and steaks.

If your ship docks at St. George, you will find numerous souvenir shops and boutiques right at the harbor. The most interesting and accessible beach is at Tobacco Bay. The mile-and-a-half path that runs along the harbor and ocean between the dock and Tobacco Bay past Fort St. Catherine is scenic and worth exploring.

THE CAYMAN ISLANDS

The Cayman Islands, peaceful little islands lying 100 miles northwest of Jamaica, have a colorful history dating to their discovery by Columbus on his fourth voyage to the West Indies. They are now a crown colony of the United Kingdom, and their favorable tax policy makes these islands one of the world's most attractive tax havens. Several cruise ships tender to **Georgetown** on Grand Cayman to permit their passengers to enjoy a day exploring one of the most beautiful stretches of white-sand beach in the Caribbean. Although Grand Cayman is only 22 miles long and 8 miles across, it boasts a 7-mile strand of beach lined with pines, palms, and small cottage-like hotel complexes. You can spend your day swimming and snorkeling in the crystal-clear waters; visiting a turtle farm where turtles are bred and raised; playing with stingrays at Stingray City (available by motor launch); golfing at the Britannia or Safe Haven courses; or browsing through the duty-free shops in Georgetown in search of bargains in china and crystal imported from all over Europe, Swiss watches, black coral jewelry, and French perfumes.

Should you be docking in the evening, you can dine at Chef Tell's Grand Old House on a broad veranda and watch the sun set over the beautiful blue waters of the Caribbean while enjoying some of the best food on the island. Hemingway's at the Hyatt Regency; Lantanas at the Caribbean Club; Pappagallo, an Italian and seafood restaurant set in a bird sanctuary overlooking a lagoon; and Ottmars are also excellent. The Holiday Inn, the Hyatt, the Westin, and the Radisson are the largest hotels on the island, and each offers tennis courts, a swimming pool, and beaches with full facilities. Those who wish to scuba or snorkel can make arrangements in Georgetown or at any of the larger hotels.

COSTA RICA

Cruise ships traversing the Panama Canal often stop at Central America's most developed democratic republic, which is bordered by Nicaragua on the north and Panama on the south. The beauty of the country is its varied scenery, which includes lush green mountains and valleys, volcanoes, ranches, farmland, rolling hills, lovely streams and waterfalls, jungles, and beaches.

In the center of the country, surrounded by mountains, sits San Jose, the capital, where tourists may wish to visit the many parks, the lavish Teatro National (an architectural jewel built in the nineteenth century that presently offers concerts, ballet, opera, and theater), the National Museum with its archeological and historical artifacts, the Museum of Contemporary Art, the Museo de Oro with its displays of all kinds of gold, the Jade Museum, and the president's home.

Ships call at either the Atlantic port of Limon or the nearby Pacific ports of Caldera and Puntarenas. On the Atlantic side, the best beaches are at the National Park of Cahuita; on the Pacific they are on Nicaya Peninsula. From Puntarenas ferries traverse the gulf of Nicaya to Tambor and Paquera; however, timetables for returns can be unreliable and anyone wishing to visit this area is advised to be certain about the timing of their return. From Tambor or Paquera, you can take a taxi to the beaches and hotels at Playa Tambor, Playa Montezuma, and Cabo Blanco.

Cruise ships generally offer excursions to San Jose, Sarachi (the handicraft town where you can purchase the famous Costa Rican hand-painted oxcarts, as well as wine glasses and decanters), the rain forest at Carrara Biological Reserve, horseback rides through tropical valleys and forests, river rafting, Poas Volcano National Park, and offshore islands. Those venturing out on their own can hire a taxi at the port (maximum four passengers) and for about $150 for three to five hours see the beautiful countryside, visit the Carrara Rain Forest, and explore Jaco, where there is a long stretch of black-sand beach, horseback riding, souvenir shops, and several local restaurants. Unfortunately some of the more popular resort communities cannot be accessed during a one-day visit.

DEVIL'S ISLAND

Lying 9 miles off the coast of French Guiana are three small islands that were known as the Devil's Islands until 1753, when they were renamed the Salut Islands (islands of salvation).

The largest is L'ile Royale. Saint Joseph to the east is the most beautiful, and Devil's Island to the north is the wildest. These islands were the site of the notorious French penal colony.

Cruise ships send tenders to **L'ile Royale,** where there is a small rustic inn offering limited shopping and cold drinks. Around the island are some of the vestiges of the prison colony, including the prison cells, chapel, death row cells, warden's accommodations, hospital, morgue, and children's cemetery.

L'ile Royale receives a lot of rain and as a result is very lush and verdant. There are numerous paths around the island, rewarding visitors with magnificent views of palms, rocky ocean coastlines, and the two neighboring islands. It is possible to walk or jog around the island. A protected sea area known as the Prisoner's Pool is located directly across the island from the dock. However, the waters in the vicinity are infested with sharks, and I do not know how safe it would be to swim here.

THE DOMINICAN REPUBLIC

The Dominican Republic shares the island of Hispaniola with Haiti. Although this Spanish-speaking island boasts some majestic mountains and jungle rivers, your ship will probably not dock for a sufficient time to permit you to explore the island. If the ship drops anchor at **Santo Domingo,** you may wish to visit such historical landmarks as Alcazar de Colon, the restored sixteenth-century palace built for Columbus's son Diego, and the 400-year-old Cathedral Santa Maria La Menor, site of the Christopher Columbus tomb. The National Museum of the Dominican Republic offers some interesting Indian artifacts, while the National Museum of Fine Arts features the work of more recent painters and sculptors. The 445-acre Botanical Gardens at Arroyo Hondo are the largest in all of Latin America and can be toured on foot, by horse carriage, or by boat. The best buys are in amber, which is mined and crafted on the island. You can swim at the pool, play tennis, and gamble at El Embajador Hotel, Jaragua Renaissance, Intercontinental, or the Sheraton; or, if time permits, drive out to the Caribbean's largest full-facility resort, Casa De Campo at La Romana, where there are three challenging golf courses, thirteen tennis courts, a riding stable, water sports, a picturesque

Romanesque-designed artist's village with shops and restaurants, a shooting range, numerous restaurants, and a beautiful beach. Ships of Costa Cruises currently offer beach parties on a private island, with optional excursions to Casa De Campo.

If your ship docks in **Puerto Plata,** there is little to do other than shop for amber in the local market; but if you feel adventurous, rent a horse at the dock and ride through the countryside to the beach. Several new hotels have been built at Playa Dorado, the site of a Robert Trent Jones-designed golf course. Properties with the most facilities include Jack Tar Village, Caribbean Village Club on the Green, and Plaza Dorado Hotel and Casino. The best beach is located 15 miles east of town at Sosua.

THE DUTCH ISLANDS

The Dutch Islands of Aruba, Bonaire, and Curaçao represent the Netherlands in miniature, with gabled, pastel-colored buildings along picturesque streets. Dutch is the official language, although employees in the shops, hotels, and restaurants all speak English. The climate is sunny and dry, cooled by pleasant trade winds with temperatures ranging from a mean of eighty degrees in the winter to eighty-four degrees in the summer.

In **Curaçao,** you will find a fair selection of merchandise in a number of shops offering bargains in jewelry, watches, china, and antiques. Willemstad is no longer the shopping haven it used to be. You can see the world-famous floating pontoon bridge in Willemstad swing open to allow ships into the harbor, or from atop the 33-foot-thick fortress walls you can watch the ships sail into the harbor. One of the oldest synagogues in the Western world still in use, the Mikve Israel Emanuel Synagogue, is right in town, and on the outskirts of town you can visit the Jewish cemetery, which is one of the oldest Caucasian burial places in the New World. You can sample Curaçao liqueur at the distillery where it is made in Chobolobo, or eat *rijsttafel* (rice with forty or more exotic complements) at the Rijsttafel Indonesia Restaurant, or you can try *kapucijners* (meat, chick peas, beans, bacon, onions, and sauces) at the historic Fort Nassau Restaurant, a renovated military fort on a hill overlooking the city. Try the French and Swiss cuisine at Bistro le Clochard and L'Alouette, or international offerings with a view at Le Tournesol, atop the Plaza Hotel in town. For tennis or swimming, your best bets are Sonesta Beach Hotel and Casino, Princess Beach Hotel and Casino, or the newly renovated Curaçao Sheraton Hotel and Casino. Other attractions include Christoffel National Park, Curaçao Seaquarium, Curaçao's Ostrich Farm, Curaçao Underwater Marine Park, and Hato Caves.

Bonaire boasts 18 miles of reef that surround the island, offering some of the most spectacular scuba diving, spearfishing, and underwater photography in the Caribbean. At many of the larger hotels, arrangements can be made for these activities, as well as for swimming, water-skiing, sailing, and glass-bottom boat rides. Hotels with the most facilities include Captain Don's Habitat, Harbour Village Beach Resort, Divi Flamingo Beach Resort & Casino, and Sand Dollar

Condos and Beach Club. The best dining is at Jardine Tropicale and Capriccio and the best beach for windsurfing is at Lac Bay. This is also the island of the flamingos, and in the late afternoon bird watchers can see these graceful birds as well as thousands of herons, snipe, pelicans, parrots, parakeets, and others making their way across the blue Caribbean skies.

Aruba's capital is Oranjestad, where you can see many traditional Dutch multicolored houses with red-tile roofs, as well as a charming deep-water harbor. Don't miss the strange Divi-Divi tree and the huge monolithic boulder formations at Casibari. Swim at the beautiful, wide Palm Beach, which services the Aruba Marriott, Americana, Hyatt, Radisson, Sheraton, and Holiday Inn hotels. These hotels also contain casinos. Taste Indonesian *rijsttafel* while dining on a houseboat at Bali Floating Restaurant, or try Dutch food inside an old windmill at De Olde Molden. For more upscale dining, Chez Mathilde near the Sonesta, Escale in the Sonesta, Brisas del Mar, Papiamento, or La Dolce Vita (Italian cuisine) at Palm Beach are recommended. The town is near the harbor and contains numerous shops offering international bargains.

GRENADA

Grenada, which became an independent nation in 1974, is known as the "Spice Island" because it is here that cloves, mace, cinnamon, ginger, and nutmeg are produced and shipped throughout the world. The 133-square-mile island has a population of 105,000 and an average year-round temperature of eighty degrees. The capital, **St. George,** is often referred to as the most picturesque harbor in the Caribbean, and you will want to climb up one of its quaint cobblestone streets to get a panoramic view of the magnificent waterfront. You may wish to swim at one of the hotels located on the beautiful Grand Anse Beach, such as Spice Island Inn, Coyaba Beach Resort, and Grenada Renaissance. Or you may prefer to drive to Annandale Falls or Concorde Falls to picnic and swim in tropical pools beneath cascading waterfalls. You can visit the nutmeg factories at Gouyave and Grenvelle and purchase samples of the island's spices either at the factory or almost anywhere in town. Although the island and the beaches are lovely, you will be harassed constantly by vendors and beggars to the point of distraction. The highest-touted restaurants are La Belle Creole, Canboulay, and Spice Island Inn. LaBelle Creole and Canboulay both serve West Indian cuisine with hillside panoramic views. Spice Island Inn overlooks the beach and sea.

GUADELOUPE

Guadeloupe is a French department made up of two islands separated by a narrow channel—giving the appearance from the air of being a butterfly. Pointe-à-Pitre is in **Grande-Terre,** which is the flat, developed island with fine beaches. **Basse-Terre** is mountainous, with volcanic peaks, tropical green forests, lush vegetation, mountain streams, and waterfalls. The 327,800 inhabitants speak French and live in a basically warm climate that has a great deal of rain from July to November. You may wish to sample some French or Creole cooking at one of the hotel restaurants or in town, or shop for some of the excellent bargains in French perfumes, linens, and wines.

Good beaches include Anse de la Gourde between St. Francois and Pointe des Chateaux, Caravelle Beach near St. Anne, and Le Grand Anse north of Deshaies on Basse-Terre; there are nudist beaches at Place Crawen, Pointe Tarare, Illet du Gosier, and Pointe des Chateaux. However, you will find the most facilities at the beautiful, tree-lined, white-sand beach of the Club Med Caravelle Hotel, where you can water-ski, play tennis, and have lunch. You may have to pay to get on the premises. Other large hotels with facilities include La Plantation Ste-Marthe and Le Meridien at St. Francois and Canella Beach, Arawak, and Auberge de la Vieille Tour, located on the 5-mile beach at Gosier. The highest-rated restaurants on Grand Terre include Auberge de la Vieille Tour, La Balata, La Canne a Sucre, La Louisiane, Les Oiseaux, and the restaurant at La Plantation Ste-Marthe.

If you have enough time, you can drive 40 miles from Pointe-à-Pitre to Basse-Terre and pass through sugarcane plantations, tropical forests at Guadeloupe's National Park, banana trees, beautiful hibiscus, and the high volcanic peaks of La Soufriére with its waterfalls, lakes, and streams. Crayfish Falls at the National Park is one of the most popular sites on the island.

HAITI

Haiti is a tropical country occupying the western portion of the island of Hispaniola. French is the official language, but the majority of the inhabitants speak a Creole tongue that is difficult to distinguish.

Port-au-Prince is an unusual town with a blend of African and French cultures exhibited in the exquisite native paintings and crafts. You may wish to visit one of the luxury hotels located in the cooler heights of Petionville. Here again, the most facilities will be found at the Club Med; however, you must make advance arrangements to be admitted. You will enjoy tasting some of the French-Creole delicacies as well as the local Barbancourt rum and liqueur. If you have time, you can take a taxi up into the mountains and visit the Barbancourt factory to sample their many different beverages. At night you can dance at a local club, witness a fairly authentic voodoo ceremony, or gamble at the International Casino on the waterfront.

Several ships dock at **Cap Haitien,** 200 miles from Port-au-Prince. This picturesque but poor little city once was the richest colonial city in the French empire. Here you can explore the ruins of the Sans Souci Palace and Christophe's Citadelle atop a donkey, or you can browse through the native market. Whether you are in Port-au-Prince or Cap Haitien, the things to buy are native paintings and sculpture. Much of the arts and crafts sold throughout the other Caribbean islands are produced in Haiti.

JAMAICA

Jamaica is one of the lushest and most beautiful of the Caribbean islands. It is a land of white-sand beaches, emerald-blue still waters, green forests, jungle rivers, and Blue Mountains. The climate is warm and sunny throughout the year, with little seasonal variation in temperature. Montego Bay, Negril, and Ocho Rios are the fashionable resort areas with numerous fine hotels on long stretches of white-sand beach. Unfortunately, because the attitude and aggressive behavior of some of the citizens have turned off prospective visitors, fewer cruise ships have chosen Jamaica as a port of call.

If your ship docks at **Montego Bay,** you can take a short taxi ride to town and browse through the shops displaying the local crafts, jewelry, watches, and foreign imports. You may wish to tour Rosehall or Greenwood Great Houses, visit Croydin Plantation, take a donkey ride, or go for a swim at Doctor's Cave Beach, Walter Fletcher Beach, or Cornwall Beach, where there is an underwater marine park. You may also wish to take the drive to raft down the tropical Martha Brae River or at Mountain Valley from the Lethe Plantation 10 miles south of town. Perennially, the best resort hotels here have been Round Hill; Tryall Golf, Tennis, and Beach Club; Half Moon Golf, Tennis, and Beach Club; and Sandals.

Many cruise ships dock at **Ocho Rios.** Within walking distance of the dock are numerous shops, a public beach, and two semi-high-rise hotels that have changed ownership numerous times over the years and are presently operated as the Grande Renaissance Resort. If you wish to spend the day at one of the better hotels or resorts such as San Souci Lido, Plantation Inn, Jamaica Inn, Ciboney, Sandals Dunn's River, Boscobel Beach, or Couples, you must make arrangements in advance because you will have difficulty getting past the front gates.

Probably the most unusual tourist attraction here is Dunn's River Falls, about a 5- to 10-minute taxi ride from the port. You can take photos and wander around the park that surrounds these incredible multilevel falls that descend to the sea, or you can experience climbing them with the assistance of a trained guide. Climbing the falls is a sensational experience; however, it is rather dangerous and not advisable for pre-teenage children. Wear a bathing suit and either waterproof athletic shoes or sandals that will not fall off.

From Ocho Rios, you could drive to Kingston via beautiful Fern Gulley and the breathtaking Blue Mountains. This is a beautiful, but somewhat dangerous drive that should be attempted only if you are not in a hurry. You would need at least ten hours in port at Montego Bay to have sufficient time to raft down the Martha Brae, visit Dunn's River Falls and Fern Gulley at Ocho Rios, and have lunch and a swim at a hotel. If time allows, you may wish to drive in the opposite direction to explore the beautiful beaches at Negril, also the location of numerous, full-facility resorts. The most facilities will be found at Negril's all-inclusive resorts such as Grand Hotel Lido, Hedonism II, and Sandals, or the more upscale Poinciana Beach Hotel. You will enjoy walking along Negril's 7-mile beach.

Should your ship drop anchor at **Port Antonio,** you will want to take the fabulous raft trip down the Rio Grande. The best hotel here is Trident Villas and the best beach is San San.

Should you be in Jamaica during the evening, don't miss taking in a native calypso or limbo show at the local clubs or hotels. There are no outstanding restaurants around the island and you are best off dining at one of the better hotels. Best items to purchase are Tia Maria liqueur and the local rums.

KEY WEST, FLORIDA

Key West is not in the Bahamas or the Caribbean, but it is becoming a popular stop for many cruise ships. Technically the southernmost point in the continental U.S., Key West is about 80 miles farther south than the southernmost point in Texas. Lying between the Gulf of Mexico and the Atlantic Ocean, this final vestige of the Florida Keys will remind visitors of the Bahamas, New Orleans, and south Florida rolled into one. Only 2 miles by 4 miles in size, the island is easy to navigate on foot or bicycle.

Adjacent to the harbor, visitors can pick up the Old Town Trolley or the Conch Tour Train, both of which provide an excellent overview of the island. Points of interest include Mel Fisher's Maritime Heritage Society Museum; the Ernest Hemingway House, where the famous author wrote many of his novels; the Audubon House, a museum displaying many works of art by the famous artist and naturalist; and the Curry Museum, a turn-of-the-century National Historic Register Museum with three stories of period furnishings. If you elect to walk from the harbor into town (about a mile and a half), you will pass through a lovely residential area.

Arrangements can be made for glass-bottom boat rides to a living coral reef, for snorkeling and scuba tours, and for sailboat racing.

Most tourists enjoy browsing through the hundreds of souvenir shops and colorful bars that line Duval and neighboring streets—Sloppy Joe's (Hemingway's favorite bar) and Jimmy Buffet's Margaritaville are the best-known drinking establishments. There are numerous small restaurants featuring fresh fish and seafood. The largest hotels are the Hilton, Hyatt, and the Ritz-Carlton.

MARTINIQUE

Martinique, like Guadeloupe, is a department of France, and its 340,000 inhabitants speak French and a Creole dialect. The weather is generally very warm throughout the year, with considerable rain from July through November. Here, you can see the black-sand beaches that inspired the paintings of Gauguin, visit the birthplace of Empress Josephine at Trois Ilets, walk through a petrified forest, drive out to the Mont Pelée Volcano and see the lava-drowned town of St. Pierre (sometimes referred to as the Caribbean Pompeii), swim at Meridian or Bakoua Beach (watch out for sea urchins), or just stroll around the old, quaint harbor town of Fort-de-France. You will want to save time to visit the shops along Rue Victor Hugo (Roger Albert's is the largest and most popular), where you can pick up some excellent bargains in French perfume, Lalique and Baccarat crystal, Limoges china, gloves, and other French imports. You can sample French-Creole cooking in town or take a motorboat out to the hotels Meridian or Bakoua-Sofitel across the bay at Trois Ilets/Pointe Du Boute. If time permits, you may prefer to take the 50-kilometer ride to the Club Mediterranean's vacation village at Buccaneer's Creek. Here you will find the island's best beach and water sports. However, you may have great difficulty getting on the premises, so it is best to call before you undertake the long drive. Noteworthy restaurants include Leyritz Plantation at Basse-Pointe (Creole), La Grande Voile in Fort-de-France (Creole), Le Planteur in Forte-de-France (French and Creole), Le Verger at La Mentin (French), and La Villa Creole at Les-Trois-Ilets.

MEXICO (EAST COAST)

Cancún is a man-made resort area created on the northeast tip of Mexico's Yucatán Peninsula. Ships generally dock at Playa del Carmen, from which it is a 30-minute ride to Cancún or at the recently built port of Calica, which is 15 minutes further away. Here you will find 14 miles of white-sand beaches, crystal-clear waters, and an average year-round temperature of eighty degrees. You can spend your day swimming, sunning, snorkeling, or playing tennis at one of the posh resort hotels such as the Ritz-Carlton, Fiesta Americana, Hyatt, or Marriott. You can enjoy 18 holes of championship golf at Pok-Ta-Pok, water sports at Aqua Bay Marina, snorkeling at Xel-Ha River near Tulum, a day of horseback riding through the jungle and beach trails at Rancho Bonita, or the incredible experience of swimming for 30 minutes down an underground river through prehistoric caverns and grottoes at the picturesque Xcaret Archeological Park adjacent to Calica. Xcaret is a unique attraction. In addition to two exotic, underground rivers, visitors can swim with dolphins; snorkel and relax at a picturesque beach; browse through an indoor/outdoor aquarium; visit a wildlife refuge, a bird sanctuary populated with exotic local birds, a butterfly pavillion, an orchard and mushroom nursery, a botanical garden, and many archeological treasures; go horseback riding through jungle trails; and enjoy lunch at one of several restaurants spread around the property.

Most cruises that stop at this area offer optional side trips to **Tulum** or **Chichen Itza** to explore the ruins of these ancient Mayan civilizations.

Cozumel is a small island off the southeastern coast of the Yucatán with fine beaches for swimming, snorkeling, and scuba. The best beach to swim and enjoy a snack or drink is Playa del Sol, about 10 miles from town. For snorkeling, Chankanaab Lagoon Park is only about 5 miles from town. You can spend the day at Stouffer's Presidente Hotel or Fiesta Americana's Sol Carib, both only a short distance from town with nice pools and restaurants, but no outstanding beaches. In town, there are many typical restaurants and art, crafts, souvenir, and jewelry shops. Lunch or drinks at Carlos 'n Charlie's is always wild and fun.

NEW ORLEANS

New Orleans is the home port for Delta Queen Steamboat Company's three river-boats as well as various cruise ships of the major cruise lines. Passengers frequently opt to spend a few days before or after their sailing in this colorful, historic city. Located at the junction of 19,000 miles of inland waterways created by the Mississippi River, its tributaries, and the Gulf Intracoastal Waterways with access to the Gulf of Mexico, New Orleans has developed into one of the United States' major international sea ports.

Tourists most frequently gravitate to the French Quarter, drawn to its centuries-old buildings with unique ironwork and courtyards and its concentration of fine restaurants, nightclubs, bars, shops, and cafés. When touring this area by foot, you may wish to visit historic Jackson Square to see Clark Mill's equestrian statue of Andrew Jackson; nineteenth-century St. Louis Cathedral and the Cabildo, which now houses part of the Louisiana State Museum; the Pontalba Apartments, which include the 1850 House and the Le Pétit Théâtre du Vieux Carré; the Manheim Gallery in the old Bank of Louisiana building; Casa Faurie (which houses the famous Brennan's Restaurant); the 1792 Merieult House, location of the Historic New Orleans Collection; picturesque Brulator Court and the Court of the Two Lions; Preservation Hall; Pirates Alley; Père Antoine Alley; Cathedral Garden; Gallier House; and the Haunted House—all located on, or just off of, Royal Street; Soniat House, Beauregard-Keyes House, Old Ursuline Convent, the Pharmacy Museum, and Napoleon House on Chartres Street; as well as the French Market on Barracks Street, where you can sample freshly prepared beignets and chicory coffee, a Louisiana culinary tradition. It would be best to purchase a map of the French Quarter to assist you in your exploration.

Other areas of interest located throughout the city include: the Faubourg-Marigny Historic District, just east of the French Quarter, with its varied collection of eighteenth- and nineteenth-century Creole-style structures built on narrow lots; the elegant Garden District; the Aquarium of the Americas with its underwater walkway; and the shops and restaurants along the Riverwalk and connecting Ernest N. Morial Convention Center proximate to the cruise ship terminal.

If you wish to stay overnight in the French Quarter, the most highly rated hotels include the Omni Royal Orleans, Royal Sonesta, Hotel Maison de Ville, Holiday Inn French Quarter, and Marriott. Best choices nearer to the Central Business District and convention center include the Fairmont, Hyatt Regency, Hilton, Sheraton, Westin, Radisson, and Windsor Court (the most elegant in the city).

Extraordinary dining is New Orleans' tour de force. Although new restaurants surface from time to time, the traditional establishments are the most reliable and world-renowned. Commander's Palace, set in an 1880s restored building with lush green patios and gardens and a jazz band on Saturdays and Sundays, is a must for visitors seeking typical Creole dishes. Other perennial favorites include Brennan's, Broussard's, Antoine's, Galatoire's, Louis XVI, Arnaud's, and Pascal's Manale Restaurant. K-Paul's Louisiana Kitchen, in the French Quarter, is an unpretentious establishment where New Orleans' most famous chef, Paul Prudhomme, dispenses his special interpretations of Creole, Cajun, French, and New Orleans cuisine. For more elegant Continental and French dining, you may wish to try the Caribbean Room at the Pontchartrain, Le Jardin (especially for Sunday champagne jazz brunch), Sazerac at the Fairmont, Winston's at the Hilton, and the Windsor Court Grill Room. Of course, any respectable tourist would not miss the compulsory pilgrimage to Café du Monde in the French Market for café au lait and beignets.

For nightlife, you will want to stroll through the streets of the French Quarter (especially Bourbon Street) to bar hop, listen to jazz bands, browse through souvenir shops, and experience the after-dark sounds, smells, and exuberant vitality most associated with this city. Many of the larger hotels have quiet piano lounges, as well as music for listening and dancing. Another nighttime possibility would be to take in the riverfront attractions along the Moonwalk and Riverwalk.

New Orleans is also a shopper's paradise where you can search out bargains in antiques or peruse designer shops. The best shopping areas for tourists include Canal Street, the French Quarter, and the complexes at One Canal Place and Riverwalk.

PUERTO RICO

Puerto Rico is a commonwealth voluntarily associated with the United States. Spanish is the native tongue of the 2,690,000 inhabitants, although many also speak English. The climate is reliably sunny and warm throughout the year. Cruise ships dock at the harbor in **San Juan,** the colorful cosmopolitan capital of the island. During the day, you can explore the quaint, authentically Spanish section of town known as "Old San Juan." Here you walk through cobbled streets surrounded by pretty plazas, Spanish-style buildings, shops, art galleries, restaurants, and museums. You can visit the El Morro Fortress and the San José Church, and try some arróz con pollo, paella, asopao, or black bean soup at one of the Spanish restaurants.

In new San Juan, you can visit the sea museum and botanical gardens, or just relax, swim, play tennis, or sip a piña colada at one of the large oceanfront hotels. Perhaps you will have time to drive out to the tropical El Yunqué rain forest and witness the beautiful lush vegetation and impressive variety of birds.

If you drive west from San Juan for about 20 miles, you will come to the Hyatt Dorado Beach and Hyatt Regency Cerromar hotels, two upscale establishments. Both of these resorts feature Robert Trent Jones golf courses, beautiful tennis courts, swimming pools, and powder-sand beaches. The pool at the Cerromar is one of the most spectacular water playgrounds in the world. The spectacular El Conquistador Resort is located 31 miles east of San Juan. This mega-resort descends down a cliff and offers an 18-hole golf course, seven tennis courts, several pools, and its own private beach on Palomino Island, a 20-minute motor-launch ride from the hotel marina.

In the evening, you can stroll through Old San Juan, take in top-name entertainment, dance at the many nightclubs, or try your luck at the elegant hotel casinos. In San Juan, there are casinos and nightclubs at the Caribe Hilton, El

San Juan, the Ritz Carlton, the Holiday Inn, the Condado Beach, the Sands, and the Radisson.

ST. BARTHELEMY

Located 15 miles southeast of St. Martin and 140 miles north of Guadeloupe, St. Barts, a political dependency of Guadeloupe, is the most unique of the French West Indian islands. Its predominantly white population is of French and Swedish descent, and the atmosphere is more akin to a small French village on the Côte d'Azur than an island in the heart of the Caribbean.

Most visitors rent jeeps, mokes, or small cars, and enjoy visiting the numerous white-sand beaches, small hotels, guesthouses, atmospheric open-air restaurants, and cafés spread around this 8-square-mile island. **Gustavia,** the capital, is a quaint town with numerous cafés, restaurants, souvenir shops, and boutiques featuring a wide selection of imported goods.

Of the fourteen white-sand beaches spread around the island, Baie De St. Jean is the most popular and a colorful strand on which to people-watch or take a stroll. Grand Cul-de-Sac on the northern shore is another local favorite. The most scenic beaches are Anse du Gouverneur, Anse de Grand Saline, and Anse de Colombier. Shell Beach, which is not very attractive, is within walking distance of town.

The two hotels boasting the most facilities on St. Barts are Guanahani at Anse de Grand Cul-de-Sac and Manapany at Anse des Cayes—both offering pools, good beaches, tennis, gourmet restaurants, and expensive exclusivity. In Gustavia, the most highly touted restaurants are Carl Gustav, Sapotillier, La Cremaillère, and Aux Trois Gourmands. Other restaurants of note outside of town include Francois Plantation, Adam, Maya's, and Le Tamarin.

ST. KITTS AND NEVIS

This two-island nation was an associated state of Great Britain until it chose independence in 1983. St. Kitts covers 65 square miles and has a population of 40,000, while Nevis is only 36 square miles with 9,000 inhabitants. Jets can fly into St. Kitts, but Nevis is only accessible by smaller craft or by a 40-minute ferry ride from its sister island. The islands were first settled by the English and French in the early seventeenth century and became important producers of tobacco, ginger, cotton, and sugar, as well as a major hub for slave trading.

Today the islands offer an ideal climate with warm Caribbean sunshine cooled by trade winds. There is sufficient rain to keep the interiors lush, verdant, and tropical.

St. Kitts is dominated by Mt. Misery with its crater lake that rises 4,000 feet amidst rolling hills of sugarcane and palm trees. Cruise ships can dock at Deep Water Harbor, which is only a five-dollar taxi ride or a 30-minute walk from the main town of **Basseterre** with its shops specializing in batiks. About 3 miles from the harbor is Frigate Bay, where there are shops, restaurants, "so-so" Atlantic and Caribbean beaches, and a Jack Tar Village that has an eighteen-hole Robert Trent Jones golf course, tennis courts, two pools, shops, a casino, and restaurants. Because guests pay an all-inclusive price to stay there that includes food and drinks, visitors have a difficult time getting in. However, in the evening, the casino is open to the public. A typical, casual place for a seafood lunch or dinner would be Fisherman's Wharf. For West Indian and Continental dishes try the restaurants at the Golden Lemon, Ottley's Plantation, and Rawlins Plantation hotels.

Points of interest include Brimstone Hill, an imposing fort situated seven hundred feet above the sea affording views of Statia, Saba, St. Martin, and St. Barts; Romney Manor, a seventeenth-century plantation producing batik handicrafts; and an impressive tropical rain forest. The best beaches are at Banana Bay, Cockleshell Bay, and the Caribbean side of Friar's Bay.

The main town in Nevis, **Charlestown,** is a small, unusually clean Caribbean town with a few guesthouses, small inns and hotels, restaurants, and shops. There is a nice strand of beach about 3 miles from town that is used by some cruise ships for beach parties.

Nesbit Plantation on the north of the island also has a good beach, a restaurant, tennis courts, horseback riding, and water sports. In the early nineties, the Four Seasons Hotel chain opened Four Seasons Resort Nevis (one of the most luxurious resorts in the Caribbean), which features an eighteen-hole Robert Trent Jones II golf course, ten illuminated tennis courts, long stretches of sand on Pinney's Beach, water sports, horseback riding, and several restaurants. From St. Kitts, visitors must take the resort's private shuttle boat from its dock in Basseterre.

ST. LUCIA

St. Lucia, an independent member of the British Commonwealth, 21 miles south of Martinique, has a population of 101,000. The climate is dry and sunny in the winter, but a bit warmer and a great deal wetter during the summer months. The capital, **Castries,** is a picturesque town with a beautiful landlocked harbor where you can shop for duty-free bargains in crystal, jewelry, cameras, watches, perfume, and liquor, or sample the island's famous lobsters at a local restaurant. You can drive to Morne Fortuné, one of the two hills behind the town, and at the top explore the remains of Fort Charlotte, a typical eighteenth-century stronghold. You can take a two-hour voyage by launch to the fishing village of Soufrière, which is located at the base of St. Lucia's famous twin mountains, the Pitons. Here you can drive up Mount Soufrière, the only "drive-in" volcano in the world. You can actually drive right up to the lip of the smoldering crater and look in. Nearby, you can take a dip in sulphur springs, which are said to be therapeutic for sufferers of arthritis and rheumatism.

There is excellent swimming at all the public beaches; however, I would recommend spending the day on one of the hotel beaches at Jalousie Plantation, Sandals St. Lucia and Sandals Halayon, Anse Chastanet, Le Sport, The Royal, and Rex St. Lucien. The restaurants touted to be the best on the island are Green Parrot (seafood), San Antoine (Continental), Piton Restaurant and Bar (Caribbean), and Dasheene Restaurant and Bar (Caribbean).

ST. MARTIN

St. Martin (Saint Maarten) is a 37-square-mile island that was divided by the Dutch and French in 1648. **Philipsburg** is the capital of the Dutch section (Saint Maarten), and **Marigot** is the capital of the French (St. Martin). In addition to Dutch and French, the 14,000 inhabitants also speak English. The climate is dry and pleasant, with temperatures varying from seventy-one to eighty-six degrees. In Philipsburg, you can try numerous Continental and ethnic restaurants and shop for duty-free bargains in delft and Royal Dutch pewter. In Marigot, you can sample French cuisine and purchase duty-free bargains in French wines, perfume, and gloves. Other than the scenery, there are not many attractions of significant interest to tourists. There are casinos in many of the hotels, and swimming is best at the beautiful beaches at the Mullet Bay Resort, where you will also find tennis courts, an 18-hole golf course, numerous shops, and restaurants. Orient is a very colorful beach, a 15-minute drive from Philipsburg. It is reminiscent of Tahiti Beach in St. Tropez, France, and offers topless and nude bathing, as well as numerous small, beachfront restaurants and boutiques. Spartico is an excellent Italian restaurant located on the road between the airport and Marigot. Other good restaurants include LeBec Fin (Continental), Oyster Pond Beach Hotel (Continental), Le Perroquet (French), Chez Martine (French), Rainbow (Continental and West Indian), La Vie en Rose (French), Alizea (French), and L'Auberge Gourmande (French). LaSamanna is the most exclusive resort on the island and is located on Baie Longue, one of the best beaches. If you make arrangements to have lunch at its highly acclaimed restaurant, chances are you can have access to the beach.

ST. VINCENT AND THE GRENADINES

Lying south of St. Lucia, north of Grenada, and west of Barbados in the southern part of Caribbean's Windward Islands is the nation of St. Vincent, which is composed of thirty-two islands and cays. The largest island is named St. Vincent and is the site of the Caribbean's most active volcano, La Soufrière, which last erupted in 1979.

South of the island of St. Vincent are the islands of Bequia, Mustique, Canouan, Mayreau, Palm Island, and Petit St. Vincent, all low-keyed tourist destinations occasionally visited by cruise ships.

If your ship stops at the island of St. Vincent, the best beach for swimming is Buccament Bay, a black-sand beach on the west coast. A favorite excursion is the boat trip to Baleine Falls, where you can swim in a freshwater pool, climb under the 63-foot falls, and enjoy scenic views of the island. Hotels with the most facilities include Grand View Beach Hotel and Young Island. The most highly recommended restaurants are the French Restaurant and Dolphins, both on Villa Beach.

Nine miles south of the island of St. Vincent is Bequia, known for its good beaches, snorkeling, and diving. The best beaches are at Friendship Bay, Industry Bay, Lower Bay, and Hope Beach (the waters can be rough here). Located near both Princess Margaret and Lower Bay beaches is Plantation House Hotel, the best place to dine and spend the day.

On Canouan your best bet is the Tamarind Beach Hotel and Yacht Club; on Mayreau, Salt Whistle Bay Club and Salt Whistle Bay Beach; on Mustique, Cotton House; and on Palm Island, Palm Island Resort. Petit St. Vincent is a 113-acre private island, the location of one of the Caribbean's highest-rated resorts.

TORTOLA, PETER ISLAND, AND VIRGIN GORDA (THE BRITISH VIRGINS)

Several of the cruise ships traversing the Virgin Islands spend a day at **Tortola.** From Tortola, passengers can take a ferry to St. John and to most of the British Virgin Islands. Unspoiled **Peter Island Resort and Yacht Harbor** is only a 20-minute ride away. There you can sunbathe and swim at one of the resort's lovely pristine beaches, have lunch, play tennis, and participate in numerous water sports.

Your ship will tender you into **Road Town,** the main city of Tortola and capital of the British Virgin Islands. Road Town is not a duty-free port; however, there are bargains on imported British goods and local handicrafts. You can take a taxi ride west to Mount Sage, the island's highest peak, where you will be rewarded with a view of Peter, Salt, Cooper, and Ginger islands. Another excellent view is at Skyworld, a mountaintop restaurant and Tortola's most popular luncheon spot.

There are good beaches with white sand and clear warm water at Smuggler's Cove, Long Bay, Apple Bay (where there is good surfing), and Cane Garden Bay. The last one is the most pristine, and if you spend the day there, you can lunch at the colorful Rhymer's.

Scuba diving and snorkeling are popular here. The wreck of the *Rhone* is one of the most famous dive sites in the Caribbean and the location for the filming of *The Deep.* The *Rhone* was a British mail steamer that sank in 1867. Snorkelers and divers will want to visit the many reefs that follow the coastal beaches on the north side of the island, Smuggler's Cove being most snorkelers' favorite.

Those not opting to take the ferry to Peter Island can enjoy a day at one of the resorts on Tortola, which include Long Bay Hotel on the north shore and Prospect Reef Resort and Frenchman's Cay Hotel and Yacht Club on Frenchman's Cay, which is connected to Tortola by a bridge.

Virgin Gorda is one of the more picturesque and quaint of the British Virgins. Visitors will enjoy meandering through the shops and pubs in the small town near the harbor, visiting the unique "baths" where they can explore caves and natural pools formed by large boulders while snorkeling in aqua-blue waters, or spending the day at world-famous Little Dix Bay resort with its magnificent beach and lovely grounds. Some ships drop anchor at the opposite end of the island, so passengers can spend the day at Bitter End Resort or nearby Biras Creek.

TRINIDAD AND TOBAGO

Trinidad and Tobago compose a two-island republic 9 miles off the coast of Venezuela that became an independent member of the British Commonwealth in

1976. Trinidad is the largest island in the southern part of the Caribbean, having an area of 1,980 square miles and a sunny, pleasant climate. Its more than one million residents are a mixture of African, East Indian, Middle Eastern, and Asian cultures. Trinidad is said to be the birthplace of the calypso, steel band, and limbo, and should your ship be in port during the evening, don't miss an exciting and colorful native show. In **Port-of-Spain,** the capital, there is "in-bound" shopping for numerous duty-free bargains that are sent by the storekeeper directly to your ship. Tobago offers lovely beaches, unspoiled rain forests, and coral reefs.

Trinidad boasts beautiful mountains, tropical jungles, lush plantations, and sweeping white-sand beaches. You can drive to Pitch Lake near La Brea, where tons of asphalt are excavated and shipped throughout the world, or you may wish to take the Skyline Highway to the beautiful white-sand Maracas Beach, which is surrounded by palm trees and mountains. (The major hotels are not located near the beaches.) Additionally, you can visit a sugar or coconut plantation, the Caroni Bird Sanctuary, and the Royal Botanic Gardens.

If you wish to dine in Trinidad, you may enjoy the Italian food at Lucianos and Topo Caro, the East Indian food at Gaylords or Mangals, Chinese cuisine at Tiki Village, or French-Continental food in the restaurants at the Trinidad Hilton and the Normandie hotels.

In Tobago, the best resorts are the Grafton Beach Resort, Coco Reef, Arnos Vale Hotel, Le Grand Courlan, and Rex Turtle Beach Hotel. Best restaurants outside the hotels include Dillon's, Kariwak Village, and Rouselle's. The best beaches are found at Englishman's Bay, Great Courland Bay, King's Bay, Pigeon Point, and Stone Haven Bay.

U.S. VIRGIN ISLANDS

The U.S. Virgin Islands were purchased from Denmark in 1917, and they offer the finest shopping and possibly the most beautiful beaches and most desirable climate in the Caribbean. Cruise ships dock at the islands of St. Thomas and St. Croix, and those wishing to explore St. John catch a ferry from the center of town or Red Hook Beach in St. Thomas. (Watch your time here, so you don't miss the ship.) In both St. Thomas and St. Croix, you will want to leave ample time for duty-free shopping at the hundreds of attractive stores that line the main streets. Remember that when purchasing merchandise in the U.S. Virgin Islands, your duty-free allowance increases to $1,200 and your liquor quota increases to a gallon.

In **St. Thomas,** you can swim in crystal-clear waters at one of the truly beautiful beaches such as Magens Bay, Coki Point, Sapphire Bay, Red Hook, Morningstar Beach, and Limetree Beach. You may wish to visit Fort Christian, Bluebeard's Tower, and take a glass-bottom boat ride. At night, go to one of the hotels and see a local limbo show. For those who wish to play tennis and swim at one of the outstanding beaches, I would recommend spending the afternoon at the Virgin Grand Resort, which has a pool, private beach, restaurants, and tennis courts and is across the road from the fantastic Coki Beach and Coral World. Marriott recently took over and renovated Frenchmen's Reef, which also has tennis courts and is only a few minutes from where you dock; however, it is located on Morningstar Beach, which is fine for swimming but is not quite as beautiful or unspoiled as the others. The most luxurious resort is the Ritz Carlton, which has a nice pool and small beach. There are numerous restaurants in town and in the hotels. Many cruisers have indicated that L'Escargot on the waterfront is the best.

Shoppers will enjoy exploring the hundreds of stores lined up for a mile along the main drag in town. I have found the best selections at Continental (for crystal, jewelry, imported woolens, and European goods), A. H. Riise (for perfume, china, crystal, watches, jewelry, and liquors), Sparky's (for liquor), and Little Switzerland (for watches and jewelry). Branches of these shops and many others are located in the shopping mall adjacent to where your ship docks. Therefore, it is not necessary to go into town if time is limited.

From **St. Croix** you can sail out to **Buck Island** for some of the best underwater snorkeling in the Caribbean, or you can swim at one of the excellent beaches at the various hotels. The Buccaneer Hotel has a fair beach, a golf course, and excellent tennis courts. Westin Carambola Resort has a lovely beach and good restaurants, and its golf course—4 miles from the resort—is considered one of the best and most picturesque in the Caribbean. Don't miss walking through the charming town of **Christiansted,** where Danish architecture is evident in the little pastel-colored homes and stores. Unfortunately, most ships dock at **Fredericksted,** and you must take a long bus or taxi ride to get to Christiansted, which is on the other side of the island.

For those travelers who have already been to St. Thomas and first-time cruisers seeking "heavenly perfection," I recommend spending the day at Caneel Bay Resort or the Westin on the island of **St. John.** To get there, you must take a 30-minute taxi ride from your cruise ship to Red Hook Bay, where you catch a ferry for a pleasant 30-minute boat ride to the island of St. John, followed by another 10-minute taxi or bus ride to the hotels. A few times each day boats leave from the center of town and go directly to St. John. This may sound like a long trip, but it is well worth it. At Caneel Bay, you can explore six virgin horseshoe-shaped, private white-sand beaches studded with palm trees; lie out on a secluded hammock overlooking the sea; swim in clear, warm waters with beautiful tropical fish weaving between your legs; play tennis on one of seven excellent courts; and have a drink and buffet or à la carte lunch in the main building or at Turtle Beach. Joggers will want to scurry down the miles of paths connecting the various beaches, facilities, and cottages; and snorkel enthusiasts will wish to head out for the nearby Trunk Bay, where appropriate equipment can be rented to explore an underwater trail of flora and coral formations. Few resorts in the Caribbean surpass the beautiful grounds of Caneel Bay.

Several smaller vessels now offer regular cruises to St. John as well as some of the more remote British Virgin Islands.

South America

Cruising to foreign lands offers you an opportunity to sample numerous ports to determine whether or not you would wish to return for a longer, in-depth vacation. Just as you can cruise to several Caribbean islands, different countries in the Far East, or various ports in the Mediterranean, so can you cruise to many of the major cities of South America. Because air travel to South America is so expensive, cruising represents an economical yet pleasurable alternative.

Most of the major cities in South America are close enough to the equator to afford year-round sunshine and mild climates. Inasmuch as the seasons are reversed in the Southern Hemisphere, even Buenos Aires has warm weather between December and April.

In recent years, several cruise lines have been tapping the wealthy South American market, promoting trips to many of the major cities including Rio de Janeiro, Montevideo, and Buenos Aires, as well as cruises up the Amazon River. Each year, vessels of the Cunard, Costa, Seabourn, Renaissance, Holland America, Silverseas, and Crystal lines stop at a number of South American ports. Caracas, located at the tail of the string of Caribbean islands, often receives visits from ships doing southern Caribbean itineraries. It is also possible to explore the Galapagos and the west coast of South America on ships of Metropolitan Touring and Odessa America Lines.

AMAZON RIVER CRUSIES

The Amazon River, the largest river in the world and estimated to contain one-fifth of all the fresh water on earth, stretches 4,000 miles from its source in the Andes to the Atlantic Ocean. Although oceangoing ships can navigate inland for some 2,300 miles, many of the regular cruises offering Amazon itineraries enter at Belem, the 200-mile-wide mouth of the river, traverse the Narrows of Breves, stop at Santarem, and conclude their exploration at Manaus. The river is so wide at spots that you will be unable to see the other side; however, when passing through the Narrows of Breves you are treated to miles of beautiful green flora and tributaries located on both sides of your ship. The Amazon hosts 1,500 species of fish, 14,000 species of mammals, 15,000 species of insects, and 3,500 species of birds, although few of these will be visible on your cruise.

Many cruisers opting for an Amazon River itinerary expect to experience a ride up a picturesque jungle river right out of the Tarzan movies. Unfortunately, most cruises do not afford an opportunity to explore the more primitive areas, and most of your time will be spent sailing up a brown-colored river with ever-changing scenery and some unusual, but not fascinating ports of call.

Belem is situated on Guajara Bay at the gateway to the Amazon and is often the first or last stop for cruise ships exploring the river. The town thrived during the rubber boom of the early 1900s and is still the great trading center of the Amazon.

Your ship will either dock adjacent to the downtown area, where everything is within walking distance, or anchor at Scoraci and tender passengers ashore.

The Hilton Hotel is located in the center of the town and is a good focal point for your explorations. Points of interest include: The Jungle Park, a zoo filled with local animals in their natural habitat; the Goeldi museum, with its extensive collection of Indian artifacts; the neoclassical Teatro de Paz, built in 1874; the Basilica de Nossa Senhora de Nazere, built in 1909 as a replica of St. Peter's; the cathedral in the old colonial section of town, built in the eighteenth century and restored in 1887; Fort de Castelo; and Ver-o-Peso market on the waterfront.

Numerous little shops offering handicrafts and souvenir items are spread along President Vargas Street between the Hilton and the waterfront.

Many ships also commence or conclude their Amazon River cruises at **Manaus** because its airport can service large planes, affording passengers access to the middle of the Amazon by air. Although it was a thriving commercial metropolis in the late 1800s during the rubber boom, today one might refer to Manaus as the armpit of South America. However, that reference may be unfair to numerous other South American cities that deservedly have received the same accolade, yet by comparison look like Beverly Hills. Rarely can one find a city where every building, street, and sidewalk is in total disrepair and cluttered with garbage.

The city bus tour visits Sao-Sebatiao Square, the nineteenth-century Palacio Rio Negro, the Opera House that dates back to 1896, the Indian Museum, and the military zoo. Branches of the two largest South American jewelry chains, H. Stern and Amsterdam Sauer, offer transportation from your ship to their shops.

A more interesting option would be the riverboat ride down the Rio Negro to Lake January. Here the boat docks, and you can take a walk on a wooden bridge into a jungle swamp to a pond filled with giant lily pads and an occasional alligator. The night tour to Lake January is dedicated to seeking out alligators by flashlight. Our guide was supposed to wrestle one; however, the match never took place. Although not as picture-perfect as the all-inclusive jungle ride at Disney World, these tours are through an authentic jungle and provide an opportunity to take some unique photographs to show the fans back home. If you are more adventurous, you can attempt to hire your own boat and guide and possibly get deeper into the jungle.

Halfway between Belem at the mouth of the Amazon and Manaus lies the third-largest town in the Brazilian Amazon—**Santarem.** The population grew to 50,000 during the years of the gold rush in the 1920s.

Buses meet ships at the harbor to transport passengers to either the marketplace (*mercado*), which lies about a mile and a half downstream, or inland about a mile to the Hotel Tropical, where you can relax by the swimming pool and enjoy a local beer or a *caipirinha,* the traditional drink of the region consisting of smashed lime, sugar, and rum. Santarem is less crowded and in better repair than Manaus and is therefore a more comfortable place to shop for local crafts, many of which can be purchased from the artisans right at the gangway to your ship.

Alter do Chao is a sandy beach 15 miles from Santarem on the Tapajos River. Some ships offer beach parties here.

ARGENTINA—BUENOS AIRES

Most ships that call at Buenos Aires only remain from 8 to 24 hours, not permitting sufficient time to explore this cosmopolitan metropolis that is the only place in South America reminiscent of European cities in France, Spain, and Italy. Because your time will be limited, you will want to take an organized morning tour of the city, where you can visit the principal square, Plaza de Mayo; La Cathedral, where you can see the tomb of General José de San Martin, the obelisk which is the symbol of the city; the Teatro Colón, an important opera house; La Boca, an Italian district near the old port area; the botanical gardens; and the residence of the president.

During the afternoon, you will want to stroll down Florida and Lavalle, the major shopping streets, where you will find excellent bargains on leather shoes and purses as well as a good selection of European-style boutiques. The quality of the merchandise and inexpensive prices make Buenos Aires the best shopping city in South America. Visitors often enjoy having a steak with all the trimmings and bottle of local beer or wine at a typical Argentine restaurant. Due to the weakness of the currency, this could cost less than a hamburger and Coke at a stateside McDonald's.

BRAZIL

When taking a cruise from **Rio de Janeiro,** you'll want to arrange to stay over in this unique city for a few days at the beginning or end of the cruise. Rio's beauty is due to its natural environs in which green-clad mountains border a city of high-rise apartments and hotels situated across from a string of beaches on the Atlantic Ocean. The hotel-beach-restaurant area starts in the north at the District of Leme and continues south through the districts of Copacabana, Ipanema, Leblon, and Gavea. The best hotels in Copacabana are the Rio Palace, the Rio Othon Palace, the Copacabana Palace, and the Méridien. In Ipanema, it's the Caesar Park. The Sheraton lies at the intersection of Leblon and Gavea, and the Intercontinental Resort Hotel is still farther away in Gavea. All of these hotels are across the road from the beach and feature private pools, numerous restaurants, shops, and bars. If you desire a resort atmosphere, you will prefer either the Sheraton or the Intercontinental, which are farther away from the main part of the city.

You can eat quite inexpensively at one of the numerous pizzerias that line the beach area, or you can sample local Brazilian and Continental dishes on the second floor of the Hotel Trocadero or at most of the hotel restaurants.

Tennis buffs can rent a court at either the Sheraton or Intercontinental hotels, and joggers can wear out their "New Balance specials" along the walk that stretches for 6 miles from Leme Beach to the end of Ipanema. Don't miss the samba show at Oba Oba or Plataforma I, nor the picturesque cable-car ride to the top of Sugar Loaf Mountain, where you have a panoramic view of the entire city. A train ride to the top of Corcovada Mountain, where the statue of Christ towers over the entire city, is also a must for all visitors. If time permits, there are organized tours to Tijuca Forest, Paradise, and the Paqueta Islands.

There are many shops and boutiques on Copacabana Avenue, two blocks up from the beach, as well as in the Ipanema area, offering leather goods, jewelry, sportswear, and local handicrafts; however, I found few bargains. Gemstones and jewelry are reputed to be the best buys. H. Stern, the world's leading retail jewelry enterprise, has shops in all the major hotels.

One of the most enjoyable stops is **Salvador** (Bahia), where you can sun on one of the two beautiful beaches at Piata and Itapoa; visit numerous cathedrals and museums throughout the city; shop for silver, jewelry, and hand-carved rosewood at Mercado Modelo, silver at Gerson shops, and arts and crafts at Instituto (Mauá); play tennis at the Hotel Méridien, which has a restaurant at the top that offers the best view of the city; or take an excursion to the island of Itaparica to swim and stroll through a small, charming town filled with parks. You will want to sample the unique Bahian cuisine (combining African and European cooking styles) at Chica da Silva, Yemanja, Lampiao, and Moenda. For French and Continental cuisine, the best in town are St. Honore (at the Hotel Méridien) and Chez Bernard. With limited time, you can spend your day at either Hotel Méridien Bahia or Bahia Othon Palace, which offer good pools, shops, and restaurants.

COLOMBIA—CARTAGENA

Located on the Caribbean Coast of Colombia, this 450-year-old city of Spanish heritage has become a popular stop for ships traversing the Panama Canal.

Visitors will want to visit the seventeenth-century fortress of San Felipe with its impressive walls, tunnels, and cannons; the old walled city composed of colonial-style buildings with wood balconies and red tile roofs, parks, monasteries, and monuments; and the new city area of resort hotels, beaches, shops, and restaurants.

The best shopping is at Prerino Gallo Plaza, near the Hilton, where there are several emerald shops, leather stores, craft shops, a disco, and casino.

The beaches are crowded and dirty, and those wishing to sun and swim are best off going to the Cartagena Hilton, where there is a nice pool area, tennis courts, health club, shops, and restaurants.

Walkers and joggers may enjoy the path along the sea that starts at the old city and extends into the new city for three miles or so to the Hilton. Walking or jogging from the port to the old fortress or into the middle of town also is possible because both are only a mile or two from the harbor.

URUGUAY—MONTEVIDEO

In Montevideo you will have the best view of the city from the top of the town hall, where you can also eat lunch at Panormacico Municipal, one of Montevideo's better restaurants. Below town hall is the shopping district, where you can buy leather goods and woolens.

With only one day in port, you can take the city tour and see the obelisk, the La Carreta statue, the flea market, the natural history museum, the cathedral, and the mausoleum of José Artigas; or you can take a taxi out to the resort area of Carrasco, where you will find beautiful homes, restaurants, hotels, and beaches. Those traveling with children may wish to visit the zoological gardens and Rodo Park, an amusement park with rides, ponies, and theaters.

In the evening, there is a tango show and Uruguayan folk music at Tangueria del 40 in the Columbia Palace Hotel, dinner and dancing at El Mirador in the Hotel Oceania, and several discos including Zum Zum, Lancelot, and Ton Ton Metek.

If time allows, Punte del Este is a charming resort town with numerous excellent beaches. L'Auberge and La Posta del Cangrejo are the two best hotels on the beach with good restaurants.

VENEZUELA—CARACAS

The South American port most frequently visited by cruise ships is La Guaira (Caracas), Venezuela. This is the richest nation in South America because of its large oil production; however, the economic good fortune of the country has not passed down to the average man in the street, who appears to be living in relative poverty. The shacks of the poor offer a contrast to the opulent residences of the rich. Caracas is a city in a valley surrounded by mountains. The best view is from Mount Avila at its 6,500-foot summit. Check whether the cable car to the top is working—it is almost always out of order. You can also get a good view of the city from atop the Hilton Hotel.

A city tour will visit La Cathedral, with its artistically decorated interior; Santa Teresa Basilica, housing the oldest image of Christ in Venezuela; the capitol building, featuring the paintings of Tovar; Bólivar's birthplace, an outstanding example of colonial architecture; Los Caobos Park; Los Proceres Park; and the Museum of Natural Science, with its collection of stuffed animals.

There is little shopping that is worthwhile. The shops offer a variety of gold jewelry, but there are no bargains. Should you be in Caracas on Sunday, you can attend a bullfight at Plaza de Toros. For tennis or swimming, try the Macuto Hotel in La Guaira. The beach is not terrific, but the hotel has a large pool, shops, restaurants, a disco, theater, nightclub, and many facilities. Many cruisers not wishing to take the hectic tour of Caracas spend the day at the hotel.

Caracas also boasts many good restaurants offering French, Italian, and Venezuelan cuisines.

The Mediterranean, Greek Islands, Middle East, and Environs

Like the Caribbean, the Mediterranean, Adriatic, Aegean, and Black seas are calm, and the weather in the area is generally pleasant, except for certain winter months.

There are probably no cruise grounds that offer as representative a sampling of history, as great a diversity in cultures, or as many varied and exciting places of interest as the Mediterranean. Imagine climbing up to the ancient Acropolis in Athens, standing before the Wailing Wall of Jerusalem, strolling through the famous shopping bazaar of Istanbul, gambling at the posh casinos in Monte Carlo, sunning at the jet-set beaches of the Côte d'Azur or Greek islands, all in seven to fourteen days.

For a number of years, the ships of Epirotiki and Sun lines (Royal Olympic Cruises) have been running regularly scheduled cruises from Piraeus to the Greek islands and to the coastal cities of Turkey. Many of the vessels have seven-day itineraries calling at such ancient and legendary islands as Rhodes, Mykonos, Delos, Santorini, Crete, Corfu, and Patmos, as well as such unusual Turkish ports as Istanbul, Marmaris, and Kusadasi. Some of these ships return to Piraeus between the third and fourth day, permitting passengers with tight schedules to take only half of the itinerary.

Regular cruises to other parts of the Mediterranean and adjoining seas leaving from Genoa, Venice, Naples, Nice, Cannes, Monte Carlo, Athens, or Istanbul have recently been offered by the Costa, Princess, Renaissance, Radisson Seven Seas, Seabourn, Cunard, Crystal, Windstar, Celebrity, Silversea, Orient, Mediterranean, and Club Med cruise lines. In addition to the aforementioned Greek islands and Middle Eastern ports, these cruises may call in the western Mediterranean at Capri, Sorrento, Palma de Mallorca, Barcelona, Sicily, Malta, Sardinia, Elba, Corsica, or Algeciras; in Africa or off the African coast at Casablanca, Tunis, Dakar, Tangier, Tenerife, Las Palmas, or Funchal; in the Adriatic at Split, Bari, or Dubrovnik; in the Black Sea at Odessa, Yalta, or Sochi; and in the Middle East at Haifa, Israel, Alexandria, Egypt, Beirut, or Cyprus.

Although the majority of these ports have harbors that can accommodate only the smaller vessels, the large ships can drop anchor outside the harbor and transport the passengers ashore in small tenders. Today, a growing number of large luxury liners from the above-mentioned lines are scheduling numerous cruises each summer in the Mediterranean area. These cruises appeal to Europeans as well as to Americans, and have resulted in the development of a highly competitive Mediterranean cruise program paralleling that found in the Caribbean. Unfortunately, terrorism, local wars, and general unrest have caused ships to cancel their itineraries from time to time.

The following are the highlights of some of the more popular cruise stops in this area:

ALGERIA

Algiers, with its population of 900,000, is Algeria's capital; it is a Mediterranean seaport standing on a hillside overlooking the bay. At the bottom of the hill is the modern city, and farther up is the old Moorish section called The Casbah, named for the citadel that stands on the top of the hill. The unique Casbah is an interesting section of crowded, narrow alleys, courtyards, and shops. The climate is varied, with temperatures falling to the twenties in the winter and up over one hundred during the summer months. The best season to visit Algiers' "turquoise coast" is between April and November. Worth visiting are several distinguished mosques dating from the Ottoman era, the National Museum of Moslem and Classic Antiquities, the Essai Gardens, and the university. You can take a bus ride, which provides superb views of the city, to the chic residential suburb of El Biar past the palace of the president. Algiers is flanked by several fine beaches on the Mediterranean, where you can swim and skin-dive from March through October. The nightlife is limited largely to hotel bars and cabarets catering to foreigners.

CROATIA

Dubrovnik is a small Croatian port with a population of 26,000 located on the Adriatic Sea across from Italy. Its mild climate and medieval architecture have made it a favorite tourist attraction. As you sail into the harbor, you will note its fjordlike coastline. From the harbor you can take a boat across to the island of Lokrum, which is a botanical preserve with interesting foliage, gardens, and a natural history museum. You can drive up Zarkovica Hill for a magnificent view of the city and swim at the beaches at Lapad and Sumratin. The area called the "old town" is completely encircled by a wall built during the fourteenth century. There are no motor vehicles allowed in the old town, and you will enjoy walking through the main street, Placa, and visiting St. Blaise's Church, Sponza Palace, the colorful market in Gundulic Square, the Rector's Palace, the cathedral, the Trade Union House, the tiny shops on the nearby street called *Ulica od Puca,* and the Fortress Minceta, where you can view the city from atop a circular tower at the highest point on the wall.

At the Dubrovnik President Hotel, a five-minute ride from the harbor, there are numerous bars, a glass-enclosed indoor pool, an outdoor lounge area, both a regular and a nude gravel beach, and an excellent shopping center a block away. Visitors can opt to take a scenic walk or jog back to the harbor from here—it is about 2 miles, all downhill.

At night you can go to one of the fine local restaurants and taste such native dishes as *borec,* a kind of flaky pastry containing cheese, meat, or fruit; *djuvech,* thin slivers of pork grilled with rice, vegetables, and pepper; *raznici,* a lamb kebab; and *kruskovac,* a pear brandy. After dinner, there are numerous nightclubs, including the outdoor Labyrinth Club at the gate of the old town that offers music, dancing, and a striptease. You can try your luck at the gambling casino, dance at a discotheque, or attend Dubrovnik's summer festival, which features ballets, concerts, and various European artists.

CYPRUS

Cyprus is an island republic in the northeast corner of the Mediterranean, south of Turkey and west of Syria. The island covers 3,500 square miles, and its 650,000 inhabitants are of Greek and Turkish origin. Cyprus has lofty mountain resorts that offer skiing during the winter, some interesting hilltop monasteries and castles, and beautiful forests filled with the regal cedar of Lebanon trees. Cruise ships generally dock at the ports of **Limassol.** Limassol is a resort town bordering the sea with many fine hotels. Le Meridien, Four Seasons, Hawaii Beach, and Amathus Beach hotels offer the most facilities, large pool areas, not-so-nice beaches, water sports, tennis, and restaurants. The entire 10-mile stretch between the harbor and Le Meridien lends itself to walking expeditions with visits to luxury hotels, restaurants, shops, and tavernas. Apart from the resort hotels and sea front, there is little of interest for tourists in this city. The old city of Famagusta is surrounded by an impressive wall and fortification containing such sights of historical and architectural interest as the Venetian Palace, Othello's Tower, the Church of St. Peter and St. Paul, and the Cathedral of St. Nicholas. Modern Famagusta, called Varoska, lies a mile to the south of the walled city and is a prosperous Greek community with sandy beaches, shops, tavernas, discos, and bars.

Fifty miles from Famagusta is Nicosia, which is part Greek and part Turkish. Within the walls of the Old City, you can visit St. John's Church (built in 1662) and the Folk Art Museum (formerly a Gothic monastery of the fifteenth century). There is also the Cyprus Museum, with well-preserved artifacts from archeological excavations. If you drive on the southern coast to the monastery of Stavrovouni, located on the crest of a mountain 2,260 feet above the sea, you can enjoy a breathtaking view of Cyprus, watch the monks at their work, and perhaps break bread with them at lunchtime. Other popular excursions include exploring the Greco-Roman theater at Curium and the wine-producing village of Omodus.

EGYPT

Ships generally dock at either Port Said or Alexandria, both of which are rather dirty, polluted port cities. **Alexandria** is the chief port and second-largest city in Egypt, lying on the northeastern end of the Nile River Delta on a strip of land between the Mediterranean Sea and Lake Mareotis. The temperatures climb from the fifties and sixties in winter to the nineties in summer. The city, which was founded by Alexander the Great in 332 B.C., was a center of Greek culture and learning, but it has lost much of its former importance under the Egyptians. You may enjoy chartering a small boat to take you on a tour of the harbor, or you may prefer to relax on the 20 miles of sandy (so-so) beaches at Montaza, Maamura, or Agami. You can visit the Catacombs of Komel Shuquafa constructed in A.D. 2, the Roman Amphitheater, the Mosque of Aboual-Abaas Mursi, and the Montaza Palace with its beautiful grounds and gardens, which were a former residence of King Farouk and today have been converted to a guesthouse for government officials. The main shopping areas are Mansheya Square, Ramle Tram Station, and the Gold Souk. However, the main reason for your visit is to permit a tour to **Cairo,** Egypt's capital, where you can explore the Egyptian Museum, which houses the most important collection of Egyptian antiquities, including the Tutankhamen treasures; Coptic Museum; Abdin Palace; the Ibn Tulun Mosque; the Sultan Hasan Mosque; the El Ashar Mosque; the "Old Cairo" area (site of numerous ancient Christian churches); or the shops at Kahn al Kahlil and the Musky Bazaar.

Certainly the highlight of any visit to Cairo is the site of the Pyramids of Giza and the legendary Sphinx, located in the Sahara Desert right outside the city. You can tour these magnificent antiquities on foot, on horseback, or by camel. Those not subject to claustrophobia may enjoy walking through the steep, low passages of the interior chambers of one of the pyramids. The Pyramid of Cheops is one of the remaining Seven Wonders of the Ancient World. Built in 2650 B.C., it is still the largest and most massive stone structure in the modern world. A convenient oasis for lunch would be the historic Mena House, a deluxe hotel that was formerly a palatial hunting lodge and is located only minutes from the pyramids. You may prefer one of the river-cruising restaurants along the Nile operated by the Oberoi Hotels group.

Those wishing to visit the antiquities of ancient Egypt will want to consider one of the Nile River cruises from **Luxor** offered by ships of Sheraton Nile Cruises, Sonesta Hotels and Nile Cruises, and Abercrombie & Kent cruise lines. At Luxor, you will want to visit the awesome ruins of Karnak, the largest temple in the world, as well as the temple of Luxor. Across the river on the western bank lies the "city of the dead," with its ornate tombs and artifacts. The ships generally conclude their cruises in **Aswan,** where you can visit the Aswan Dam.

FRANCE
(Including Côte d'Azur and Monte Carlo)

Calvi, on the island of Corsica, has recently become a port for some of the smaller cruise ships. For many years an Italian island, Corsica was sold to France in 1786. However, you may find the island more reminiscent of Greece or Italy than France. The small streets that wind around the harbor offer numerous small restaurants, cafés, souvenir shops, boutiques, and food stores. Above the harbor (a five-minute walk) sits the Citadel of Calvi, which dominates the landscape when you approach the town by boat. Walking left from the town will bring you to a long strand of beach surrounded by a pine forest. There are lounges and umbrellas for rent and numerous small bars and snack shops here. Although not well known, Calvi is a charming cruise stop where you can spend a relaxed day at the beach and browsing around the quaint little village.

Cannes and **Nice** on the Côte d'Azur (French Riviera) are the most popular cruise ports in southern France. The climate is warm and sunny throughout the year, except for the winter months, when temperatures at night and in the morning can be quite chilly. You will enjoy walking down the world's most chic promenade, "The Croissette," stopping to browse in smart boutiques or to rest at an outdoor café where you can nibble on cheese and crisp bread while you watch the beautiful French women parade by in their bikinis. The beaches in Cannes and Nice are quite colorful, although not ideal for swimming. You can drive west to **St. Tropez**

and sun and swim at Tahiti Beach, which has sand and numerous rental lounges, small restaurants, bars, and facilities, but is not all that much more desirable for swimming. On all the beaches the majority of the women go topless. If your ship stops at St. Tropez, in addition to the beaches, you may enjoy exploring the numerous small boutiques and bistros in town spread along the streets and alleys around the harbor. Some of the cruise lines offer excursions from St. Tropez inland through Provence to visit the wine vineyards.

An interesting side trip would be to the old walled town of **St. Paul-de-Vence,** which rests on a hill terraced with vineyards. This charming little walled city consists of narrow, winding, cobblestone streets lined with quaint shops and villas. You can enjoy lunch and dinner at Chateau du Domaine St. Martin or Le Mas d'Artigny— two of my favorite French inns—or the Colombe d'Or, all of which are located near the city. In the evening in both Cannes and Nice, you may wish to dine at one of the many fine French restaurants, dance at a discotheque, or gamble at the elegant casinos.

The largest hotels in Cannes with the most facilities are the Majestic, the Carlton, the Martinez, and the Grand. My favorite French restaurants on the Riviera are L'Oasis, La Bonne Auberge, Moulins de Mougins, the Chanteclair at the Negresco, Eden Rock at Hotel du Cap, and Restaurant LeCap at Grand-Hotel du Cap-Ferrat, all of which are highly rated and *très cher.*

Monte Carlo in the principality of Monaco has become a popular port for smaller cruise ships that can pull right up to the docks in town. The harbor area is colorful with bars and cafés. The main tourist attraction, however, is the main square that is surrounded by the world-famous Casino of Monte Carlo, Hotel de Paris, and Café de Paris. Here you can browse through designer shops, dine at elegant restaurants in Hotel de Paris and the Hermitage, try your luck at the Casino, and soak up the ultraposh environment. Those preferring American-style gambling can be accommodated at the casino across the square from Hotel de Paris or at Lowe's Hotel. Passengers on ships stopping at Monte Carlo or Ville France may wish to take the short drive to the ancient Village of Eze, where they will be rewarded with panoramic views, a quaint, small French town, and various dining options including the acclaimed restaurant at Chateau de la Chevre d'Or.

GREECE AND THE GREEK ISLANDS

Piraeus is the port of Athens and the busiest cruise port in the Mediterranean area. You will enjoy dining at one of the smaller outdoor restaurants along the waterfront, where you can select your own fish or lobster and watch it cooked to order. It is approximately a 5-mile drive into Athens, where you can take in such historic sights as the ancient Acropolis, Hadrian's Arch, the Temple of Zeus, the great marble stadium, the Parthenon, the Byzantine Church of St. Elefterios, and the archeological museum. At the foot of the hill beneath the Acropolis are numerous charming garden restaurants where you can enjoy lunch or a cold drink. Dyogenes is especially enticing.

After a day of sightseeing, you may enjoy shopping for local jewelry, handicrafts, antiques, designer fashions and furs, or taking a short drive to Vouliagmeni Beach, which is a "so-so" public beach with decent facilities. In the evening don't miss the impressive "sound and light" program across from the Acropolis, where the story of ancient Greece is recounted while music, lights, and sound effects bring the story to life. Later in the evening, you will want to visit the charming "plaka" area, where hundreds of tavernas offer authentic *bouzouki* music, Greek dancing, ouzo, and local wines (Cava Campas, Porto Carras, and Robola Calliga being the best white wines of Greece, and Cava Boutari the best red). Most of the tavernas are on or near Mnisikleos Street. On a warm evening, one of the more scenic and romantic experiences in Athens is dining at Dionysos Restaurant at the top of Mt. Lycabettus while watching the sun set over the Acropolis.

If you are spending a day before or after the cruise in Athens, the best hotel is the Grand Bretagne on Syntagma Square; the best resort hotels are the Astir Palace resort complex at Vouliagmeni Beach; and the Hilton, only five minutes from the center of town, with its numerous restaurants and pool and garden area.

If you are driving to Vouliagmeni or staying at the Astir Palace complex, two excellent seafood restaurants with panoramic views are the Club House near the bungalows at Astir Palace and Ithaki, located on a hill about a half-mile before you reach the entrance to the Astir Palace. Ithaki is possibly one of the most romantic restaurants in Greece, serving some of the finest fresh fish and other cuisine with the friendliest, most efficient service—well worth the trip.

When taking a taxi, be certain to obtain some idea of the correct fare before embarking. Often the meters are not working, or when they are, the driver may frequently adjust the meter (up) as the trip progresses.

Corfu is the northernmost Greek island, located in the Ionian Sea, and has a population of a little more than 100,000. The best weather is in late spring and early fall, with the summers being quite hot. Its 229 square miles are covered with green mountains, beautiful flowers, and millions of gnarled olive trees. Don't miss swimming in the warm, calm Ionian Sea at one of the lovely hotels or taking a horse-and-buggy ride through the quaint little town with its winding streets and interesting people.

You may wish to spend your day at the Corfu Holiday Palace (formerly the Corfu Hilton) overlooking "Mouse Island," 2 1/2 miles from town, or the Astir Palace on Komeno Bay, 6 miles out of the city. These hotels feature lovely pools, beaches, water sports, and good restaurants. The Corfu Holiday Palace is a real charmer in a very picturesque setting. I highly recommend lunch by the pool, followed by a climb down the olive tree-clad hill leading to the azure-blue sea and the bridge over to Mouse Island.

The most picturesque area in Corfu is the beach at Paleokastritsa. It has little grottos, restaurants, and an incomparably beautiful setting. Other nice beaches more suitable for swimming can be found at Glifada on the west coast, Sidari on the north coast, Dassia and Ipsos on the east coast, and Kavos at the southern tip of the island. Those wishing to take a scenic drive, reminiscent of the Amalfi Drive in southern Italy, should start at the beach at Dassia and proceed north to the charming village of Kassiopi, passing through Ipsos, Nissaki, Kalami, and Kouloura.

Crete (Heraklion) is located 81 miles south of mainland Greece between the Aegean and Mediterranean seas. It is the largest and most important of the Greek islands, covering 3,200 square miles and having a population of 483,000. A chain of high mountains divides the island into four distinct regions, each having a different scenery combining to form the impressive beauty of the Cretan landscape. The people are friendly and hospitable and often can be seen in local costumes observing their age-old traditions. The Archaeological Museum of Heraklion has 23 halls that house the remains of the highly developed Minoan civilization, which flourished for more than 2,000 years. If you drive out to Knossos, you can see a maze of ruins, including the remarkable excavation of the partially restored palace of King Minos. You can also drive out to a fishing village in the south and spend a quiet day swimming and sunbathing.

Delos, an uninhabited island 1 1/2 miles southwest of Mykonos in the center of the Aegean Sea, was the legendary birthplace of Zeus's children, Apollo and Artemis, and the most sacred of the Greek islands during Hellenistic times. Under Roman rule, the island grew in stature and wealth, only to be ravaged later by wars and pirate raids. Today, cruise ships dock for a few hours to enable passengers to walk through the ancient ruins, visit the island's small museum, and see the most impressive remains—the lions made of Naxos marble. Delos is considered to be one of the greatest open-air archeological museums in the world.

Situated in the Aegean Sea not far from the coast of Turkey lies **Kos,** a 170-square-mile island with 20,000 inhabitants. It is rich in history, but is best known as the birthplace of Hippocrates, the "father of medicine." Most of the important sites are within walking distance of the harbor; however, many visitors opt to rent bicycles, which of course permit greater mobility for exploring the island. Surrounding the harbor are hundreds of small souvenir shops offering T-shirts, beach attire, leather goods, gold, and pottery, as well as small taverns and restaurants. There are a number of beaches near the town of Kos, including Psalidi, Lambi, and Aghios Fokas. Seven miles west of town is a somewhat better beach at Tinzaki, and 2 miles farther is a nice sandy beach at Marmari. From the harbor, charter boats offer trips to neighboring islands.

Ancient Kos has two sections. Immediately adjacent to the harbor is the famous Castle of the Knights of St. John, which is a fortress with two enclosures dating back to the fourteenth and fifteenth centuries. It is surrounded by a deep moat, and it was originally built as a medical center. Nearby are several Turkish mosques and the famous Hippocrates Tree, reputed to be the oldest tree in Europe and the site where Hippocrates treated the sick.

Southwest of the harbor in the other section of ancient Kos, you can visit impressive ruins, including a vast Roman bath, the Casa Romana, with its well-preserved mosaic floor from the third century A.D. depicting the abduction of Europa by Zeus, the fourteen-tier Odeon from the Roman period, and the remains of the old Roman Way.

Two miles south of the town of Kos is the sacred shrine of Asklepion, the god of healing. Considered the first medical school in the world, it dates back to the fifth century B.C., when Hippocrates opened the school to encourage the study of medicine. The island was the center of medical practice in ancient times.

Mykonos is the favorite island of the young, bargain travelers as well as the jet set. Here you can stroll through little whitewashed towns with windmills and winding streets, shop for bargains in handmade woolens and jewelry in its small boutiques, buy a designer dress from Galatis at his shop right off the main square, or swim and sun at one of its many excellent sandy beaches on the crystal-clear, blue Aegean Sea. The three best beaches, which can only be reached by taxi or a short boat ride, are the Paradise, the Super Paradise, and the Ilia. The first features nude bathing. Ilia is the most beautiful of the three. There is also a nice beach 2 miles from town, San Stephanos. The town is known for its windmills on the site of the ancient city, its hundreds of small churches and its mascot, Petros the Pelican, who can be found strolling near the harbor. In the evening you will want to visit the tavernas and cafés bursting with the sounds of *bouzouki* music and fragrant with the aroma of ouzo, coffee, and baklava. The three most upscale restaurants in town are Catrin, Philippi, and Edem.

Patmos is in the northern section of the Greek islands, lying close to Asia Minor in the Aegean Sea. This tiny island of only 13 square miles with 2,500 inhabitants is the most sacred of the Greek islands today. It was here that John the Apostle wrote the Apocalypse (the Book of Revelation). The site where St. John saw his prophetic visions is marked by a Byzantine-style church. You can also visit the grotto where he lived or the eleventh-century monastery nearby that houses priceless manuscripts and religious works of art. You can walk or ride up to the monastery, which offers some of the most spectacular and beautiful views you may ever experience; or you can swim at one of the colorful sandy beaches— Griko Beach and Dikofti Beach being the most popular.

Rhodes, with its area of 540 square miles and population of 64,000, is located 12 miles off the coast of Turkey in the Aegean Sea. The island's long and eventful history is represented by pre-Hellenic temples, Byzantine churches, mosques and minarets, classical monuments, medieval walled towns, fortresses, and picturesque little villages. This large, fertile island was called "Bride of the Sun" by Homer and "Island of Roses" by more recent poets. In ancient times, it was a prosperous island, and the medieval Knights of St. John of Jerusalem settled here and built a walled, fortified city that is now the best-preserved such town in the Mediterranean area. Rhodes divides into the new and the old town. The new town consists of hotels, boutiques, restaurants, and public beaches; the old town situated near the harbor behind the walls of the Castle of the Knights is a maze of narrow cobbled streets, arched facades, and antiquities. Here you will find hundreds of small tourist shops, tavernas, and restaurants as you work your way up to the historic sights. Sightseeing in the old town of Rhodes should include the fourteenth-century Castle of the

Grand Master, the remarkable Street of the Knights, the mosques built during the Turkish occupation, and the quaint Jewish synagogue.

This is possibly the most developed resort area in the Greek islands, with hundreds of hotels, the most fashionable being the Rodos Palace, 3 miles from town. All the large hotels feature desirable shops, restaurants, and swimming pools and are situated on beaches. Most of the beaches are dirty, pebbly, and hot; however, the water is clear, warm, and delightful for swimming. There are numerous good indoor/outdoor restaurants near the Grand Hotel in the center of town; and several of the outdoor garden restaurants in the old town area appear inviting.

In the evening, you may enjoy the sound and light performance in the Palace of the Knights or the wine festival at Rodini Park, where you can consume all the wine you can drink for a few drachmas.

Beach enthusiasts will prefer to take the scenic 32-mile drive across the east coast of the island past charming villages set among orchards and olive trees to the town of Lindos, where there are sandy beaches that offer excellent swimming. Here you also can ride a donkey up to the ancient acropolis situated on top of a scenic hill, browse through souvenir shops, and have a beer at a local Taverna.

Santorini, the site of Greece's active volcano, is located on the Aegean Sea, north of Crete and south of Mykonos. The bay on the west coast was once part of the island that sank after a violent eruption of the volcano. Your ship will anchor in the harbor and you can either take a donkey ride or a cable car to the whitewashed town of Thira, with its narrow streets perched on the edge of a steep cliff rising from the sea and offering a superb panorama. An important site is the ancient ruins of Akortiri. The excavations date back to 2000 B.C., when the town was destroyed by earthquakes and volcanic eruptions. Akortiri is one of the best-preserved ruins of a Greek town in existence. You can visit the Boutari Winery, located midway between Thira and Akortiki, where you can tour the winery and taste a selection of Boutari wines. Strolling through the winding streets of Thira, with its small shops, rooftop restaurants, small hotels, and outside cafés overlooking the sea, is a delightful experience. Kastro and Zafora, near the cable-car station, offer a nice selection of Greek dishes and beverages and afford an excellent panorama of the town and harbor.

Skiathos is an incredibly charming, pine-studded island that has not yet suffered the effects of the hordes of European tourists that inundate Mykonos, Rhodes, and Corfu. This beautifully pristine haven in the Northern Aegean boasts colorful shops and cafés that line the waterfront's cobblestone streets, and sandy strands that beckon beachgoers to enjoy the warm waters of the azure sea. The best beach is at Koukounaries, situated at the foot of the Skiathos Palace Hotel, a 20 minute bus or taxi ride from the harbor. Unusual rock formations and a secluded beach can be found at Lalaria, which is accessible by boat. In addition to the beaches, tourists will enjoy strolling through the streets that emanate from the harbor, browsing through the small shops, and having a drink or light meal at one of the numerous outdoor cafés.

ISRAEL

Israel is the small nation on the eastern shore of the Mediterranean founded in 1948 as a homeland for Jews from all parts of the world. The weather is most pleasant in the spring and fall, when the days are warm and the evenings cool. Your ship may dock at **Haifa,** where lovely Mount Carmel descends to the sea. If you only have a short time in port and cannot drive to Jerusalem, you can spend a delightful day in the vicinity of Haifa, where you can visit the Bahai Temple, Elijah's cave, the artist colonies at Ein Hod and Safad, the Druze villages, and a nearby kibbutz (a communal farm where the residents grow the food they eat and lead an industrious, self-sufficient life, seldom leaving their own community). You may wish to relax and have lunch or dinner at the Rondo Grill in the beautiful Dan Carmel Hotel, which offers a spectacular view of the city and harbor, or at the nearby Dan Panorama Hotel. If you have time, take in a local folkloric show with Israeli dancing and singing, and try Israel's delicious answer to the hot dog—a *felafel* sandwich, hummus (mashed chick peas and olive oil), vegetables, and spicy yogurt sauces stuffed into pita bread.

If your ship docks at Ashod or anchors overnight in Haifa, you will have time to drive down the coast to **Tel Aviv,** a modern, industrious Israeli city. There are lovely beaches here and in the nearby suburb of Herzliya. In the evening, you will enjoy walking through the quaint streets and shops in the old town of Jaffa, where there are good Continental and Israeli restaurants and nightclubs. The most highly acclaimed French-Continental-Israeli restaurant in Tel Aviv is Twelve Tribes at the Sheraton, and for typical Middle Eastern specialties, your best bet is Shaul's Inn near the Carmel market. If time allows, you may want to stay overnight at one of the deluxe seashore hotels such as the Hilton, Dan Panorama, Sheraton, Carlton, or Holiday Inn. A new Intercontinental and Hyatt are presently under construction.

You can drive to **Jerusalem** in about an hour from Tel Aviv. Within the walls of the old city are contained some of the holiest sanctuaries of Christianity, Judaism, and Islam. After entering one of the historic gates, you will walk through winding, narrow streets lined with shops and intriguing passageways to the Western Wall or "Wailing Wall," the holiest of Jewish sites and the only remnant of the walls surrounding the temple of biblical times. You can walk down the Via Dolorosa, with its fourteen Stations of the Cross, to the Church of the Holy Sepulchre, which stands on Golgotha, the traditional site of the crucifixion of Jesus. The Dome of the Rock nearby marks the spot where Mohammed is said to have ascended to heaven. While in Jerusalem, you may also wish to see the Chagall windows at the Hadassah Hospital, the Kennedy Memorial, Yad Vashem, the memorial to the Holocaust, the Dead Sea Scrolls at the Shrine of the Book, the Knesset building, and the views of the city from the Mount of Olives and Mount Scopus. If you wish to sample typical Middle Eastern dishes in a comfortable atmosphere, you will enjoy Minaret Restaurant at Eight King David Street, where four generations of Abo Salah's family have entertained locals, tourists, and dignitaries since 1960. Start off with a tasting of mixed salads including hummus, tahina, baba ganush, and several other varieties followed by a sampling of grilled meats and poultries on skewers. Currently popular French-Continental restaurants include Arcadia, Mishkenot Sha'anim, Katy's, Darna (Moroccan/ French/Kosher), and Ocean (seafood); however, in Israel many upscale restaurants frequently come and go. The best hotel facilities are at the King David Hotel, which is a centrally located hotel with a great deal of old-world charm; the Hilton next door; Laromma; the Sheraton; and the Hyatt, which sits on Mount Scopus near Hadassah Hospital overlooking the old city.

Bethlehem is only a short drive from Jerusalem, and you can continue on to the famous Dead Sea. Here you can float in hot water so dense with salt that it is impossible to sink. If time allows, you will want to visit historic **Masada,** the recently uncovered ruins of the mountaintop fortress where an entire city of Jews made a last stand against the Romans in A.D. 70, all preferring to take their lives rather than surrender. Continuing back to Haifa, you can take a lovely drive past the Sea of Galilee, Tiberius, and the Golan Heights.

ITALY

Elba is a small Italian island with 91 miles of coastline lying in the Mediterranean between Corsica and mainland Italy, and is best known as Napoleon's place of exile in 1814. His residence in Portoferraio and country home in San Martino are still open today as museums for visitors to Elba. Ships dock at the capital, Portoferraio. This is a busy, not-too-beautiful port town with a few shops, restaurants, a fortress, and a decent public beach (with pebbles and no sand). The best restaurant in Portoferraio is touted to be La Ferrigna, with its emphasis on Elban cooking, fresh fish, and seafood. After taking a tour around the island, which should include Napoleon's country home in San Martino, the port town of Porto Azzurro, and the fishing village at Marciana Marina, you may wish to have lunch and spend the afternoon at the beach areas at Procchio, Marina di Campo, or the bay of Biodola. The bay of Biodola is only a 10-minute drive from Portoferraio, has a nice brown-sand beach, lovely setting, and numerous upscale hotels with private beach areas, pools, and restaurants. The Heritage is probably your best bet.

Genoa, Italy's largest port, ranks second in size only to Marseilles among Mediterranean ports. It has been said that Genoa is a city of layers or levels: the lowest level is the noisy and dirty harbor area with its ships, dance halls, and bars; the middle level contains large hotels, bright shops, good restaurants, cinemas, the opera house, and the Via Garibaldi, with its chain of late Renaissance palaces; and the upper level is a series of hills, winding streets, and funiculars. Genoa lies in the middle of Italy's two Rivieras, and you can drive to such seaside resort towns as San Remo, Rapallo, Santa Marguarita Linguere, La Spezia, and Viareggio.

With only limited time, you may enjoy driving to **Portofino,** 50 miles southeast of Genoa. After exploring the town, with its excellent shops and restaurants, you may enjoy relaxing, sunbathing, and having lunch or dinner at the fashionable Splendido Hotel, a yachtsmen's rendezvous perched on the side of a mountain overlooking the harbor. Many ships now anchor in the harbor at Portofino and tender passengers into town. There are additional shops and restaurants at the seaside town of Santa Marguarita Linguere, 3 miles from Portofino.

Naples, the third largest city in Italy, is a major manufacturing center and one of Italy's busiest ports. Although the city itself is crowded and dirty, it enjoys a scenic location, with Mount Vesuvius rising high above a plain 10 miles to the southeast; vineyards and groves surround the city on the bay's eastern shore; and the famous Isle of Capri lies to the south across the Bay of Naples. In the city itself, you may wish to shop for bargains in silks, gloves, purses, other leather goods, and gold jewelry; or visit the National Museum to see its valuable art collections and relics from Pompeii. Also very worthwhile are the Aquarium of Naples, the San Carlo Opera House, or the many beautiful churches and castles.

You can drive south to visit the ruins of **Pompeii** and then ascend the crater of Mount Vesuvius by chairlift, or take the fantastically beautiful and breathtaking Amalfi Drive to the south, passing through the quaint seaside towns of Amalfi, Positano, and Sorrento. Stop for lunch or dinner at the Santa Catarina Hotel in Amalfi or the San Pietro in Positano and enjoy the charm and view of these seaside resort hotels. If time allows you to continue your visit, another charming city set in the hills above Amalfi is Ravello. Here you will enjoy having a fine meal on the terrace of Hotel Palumbo while being treated to an extraordinary vista of a large portion of the Coasta Amalfitano.

From Naples, you can take a hydrofoil over to the beautiful floral **Isle of Capri,** where you will be dropped off in a pretty little harbor. A funicular railway takes you up the mountain to the main square, where you can sit at an outdoor café and watch a colorful assortment of tourists in the world pass by. There is a pebbled beach at Marina Piccola, and nearby you can dine and swim in a pool at Gracie Field's Canzone del Mare. The best hotel in Capri is the Grand Quisisana. Be certain to have lunch by the pool or dinner at Restaurant Quisi for a truly elegant gourmet experience. You may enjoy browsing numerous designer shops, or taking the short bus ride up to Anacapri where there are more hotels, restaurants, and shops, as well as panoramic views down to Capri Town and the sea. At Marina Grande, you can charter a boat to take you to the famous Blue Grotto. This area south of Naples (Amalfi, Positano, Sorrento, Ravello, and the Isle of Capri) is possibly the most beautiful part of southern Europe and shouldn't be missed.

Sicily is an Italian island off the coast of Italy with an area of 9,900 square miles, making it the largest island in the Mediterranean. Its 4,800,000 inhabitants live in a mild climate, with the average temperatures ranging from forty-five degrees in winter to eighty degrees in summer. Cruise ships stop at the capital city of Palermo and at the resort area of Taormina.

In Palermo, you can browse through the fine shops on the Via Liberte, Via Roma, and Via Ruggero Settimo and visit the old royal palace, which contains a lovely chapel well known for its mosaics and marble floors, or you can see the sanctuary on Monte Pellegrino at 2,000 feet above sea level, offering a striking view of the island. From Palermo, you can drive to Syracuse to see a classical production at the ancient Roman amphitheater; or you can drive to Mondello, where there are pleasant beaches and fine seafood restaurants; or you may prefer spending the day at Citta Del Mare in Terrasini, 20 miles away, which is a lovely Club Med-style resort village complete with eleven tennis courts, a miniature golf course, an Olympic-size pool, a cinema, electronic games, a discotheque, and numerous restaurants and bars. The *pièce de résistance* is a conglomerate of water slides that connect three pools set vertically down a steep hill and finally dump you into the Mediterranean.

If your ship docks in **Messina** or **Catania,** it is less than an hour's drive to the resort town of Taormina. This picturesque village winds in and out of hills, then drops to the sea. The craggy coastline is dotted with European-style beaches, where you can rent chairs and purchase snacks and drinks. From the northern slope stretch the beaches of Isola Bella, Mazzaro, Spizzonli, and Mazzeo. On the southern slope are the beaches of Villagonia, Giardini, and Naxos. At these beaches, the water is clear but the terrain is pebbly. Those wishing to base themselves at a hotel can try the Sea Palace at Mazzaro, which has a pool, lounge area, and a nice restaurant in addition to its beach.

Any stop at Taormina should include a visit to the Greek-Roman theater, an illustrious monument built by the ancient Greeks and rebuilt by the Romans. Most of the shops are located in the center of Taormina, which lies higher up in the hills. There is little shopping on the beaches. If time permits, a nice place to visit and have lunch is the San Domenica Palace. This is an old monastery converted to an elegant hotel, replete with hundreds of original antiques and Renaissance paintings. The gardens here are beautiful and afford a breathtaking panorama of the coast and sea below. In the evening, you will enjoy the sound and light spectacle.

Above Taormina is the world-famous volcano, Mount Etna. Rising 10,784 feet from the sea, it is the highest volcano in Europe. You can take a tour to the 6,000-foot level and have lunch, then continue up to the observatory at 9,000 feet.

Venice is the unusual Italian city on the Adriatic lying on a cluster of small mud islands divided by canals. You can walk down the narrow streets where picturesque stone bridges cross the canals, or you can ride down the canals in gondolas and motorboat buses. The Rialto Bridge is in the heart of the city and crosses the Grand Canal; it has a single arch 32 feet high, with shops built along each side. The Bridge of Sighs crosses from the Doge's Palace (an example of the Italian Gothic style of architecture containing a priceless collection of paintings) to an old prison. The palace and bridge stand next to the famous Cathedral of St. Mark (a fine example of Byzantine architecture) in the world-famous Piazza of St. Mark. This square, with its old clock tower and thousands of pigeons, is one of the most photographed spots in Europe. In the evening, it is quite romantic to sit out in the square at an outdoor café overlooking the Grand Canal while listening to an Italian band. You can then charter a private gondola for a ride through the winding canals or sail over to the Lido area, where there are nightclubs and a casino.

You can visit the Murano glass factory, where Venetian glass is designed, and swim at the so-so sand beaches on the Adriatic in the Lido area. Try the beach at the Excelsior Palace. Some of the outstanding restaurants in Venice include the

Taverna La Fenice, the roof of the Royal Danieli Hotel, the Gritti Palace, Da Forno, Quadri, and Harry's Bar. Shopping opportunities are everywhere, with the best shops located near San Marco, and the best bargains near the Rialto Bridge. For a special treat have lunch by the pool or dinner overlooking the canal at the Hotel Cipriani on Guidecca Island, a 5-minute boat ride by the hotel's private water taxi from San Marco.

If your ship stops at Port Cervo on the Costa Smeralda on the island of Sardinia, you will see one of the largest concentrations of luxury yachts to be found in the world. You can browse through boutiques and shops that surround the harbor and Hotel Cervo, play 18 holes of golf at the Robert Trent Jones-designed Prevero Golf Club, or spend the day at a beach. Since all beaches are public, you can also visit the beach at the luxury resort Cale Di Volpe (about a 10-minute taxi ride from the harbor). If you are willing to drop about 180,000 lire per person, you can joint the resort's affluent clientele for one of the most lavish (and excellent) lunch buffets imaginable, which includes salads, all varieties of antipasto, imported cheeses, pastas, pastries, and fresh fish and meats grilled to your specification. Other nearby luxury resorts include Romanzzina and Pitriccia.

MALTA

Malta, an island located in the Mediterranean between Italy and Africa, previously part of the British Commonwealth, is today a self-governing constitutional monarchy. The climate is mild during the winter and dry and hot in the summer. After your ship pulls into the port city of **Valletta**, you can charter a horse-and-buggy and ride into the main section of town. You will find some fine examples of baroque and Renaissance art and architecture if you visit the Palace of the Grand Masters, the Royal Malta Library, or the Cathedral of St. John. You will enjoy stopping for lunch and a swim at the Malta Hilton or the Sheraton Malta hotels, which are a short distance from town. Lace, homespun cotton clothes, and wool rugs are the best buys. In the evening you may wish to stroll through the area referred to as "The Gut," with its dives, honky-tonks, beer parlors, and cabarets.

MOROCCO

Casablanca is a major port in North Africa, with more than a million inhabitants enjoying a mild, warm climate. Some of the more popular tourist attractions include the tiny old Medina near the harbor, which is a historical relic and site of the earliest settlement; the new Medina on the eastern side of town, where you can watch cases being tried at the local courts; and the United Nations Square, which is surrounded by tropical gardens grouped around government buildings. At United Nations Square, you can walk through the local shops and find bargains in ancient and modern carpets, leather, jewelry, and local crafts. You can stop in a Moroccan restaurant and try kabobs, *harira* (a type of chicken soup), *pastia* (layers of filo leaves stuffed with chicken, eggs, cinnamon, and exotic spices), *tajin* (a type of stew), and some local wine. If you wish to relax at a beach or pool, you will prefer to take a leisurely ride along the corniche to Anfa and Ain Diab. If time permits, you will want to travel to the ancient city of **Marrakesh,** driving through this colorful town in an open, horse-drawn carriage.

PORTUGAL

Overlooking a broad bay, **Lisbon** lies on Portugal's west coast, about 7 miles from the Atlantic Ocean. The city's 820,000 inhabitants enjoy an ideal climate where temperatures average in the fifties in January and in the seventies in July. You will want to walk through the picturesque old section of the city, where the pavements are of black and white mosaics in checked patterns or forming scenes that recall outstanding events from Lisbon's history. The narrow streets are always crowded with colorful throngs, and in Rossio Square you may see an apple peddler or a country woman with a basket on her head.

On the Avenida da Liberdade are the better hotels, and on Chiado Street you will find the fashionable shops, where you can purchase handmade shoes, fine dresses, decorative glazed tiles, beautiful pottery, copperware, and leather goods. You will want to stroll through the beautiful Alfama area. Here you can ride a donkey to an old castle enclosed by moats with reedy waters filled with ducks, fish, and flamingos. Nearby you can visit the twelfth-century Romanesque cathedral and the King's Fountain. Later you can take in a bullfight and relax at one of the many excellent restaurants that feature fish, seafood, and Portuguese wines. Those of you who wish to swim can take the short train ride or drive to the fashionable resort areas north of the city, with their posh hotels, shops, fine beaches, and gambling casino.

Funchal is the port of the Portuguese Madeira Islands, which lie in the Atlantic 500 miles off the coast of Lisbon. These volcanic islands enjoy a mild, sunny climate, with temperatures ranging from the sixties in winter to the seventies in summer. As you approach port, you will notice the rocky coastline studded with quaint lighthouses, fishing ports, and whaling villages. As you disembark, you will be greeted by the natives in rowboats filled with fruit, baskets, and embroideries welcoming you to this island covered with flowers, bushes, trees, and other vegetation.

Funchal is a resort town with a lazy holiday atmosphere, and you will enjoy walking through the main square, stopping to visit the Jesuit Church, Town Hall, and the Bishop's Palace. You can browse through quaint shops for antiques as well as for beautiful embroideries on Irish linens and French silks, or you can stroll through the open-air market. You can sip some famous Madeira wine and relax at one of the hotel pools overlooking the cliffs, since the beaches have volcanic black pebbles and are not desirable for swimming. If time allows, you can drive to Cabo Girao to visit the vineyards, to Curral las Freiras to visit a village monastery hidden from view by rocks, or to Comacha to see the house where Madeira baskets are made.

SENEGAL

Dakar is an Atlantic port and the capital of Senegal in western Africa; it has a hot climate and much rain during the summer. The city itself reflects a great deal of European style and French influence, but the people have a definite African character. Some of the more interesting sights include the graceful Presidential Palace; the elegant new Parliament Building; the university; the teeming Sandaga Market; the Ifan Museum, with its magnificent collection of West African carvings, pottery, cloth, and musical instruments; and the medina, with its colorful, cluttered market. There are nice beaches for swimming at N'Gor and Bernard Inlet. If possible, try to attend a native *mechoui,* which is a colorful feast including the barbecue of a sheep or goat. At the Craftsman's Village at Soumbedioune, you will find bargains on native jewelry, leatherwork, pottery, fili-gree, and woven goods.

SPAIN

Algeciras is a port in southeastern Spain across the bay from Gibraltar. From this town, you can take an overnight boat train to Madrid, a 2 1/2-hour ferry ride to Tangier in North Africa, or a several-hour drive to the Costa del Sol area and visit the picturesque towns of Marbella, Malaga, Torremolinos, and Porto Banus. On the Costa del Sol, you will find numerous resort hotels, beaches, boutiques, shops, good restaurants, night spots, and tourists from all over Europe. The best resorts with the most facilities are Los Monteros, Marbella Club, and Puente Romano, all located in Marbella. The most colorful harbor area is at Puerto Banus, a 10-minute ride from Marbella. Here you can stroll along the waterfront filled with giant yachts and visit some of the best shops and small ethnic restaurants to be found in Spain.

If your ship docks in the harbor of Malaga, you will be able to take the tour to Granada and visit the famous Alhambra Castle and charming surrounding parks and attractions. On your way, you may wish to stop for lunch or a drink at the magnificent La Bobadilla Resort, which is built on a hillside in the style of a Moorish village.

Barcelona is located on the Mediterranean coast of northern Spain, not far from France. This busy city with more than two million inhabitants is the largest Spanish-speaking port in the world after Buenos Aires. You will be able to capture the Spanish flavor by taking in the traditional bullfight, enjoying a flamenco show, or having some gazpacho and paella at a typical Spanish restaurant. You can visit the historic cathedral known as "La Seu" in the old town as well as the interesting building nearby; drive or take the cable car up to the top of the hill of Tibidabo, from the heights of which you can see the Pyrenees; visit the National Museum, the museum of Catalan Art in the Palacio Nacional, and the *Pueblo Españñol* (Spanish Village), built in 1929, which displays the architecture, arts, and crafts from the various regions of Spain; stop by Gaudi's famous Cathedral of the Holy Family; or walk down the Paseo de Gracia or the tree-lined Ramblas Avenue with its colorful flower stalls and shop for leather goods, linens, and souvenirs. The best restaurants in town are Atalaya (Spanish and French food and a good view of the city), Jaume de Provenca (Spanish and Continental food in a lovely setting at reasonable prices), and Via Veneto (Continental menu in a grand environment—expensive).

The **Canary Islands** are a group of seven Spanish islands in the Atlantic Ocean 60 miles off the coast of northwest Africa. The islands are mountainous and have a mild climate with temperatures ranging from the sixties in winter to the seventies in summer. Most cruise ships stop at either **Las Palmas** on the Grand Canary Island or **Santa Cruz** on the island of Tenerife. The islands are volcanic, resulting in several black-sand beaches. Although there are no famous restaurants, you will want to try the fish and seafood as well as some of the local rice dishes. At Las Palmas, you can shop at a number of attractive, duty-free stores; explore the narrow streets and plazas of the old part of the city by horse and carriage; watch the sunset at an open-air café; swim at the beaches of Las Canteras, Alcaravaneras, or La Laja; or witness a cockfight.

Santa Cruz is a lively town that may seem to be more beautiful than Las Palmas. Here you can visit the archeological and anthropological museum, the seventeenth-century Carta Palace, and the historical relics of the Church of the Concepción. There are beaches at Las Tereitas and Las Gaviotas. Tourists often take an excursion from Santa Cruz through the town of La Laguna, followed by a beautiful drive to Orotava and Porto de la Cruz, passing by beautiful coastlines, tropical flowers, and foliage. From Orotava, you ascend the Teide Mountain, which includes a funicular railroad ride to the volcano's cone, where you can witness a panoramic view of all the Canary Islands. On the way back to Santa Cruz, you may wish to swim in the warm waters and fine sand of El Medano Beach.

Palma is the main resort area and port of Majorca, one of the Spanish Balearic Islands lying in the Mediterranean 120 miles south of Barcelona. Tourists from all over the world pour into Palma each year to enjoy its mild winters and beautiful summers. In town, there are numerous Spanish-style restaurants (El Patio is among the best) and excellent shops where you can obtain bargains in pearls and leather goods. The best shopping area is along Jaime III, General Mola, and Paseo de Borne streets. The larger hotels in Palma are not on the ocean, and you will have to travel away from the city to bathe in the sea. A worthwhile trip that will take an entire day would include a visit to the Drach caves at Porto Cristo, followed by a trip to Formentor. The Drach caves are the largest in the world, with magnificent stalagmites and stalactites and a natural underground lake and auditorium where you can witness a truly unique concert. The drive up a mountain and down to the hotel at Formentor is breathtaking. Here you can enjoy a delicious lunch complete with sangria; swim at a sheltered, pine-studded bathing beach; play tennis on modern courts; and go horseback riding in the mountains. The best resorts near the town of Palma are the Son Vida, a delightful choice for an outdoor lunch by the pool, and Arabella Golf Hotel, a sister hotel on a scenic golf course.

Some cruise ships call at ports on other Balearic Islands. Most ships visiting the island of **Menorca,** anchor or tender to the port of **Mahon** (Mao). Here there is little of interest other than taking a picturesque walk along the harbor where you will find small cafés and a few souvenir shops, or walking up the stairs near the main harbor to the town where you can explore charming little streets and visit additional shops and restaurants. There are beaches located around the island accessible by taxi. **Ibiza** is a more interesting cruise stop and a major vacation destination for the British and Germans. Right off the harbor are narrow streets lined with restaurants and souvenir and leather shops. You will want to visit the fortress and castle that sit above the harbor and one of the colorful beaches (some of which include nude bathing). Salines is the most popular beach and only a short bus ride from the town.

TUNISIA

Your ship will dock at **LaGoulette** or **Bizerte,** the ports for Tunis and Carthage. Your best choice will be to take an organized tour that transports you to Tunis and visits the ruins of ancient Carthage dating back to 814 B.C. You will probably stop at the National Archeological Museum; the pretty suburb of Sidi Abon Said, with its white buildings and cobbled streets; and the interesting Casbah, with its mosques and numerous *souks* (shopping streets) featuring Oriental rugs, brass trays, gold jewelry, linens, and souvenirs.

TURKEY

Turkey has become a very popular stop for Greek island and Mediterranean cruises. Traditionally, the three ports most often visited are Istanbul, Izmir, and Kusadasi. However, several ships now offer stops at the more scenic coastal resort towns of Marmaris and Antalya.

Istanbul, formerly Constantinople, is the city of legend and history where East and West meet. This great commercial seaport is the largest city in Turkey, stretching along both the European and Asiatic sides of the Bosporus, which connects the Sea of Marmara with the Black Sea. You will not want to miss the Grand Bazaar in the heart of the old city, which is one of the most unique shopping areas in the world. Here you can browse through four thousand tiny shops spread along 92 winding streets and see bargains in gold, copper, ceramics, jewelry, rugs, leather, suedes, handicrafts, and just about anything else you could imagine. There are a number of stores both in the bazaar and nearby where you can have leather and suede outfits made to order while you wait. You will want to visit the famous Topkapi Museum, formerly the Palace of the Sultans, where today you can view some of the world's most valuable and beautiful works of art, rare stones, jewels, ancient weapons, furnishings, other antiquities, and the harems of the Sultans.

One of the most unique sights when sailing into Istanbul is the skyline filled with beautiful mosques with their domes, semidomes, and minarets. The most famous is the Blue Mosque or Sultan Ahmed Mosque located near the Topkapi Museum. You will also want to visit St. Sophia, which was built by Emperor Justinian in the sixth century as a Christian church, altered to a mosque, and later turned into a museum with its magnificent architecture, important mosaics, and unusual chandeliers. Aghia Sophia (as it is now called) is said to be the world's finest example of Byzantine architecture. You can stop at a restaurant where the locals eat in the Cicok Pasaji, Kumkapi area, or atop the fourteenth-century Galeta Tower, not far from the pier, for simple versions of Turkish appetizers and salads, fish, seafood, shish kebab, baklava, and coffee; or you may wish to have a drink or dine at one of the magnificent Istanbul hotels such as the Ciragan Palace, Hilton, Four Seasons, Intercontinental, or Conrad. All of these make excellent pre- or post-cruise headquarters with central locations, panoramic views, numerous restaurants, large health clubs, and pools. The top epicurean dinner restaurants in Istanbul include Ulus 29, Safron at the Intercontinental and Körfez for seafood, accessible by a short ferry ride.

Some ships stop at the small port town of **Dikili** to enable passengers to take the short drive through rolling hills, pine trees, and vineyards to Bergama and the ruins of Pergamon. Pergamon was an ancient Greek city in Asia Minor that dates back to the third century B.C. The city was built on terraces of steep mountains and is composed of an acropolis with ruins of several temples and a sanctuary to the god of medicine. After the tour, you can wander through the small shops and outdoor markets near the harbor or enjoy fresh fish right off the boat at a local restaurant.

Izmir and **Kusadasi** are other ports in Turkey where cruise ships often stop. Izmir is an important, colorful port and the headquarters for the NATO Command guarding the eastern Mediterranean. Kusadasi is a summer resort town where you can swim at small beaches, ride a camel on the sand, or shop for gold, jewelry, rugs, leather, suede, and antiques at one of its many stores. Bargains on leather are probably among the best in the world. Kusadasi has several excellent resort hotels with lovely pool areas, including the Fantasia, Onur, and Koru-Mar. The Koru-Mar is only a mile away from the harbor and affords picturesque views of the city and sea. **Ephesus** is inland from Izmir or Kusadasi. This ancient city, uncovered by Austrian archeologists, has some of the most impressive archeological ruins in the world, including a mile-long marble road, restored buildings, the Arcadian Way, Temple of Hadrian, the Library, the Odeon, the public toilets, the ruins of the Temple of Diana, the site of the Temple of Artemis (considered one of the Seven Wonders of the World), and the Last Abode of Mary. There are numerous restaurants spread throughout the town, most specializing in fresh fish and seafood.

Once a tiny sleeping village leveled by a devastating earthquake in 1057, **Marmaris** has been resurrected as Turkey's most beautiful, upscale resort area and yacht haven. Fringing a protected bay surrounded by rugged pine-forested mountains, the town has a floral beach walk that meanders along the harbor and bay past numerous hotels, posh resorts, restaurants, tavernas, and shops. The harbor where the cruise ships generally dock is dotted with private yachts and sailing vessels and is only a 10-minute walk from the town center, where you will find dozens of restaurants, bars, and tavernas reminiscent of St. Tropez and Puerto Banus. In the town center, there is also a covered bazaar that offers many of the same bargains in gold, jewelry, leather goods, carpets, and other merchandise as found in the Grand Bazaar of Istanbul or in the shops of Kusadasi, except in a less crowded, more pleasant surrounding. Extending for about 5 miles from the town center is the beach walk mentioned above. The most beautiful resort is the Marmaris Palace, which has private bungalows and hotel rooms with pools, restaurants, and lush grounds that run down pine-clad hills to the beach area. The clientele is mostly German. Other nice beach resorts in the area include Mares Marmaris and Grand Azur. Side trips can be taken to the typical Turkish seaside villages of Icmeler, Tarunc, and Kumlubuk, and tours are also offered to the graves of Likya and the ruins of Caunos.

Antalya, set on a majestic coastline of beaches and rocky caves, is a very attractive resort city with shady, palm-lined boulevards, a picturesque marina, and an old quarter called Kaleici with narrow, winding streets and quaint, old wood houses next to the city walls. Places of interest include the Archeology Museum, the clock tower, Hadrian's Gate, Hidirlik Tower, Kesik Minaret complex, and the Turban Kaleici Marina. There are several full-facility resort hotels, the Sheraton Voyager being the most upscale. Other choices overlooking the sea include Talya, Falez, and Cender. The beaches, although picturesque, are pebbly and uninviting. Excursions away from the city may include the upper and lower Dudden waterfalls, the restored archeological ruins at Perge, or the archeological sites and beaches at Patara. Golfers may wish to opt for the 24-mile drive to the National Golf Club in Belek, where they will find both a 9-hole and a championship 18-hole course situated amongst shady pine forests near pretty beach areas.

FORMER U.S.S.R. (SOUTH)

A number of ships cruise the Black Sea, stopping at such Russian ports as Odessa, Sochi, and Yalta.

Odessa is called "the pearl of the Black Sea," with its picturesque seascape, streets, and marketplaces. To the landlocked Russian, this is a town of sun, golden-sand beaches, and green parks. You can stroll from one end of the seafront to the other, visiting the Pushkin Statue, the Opera House, the Vorontsov Palace, the Square of the Commune, and the archeological museum. You may wish to visit one of the city's beaches at Arcadia, Luzanovska, and Chernomorka.

Sochi is the largest seaside resort in the former U.S.S.R., protected from cold winds and sudden temperature changes by the Caucasus Mountains. There is a large central bathing beach as well as many smaller beaches with adjoining sanatoria (Russian health resorts with clinics, solarium pools, beaches, public rooms, and sports facilities). You may wish to visit the famous Dendrarium Botanical Gardens, containing fountains, statues, subtropical flora, and trees and shrubs from all over the world.

Yalta is a Black Sea port on the southern coast of the Crimean Peninsula at the southern foothills of the Yaila Mountains. The city is also sheltered by mountains and enjoys a temperate climate. This seaside resort town is surrounded by woods, vineyards, and fruit farms where pear, almond, peach, apple, and apricot trees are grown. There are three main beaches and numerous sanatoria. You can walk along the Lenin Quay, where you will find the main shops, hotels, cafés, and restaurants. Places and points of interest include the Ethnographic Museum (devoted to Eastern art), the Tchekhov Museum (which was once the author's house), Yuri Gagarin Park, Massandra Park and Combine (famous for its wines), and the Nikitsky Botanical Gardens.

Northern Europe, the Baltic, the North Sea, the Fjords, and the Rivers of Europe

During the late spring and summer, a number of ships offer cruises to Northern European ports in the Baltic and North seas as well as up to the picturesque fjords of Norway and down the rivers of Germany, Austria, Hungary, and France. Although the climate may not be as ideal as in the Caribbean or Mediterranean, the weather is generally mild enough at these times of year to permit you to sit out on deck and take in the magnificent sights and scenery.

The cruises are generally longer (at least ten to fourteen days) and more expensive than those found in the Mediterranean; however, they afford you an opportunity to visit a large number of interesting ports while sampling a variety of cultures all in one trip without the inconvenience of flying from place to place.

These cruises usually initiate from Southampton, Tilbury, Le Havre, or Copenhagen, and the ships either sail up the coast of Norway to the fjords and "Land of the Midnight Sun" or stop at such interesting northern European ports as Amsterdam, Oslo, Helsinki, Stockholm, Hamburg, Gdynia, Tallinn, Visby, and St. Petersburg.

The ships of most major cruise lines cruise the northlands.

For a totally different experience, seasoned cruisers will enjoy a leisurely riverboat trip on the Rhine, Moselle, Danube, Elbe, Seine, Saône or Rhône rivers with visits to historic cities and charming villages.

The following are the highlights of some of the more popular northern ports:

DANUBE RIVER

The Danube River emanates in the southeast portion of Germany and passes through eight European countries before it connects with the Black Sea. Most riverboats embark passengers in **Passau**, the location of the confluence of three rivers: the Danube, Inn, and Ilz. Quite close to the point where the rivers converge is the old town area, where you can walk through narrow cobblestone streets and alleys; visit St. Stephan's Cathedral with its baroque stuccoed ceiling, Gothic architecture, frescoes, and the world's largest church organ; and see the town hall and the thirteenth-century Castle Oberhaus—the location of a museum, art gallery, and observatory. You can rest along the way at an outdoor café overlooking the river and sample a local beer, ice cream, or pastry.

The stretch of the river extending between Passau and Vienna is the most picturesque, meandering through verdant hills and symmetrical forests. Each evening, passengers are mesmerized by the sunset over the smooth waters of the Danube, creating the appearance of a bright orange ball melting into the river.

After Passau, your boat will pass through the **Wachau** region, a wine-producing area with vine-clad rolling slopes. The round towers of fortified churches and the battlement turrets of ancient castles frequently emerge as the river winds its way through Austria.

Prior to reaching Vienna, most boats visit **Dürnstein,** a charming Austrian village dominated by the beautiful baroque tower of an early eighteenth-century convent. You can visit the cathedral, stroll the narrow streets of the town as they wind up a hill, taste wine at a local vintner, or walk along the paths bordered by vineyards that follow the river. You can even enjoy the panoramic view from the twelfth-century castle that sits on a steep hill, 520 feet above the town, and is connected by an ancient wall. This castle is where King Richard the Lionhearted was said to have been incarcerated.

The next major stop is one of the highlights of any cruise on the Danube, Austria's famous capital, **Vienna.** From the river, you will want to take a taxi or the metro (train No. 1) to Stephansplatz, which is in the middle of the historic and commercial core of the city, as well as the site of the soaring St. Stephan's, an impressive Gothic cathedral with a steeple that rises 450 feet. In this area are numerous traditional Viennese coffeehouses, outside cafés, and pedestrian-only shopping streets. Within easy walking distance are the 700-year-old, 2,600-room Hofburg Palace (about two dozen rooms are open to the public, as is the crown jewel collection); the Museum of Fine Arts; the State Opera House; the 1,441-room early seventeenth-century Schonbrunn Palace; and the city park with its statue of Johann Strauss.

There are highly rated, more formal restaurants in the deluxe hotels such as the Bristol, Sacher, Hilton, and Imperial. Less expensive typical Viennese restaurants are spread throughout this area. I especially enjoyed lunch on the protected patio of the Sacher Hotel dining room, where Viennese specialties reach top gourmet level, embellished by the excellent service staff. Another highly esteemed dining establishment is Zuden Drei Hussarin, located right off of St. Stephan's Square. If you do not have time for a meal, a must is sampling a coffee and pastry, or at least an Austrian beer, in a coffeehouse. Although a version of Sacher Torte is available throughout the city, purists can enjoy a slice of the rich chocolate delight in the café connected to the Sacher Hotel.

On your way back to the river in the evening, you can visit the amusement park at the Prater, where a Ferris wheel with large enclosed gondolas offers a scenic 10-minute ride affording the best views of the city. Another spot to enjoy the view of the city while having a coffee is the café that revolves 590 feet above ground on the Danube Tower.

Another port of call on most itineraries, **Bratislava, Slovakia,** is of interest to tourists mostly due to its political history and the evolution of its varied governments. The Bratislava Hrad (castle) houses a historical museum and sits on a hill overlooking the city above the old town. Other scenic views of the town and river are possible from S.N.P. Bridge and Tower. The Danube is a new, modern hotel on the river with an open-air bar at the top, and numerous shops, cafés and restaurants have opened during the past few years.

The shorter cruises that do not extend to the Black Sea generally turn around at **Budapest,** one of the most picturesque and interesting cities along the Danube. The capital of Hungary with a population of three million is actually composed of two cities, Buda and Pest, which are connected by a series of bridges that span the river.

The most popular tourist areas on the Buda side are Castle Hill and Gellert Hill. Castle Hill was the center of Buda during the Middle Ages; today it is composed of small souvenir shops, cafés, restaurants, the Hilton Hotel and Casino, the thirteenth-century Matthias Church, and the Royal palace, which houses a historical museum and national art gallery and numerous statues and structures of historical interest.

Although Castle Hill is an excellent location from which to look across to the Pest side of the city and the Houses of Parliament, the panoramic vista of the Danube from 770 feet above on Gellert Hill is the most awesome. The Citadel on Gellert Hill was built in 1849 as a prison and is now a tourist attraction with restaurants, shops, and nightclubs. Also located here is Liberty Statue. Visible throughout the city, it was built as a tribute to the Soviet liberators.

On the Pest side are many of the larger hotels, restaurants, pedestrian shopping streets, the Houses of Parliament, St. Stephan's Basilica, the statues and monuments at Hero's Square (constructed in 1896), the oldest synagogue in Europe, and several museums. The Atrium Hyatt enjoys an excellent location and provides many facilities, making it an excellent choice for a pre- or post-cruise overnight stay.

Margaret Island, which is connected by a bridge to both Buda and Pest, is a large, attractive park with tennis courts, soccer fields, children's playgrounds, small restaurants, a public swimming pool, and a garden theater. It is a very popular recreational area for the citizens of the city.

Gundel's, which occupies a palatial mansion in City Park, is the home of "pancakes Gundel" and offers the finest dining experience in Budapest.

The largest, most elegant riverboat cruising on the Danube is the 212-passenger M/S *Mozart* (for Peter Deilmann EuropAmerica Cruises). Other popular riverboats with similar itineraries include the *Danube Princess, River Cloud, Wilhelm Tell, Volga, Blue Danube I* and *II, Amadeus II, Prussian Princess, Swiss Pearl, Rousse, Danube Star,* and *Delphin Princess.*

DENMARK

Copenhagen, the capital and chief port of Denmark, is a friendly, charming, cosmopolitan city with some of the finest restaurants and shops in Europe. From the Raadhuspladsen, the main square with its towering town hall, you can walk (or ride a rented bicycle) down the winding Strøget street toward Kongens Nytorv and the harbor area of Nyhavn. On the Strøget, you can browse through such famous shops as Illums Bolighus (modern design center), Georg Jensen (silver), Hans Hansens (silver), Royal Copenhagen (china), and Birger Christensen (furs). From Nyhavn, you are only a short distance from Langelinie Pavillion, where you can have an outdoor lunch or dinner in a park overlooking the *Little Mermaid,* a statue inspired by Hans Christian Andersen's fairy tale that gracefully sits on a rock overlooking the harbor.

If you head in the opposite direction from the main square (Raadhuspladsen), you can visit the Glyptothek Museum, with its excellent collection of French paintings and Egyptian sculpture, and the fantastic Tivoli Gardens, with its flowers, open-air theater, concert hall, amusement rides, restaurants, nightclubs, and nightly fireworks. You may also enjoy visiting the lovely Copenhagen Zoo, Rosenborg Palace with its crown jewels, the National Art Museum, or the Carlsberg Beer factory. You will want to try one of the delicious open-face sandwiches called *smörbrod,* as well as the great Tuborg and Carlsberg beers.

Inside the Tivoli Gardens are three excellent restaurants: Divan I, Divan II, and Belle Terasse, as well as the more informal Groften. For fish and seafood, you will want to try Krogs, Fiskekaelderen, and DenGlydne Fortun. Gourmets will enjoy Kommandanten; Kong Hans Kaelder; Lenore Christine, Les Etoiles, or one of the exceptional restaurants in the Royal, Plaza, D'Angleterre, Kong Frederik, Scandinavia, and several other hotels. Actually, it would be difficult to have anything but a good meal in Copenhagen, wherever you might stop.

Possible excursions would include visits to Frilandsmuseet, an open-air museum set in the pastoral countryside to the north, where there is a display of Danish farmhouses from various regions set in their natural environs; a visit to Kronborg Castle at Helsingor, famous as the setting of Shakespeare's *Hamlet* and 45 minutes north of Copenhagen; or Denmark's National History Museum, housed in Frederiksborg Castle in Hillerod, where you can boat on the castle's lake.

ESTONIA

Tallinn is the major port city with a population of 500,000. Dating back nine centuries, almost every building in the Old Town has some historic or architectural interest. Cruise ships on their way to Helsinki and St. Petersburg have found this a convenient stop where passengers can stroll through cobblestone streets while viewing Gothic architecture, a variety of churches and museums, numerous historic sites, and lovely parks.

It is recommended that visitors tour Tallinn by foot in order to take full advantage of the many places of interest. You may wish to start your tour at Toompea, the upper town, which is situated on a hill that affords a panoramic view of the city and harbor. Here you can visit the sixteenth-century Cannon Tower, Toompea Palace, St. Alexander Nevski's Cathedral, the thirteenth-century Dome Church, and take a walk through narrow Kohter Street to the observation platform, where you will enjoy the best view of the lower Old Town. There are several souvenir shops here and refreshments can be purchased at the café adjacent to the Virgin's Tower.

In the lower town you can visit the Town Hall constructed at the beginning of the fifteenth century; the homes and guild halls along Pikk Street; the thirteenth-century spire of St. Olan's Church, which dominates the Tallinn skyline; and the Maritime Museum housed in the sixteenth-century Cannon Tower known as Fat Margaret.

Tours are generally offered to farms in the countryside. The largest hotel in town is the Viru Hotel, which is located near numerous restaurants and shops. Shuttle buses from your ship will generally leave you off in front of this hotel.

FINLAND

Helsinki is the capital, largest city, and chief port of Finland, and it lies on the southern coast on the Gulf of Finland. Tourists will find this a refreshing, clean city with its new buildings, lovely parks, and spacious walks and streets. You will enjoy shopping for Finnish-designed household items, reindeer slippers, boots, clothing, Marimekko, ceramics, and furs, either at Stockmann's (Helsinki's largest department store) or at one of the many friendly shops at the Forum Shopping Center, the Senate Center, or along the Esplanade. In the morning, there is an open-air market right at the harbor with numerous stalls featuring flowers, vegetables, fish, wearing apparel, and handicrafts. Behind the market is the Esplanade that not only is lined with shops and boutiques, but also is the location of numerous restaurants and outdoor cafés. Places of interest include the Finnish Design Center, the cathedral, the State Council Building, and the university library in Senate Square, the monument to Sibelius, Temppeliaukio Church built into solid rock, the town hall, the Empress Stone Obelisk, and the Fountain of Havis Amanda in the Market Square. Other excellent places to visit are the parliament house, the national museum, the National Art Gallery, the magnificent new Finlandia Concert Hall, the botanical gardens and their water tower, Linnanmäki (Helsinki's permanent amusement park); and the Open-air Museum of Seurasaari, which contains specimens of various types of wooden houses built by the Finns over the centuries. You will want to try a Finnish sauna as well as a Finnish smörgasbord, which will include many native Finnish dishes in addition to the usual fare. A list of the best restaurants in Helsinki will include Motti, Karl König, Havis Amanda Fish Restaurant, Savoy, and Esplanadikappeli.

FINLAND–STOCKHOLM CAR FERRY CRUISES

Several large cruise ships with capacity to carry automobiles offer overnight cruise experiences between Stockholm, Sweden, and either Helsinki or Turku, Finland. The largest and most upscale ships with this itinerary include *Silja Europa* (Silja Line, 3,000 passengers, entered service 1993), *Silja Symphony* (Silja Line, 2,700 passengers, entered service 1991), *Cinderella* (Viking Line, 2,500 passengers, entered service 1989), and *Mariella* (Viking Line, 2,500 passengers, entered service 1985). Most passengers utilize these ships as a means of transportation from one country to the other, and many take their families and automobiles. These ships offer numerous alternative restaurants and dining is generally not included in the cruise fare. There are theaters, live entertainment, casinos, and an array of facilities on these ships where passengers party into the wee hours. Departures are generally in the late afternoon and arrivals early the following morning. Do not expect the quality of comfort, food, service, or entertainment found on most cruise ships.

FRANCE

Your ship will dock at **Le Havre,** an important French harbor at the mouth of the Seine River on the English Channel. From here, you can take a train to **Paris,** where you will want to visit as many of the following sites as time allows: the colossal Arc de Triomphe; the famous Eiffel Tower, standing a thousand feet high; the magnificent Théâtre de l'Opéra; the fashionable Champs-Elysées; the beautiful Place de la Concorde; the Tuileries; Notre-Dame de Paris; the world-famous Louvre, home of the *Mona Lisa, Winged Victory,* and the *Venus de Milo;* the Left Bank area with its small cafés, artists, and colorful crowds; the basilica of Sacre Coeur on the top of Montmartre; the palace at Versailles, and a boat tour down the Seine on the *bateaux mouches.* You can shop for crystal at Lalique and Baccarat; jewelry at Cartier and Boucheron; menswear at Pierre Cardin, Givenchy's, and Laroche's; handbags at Morabito and Gucci; gloves at Hermes; and French perfumes at most department stores, shops, and *parfumeries.* You can also visit one of the couture houses such as Balenciaga, Yves Saint Laurent, Givenchy, Pierre Cardin, Balmain, Carven, Courreges, Guy Laroche, Jean Patou, Lanvin, Madeleine de Rauch, and Nina Ricci.

You will not want to miss having a meal at a French restaurant in Paris. The most famous and most expensive gastronomic palaces are the Tour d'Argent, Lucas Carton, Jamin, Rostang, Taillevant, Le Pré Catelan, Laurent, Amboissie, Apicius, Jacques Cagne, Jules Verne (on the Eiffel Tower), Maxim's, and Lasserre; however, there are many excellent, less expensive establishments where you can obtain a meal in the true French fashion. Later in the evening, you may wish to take in the Folies Bergère, the lavish production at the Lido, the Moulin Rouge, one of the many other night spots in the Montmartre area, or one of the many discotheques, jazz spots, or cabarets along the Saint-Germain-des-Pres.

If time allows, an overnight or several-day trip to the Burgundy country between Paris and Lyon or the Château country in the Loire Valley could prove to be a most charming and rewarding experience. I would recommend staying at one of the charming French inns that are owned and run by today's great chefs of France. My favorite is George Blanc's in Vonnas. Other superior choices would be Château d'Esclimont (only a short drive from Paris), Auberge des Templiers (Les Bèzards), Boyers Les Crayères (Reims), Château d'Artigny (Tours), and Domaine des Hauts de Loire (Onzain).

RHÔNE AND SAÔNE RIVERS

The *Arlene* of French Cruise Lines, *Cezanne I* and *II, Princess de Provence*, Continental Waterways, and French Country Waterways offer cruises up and down the Rhône and Saône rivers and visit some of the more interesting and historic cities and villages along the way. These cruises afford excellent opportunities to visit the famous vineyards of the Rhône and Burgundy regions as well as some of the most famous restaurants in France.

Arles is a charming town, originally inhabited by the Greeks and Romans. It boasts numerous imposing ancient ruins including a Roman amphitheater that seats 21,000 spectators and the Theater Antique, both of which were constructed in the late first century. The quaint "Old Town" area includes art museums and Romanesque cathedrals, as well as bars, bistros, restaurants, and shops. Arles was the site for many Van Gogh works, including his masterpiece, *Pont de Trinquetaille* (The Bridge). The ancient Roman cemetery at Alyscamps was the subject matter of paintings by both Van Gogh and Gauguin.

Avignon is another quaint city surrounded by 3 miles of totally preserved ancient ramparts with their original seven entrances and thirty-nine protective towers. Inside these walls are shops, restaurants, hotels, apartments, and such famous historic monuments as the fourteenth-century Pope's Palace, one of the largest medieval palaces in the world and residence of numerous popes during the Renaissance period, when the Vatican was moved here from Rome. In the evening, your boat or barge may pass by the remains of the St. Beneget Bridge, made famous by the song "Sur le Port d'Avignon" and a marvelous vantage point from which to view the Pope's Palace and ancient walls. You may wish to visit the vineyards of Chateauneuf-du-Pape, which are only a short drive from the city. The most famous restaurant here is Hiely, located in the center of town.

Viviers is a small medieval village rich in history, typical of many French towns in the countryside. Visitors can walk narrow cobblestone paths past restored buildings and ancient gates to the interesting Cathedral of Viviers, which was built in the twelfth to fifteenth centuries in a combination of Romanesque, classical, and Gothic styles. From the top of the hill behind the cathedral, you have a panoramic view of the region. You can take a tour that drives through the rolling hills, green valleys, and vineyards of the Ardéche countryside with a visit to the nearby vineyards of Côte Vivarais for a wine tasting.

Tournon is a small village that sits across the Rhône from the famous vineyards of the Hermitage. Here you can explore such wine houses as Chapoutier and Jaboulet. Your boat will dock across the road from the historic fourteenth-century castle, and you can stroll or cycle along the river Doux, a tributary of the Rhône. Also from Tournon, you can take a two-hour train ride on a turn-of-the-century steam train along the Doux and Ardéche valleys.

Vienne is yet another historic city founded by the Roman legions in A.D. 50. Of interest are the Gothic Cathedral of St. Maurier, dating back to 1200; the excavations at St. Romain en Galle; the old Amphitheater; the Pyramid; and the Temple of

Augustus. Nearby are the vineyards of Côte Rotie, considered the very finest wine of the Rhône region. In town, across from the Pyramid, is the famous restaurant of Ferdinand Pointe, who was the teacher for many of the best chefs in France. Pointe died many years ago, and although the restaurant is excellent, it no longer receives the same acclaim as in the past.

Lyon, the second-largest city in France, is set along the Rhône and Saône rivers and has much to offer its visitors. Stroll thorough one of the lovely parks or through the cobbled streets of old Lyon on the right bank of the Saône with its numerous shops, boutiques, restaurants, and bistros.

Musée des Beaux-Arts is France's second-largest fine arts museum with an outstanding collection of nineteenth- and twentieth-century paintings. Musée de la Civilisation Gallo-Romaine, which is built into the Fourvière Hill, has ancient Roman relics and is located next to the old Roman Theater—the oldest in France—built in A.D. 19. Another Roman amphitheater is located at Croix Rousse.

The region of Lyon is a gastronomic paradise and gourmet heaven, being the location of many of the very best restaurants in France. In the city, you can dine at the famous Leon de Lyon and Orsi (both Michelin two-star establishments). Only minutes from the city is the world-famous restaurant of Chef Paul Bocuse in Collange Mount d'Or (Michelin three-star). Within an hour's drive are George Blanc in Vonnas, Troisgros in Roanne, and Alain Chappel in Mionney.

Some of the cruises go up to Macon, in the heart of the Burgundy region, where a short drive will bring you to all of the famous vineyards of the Côte de Nuit, Côte d'Or, Beaujolais, Maconnais, and Chablis wine regions.

GERMANY

Bremerhaven, located on the North Sea between Denmark and Holland, is the outer port of Bremen, which is one of Germany's largest ports, with excellent harbor facilities. In Bremen, you may wish to visit the Old Town, which lies on the right bank of the Weser, with its historic old Gothic buildings, the Roland Monument, St. Peter's Cathedral, and the Rathaus. You can try a German meal at the Rathskeller, Essighause, St. Petrus Weinstuben und Flett, and the Atles Bremer Brauhaus.

You can drive to Travemünde, a Baltic beach resort with sandy dune beaches, surrounded by thick pine forests. There you can visit its casino, nightclub, and restaurant. You can also take the short trip to Hamburg and visit the Renaissance Rathaus with its tall clock tower, the Kunsthalle, the Stadtpark, the Musikhalle, the Historical Museum, the Schnapps Museum, the Bismarck Monument, and St. Michael's Church. Here you may wish to browse through the shops along Jungfernsteig, Grosse Bleichen, Neuer Wall, and Ballindamm; take an hour-long boat ride on the beautiful Lake Alster; eat in one of its many excellent restaurants; or partake in the city's roaring nightlife along the Reeperbahn (undoubtedly the naughtiest street in the world). Some ships travel down the Elbe River and dock at Hamburg. During the evening, the two-hour twilight boat ride around Lake Alster and its tributaries is especially enjoyable. Afterwards, a typical Hamburg dinner at Friesenkeller (opposite the Lake Alster dock) is a good bet.

Some ships stop at Lübeck, which has been an important port and city of trade since the twelfth century. If you do not opt to take the one-hour drive to Hamburg, you may wish to browse through this somewhat quaint town. Places of interest include St. Mary's Church, the third largest in Germany, housing the world's largest mechanical organ; the Town Hall, featuring Gothic and Renaissance styles; and St. Anne's Museum, an old monastery that displays local handicrafts. Schiffergesellschaft is a very atmospheric, typical German restaurant housed in a sixteenth-century sailor's guild house, an excellent choice for lunch ashore.

RHINE AND MOSELLE RIVERS

Five vessels of the K D River Cruises of Europe line offer two- to five-night cruises down the Rhine or Moselle rivers, passing castles and vineyards and stopping at little villages and cities along the way. These riverboats are considerably smaller than most cruise ships, and they offer fewer amenities. However, on the first-class vessels, the food and service are Continental and impeccable. On all the ships, each public room and cabin is designed to permit a panoramic view of the scenery as your boat lazily sails along the river. Similar itineraries are offered on the *Rhine Princess, Ursulla, Switzerland,* and *Prussian Princess,* which are owned by other cruise companies.

Most of the Rhine cruises travel between Amsterdam or Rotterdam in the Netherlands and Basel, Switzerland, stopping at Düsseldorf, Cologne, Speyer, Braubach, Rüdesheim, and Heidelberg in Germany and Strasbourg in France. The most scenic area of the Rhine is the portion extending between Rüdesheim and Koblenz, which offers the greatest concentration of historic castles and fortresses, as well as the legendary Loreley cliff. The Moselle River itinerary runs between Koblenz at the mouth of the Moselle and the ancient village of Trier, with stops at such villages as Alken, Cochem, Beilstein, Zell, and Berkastle-Kues. Overall, the Moselle itinerary is the more scenic and romantic.

Basel is a moderately large cosmopolitan city in northern Switzerland, a short distance from both the French and German borders. You will want to visit the Kunstmuseum of art, the zoo, the university, and shops and restaurants in the old town area. Although the Drei Könige is the best hostelry in town, if you are only staying overnight waiting to board your boat, you may prefer the Hilton, which is modern, very comfortable, has a pool and sauna, and is right near the harbor and railroad station. Hans Stucki's Bruderholz Restaurant vies for top honors in Switzerland and is a good choice for excellent haute cuisine.

Strasbourg is a charming French town on the Rhine that is definitely affected by the German influence of its neighbor. Its Gothic cathedral is one of the most impressive in existence, and the area around the cathedral is perfect for having a drink in an outdoor café, people watching, and browsing through shops. For a special treat, you can have lunch or dinner at the world-famous Beuerehiesel

Restaurant, which sits in the middle of the lovely Orangerie park and commands two stars from Michelin. A Michelin three-star favorite here is Au Crocodile. At Au Crocodile, amiable Monique and Emile Jung will escort you through a degustation of Alsatian specialties and fine wines. Although reputed by authorities to have one of the finest wine cellars in the world and to offer one of the best all-around dining experiences in France, Emile, Monique, and their dedicated staff are gracious, humble hosts who make their guests feel welcome and special. This is a must for every aficionado of fine dining. Joggers and hikers will want to run or walk along the quay of the river (to the right as you disembark from the ship) for about a mile to Orangerie and run along the paths of the park past a children's zoo, pretty lake, and outdoor musical performances.

Heidelberg is a picturesque university town with lovely old homes and buildings built on hills along the banks of the River Neckar. The old town area consists of shops, hotels, and restaurants surrounding the university. It is quite atmospheric and dates back to the Roman era. Have lunch or a drink at the historic Ritter Hotel, which exemplifies Heidelberg in the days of *The Student Prince.* Performances of this operetta in English as well as concerts are performed on the grounds of the famous fourteenth-century Heidelberg Castle, which is located directly above the town overlooking the Neckar. This is also the site of the largest wine cask in existence.

Rüdesheim is in the middle of the Rheingau wine area. You will want to visit the gardens and impressive monastery at Eberbach that date back to 1136, where you can enjoy a tasting of wines from the Rheingau and explore the ancient Gothic chapel, cloisters, and wine cellars. In the evening, you can wander through the numerous, typical restaurants, inns, wine and beer halls, and shops located up and down the streets along the river. The most activity will be found along Drosselgasse. This is one of the best towns in Germany to partake of the colorful nightlife. Many of the wine gardens have orchestras specializing in folk dancing. This is the spot to watch (and join) the people having fun. Next to where the boat docks are tennis courts, a park, and a giant swimming pool. You will also enjoy the scenic 10-minute cable-car ride to Niederwald Monument.

Cologne is a lovely historic city with a picturesque vista of the Rhine. Dominating the town in the center stands the beautifully preserved cathedral, which is the largest Gothic building in the world. If you are able to negotiate the 360-step climb up a spiral staircase to the top of the cathedral, you will be rewarded with a splendid view of the city. Among the top-rated restaurants are Die Bastei, located in an elevated, glassed-in, three-quarter-circle building jutting out over the waters of the Rhine; the elegant Stüben House at the Excelsior Ernst Hotel; the Schweizer Stübe, a Swiss eatery near the cathedral; and the Alt Köln and Sion, which feature typical German fare. The most interesting area to take a walk or stop for a drink is located between the three bridges on the west bank of the river. Immediately behind the river walk are several streets filled with shops, as well as outdoor shopping stalls.

You can take an organized bus tour around **Düsseldorf,** a large, modern metropolis with tall buildings, elegant shops, and a good mass-transportation system. You will enjoy roaming around the colorful old town section, where you will find hundreds of little bars, shops, restaurants, and discotheques. Riverboats generally stop here only in the evening to permit passengers to partake of the nightlife in the old town area. The most highly rated restaurant in Düsseldorf is Im Schiffchen (French). For German cooking, try Aalschokker, Victorian, and Zum Schiffchen.

Koblenz, a charming city at the confluence of the Rhine and Moselle rivers, dates back to the Roman era and contains numerous historic landmarks. You will want to visit the Deutsches Eck monument (nineteenth century) at the point where the rivers meet; the pillars, towers, balconies, and dormer windows of the Balduin Bridge (fourteenth century); the Elector's Palace (eighteenth century), a neoclassical building; the "Plan," a square with shops and restaurants surrounded by old mansions; the Florinsmarket in the old town with its old buildings, alleyways, and wine taverns; Stolzenfels Castle (nineteenth century); the Church of Our Lady, a combination of Romanesque, Gothic, and baroque architectural styles; St. Castors Church (twelfth century); and of course, the little restaurants and taverns along the riverfront.

Cochem enjoys an enviable position in the heart of the Moselle wine country and is the most inundated with tourists. Many of the day boats stop here, and it is an excellent place to bed down for the night for those exploring the area by car. You can try Hotel Alte/Thorschenke (a historic inn from the fourteenth century), Lochspeicher, or the Landenberg. Cruise boats stop here to allow passengers to explore the many shops, restaurants, wine stores, bars, and guesthouses along the river. Excursions to the famous Eltz castle emanate from here also.

Bernkastel-Kues is undoubtedly the most charming, picturesque village on any of the rivers. When you step off the boat and see the river filled with ducks and swans beneath the old bridge and the gingerbread timbered houses and colorful dormers and steeples with a backdrop of green forests and steep vineyards as far as the eye can see, you will believe that you have just entered the world of *Hansel and Gretel.* This is also the site of the famous Bernkasteler–Doktor vineyards, and bottles of what is possibly the best of the Moselle wines can be purchased in shops here for far less than they are offered throughout the rest of the world. You will enjoy strolling down the cobblestone streets, visiting the shops, sampling the wine, and dining in one of the old inns or taverns.

Trier, a 2,000-year-old Roman town, sits near the end of the Moselle River, right after the junction of the Ruwer and before the Moselle splits into the Saar and tapers off. This is an important center of the Moselle wine industry and is surrounded by vineyards. You will want to visit the Roman amphitheater, the Basilica, Imperial thermal baths, Porta Nigra, the ancient black gate, the Landesmuseum (wine artifacts), and take a stroll down one of the wine-paths (weinlehrpfad) that pass by numerous vineyards. Moselle River cruises either embark or terminate in Trier. Overnight accommodations are available at the Europa Park Hotel, Holiday Inn, or Hotel Petrisberg.

GREAT BRITAIN

Your ship may dock at **Southampton,** where you will board a train to London, the capital and great historical city of Britain. Some ships dock at **Tilbury,** which is only a 45-minute ride from London. Smaller ships can negotiate the Thames and dock right near the Tower Bridge. Since there are hundreds of points of interest here, you will have to budget your short time in port carefully. Places of interest, history, and importance include: Westminster Abbey, where kings and queens are crowned and important personages buried; the Houses of Parliament, Big Ben, and the Palace of Westminster; Piccadilly, which is the Times Square of London; the fine shops on Bond Street, Oxford Street, and Regent Street; Trafalgar Square, with its statue of Nelson and the National Gallery; St. Paul's Cathedral, built by Sir Christopher Wren; the historic Tower of London, which now houses the crown jewels; Grosvenor Square, which is the site of the American embassy and Roosevelt Memorial; the fashionable Mayfair area, with its fine homes, hotels, and shepherd's market; beautiful Hyde Park; the law courts and Inns of Court; the British Museum; the Wax Museum; the restaurants and clubs in the Soho district; Kensington Palace; the artists' area of Chelsea; and Buckingham Palace, with its changing of the guard.

There are many well-known, excellent restaurants in London, including La Gavroche, Tante Claire, Chez Nico, the Chelsea Room and Rib Room at the Hyatt, Connaught Grill, and the Savoy Grill. At lunchtime, you may enjoy trying one of the atmospheric local pubs or perhaps the historic Cheshire Cheese, built in 1667. In the evening, you may wish to take in a play or a musical at one of London's many theaters, dine and dance at one of the fine nightclubs, or gamble at a gaming club (you must arrange in advance for membership). London also offers several world-famous department stores, including Harrod's in Knightsbridge, Selfridge's on Oxford Street, and Fortnum and Mason in Piccadilly.

A short distance from Southampton, 90 miles south of London, near New Milton, is England's most charming and luxurious resort, Chewton Glen. You will enjoy dining at this uniquely beautiful and elegant country manor house and taking a stroll around its magnificent parks, nearby forests, and seaside. Another rewarding deviation, a 40-minute drive from London in the Cotswold area, is Le Manoir aux Quat' Saisons—Raymond Blanc's gastronomic temple set among beautiful gardens. This is considered by many to be Great Britain's finest dining experience.

HOLLAND

Amsterdam is the capital and largest city in the Netherlands and one of the chief commercial ports of Europe. This city is made up of numerous islands surrounded by circular canals with bridges that connect the islands. You can obtain a good overall picture of the city by taking one of the glass-roofed boat tours of the canals. This is a charming, colorful city with friendly people, and you will enjoy exploring many of the areas on foot. You can visit the Royal Palace, the Tower of Tears,

Rembrandt's House, the tropical museum, the Van Gogh Museum, the Amsterdam Historical Museum, the Jewish Historical Museum, Anne Frank House, and the world-famous Rijksmuseum, which houses many Dutch and European masterpieces, including Rembrandt's *The Night Watch*. You will want to shop for fine porcelains, pewter, delft, jewelry, and the antiques of Kalverstraat, Rokin, and the Leidsestraat.

There are several good cabarets and nightclubs and numerous fine Dutch and cosmopolitan restaurants. On the various narrow streets that emanate from the Leidseplein and Leidestraat, you will find hundreds of excellent ethnic restaurants including French, Italian, Greek, Argentinian, Indian, Indonesian, and even a Hard Rock Cafe. For something different, try *rijsttafel* at one of the Indonesian restaurants such as Sahid Jaya, Djawa, Samba Sebo, Speciaal, or Tempo Doeloe. After dinner you may enjoy the numerous jazz clubs or the discos in the hotels.

NORWAY

Norway is a long, narrow country on the northwestern edge of the European continent whose coastline is marked by long, narrow inlets called "fjords." The northern part of the country lies above the Arctic Circle and is called the "Land of the Midnight Sun" because it has long periods every summer when the sun shines twenty-four hours a day. Many cruise ships traverse the rocky western coast of Norway, where there is surprisingly mild weather due to the warm North Atlantic current of the Gulf Stream.

Bergen sits on the natural harbor of a sheltered fjord where mountains rise majestically around a valley. This is Norway's second largest city, where you will want to visit the colorful fish, flower, and fruit markets along the quay, Rosencrantz Tower, Bryggen (a group of wooden medieval-style warehouses along the wharf), the Hanseatic Museum, the new aquarium, Lungegardsvann (a lake surrounded by trees and flowers), Trollhaugen (the home of composer Edvard Grieg), and the Bergenhus Fortress and Haakon's Hall. A must for every visitor (when weather permits) is the funicular railway ride up 1,000 feet to the top of Mount Floyen where you can enjoy a spectacular panorama, have a snack, and hike on mountain trails. You can shop and have lunch at Bryggen or the Galleriet shopping center. The best buys are Norwegian-style sweaters. The best restaurants are the Bellevue, which has excellent views, service, and cuisine; **Enfjorinen,** a wharfhouse specializing in fish and seafood; To Kokker, next door; Fiskeroyen; Augustin; and Bryggestuen. For a traditional Norwegian evening, you will enjoy Fana Folklore for dining, dancing, and singing.

Stavanger is an interesting town where the major industries are sardine exporting and shipbuilding. Its marketplace is a colorful spot where peasants come from miles around to shop for fish, vegetables, and fruits. Nearby is the famous Lysefjord, thought to be one of the most spectacular fjords in the country, with its towering mountains, farms, and Pulpit Rock, which hangs 1,800 feet above the fjord. Two good restaurants are Restaurationen and Prinsen.

Trondheim is a delightful colonial city where you may want to visit the famous Nidaros Cathedral, which is one of Europe's finest Gothic buildings; the Stiftsgarden, which is a royal residence dating from the eighteenth century and made of wood; the Bishop's Palace; and the Museum of Music at Ringve, with its remarkable collection of musical instruments. Try the restaurant at the Britannia Hotel.

Hammerfest is one of the most northerly cities in the world, lying north of the Arctic Circle in the Land of the Midnight Sun. Here the sun does not set from May through July. From Hammerfest, your ship will proceed to Skarsvog, the North Cape, and Honningsvaag.

Oslo, located in the southern part of the country, is the capital and the largest city in Norway. Here you will want to walk down the charming main street, Karl Johansgate, to the Royal Palace, past the National Theater, the University of Oslo, the statues of Ibsen and Björnson, the cathedral, and the National Art Museum. You may also wish to visit the town hall, Akershus Castle (dating back to A.D. 1300), Frogner Park (scene of 150 groups of bronze and granite sculptures by Gustav Vigeland), the Viking Ship Museum, and the Kon Tiki Museum at Bygdøy. At lunchtime, you will want to stop at a Norwegian restaurant and partake of the *koldtbord* (cold table), featuring fish, seafood, cheeses, meats, and salads. The Norwegians also serve *smörbrod* (open-face sandwiches) in many varieties. You may wish to shop for local handicrafts in ceramics, woven textiles, and carved woods, as well as in silver, pewter, and glass. You can see a permanent exhibition of Norwegian arts, crafts, and furniture at the Forum and at the Norwegian Design Store. The restaurants in the Grand, Scandinavia, and Continental hotels are all excellent.

PASSENGER AND CAR FERRY SERVICE BETWEEN EUROPE AND NORWAY

Since 1990, the cruise ships of Color Line have provided transportation between Europe and Norway on comfortable vessels that accommodate both passengers and automobiles. Cabins vary greatly in size, price, and creature comforts. The least expensive are generally located below the car deck, can accommodate up to four persons in upper and lower berths, and have wash basins but no shower or toilet. The most expensive luxury suites include small lounge areas, desks, mini-bars, televisions, radios, telephones, full bathrooms with robes, and hair dryers.

Public areas on all ships include vast duty-free shops, several bars, show lounges, indoor pools, saunas, movie theaters, and a variety of restaurants ranging from cafeterias and coffee shops to Norwegian buffets and Continental à la carte restaurants. Meals are not included in the cruise fare.

Service between Hirtshals, Denmark, and Kristiansand, Norway, which takes 4 1/2 hours, and to Oslo, Norway, which takes 8 1/2 hours, is offered on either the *Color Festival* (entered service 1985; 34,314 G.R.T.; carrying 2,000 passengers in 588 cabins, 340 cars), the *Skagen* (entered service 1975; 12,333 G.R.T.;

carrying 1,238 passengers, 430 cars), or the *Christian IV* (entered service 1981; 15,064 G.R.T.; carrying 2,000 passengers, 530 cars).

Service between Kiel, Germany, and Oslo, Norway, which takes 19 hours, is offered daily on either the *Prinsesse Ragnhild* (entered service 1981 and was renovated in 1992; 38,500 G.R.T.; carrying 1,875 passengers, 770 cars) or the *Kronprins Harald* (entered service 1987; 31,914 G.R.T.; carrying 1,432 passengers, 700 cars).

Service between Newcastle, Great Britain, and Bergen, Haugesund, and Stavanger in Norway, which takes about 23 hours, is available three times each week on the *Color Viking* (entered service 1975 and was stretched and renovated in 1989; 20,581 G.R.T.; carrying 1,250 passengers in 420 cabins, 320 cars). Cost-conscious passengers can spend the night in a reclining airplane-style chair instead of a cabin (not recommended).

During the summer season, these ships can be quite crowded with families. The primary purpose of the line is to provide transportation for tourists, families, and those on automobile vacations with numerous diversions during the crossings. You cannot compare the level of comfort with cruise ships where passengers come to relax and luxuriate.

The general agents in the United States are Bergen Line at 505 Fifth Avenue, New York, NY 10017, telephone 1-800-323-7436.

Bergen Line, Inc. also markets Norwegian Coastal Voyages, a company that has been operating for more than 100 years and calls at 34 Norwegian ports daily. The line presently has 11 ships, half of which were built since 1993, with passenger capacities between 169 and 490. Each ship has lounges, dining rooms, 24-hour cafeterias, and souvenir and sundry shops. The newer vessels have children's play-rooms, conference facilities, elevators, and cabins for disabled passengers. Fares for outside cabins range from $120 to $230 per person per day, with suites costing more and inside cabins less.

The six ships built since 1993 average 11,300 G.R.T. and 485 berths and include M/S *Nordnorge* (1997), M/S *Polarlys* (1996), M/S *Nordkapp* (1996), M/S *Nordlys* (1994), M/S *Michael With* (1993), and M/S *Kong Harold* (1993).

The ships offer cruises 6-days southbound, 7-days northbound, and 12-days round-trip. Itineraries include the cultural cities of Bergen and Trondheim; small arctic towns such as Tromso, Oksfjord, and Hammerfest; and passages through narrow straits and past magnificent fjords.

POLAND

Gdynia is the Polish port where most cruise ships stop, and it is only a few miles from the popular seaside resort of Sopot, with its beautiful beaches and festivals. Here you can sun, swim, and dance. The weather is generally moderate, with temperatures ranging from the thirties in the winter to the seventies in the summer. You are also only a short distance from **Gdansk** (Danzig), the hub of the Polish shipping industry. Here you can see a rebuilt city that was nearly destroyed during World War II, and you can try one of the several good restaurants where you can consume sausages, cabbage, *czarzy chleb* (coarse rye bread), *bigos* (sauerkraut and smoked meats), *barszcz* soup, and some delicious pastries and wash it all down with one of the domestic beers.

SWEDEN

Stockholm is the beautiful capital of Sweden, built on more than fourteen islands connected by bridges. You can walk through the cobbled, winding streets of the old town, with its ancient buildings crowded together in medieval fashion and the site of the Royal Palace and Museum. Here you can also visit antique shops, fashionable boutiques, cellar bars, and nightclubs. You will want to shop in the modern department stores such as Nordiska Kompaniet, Paul U. Bergström, and Ahlen, where you will find quality furs, Orrefors and Kosta Swedish crystal, and beautiful silver and stainless steel. You will also want to visit the town hall, one of the major architectural works of our time; Drottningholm Castle, the home of Swedish sculptor Carl Milles and filled with his own works of art; the National Museum, with its huge collection of Swedish and foreign art; and the Opera House.

You may enjoy a short trip to **Skansen,** with its zoological and botanical gardens, its charming old homes, concerts, restaurants, nightclubs, discotheques, and open-air dancing on warm summer evenings. There are opera and ballet performances at the Royal Opera and concerts at the Stockholm Concert Hall. Some of the local restaurants offer Swedish *smörgasbord,* with its large variety of fish, meat, and cheese courses. This is most often accompanied by Swedish, Danish, or German beer. Operakällaren has been considered the outstanding restaurant in Stockholm for decades. Other distinguished establishments include Restaurant Riche, the restaurants at the Grand and Strand hotels, and the Stalmästaregarden, Diana, Kallaren Aurora, Fem Sma Hus, and Stortorgskallaren.

FORMER U.S.S.R. (NORTH)—RUSSIA

Most of the ships that cruise to the Northern European capitals stop for several days at **St. Petersburg,** formerly Leningrad, offering Western tourists an opportunity to look at the lifestyle of the Russians. St. Petersburg is the second-largest city in Russia, lying on the Baltic Sea at the eastern end of the Gulf of Finland, 400 miles northwest of Moscow. This city was built by Peter the Great in the eighteenth century and originally called St. Petersburg, then renamed in 1924 after V. I. Lenin, the founder of the Communist party, and then returned to its original name after the breakup of the U.S.S.R. Most of the city is on the southern bank of the Neva River, but it also covers many islands spanned by more than one hundred bridges. St. Petersburg is a city noted for its splendid palaces, fountains, parks, monuments, and eighteenth- and nineteenth-century baroque and neoclassical architecture.

The main part of the city is divided by three long avenues that meet at the Admiralty Building, which stands in the center of the city and dominates the skyline. Close to the Admiralty stands the Winter Palace, which was built in the baroque style during the eighteenth century and served as a winter residence for the czars until 1917. Today, it is part of the Hermitage Museum and houses many famous masterpieces from the ancient Greeks, the Italian Renaissance, and the French moderns. Nearby you can also see the Alexandrovskaya column, commemorating the Russian victory over Napoleon; the massive St. Isaac's Cathedral, with its 112 monolithic columns and 300-foot gilt cupola; and the monument to Peter the Great known as the Bronze Horseman.

In addition to the many stores, restaurants, and cafés that line the principal thoroughfare, Nevsky Prospekt, you will also want to see the Smolny Monastery and Institute, built in the nineteenth century, the Kazansky Cathedral (which now houses a museum), the Pioneer Palace (a children's recreational center), the Russian Museum, the public library, and the Kirov Theater. You may also wish to visit the Park of Culture and Rest, the Leningrad Mosque, Peter-Paul Cathedral, and Kirov Stadium. Or you can take a short drive to Petrodvorets, the summer residence of Peter the Great, where there are a number of beautiful palaces, parks, pavilions, fountains, and statues created during the eighteenth and nineteenth centuries.

On Nevsky Prospekt is the Grand Hotel Europa, a very clean, elegant European-style hotel with numerous restaurants. This is a desirable place to stop and break up your tour.

Seventeen miles south of St. Petersburg is an area formerly known as the Czar's Village and the site of the Catherine Palace, named in honor of Peter the Great's wife, Catherine I. Nearby is the town of Pushkin, where the noted poet Alexandra Pushkin studied in the early nineteenth century. On your return, you could visit Pavlovsk, one of Russia's most beautifully restored palaces.

Although Russian restaurants are a far cry from those of Western Europe, you may wish to stop in and soak up some local atmosphere while drinking vodka and sampling some caviar, borscht, *kasha,* or *zakouski* (highly seasoned hot hors d'oeuvres). Don't drink the water, and be prepared for very slow service. Recommended Russian restaurants include Astoria, St. Petersburg, and the restaurants in the Grand Hotel Europa. If your time is limited, you may be wise to book a tour through St. Petersburg's "Intourist" travel service. They will supply you with a car and an English-speaking guide who will escort you through all of the above sites while offering some local history along the way. With the massive changes taking place in East-West relations, you can expect vast improvements in this part of the world as a tour destination.

Cruises from the West Coast, Mexico, the South Seas, Hawaii, and the Far East

To accommodate potential cruisers living on the West Coast and in the southwestern states, a number of cruise lines have based their ships in Los Angeles. Vessels of most of the major cruise lines offer a variety of cruise vacations departing from Los Angeles or San Francisco.

A number of the cruises follow the southwestern coast, calling at such Mexican ports as Cabo San Lucas, Mazatlan, Manzanillo, Puerto Vallarta, Zihuatanejo-Ixtapa, and Acapulco. Many of the ships extend their itineraries through Central America, crossing through the Panama Canal, cruising in the Caribbean, and terminating at either San Juan, Puerto Rico, or Port Everglades, Florida. During the spring and summer months, most of these same ships shift their itineraries, sailing to Canada and Alaska.

America Hawaii Cruises' *Independence* provides regular weekly cruises around the Hawaiian Islands, stopping at the islands of Oahu, Hawaii, Maui, and Kauai.

Several of the lines have scheduled longer cruises from California that stop at such exotic South Sea islands as Tahiti, Bora Bora, Moorea, Tonga, Samoa, New Caledonia, Vanuatu, and Fiji. Many of these ships go on to New Zealand, the Great Barrier Reef, and Australia, and even as far as Japan, Hong Kong, the Philippines, Indonesia, and Malaysia. *Paul Gaughin* of Radisson Seven Seas Cruises and two Renaissance "R-Class" ships offer regular cruises around Tahiti and French Polynesia. The Radisson Seven Seas, Crystal, Silversea, Royal Caribbean, Princess, Renaissance, Royal Olympic, Celebrity, and Cunard cruise lines offer several cruises each year in the Far East. Star Cruises, based in Singapore, is a relative newcomer to the cruise business, specializing in diverse Asian itineraries geared for an Asian clientele.

The following are the highlights of some of the more popular Alaskan, Mexican, Hawaiian, South Pacific, and Far Eastern ports:

ALASKA

Alaska and British Columbia have become cruise grounds for a number of ships departing from the West Coast.

Juneau, the capital of Alaska, is also the third-largest and one of the most colorful cities in the state, with a history dating back to the discovery of gold in 1879. You will enjoy cruising the myriad of fjords, straits, sounds, and passages of the Tongass National Forest, with its unsurpassed scenery and abundant wildlife. Other points of interest include the aerial tram ride that takes visitors from the cruise terminal to the top of Mt. Roberts, the incomparable Glacier Bay National Park, the Mendenhall Glacier, the Alaska State Museum, and the Golden Creek Mine Town. Most ships offer a variety of tours to Mendenhall Glacier, to the Golden Creek Mine Town, and to an Alaska salmon bake to sample the area's most famous delicacy. Other shore excursions offered by many of the cruise ships include a rafting trip down the Mendenhall River, a helicopter flight over the Mendenhall Glacier and other glaciers with a landing on an ice field, and a float plane ride to Taku Lodge through the glaciers to a wilderness habitat where visitors can gorge themselves with barbecued salmon and take a nature walk. Most ships cruising this area meander into Glacier Bay. This affords passengers an opportunity to photograph both the mirrorlike blue waters with bobbing ice formations, all surrounded by jagged wilderness, mountain peaks, and fjords interlaced with gleaming white glaciers.

Ketchikan is known as Alaska's first city because it is the first major community travelers see as they journey north. The city is located on a large island at the foot of Deer Mountain with fishing, timber, and tourism comprising the major industries. The city is known for its outstanding collection of native totem poles located at Totem Heritage Center, Totem Bight Historical Park, and Saxman Village. Excursions include tours of the town and totem poles; a visit to Saxman Village to explore a native community and to view totem carvers at work and folkloric performances; a float plane ride to Misty Fjord National Monument, a 2.2-million-acre wilderness area, home to brown and black bear, mountain goats, moose, and bald eagles; a hike up the 3-mile trail from town to the top of Deer Mountain to enjoy a spectacular panorama of the harbor and wilderness; a mountain-bike tour along the shore of the Inside Passage; canoe and kayak tours; and sport fishing for salmon.

Sitka is a picturesque little city reflecting the early Russian influence of its first European settlers. You will see harbors filled with little fishing boats, roofs lined with gulls, and a backdrop of snow-peaked mountains. In the summer you can take a three-hour jet boat cruise past little islands to view bald eagles, sea otters, and humpback whales. You may wish to visit the Sitka National Monument to see its museum, totem poles, craft shops, and spruce forest paths; the Alaska museum; and St. Michael's Cathedral; or see the scenic Harbor Mountain or Mt. Verstovia and the Mt. Edgecumbe Crater. The helicopter tour, weather permitting, is a good way to see many of these sites. Possible options include a catamaran tour of Sitka's islands combined with motorized raft rides to a wildlife sanctuary, the scenic Silver Bay Cruise, or a fishing charter.

Skagway, dating back to the Gold Rush days of Alaska, is presently a tribute to that era. From the pier where your cruise ship docks, you can walk to downtown Skagway, or you can take a horse-drawn carriage or antique bus on a tour. Options for tourists include a spectacular helicopter ride landing on a glacier, a glider ride over ice fields and Glacier Bay with a float trip through a bald eagle preserve, a city and historical tour on a streetcar, a tour to an 1898 gold miners' camp, a cruise on the *Glacier Queen* to Smuggler's Avenue and the old Gold Rush town of Dyea, a bicycle or horseback ride on the Dyea Plains, a railroad tour to White Pass Summit, or a hike from town to Upper Dewey Lake.

AUSTRALIA

Australia is a young, growing country. Its location south of the equator results in the seasons being reversed, with the best weather coming in September through April. Many cruise ships dock at **Sydney,** where you will pull into a magnificent harbor and see the Sydney Harbor Bridge, the largest arch bridge in the world. You may want to browse through the shops at Centrepoint Shopping Center and look for woolens, Australian opals, jewelry, and kangaroo furs, followed by lunch or dinner at its revolving tower restaurant, which affords a spectacular view of the city and surrounding area.

Perhaps you would prefer to test your skills at surfing and skin-diving at one of the many beautiful beaches. There are numerous small, sheltered, romantic coves hemmed in by high rocky cliffs, as well as wide strands of white-sand beaches with magnificent surf. Bondi Beach, 5 miles south of town, offers good surf, restaurants, a pavilion, and swimming pool; Manly Beach is a resort with a lovely park, pool, and numerous restaurants reached via a 20-minute ferry ride; and Palm Beach, the most beautiful of all, is an hour-and-a-half drive north from the city. You can see the koala and the duckbill platypus at the famous Taronga Park Zoo or visit Parliament House, the botanic gardens, Hyde Park, Randwick Racecourse, and the unusually designed Sydney Opera House.

If you have time, you can take a trip through the Blue Mountains to the limestone caverns and wildlife sanctuaries at Jenolan Caves. You can go down to Circular Quay in the harbor and take a boat trip, or visit "The Rocks," an atmospheric, old town area with pubs, restaurants, souvenir shops, and art galleries. In the evening, you may want to see the theaters, bars, and nightlife in the King's Cross area, or take in a concert, opera, play, or ballet at the Sydney Opera House. If you have time to eat dinner off of the ship, you may wish to try You and Me on King Street (French), Fifth floor of Wentworth (Continental), Bulicinella at King's Cross (Italian), Doyles at Watson Bay (seafood), or the Summit Restaurant on the forty-seventh floor of the Australia Tower.

Several ships traverse the Whitsunday Islands area near Cairns and the Great Barrier Reef. Generally, passengers participate in organized tours on smaller crafts to see the reef. If time allows, you would enjoy visiting Hayman Island Resort, located on its own private island and considered one of the most exclusive properties in this part of the world. Visitors fly into Hamilton Island Airport and are transported to Hayman Island by one of the resort's private launches.

BRITISH COLUMBIA

Vancouver, with a population of more than one million, is Canada's third-largest and most scenic city, as well as her busiest and most famous seaport. Located just 25 miles from the U.S. border, Vancouver is the center of Canada's fishing, mining, and lumber industries. The mild climate is due to the protective mountains and warm winds from the Pacific. Places of interest to the tourist include spectacular Stanley Park, the 1,000-acre-wilderness woodland set on a peninsula with its famous zoo, aquarium, totem poles, children's amusements, and Evergreens, 5 1/2-mile seawall path ideal for long walks, jogging, cycling, and in-line skating, and the 1 1/2-mile walking/jogging path around lovely Lost Lagoon; Chinatown along Pender Street; the historic gaslight district known as Gastown; shops, restaurants, and cafés on Robson Street; the botanical gardens and arboretum in Queen Elizabeth Park; the fountain display in front of the City Courthouse, with its changing patterns of water and lights; and the skyride up to the top of Grouse Mountain, where there is a restaurant with a beautiful view of the environs. Shop for English woolens, china, and imports. The best shopping center is the Pacific Center Mall and boutiques on the adjoining streets.

The best hotels are Four Seasons, Pan Pacific, Sutton Place, and Hyatt for luxury and proximity to the business district and the cruise ship docks at Canada Place. However, those opting for a pre- or post-cruise stay may prefer Westin Bayshore at the entrance to Stanley Park, where the tower rooms enjoy spectacular views of the park, harbor, and snowcapped mountains. Although there are numerous restaurants featuring cuisine from around the world, for a very special gastronomic dinner, Chartwell's at the Four Seasons is a don't-miss. Here preparation, presentation, ambiance, and service blend to offer a world-class experience.

Victoria, the capital of British Columbia, is the largest city on Vancouver Island. It can be reached only by ferryboat from Vancouver. Vancouver Island is the largest island on the Pacific Coast of North America, lying directly west of Vancouver and the state of Washington. Victoria is often referred to as Canada's most British city, with its flower gardens, narrow winding streets, Parliament buildings, Provincial Museum, and Empress Hotel (an excellent choice for an Indian buffet lunch). Lumbering is the city's chief industry, and you will see beautiful forests of fir, cedar, and hemlock on mountain slopes. You may wish to see the 35-acre Butchart Gardens; one of the tallest totem poles in the world at Beacon Hill Park; numerous other totem poles at Thunderbird Park; Oak Bary Marina and Sealand; Dunsmuir Castle; the Pacific Undersea Gardens, a natural aquarium with an undersea theater; The Royal London Wax Museum; or Chaucer Lane, with its replicas of Shakespeare's and Ann Hathaway's English cottages.

BORNEO

Borneo is the name of the large island located south of the Philippines and northeast of Indonesia that is surrounded by the South China, Sulu, and Java seas. The southeast portion of the island, known as Kalimantan, is a province of Indonesia. The northwest section is made up of the tiny Sultanate of Brunei, which is bordered by the Malaysian states of Sabah to its north and Sarawak to its south.

Cruise ships most commonly visit **Kota Kinabalu,** the capital city of Sabah, or Brunei. The city, known as Jesseltown prior to 1968, has a population of approximately 150,000 people of Chinese, Malay, Filipino, and Indonesian origins. Your tour of the city should include the State Mosque with its 216-foot-high minarets and lavish furnishings, the Sabah Museum, the outdoor market at Kampong Ayer Square, the thirty-story cylindrical tower of the Sabah Foundation, the view of the town and offshore islands from Signal Hill, and the resort area at the Tanjung Aru Beach Hotel.

Excursions outside the city may include a visit to a tribal community at Mengkabong water village, where thatch-roofed homes built on stilts over the sea are inhabited by the Bajous. Penampang Village is where the Kadagan tribe lives today in modern stilt houses furnished with electricity, water, and hi-fi's. Here you will also see skulls wrapped in palm leaves hung from living room ceilings like wine bottles as heirlooms of the families' head-hunting ancestors. A popular all-day tour will take you to the National Park to view hundreds of varieties of wild orchids and other flora, as well as birds, monkeys, deer, a rain forest, and the famous Mt. Kinabalu, which towers 13,455 feet above the sea and is the tallest mountain in Southeast Asia.

Beach people will enjoy spending a perfect day at the lovely Tanjung Aru Beach Resort, 10 minutes from town. At the hotel, visitors can sunbathe and swim in the sea or in a large, picturesque pool, play tennis and golf, sample excellently prepared Malaysian and Chinese cuisine, and visit one of the unspoiled pristine islands that sit in the bay. For approximately $8.00 per person, the hotel's motor launch will transport you to Sulug, Memutik, Gaya, Manukan, or Sapi. These islands, reminiscent of the Yasawa Group off Fiji, boast white-sand beaches, lush tropical forests, rare varieties of sea shells, clear waters, good swimming and snorkeling, and few, if any, other visitors.

Brunei gained its independence from Great Britain in 1983 and today is an independent Islamic sultanate covering only 2,230 square miles. Most of its Malay and Chinese population enjoy a somewhat higher standard of living than their neighbors due to the large production of oil and gasoline in this country. There are no income taxes, and there is universal education, free medical care, and pensions for the old and needy. However, many of the people still live in stilt houses and follow the traditional customs, despite having one or two new automobiles parked outside their primitive dwellings. Brunei is not too different from the oil-rich Middle East sheikdoms and is often referred to as a "Shellfare state" (after Shell Oil).

From the port of Muara at the mouth of the Brunei River, you can take the 17-mile drive to the capital city of Bandar Seri Begawan (BSB), or you can take a boat up the river past mangrove swamps and tie up at a wharf in the city. Across from the center of the city, connected by water taxis, is Kampang Ayer, the water village of stilt houses that encircles the Omar Ali Saifuddin Mosque, one of the largest mosques in Asia. The golden dome of the mosque dominates the view of BSB.

You will want to include a visit to the Churchill Memorial and museum; the billion-dollar Sultan's Palace, with its minarets, extensive grounds, 2,000 rooms, and 1,000 servants; and the ruins of the Stone Fort at Kota Batu, once the palace of the sultans. The Sheraton is the deluxe hotel in BSB, and you will find numerous good Malay, Chinese, and Indonesian restaurants around town. An interesting 45-minute boat ride will take you to visit a communal long house in the Temburong district, where Iban tribal people will greet you with dancing, and where you can see shrunken heads hanging from roofs.

There are good beaches at Maura, 17 miles from BSB, and Panajing, 29 miles away.

THE FIJI ISLANDS

The Fiji Islands consist of more than five hundred scattered islands northeast of Australia in the South Pacific, with temperatures ranging from the mid-eighties during the day down to the low seventies at night, and with much rain from June through October. Fiji was a British Crown Colony until 1970, when it became independent. The population of approximately 550,000 is 40 percent native Fijians (originally from Africa), 10 percent miscellaneous, and 50 percent descendants of laborers brought to the island from India. Most of the islands were formed by volcanoes and have high volcanic peaks, rolling hills, rivers, tropical rain forests, and coral reefs.

Your ship will dock at the largest island, **Viti Levu,** at either Suva or Lautoka, the port nearest to Nandi. The towns themselves are of little interest, and the real beauty is in the scenery and beaches. Depending upon your time limitations, you may wish to take a boat ride to one of the lovely, unspoiled outer islands in the Mamanuca group that lies off the coast of Lautoka. One-day trips can be arranged to Plantation, Mana, Beachcomber, Castaway, or Treasure islands, all of which offer water sports and small resorts with facilities.

If your time is more limited, you will want to spend your day at either The Fijian, Sheraton Royal Denarau, or Sheraton Fiji Resorts. The Fijian offers a lovely beach, tennis, horseback riding, golf, numerous shops, restaurants, and other facilities. The two Sheratons are newer, more lavish, have nice pool areas, and are closer to Nandi; however, the beaches are not as desirable and they have fewer facilities. In the evening, you may enjoy attending a Fijian *mangiti,* where meats, vegetables, and seafood are wrapped in banana leaves and steamed in an oven of hot stones in the ground. After dinner, you will be entertained by native dancers in a *meke* performance (all of which is similar to the Hawaiian luau).

The most picturesque and pristine outer islands are in the Yasawa group, which includes Turtle Island and Sawa-I-Lau cave, where the movie *Blue Lagoon* was filmed. Presently, Blue Lagoon Cruises and Seafarer Cruises, Ltd., offer three- and four-night cruises to the Yasawas from the dock at Lautoka; and Captain Cook cruises from the marina at the Denarau Resorts. These are very small boats on which the accommodations, food, and service were historically a far cry from your usual cruise ship; however, newer more upscale vessels were built in the 1990s and offer more comfortable surroundings.

For a very special, tropical-island experience before or after your cruise, the Wakaya Club and Vatulele Island Resort, each located on its own private island, offer the ultimate in casual luxury.

THE HAWAIIAN ISLANDS

Hawaii, composed of more than twenty islands and atolls 2,300 miles southwest of California, has a total population of approximately 800,000 and a year-round average temperature of seventy-five degrees. Cruise ships dock at the harbors of Honolulu in Oahu, Hilo and Kona on the big island of Hawaii, Nawiliwili in Kauai, and Lahaina in Maui.

In **Honolulu,** on the island of Oahu, you will want to walk along the famous Waikiki Beach, lined with giant hotels and crowds of sunbathers, swimmers, and surfers. You can shop for your *muumuu* and other items in the mall at the Ala Moana

Shopping Center, and later sail out to the *Arizona* Memorial at Pearl Harbor. If you drive past Diamond Head to the posh Kahala section, you can see beautiful homes and landscaping and finally stop at the lovely Kahala Mandarin Oriental hotel for a cool drink, a dip in the ocean, or just to watch the feeding of the dolphins and tropical fish in the hotel lagoon. If time allows, attend a "luau" at one of the large hotels or drive around the island to the Polynesian Cultural Center, where you can see exhibits, clothes, dances, and crafts, as well as sample foods from six different Polynesian islands. There are many exceptional restaurants on Oahu, including Hoku's at the Kahala Mandarin Oriental, La Mer at Halekulani, Micheles at the Colony Surf, and Nicholas Nicholas. The newest and most modern resorts on Oahu are the Kahala Mandarin Oriental and Ihilani in the Ko Olina development, both 20-minute drives from the airport.

When your ship pulls into the town of **Hilo** on the big island of Hawaii, you can rent a car at the airport only 10 minutes' drive from town and purchase a map of the Hilo area. If you take Hawaii Highway 19 north for a 15-minute drive, you will reach Akaka Falls, where you can take a half-hour walk through banyan trees, ti plants, ginger plants, and other tropical vegetation to view two different waterfalls. On your drive back toward Hilo, look for the "Hawaiian Warrior Marker" on Waianunue Avenue, which will direct you to the lookout above the Rainbow Falls that flow into the Wailuku River gorge. Early in the morning you can see a rainbow on the mist of the falls.

At the north end of Banyan Drive, you can visit the thirty-acre replica of Japanese gardens. If you drive for 30 miles on Hawaii Highway 11, you will arrive at Hawaii Volcanoes National Park, where you can have lunch overlooking the crater of Kilauea, an active volcano that periodically pours out molten lava. Head back by way of Chain of Craters Road to Hawaii Highway 130, following the Kalapana coastline to Kaimue black-sand beach (near where Hawaii Highway 130 intersects Hawaii Highway 137). Here there is a small cove dramatically lined with a dense grove of tall coconut trees. On the way back to Hilo on Hawaii Highway 11, you can visit the macadamia nut factory.

If you are in the area of **Kona,** on the West side of the island, you can visit coffee plantations and the Parker Ranch (second largest in the United States), or partake of the famous buffet lunch at the fabulous newly renovated Mauna Kea Beach Hotel near Kamuela (a 45-mile drive north of Kona) or at its sister property, Hapuna Beach Hotel. At these hotels you can play tennis on championship Lay-Kold courts, golf at the Robert Trent Jones-designed championship course, or sun and swim in the crystal waters of the two best beaches on the island. Nearby is the equally excellent Mauna Lani Resort, which also boasts a lovely beach, pool, tennis courts, golf courses, a diversity of good restaurants, and lovely grounds. The Hilton Waikoloa features one of the most exotic swimming-pool complexes in the world, as well as vast facilities and excellent restaurants. Four Seasons Hualalai is perhaps the most elegant resort in the Kona area and offers golf, tennis, a health spa and fine dining. All over the island you will be able to see the towering peaks of the Mauna Kea and Mauna Loa mountains. There is shopping in Kona at the Kona Inn

Shopping Village and Akona Kai Mall. There are a number of short cruises offered that explore the Kona coast, such as Capt. Bean's sunset cruise or moonlight cruise, the *Capt. Cook VII* glass-bottom boat cruise, and the Fairwind Tours' fifty-foot trimaran (snorkeling) cruise. There is a beach at Kahaluu Beach Park, 4 miles south of Kona.

Kauai is the lushest and greenest of the islands. Here you will want to drive up to the top of Waimea Canyon, which is reminiscent of the Grand Canyon in Arizona; body surf at Poipu Beach; take a boat down the Wailua River to visit the famous Fern Grotto; and swim at Lumahai Beach, possibly one of the more picturesque golden-sand beaches in the world. The finest resort on the island is the Hyatt Regency Kauai near Poipu Beach. The pool complex and health spa are awesome, as are the setting and decor. Another good choice is at Princeville on Hanalai Bay.

On the island of **Maui** you can visit the Halekala Crater, which is the largest dormant volcanic crater in the world; see the 2,000-foot Iao Needle, which rises from the beautiful Iao Valley; walk through the historic and charming whaling village of Lahaina, with its shops, pubs, and restaurants; swim, golf, play tennis, and shop at the hotels in the posh Kaanapali area, such as the Hyatt, Sheraton, Westin, and Royal Lahaina; or take the picturesque, winding drive to heavenly Hana, stopping to explore the Waianapanapa Cave and black-sand beach, the unique Hana Ranch Hotel, Hamoa Beach, and the Seven Sacred Pools. Excellent resorts with full facilities include the Hyatt Regency Maui in Kaanapali, the Four Seasons and Grand Wailea in Wailea, and Kapalua Bay Resort and the Ritz-Carlton in the Kapalua area.

Although ships do not presently visit Lanai, this small island, proximate to Maui, is the home of two of Hawaii's finest resorts and golf courses. The Lodge at Koele and Manele Bay are two upscale properties with reciprocal privileges that offer the ultimate vacation experience for the well-heeled traveler.

HONG KONG

Hong Kong, a former British crown colony and now a part of the People's Republic of China, is composed of 236 islands with five million inhabitants. Most of the population, industry, and commerce are concentrated in the city of **Kowloon** and on neighboring Hong Kong Island. These teeming metropolises are separated by lovely Victoria Harbor, which can be crossed in seven minutes on the local *Star Ferry* at a cost of approximately fifteen cents. You can capture the magnificence of the harbor, with its imposing skyline of high-rise buildings, while crossing on this ferry or from the top of Victoria Peak, which is accessible by an eight-minute ride up the "Peak Train" (located on Hong Kong Island a mile from the ferry station). The weather is best during the dry season from July to March. In the summer, temperatures vary from the mid-seventies to the high eighties, but winter temperatures are usually in the fifties and sixties.

You can arrange for various sightseeing tours that visit the floating city of Aberdeen, where people live on junks and sampans (this is where the floating restaurants of Hong Kong are located); the Tiger Balm Gardens, with its pagodas, grottos, and paths studded with weird creations depicting Chinese mythology; the Botanical Gardens; a so-so beach and semiresort area at Repulse Bay; the Sung Dynasty Village, a full-size model village reproducing houses, shops, temples, and gardens from the tenth through the twelfth centuries; and the New Territories, with their industrial complexes, farming villages, and skyscraper towns. Within a five-minute walk from the dock are the Hong Kong Center for the Performing Arts; the Space Museum, which is a large planetarium; Kowloon Park; the *Star Ferry* terminal; and a giant indoor shopping mall. For an interesting view across to Hong Kong Island, as well as an opportunity to sample the flavor of Kowloon, take the walk along the path that borders the harbor and extends from where your ship docks at Ocean Terminal, past the Clock Tower, Space Museum, and waterfront hotels, and ends at the post office.

With most visitors, however, sightseeing generally plays a subordinate role to the main order of the day: shopping and bargaining. Nowhere in the world can one find as vast an array of shops and quality merchandise at such incredibly low prices (sometimes one-third to one-half of the prices in the United States). No matter where you are, you will find shopping centers with an assortment of shops that make the major shopping malls in the United States seem like dime stores. The shops in the side streets that intersect Nathan Road (Kowloon) are touted to offer the best bargains, although you may find it easier to maneuver in the shopping centers that are found in the large office buildings and hotels and adjacent to the *Star Ferry* (Kowloon side) and those connected to the New World Hotel. The best bargains are in gold, jewelry, European designer clothes, ivory, oriental furniture and antiques, cameras, optical goods, linens, watches, pearls, jade, and leather. If you have a few days, thousands of tailor shops will provide you with a tailor-made suit at a reasonable price (the fabrics are quality but the tailoring is not).

If all of this shopping drains your energy, you can rejuvenate at one of Hong Kong's thousands of fine restaurants, which offer cuisine from every country of the world and every region of China. Western-style steak houses, fast-food franchises, and gourmet Continental establishments also abound here. It would be impossible to list all of the good restaurants; however, if I had to pick the three best (and most expensive), I would recommend Petrus at the Island Shangri-La as the best French restaurant in Hong Kong and perhaps all of Asia (Chef Alain Verzeroli, formerly executive sous-chef at Restaurant Joel Robuchon [three-star Michelin] in Paris, has settled in to provide gourmet visitors to Hong Kong with exquisite French cuisine accompanied by an impressive variety of international wines); Lai Ching Heen at the Regent provides a most satisfying opportunity to experience the ultimate in presentation and service while sampling gourmet Chinese cuisine; and Man Wah's at the top of the Mandarin Oriental is another established tradition for gourmet northern Chinese dishes with a view. Other restaurants of note include the Plume (Continental) at the Regent, Mandarin Grill (Continental) at the Mandarin Oriental, Gaddis (Continental) at the Peninsula, Chang Palace (Chinese) at the Shangri-La, One Harbour Road (Cantonese) at the Grand Hyatt, and China (Cantonese), Va Bene

(Italian), and Tuto Meglo (Italian), all three being in the Lan Kwai Fung Area, a 10-minute walk from the Mandarin Oriental Hotel.

There are many excellent luxury hotels, the largest and best being the Mandarin Oriental, Ritz-Carlton, Island Shangri-La, Grand Hyatt, Conrad, and Marriott on Hong Kong Island and the Regent, Peninsula, Shangri-La, Hyatt Regency, and Nikko on Kowloon. The Grand Hyatt is the most convenient to the new convention-trade show center and offers very comfortable, elegant accommodations, fine dining, and an adjoining garden plaza, as well as a lovely pool and health spa complex. The Peninsula, Regent, Mandarin Oriental, and both Shangri-La hotels are extremely comfortable, with numerous amenities, and provide a more typical Hong Kong atmosphere with some of the best dining possibilities. Tourists wishing to devote their time to shopping and dining may find residing on Kowloon more convenient.

If time allows, you may wish to arrange a one- or two-day side tour to the Portuguese territory of Macau or to other border cities of the People's Republic of China.

INDIA

Bombay, (now officially known as Mumbai) India's major harbor city and one of the largest ports in the world, sprawls over seven islands linked by causeways and bridges. The city is an industrial and commercial center and the country's film capital. Your ship will dock in the Fort District near Victoria Terminus train station, the Gateway of India arch, and the famous Taj Mahal Intercontinental Hotel. This is an extremely crowded and dirty city and most streets and walks are in bad condition, which results in very slow traffic. Allow yourself plenty of time when venturing out on your own.

Major tourist attractions include The Prince of Wales Museum with its fine display of Asian art, archeology, porcelain, and jade; the Jahangir Art Gallery; Rajabai Clock Tower, a semi-Gothic monument rising 260 feet; Crawford Market, erected in 1867, where cloth, meat, fish, and vegetables are sold; Javeri Bazaar; the Jewelers Market; and Chor Bazaar, the flea market; Victoria Museum and Victoria Gardens, where elephant, camel, and pony rides are available. The Aquarium, the elegant residences, Hanging Gardens, and Kamala Nehru Park are all on Malabar Hill, an excellent locale to observe a panorama of the city, especially at sunset.

Excursions from Bombay could include Elephanta Island, 6 miles across Bombay Harbor. There you can view caves with impressive displays of early Hindu religious art, including the 18-foot-high panel of Siva Trimurti (a three-headed statue depicting the triple aspect of Hindu divinity); the Kanheri Caves, located in a national park 28 miles from the city, where more than 1,000 caves were carved between the second and fifteenth centuries. Or you can take a two-hour flight to Agra for a visit to the world-renowned Taj Mahal, built in the seventeenth century by the Mogul emperor Shah Jahan in tribute to his wife.

When dining in Bombay, you will want to sample authentic Indian curries (spicy stews), prawn patia (a combination of prawns, tomato, and dried spices),

Dahi Maach (fish in a yogurt-ginger sauce), Biriani (saffron rice with chicken or lamb), tandoori (clay-oven prepared) chicken marinated in yogurt and seasonings, and tandoori naan bread (leavened bread cooked in a clay oven). All of the better hotels, such as the Oberoi and Taj Mahal Intercontinental, have excellent Indian-style and Continental restaurants. My favorite for tandoori Indian cuisine with a great view is the Kondahar on the second floor of the Oberoi, where Vinod Kumar supervises a superb kitchen.

You may enjoy bargaining in the shops for gold and silver jewelry, precious stones, marble from Agra, embroidered silks, leather goods, pottery from Jaipur, Tibetan-style carpets, and Mogul paintings reproduced on silk. The shopping arcade at the Oberoi Hotel offers several floors of shops in a clean environment away from the clamor of the streets and markets. Bargains abound and prices are as cheap as can be found anywhere in the world for this type of merchandise.

Madras, (known as Chennai since 1997) is India's fourth-largest city, featuring an abundance of squalor, pollution, dense street traffic, and aggressive, annoying vendors and taxi drivers. Although this is a most disappointing port of call, many ships still visit Madras on extended world cruises because it is one of the only options en route to break up the journey from Bangkok or Singapore to the Middle East and Africa.

The city's maze of streets is easy to get lost in. You are best advised either to take an organized tour or hire your own taxi. There are three upscale hotels in the city in which to have lunch or to use as your headquarters: the Taj Cormandal, Park Sheraton, and Chola Sheraton. Although there are shopping emporiums, you will not find the selection that exists in Bombay and Delhi. If you wish to take a walk, the least-polluted area is along Marina and Elliot's Beach, which are located about a mile to the left (south) of the harbor. You will pass by the War Memorial, Madras University, Senate House, the Moorish-style Cepauk Palace, Presidentia College, the Auna Memorial, and the Marina Swimming Pool and Aquarium.

Tours outside of Madras should include the ruins at Mahabalipuram, which date back to the seventh century A.D. and include the "Rathas" carved out of rocks in the form of temple chariots decorated with pillars, stone elephants, and guardian animals. If you prefer to spend your day at a beach resort, Taj Fisherman's Cove on Covelong Beach and V.G.P. Golden Beach Resort can be accessed south of the city on the road to Mahabalipuram.

INDONESIA

Indonesia is the world's largest archipelago, consisting of 13,677 volcanic verdant islands straddling the equator, nine hundred of which are settled. **Jakarta,** the nation's capital, is located on the northwest coast of Java. Its seven million inhabitants consist of many races, ethnic groups, and varied cultures. You will want to visit "Taman Mini Indonesia," a 300-acre cultural park with twenty-seven full-scale houses from the twenty-seven Indonesian provinces and displays of regional crafts at the Museum Indonesia. The National Museum at Jalan Merdeka Barat is considered to be one of the top archeological museums in Southeast Asia, with a rich collection of Indonesian cultural, historical, and art relics and one of the world's finest Chinese ceramic collections. Ancol Dream Land, located on the Bay of Jakarta, is a 137-acre recreational resort area with hotels, theaters, nightclubs, art markets, water sport facilities, a golf course, and an amusement park. Shoppers can browse through the open-air market called Jalan Surabaya, the Sarinah and Matahari department stores, the Sarinah Jaya shopping center, or the shopping arcade attached to the Hyatt. There are pools and numerous restaurants at the luxury hotels such as the Hyatt, Hilton, Mandarin, and Bobodur Intercontinental. The Oasis is an elegant landmark dinner restaurant in which to sample Indonesian specialties or Continental cuisine.

Beautiful **Bali,** one of Indonesia's islands, is a tropical land with lush vegetation, rice paddies, soaring volcanic peaks, sandy seacoasts, and dense jungles of palms, bamboo, rattan, and banyan trees. The best time to visit Bali is during the dry summer season or in very early fall before the monsoons. On your tour of the island, you will want to include a visit to the most sacred Balinese temple, Pura Besakih, on the slopes of Mount Agung; the village of Ubud for paintings and the Museum of Modern Balinese Art; the village of Mas for woodcarvings; the village of Celuk for gold and silver work; the village of Klungkung for wood and bone carvings; and the Nusa Dua Beach area, with its shops and resort hotels (the Bali Grand Hyatt, Sheraton, Bali Hilton, and Nusa Dua Beach being the largest).

If your time is limited, you may wish to use one of these hotels as the focal point of your visit. Each is a lovely hotel capturing the Balinese atmosphere, offering an interesting pool area, tennis courts, a sandy beach, beautiful grounds, representative shops, and an outdoor dining area where in the evening you can watch Balinese dancers and sample such Indonesian cuisine as *rijsttafel* (numerous dishes of meats, vegetables, and condiments with rice), *satay* (meat or chicken barbecued on skewers with peanut-coconut sauce), *babi guling* (baked pig), and *nasi goreng* (Indonesian fried rice). From here you can take side tours to the various villages to shop for native crafts.

You will want to witness a performance of the Balinese dances. The "Kejak-monkey dance" is performed most evenings in several villages where groups of nearly two hundred men sit in concentric circles and act out a Balinese mythological story. There are also the "Legong," performed by three girls; the "Djoged Bumbung"; and the colorful "Barong," with its costumed characters portraying the fight between good and evil. I found the Barong dance to be the most interesting. If you prefer to spend your day at a uniquely picturesque luxury resort, there are six exquisite choices: The Four Seasons and Ritz-Carlton at Jimbaran Bay, Amandari or Four Seasons-Sayan near Ubud, Amanusa above Nusa Dua Beach, and Amankila on the east side of the island.

JAPAN

Japan consists of a group of islands off the coast of Asia with a population of more than one hundred million people in an area about the size of the state of California.

The weather is similar to the central United States, with cold winters, rainy springs, hot summers, and lovely autumns. Your ship will dock at **Yokohama**, the port of Tokyo, where you will disembark and then proceed up to **Tokyo**, a modern, busy, crowded, energetic city. The best values are Japanese cameras, binoculars, transistor radios, watches, jewelry, and pearls. Be sure to bring along your passport to take advantage of the fact that many items are sold tax-free to tourists, although actually there are few real bargains today, and most of the Japanese goods can be purchased for less in Hong Kong. The best shopping can be found in the department stores located along the Ginza area or in the arcades of the large hotels.

You will want to try such traditional Japanese dishes as *sukiyaki* (meat and vegetables sauteed in soy sauce and sake), *teriyaki* (slices of beef marinated in soy sauce), *tempura* (seafood or vegetables dipped in batter and deep fried), *yakitori* (bits of chicken barbecued on a skewer), *oil-yaki* (steak broiled in oil), and *shabu-shabu* (beef and vegetables cooked in a hot broth). All of these can be washed down with *sake* (rice wine) or Japanese beer. If you prefer, there are also excellent Italian, German, Chinese, and French restaurants in Tokyo. All food, especially beef, is outrageously expensive in restaurants. Plastic models of the food served in the restaurants are displayed outside the window of each establishment.

You may wish to attend a geisha party, where local geisha girls in kimonos serve dinner and drinks, play guitars, sing, and entertain; or you may enjoy a Noh performance, which is a historical Japanese play with music and dancing where the actors wear masks; or perhaps you will want to try a Japanese bath, where a pretty Japanese girl guides you through the ritual of steam bath, water bath, and massage, the best being at the Tokyo Onsen.

Getting around in Tokyo is difficult because many of the streets have no names or street numbers. Therefore, it is best to take a tour or have a local draw you a map with landmarks. Places of interest to visit in Tokyo include the Imperial Palace, Yasukuni Shrine, the Tokyo Tower, Shinjuku Gyoen Gardens, Zojoji Temple, Sengakuju Temple, and National Museum; or drive out 30 miles to Kamakura and visit the Hachiman Shrine and the site of the great 700-year-old bronze Buddha, which stands forty-two feet high and is considered one of the world's great sculptural masterpieces. If time permits, you may wish to take a train to the Fuji Lake area and see Mount Fujiyama and one of Japan's summer resort districts offering good fishing and hunting, or you may wish to proceed on to Kyoto and visit its beautiful gardens, parks, palaces, and shrines.

MALAYSIA

The country of Malaysia as we know it today was formed in 1963. Its eleven million inhabitants, living in eleven states that constitute the Federation of Malaya, Sabah, and Sarawak, are made up of Malays, Chinese, and Indians. It is a country with a warm, tropical climate, much rain, and lush forests where palms, rubber trees, orchids, and hibiscus abound.

Many ships stop at the lovely tropical island of **Penang,** which offers wide expanses of golden-sand beaches with calm, warm waters, dense forests, excellent tourist resort hotels, and a relatively high standard of living for its residents. This is one of the major resort areas in Asia. Tourist attractions include the Buddhist Temple, the Snake Temple, Botanic Gardens, a visit to a batik factory, and a ride on the funicular railway up Penang Hill. You may enjoy spending the day at the Rasa Sayang Hotel, which contains most of the facilities and amenities of luxury-class Caribbean resort hotels, including a beautiful beach with all water sports; two pools; four tennis courts; a putting range; a disco; Japanese, Malay, and Continental restaurants; shops; and lovely grounds. Similar facilities can be found nearby at the Golden Sands Hotel or at the Matiara.

Some cruises dock at Port Kelang, 28 miles from **Kuala Lumpur,** the capital of Malaysia, where you can drive to the outskirts and visit rubber estates, palm plantations, and tin mines. Seven miles north of the city are the Bata Caves, where you take a funicular cable car to see some excellent limestone caverns with illuminated stalagmites. On your drive into the city, you can visit the beautiful Blue Mosque and gardens. In and around the city you can visit the National Museum, with displays relating to Malaysian history, arts, crafts, and commerce; the Sri Mahamariamman, a large, ornate Hindu temple; the National mosque; the Lake Gardens; Chinatown; the gambling casino at Genting Highlands; the Selangor pewter factory (the largest in the world); and the Selayang batik factory. You will want to sample the many different types of Chinese cuisine as well as native Malay food, especially the delicious Malaysian *satay.* Satay is beef or chicken grilled on bamboo skewers with a hot sauce made from peanuts, coconut milk, and hot peppers. There are excellent Continental, Chinese, and Malay restaurants in the Hilton, Shangri-La, and Regent hotels. When shopping for Malaysian handicrafts, silks, batik, and pewter, you will find the best selections (but no bargains) at the TDC Bukit Nanas Handicraft Center at Jalan Raja Chulan, the Sundie Wang Shopping Complex across from the Regent Hotel, and the Sunday Market in the heart of Kumpung Bharu.

Passengers on ships stopping at Kota Kinabalu, the capital of Sabah on the island of Borneo, will enjoy spending the day at the Tanjung Aru Beach Resort and exploring the neighboring uninhabited pristine tropical islets that sit out in the bay. (Kota Kinabalu is described under Borneo.)

Another Malaysian port of call is the historic city of **Malacca,** a rather dirty, polluted port town where you can walk through a small, dilapidated commercial area to visit several Chinese temples and old Malaccan terrace houses, take a small two-person carriage ride driven by a local on bicycle, visit a history museum with a connecting restaurant, and browse through a makeshift flea market. Malacca dates back to 1400 and is the oldest city in Malaysia retaining some of the influences of all the cultures that settled there including Chinese, Dutch, Portuguese, and British. You may prefer to take a 25-minute taxi ride to the suburb of Air Keroh, where you can visit several attractions, including Mini Asia and Mini Malaysia, a theme park filled with replicas of houses and artifacts from Malaysia, Thailand, the

Philippines, Indonesia, Brunei, and Singapore. Also in Air Keroh are a butterfly and reptile farm, a zoo, an aquarium, a golf course, and several hotels—the Paradise being the largest, with nice pools, tennis courts, and restaurants.

The cluster of 104 unspoiled islands that comprise the archipelago of **Langkawi** lies off the northwestern tip of Malaysia. Many cruise ships spend a day at the largest island, Pulau Langkawi, with its mountainous interior, long sandy beaches, wildlife, marine national parks, lush vegetation, and duty-free shopping. You will enjoy spending a portion of your visit at one of the large hotels or resorts, most of which are located on lovely beaches and afford opportunities to taste Malaysian dishes at their seaside restaurants. A good choice would be the Radisson Tanjung Rhu, located on a vast expanse of white-sand beach overlooking interesting caves and rock formations. Other choices would be Pelangi Beach, Berjaya Premier, and Sheraton Langkawi. The Datai, located on the northwest tip, is a most unique property, with large bungalows set in a tropical forest that leads down to a beach, and the island's largest golf course is nearby. However, the attitude at Datai is very snobbish, and they do not permit nonguests to roam around the property.

MEXICO (WEST COAST)

Mexico is as historically interesting and as culturally different as any country in Europe or Asia. The Spanish-speaking inhabitants can trace their origins to the ancient Aztec Indians, who were conquered by Spain in the sixteenth century. Today you can see this blend of culture against a background of breathtaking landscapes, picturesque little villages, and a sophisticated range of entertainment. The most popular cruise stops on the west coast are Cabo San Lucas, Acapulco, Mazatlan, Puerto Vallarta, Manzanillo, and Zihuatanejo-Ixtapa, which are all seacoast towns with warm winters and hot summers. Although you will be able to sample such Mexican dishes as nachos, carne asada, tacos, enchiladas, and flautas at most places, the majority of the better restaurants and hotels specialize in Continental, French, and Italian cuisine.

For many years **Acapulco** has been a favorite tourist attraction of both the jet set and the average tourist because of its guaranteed good climate, large selection of hotels, restaurants, and nightclubs, and informal atmosphere. You can eat, drink, dance, sun, swim, play tennis, and golf at a number of the superdeluxe hotels. The Acapulco Princess, built in the design of an Aztec pyramid, offers four imaginative, picturesque swimming pools, an 18-hole golf course, outdoor and indoor air-conditioned tennis courts, parasailing, water-skiing, horseback riding, seven restaurants, and a discotheque. Other deluxe hotels with good facilities are the Mayan Palace, Camino Real, Acapulco Hyatt Regency, Las Brisas, and the Pierre Marques. You can shop in town for native crafts in leather, pottery, wood, and silver. You can ride a parachute high in the sky behind a speedboat (parasailing), and on Sundays during the winter months, you can watch a bullfight.

A late afternoon lunch at the open-air Paradise Restaurant on the beach (near the El Presidente Hotel) is a must. Here you can snack on grilled snapper and shrimp, sip exotic tropical drinks, dance to a lively band, haggle with vendors, and watch the locals pass by. For dinner, Acapulco boasts numerous fine restaurants, including Carlos 'n Charlie's (eclectic), Villa Demos (Italian), Chez Guillaume (French), Blackbeard's (seafood), and Le Gourmet (Continental) and Hacienda (Mexican) restaurants at the Princess. Currently the two best gourmet restaurants in Acapulco with incredibly romantic views of Acapulco Bay are Bella Vista at Las Brisas Hotel and Madieras, located about a half-mile from Las Brisas. At 8:15, 9:15, 10:30, and 11:30 each evening from the nearby El Mirador Hotel, you can watch the divers at La Quebrada leap 150 feet off a cliff past jagged rocks to the sea. The Flying Pole Dancers of Papantla perform nightly at 10:30 P.M. in a huge garden next to the Hyatt Regency Hotel. Still later in the evening, disco is in full swing at Le Club, Le Jardin, Baby O's, Bocaccios, and Carlos's Chili 'n Dance Hall. There are variety shows at most of the larger hotels and at Acapulco Centro Entertainment Complex.

Cabo San Lucas is a small village in Las Cabos at the tip of Baja California. Ships generally stop here for only a few hours. Tenders will drop you off in front of open-air shopping stalls that offer T-shirts, serapes, Mexican-style dresses, jewelry, and most of the same items you saw in the other Mexican ports. There are four hotels within a mile of the harbor: the Melia and the Hacienda, which have the best swimming beach and tennis courts; the Finistera, which sits atop a steep hill; and the Solar, which is fronted by a dramatic beach on the Atlantic that is not safe for swimming. Many visitors take the glass-bottom boat ride around "Los Arcos" to obtain a better view of these picturesque rock formations, the pelicans, and seals. There are also small boats that will transport you to and from the pristine beach that abuts the rocks and offers an ideal place to snorkel, picnic, and get away from it all. Recommended restaurants include Macambo (seafood), Mi Casa (Mexican), Seasons (Continental), and Giggling Marlin (wild and eclectic). If time permits, the best resort complex with golf, tennis, restaurants, pools, and a beach is Las Ventanas, a 20-minute drive from Cabo San Lucas.

Manzanillo is a busy Mexican port with fine beaches. If your ship docks here for a day, you may wish to take a 10-minute drive to Las Hadas. This ultraposh resort was built in 1974 for $60 million by Bolivian tin magnate Antenor Patino. Here you will find 204 charming villas and rooms built in Moorish, Mediterranean, and Mexican styles, with minarets and domes on top of all-white buildings, set off by colorful tropical plants and bougainvillea. The resort complex includes a king-size, lagoonlike pool with its own island, suspension bridge, waterfall, and swim-up bar, ten tennis courts, an 18-hole golf course, four restaurants, six bars, and a long strand of beach. This is where the movie *10* was filmed. Another excellent luxury resort also a short drive from where you dock is the luxurious Grand Bay Resort.

Mazatlan is the world's sportfishing capital, where you can charter a boat and fish for marlin and sailfish. You can take a horse-drawn *araña* along the shoreline drive or to the historic plaza and cathedral. As your ship pulls into the harbor, you can see the 515-foot El Faro lighthouse, which is the second-highest lighthouse in the world. You can shop for silver, jewelry, leather, Mexican pottery, and crafts at the Mazatlan Arts and Crafts Center, which exhibits some of the best selections of native crafts in Mexico. If you wish to spend the day using hotel facilities, you may wish to try El Cid or Camino Real. El Cid is the largest hotel, offering gigantic, picturesque pools, fifteen clay tennis courts, an 18-hole golf course, water-skiing, parasailing, and numerous restaurants. If you proceed south from El Cid, you will pass by numerous shops and restaurants. For lunch, try the Shrimp Bucket, Casa Loma, La Costa Marinara, or Señor Frog, a very happening place to chill out on margaritas.

Puerto Vallarta has been described as a sleepy little village, ruggedly beautiful and romantically placed on a superb beach. The Gringo Gulch area consists of houses inhabited by wealthy foreigners. The heart of the shopping area is Juarez Street, where you will find bargains in sandals, silver, jewelry, embroidered works, colorful skirts, and dresses. You may want to swim at the beaches at the Krystal Vallarta, Holiday Inn, or Fiesta Americana hotels and utilize their other facilities (all of these hotels are within a few minutes of where your ship docks). You can try some excellent Mexican specialties while lunching at the outdoor restaurants at these hotels, or you may enjoy Las Palomas and Carlos O'Brian's in the middle of town. Mismaloya, a more protected beach with a backdrop of verdant hills, is located 6 miles south of downtown. La Jolla de Mismaloya, an upscale hotel, is located here, as well as several secluded beaches only accessible by boat from Mismaloya Beach. Marina Vallarta, north of the harbor, in the direction of the airport, is a newly developed 445-acre resort condominium complex consisting of numerous shops, restaurants, a 400-berth marina, a 6,500-yard golf course, and numerous new hotels including the Marriott, Melia, and Villas Quinta Real.

Should you have a full day in port, a different excursion is the cruise on the yacht *Sombrero* to the village of Yelapa, leaving the marina at 9 A.M. and returning about 4:30 P.M. The boat departs, hugging the coastline and affording passengers an unparalleled view of Puerto Vallarta, and eventually winds into a sleepy cove housing the tropical village of Yelapa, where you can swim and take a horseback ride through native villages to a waterfall.

Zihuatanejo-Ixtapa is a picturesque, pristine, unspoiled fishing village surrounded by mountains on a sparkling, protected bay. The clear waters, perfect for scuba diving and snorkeling, reveal pink coral and interesting underwater life. The brilliant flowers scent the air with a delightful fragrance, and coconut palms line the shore, where peaceful fishermen sit making their daily catch. You can spend the day at one of the numerous resorts with lovely beaches that have recently been built in Ixtapa, or you can take a trip by boat to the uninhabited Ixtapa Island, where you can swim, sun, and snack on a sheltered beach facing the mainland. The hotels with the most facilities are the Camino Real, Krystal, Omni, and Sheraton. There are numerous shops across from the strip of hotels in Ixtapa and there are craft shops and boutiques near the dock in Zihuatanejo. If you are in port for dinner, in addition to the hotel restaurants, you may wish to try Bogart's or the local branch of Carlos 'n Charlie's.

MYANMAR (FORMERLY BURMA)

Situated at the crossroads of Asia with India and Bangladesh on its western border and China, Thailand, and Laos to the east, this 261,000-square-mile country is a conglomeration of people and traditions. Eighty percent are Buddhists, and visitors will view Buddhist monks in yellow-orange-colored robes walking around the country.

The capital city, Yangon (formerly Rangoon), is connected to the sea by a 20-mile stretch of the Yangon River, which can be navigated by smaller cruise ships, while others transport passengers by ferryboat. The most famous site is the golden-domed, jewel-studded Shwedagon Pagoda, one of the most dynamic and important Buddhist shrines in Southeast Asia, situated on Singuttara Hill near Royal Lake and Gardens about 2 miles north of the city center. This is an awesome conglomeration of temples, shrines, statuary, and Buddhist architecture that you must explore barefoot. You may also enjoy visiting Sule Pagoda, a shrine believed to be built in the third century B.C. and said to contain a single hair from Buddha; the National Museum; Peoples Park; and the shopping center in town. Yangon is noted for lacquerware, fine gemstones, and jewelry including blood rubies, sapphires, and jade. Beware of fakes, and although prices are higher and less flexible in government-controlled tourist stores, they may be the safest.

The Strand is the traditional, colonial hotel reminiscent of Raffles, and the Inya Lake and Thamada are two additional first-class hostelries. Visitors often opt for lunch at either the Royal Garden or Karaweik restaurants, both colorful structures that give the appearance of native boats floating on Royal Lake overlooking Shwedagon Pagoda.

NEW CALEDONIA

New Caledonia is an archipelago in Melanesia, southeast of New Guinea and northeast of Australia. Captain Cook discovered these islands in 1774 when the people still practiced cannibalism. France took possession in 1853 and created a penal colony where convicts were sent to mine nickel deposits. In 1956 New Caledonia became a French Overseas Territory, and in 1998 there was a referendum for self-determination, the results of which were unavailable at press time. Possessing 44 percent of the world's reserves of nickel together with an abundance of other minerals, these islands are among the most prosperous in the South Pacific and are the last stronghold of white colonialism in Melanesia.

Nouméa is the capital of the main island of Grande Terre, which is 250 miles long, 30 miles wide, and protected by reefs with picturesque coastal beaches and many ridges of craggy mountains in the interior. The town is near the harbor where you may wish to visit the public market, Place des Cocotiers with its flaming royal poincianas, New Caledonian Museum for native art, St. Joseph Cathedral, and the old town hall. A more scenic itinerary would include a walk commencing at Le Meridien Hotel along the waterfront at Anse Vata, past the small aquarium to the beach at Baie de Citron.

Those wishing to spend a day at a resort can choose among Kuendu Beach

Resort to the south or Le Meridien, Club Med, and Park Royal, all on Anse Vata. Two upscale (and expensive) French seafood restaurants on Anse Vata are Miratti Gascon behind the Park Royal and LaCoupole near the aquarium.

Ile des Pins, lying to the south of Grande Terre, is a lovely pine-studded island with chalk-white beaches popular with divers and sun-worshippers. You can arrange an outrigger canoe trip to the secluded beaches and warm shallow waters of Baie d'Upi and Baie d'Oro on the east coast or many of the little surrounding sandy atolls. Most cruise ships tender into Baie de Kuto, where there is an exceptional, long strand of beach lapped by aqua-blue waters. Immediately behind is Baie de Kanumera, which is more isolated and even more picturesque. Nearby are wooded forests, nature villages, camping grounds, and Hotel Kou-Bugny, a small but impressive conclave of roundevals with a pool and a restaurant a few yards off the beach at Kuto. This is one of the finest beach islands in the South Pacific.

NEW ZEALAND

New Zealand is an unusual country with green fields, tropical foliage, fjords, and snowcapped mountains. Your ship will pull into beautiful Waitemata Harbor at **Auckland,** the country's chief port, which is as far south of the equator as San Francisco is north, with similar weather, but reverse seasons. In Auckland, you can visit the crater of an extinct volcano at the top of Mount Eden, see the rare flightless kiwi bird at the zoo, look out at the city from the Intercontinental Hotel's rooftop restaurant, or take a sightseeing tour along the city's picturesque Waterfront Drive, up through the residential suburb of Tamaki Heights, and then on to Ellerslie Race Course. The best beach is Takapuna, 4 miles north of the city. Shoppers can purchase natural lambswool products at the duty-free shop near the harbor.

If you drive up to the fishing village of Russel, you can take a cruise through the **Bay of Islands,** passing through beautiful little islands, inlets, remote farms, beaches, and game-fishing waters. You will not want to miss taking the trip to Waitomo Caves to see the unique Glowworm Grotto, which is a huge cavern illuminated solely by the bluish glow of millions of tiny glowworms affixed to the rocky ceilings. If you fly or take a bus to **Rotorua,** you can see spectacular, steaming geysers such as Pohutu Geyser at Whakarewarewa, the hot waterfalls, colored pools, and deeply gashed craters at Waiotapu, the geysers at Wairakei near a resort complex adjoining Geyser Valley, or take the one-hour tour to Waiora Valley. Here you may wish to visit the Agrodome to watch a sheep-shearing demonstration, learn how sheep are raised, and purchase lambswool products.

If your ship stops at **Christchurch** you can fly, drive, or take a bus tour of the Southern Alps, visiting Mount Cook, Franz Joseph Glacier, and Milford Sound, with its waterfalls and fjords. At **Queenstown** near the southern tip of New Zealand, you can take a cable car up a mountain to view Whakatipu Glacier Lake and the Southern Alps or you can take a "jet boat" ride down the rivers past waterfalls and picturesque countryside.

PEOPLE'S REPUBLIC OF CHINA
(KUANGCHOW, FORMERLY CANTON)

Cruise ships including the People's Republic of China on their itinerary most often visit **Kuangchow** (Canton), which lies on the Pearl River 113 miles from Hong Kong (accessible by a three-hour train ride or hoverferry). Autumn is the best time of year, with the least rain and temperatures in the seventies. Summers are somewhat hotter, and in the winter the temperatures vary from the high forties to the low sixties.

Although visiting Kuangchow is an interesting and educational experience, there is no covering up the fact that this is a very dirty, polluted city where the hotels, restaurants, bathrooms, and so on are far below our concept of good hygiene. There are three new tourist hotels, China Hotel, White Swan, and the Garden, which were built in the eighties as joint ventures with private Western companies. These hotels are far superior to what existed prior to 1984. Of the other tourist hotels, only the Dong Fang would be acceptable.

On the plus side, you will be able to move around the city freely on your own. However, few of the six million inhabitants of Kuangchow and its environs speak English well enough to answer your questions. Therefore, getting from place to place is very difficult, and you will see more on an organized tour. Do not depend on the taxi drivers, hotel attendants, or service people in the restaurants to understand English. If you go off by yourself, have the name of the place you are visiting as well as the name of the place to which you plan to return written out in Chinese letters. Taxis are the best means of transportation, and they are relatively inexpensive.

Although Kuangchow is reputed to be one of the gastronomic capitals of Chinese cuisine, you will find the food in all the restaurants a far cry from the Cantonese food you have eaten at home, in Hong Kong, or in other Asian cities. The quality of most of the ingredients is so bad that it ruins many of the dishes. Most of the larger restaurants serve Cantonese "banquets" or "feasts" for groups of four or more. A banquet consists of six to ten different courses at each meal, permitting you to sample a variety of Cantonese foods. The best-known, larger restaurants are Panxi, Guangzhou, Beiyuan, and Nanyuan. Personally, I have found these "banquets" very disappointing.

You can shop for Chinese arts and handicrafts in the Friendship Stores or the People's Department Store. There is no bargaining, and prices for most of the items are lower in Hong Kong.

Thus one does not visit Kuangchow for the hotels, restaurants, or shopping, but rather to see the sights and the people. The best way to see the people and how they live is to take a tour to a commune outside the city. Here you can see their homes, their schools, their hospitals, how they spend their days, and you can ask all the nonpolitical questions you wish. I found the guides to be fairly honest and informative. Be prepared for some of the worst filth and squalor you have ever seen. The people may have enough to eat and seem happy, but their hospitals, homes, and manner of living are shocking to most Western visitors.

In Kuangchow proper, you will want to visit the "Temple of the Six Banyan Trees" and the neighboring nine-story-high "Flowering Pagoda"; the Canton Zoo, which is the home of the Chinese panda; the Guangzhou museum in Yuexiu Park; Guangxiao Temple; Dr. Sun Yat-Sen Memorial Hall; the Cultural Park; the South China Botanical Gardens; and the Orchid Garden. If you are in Kuangchow in the fall or spring, you can visit the Kuangchow Export Trade Fair.

Scenic spots to be found outside of the city are Seven-Star Crags, 70 miles west, with cliffs, caves, lakes, and Chinese pavilions; Conghua Hot Springs, 50 miles northeast, a tourist health resort; Xiqiao Hill scenic area, 40 miles west, with seventy-two peaks, stone caves, waterfalls, and springs; and Foshan City, 17 miles southwest, famous for its artistic porcelain, pottery works, art, crafts, and its 900-year-old Ancestral Temple.

PHILIPPINES

The Philippines is a mountainous country with fertile plains, tropical vegetation, and dense forests. After 350 years of Spanish rule, it became a U.S. possession and was given its independence in 1946. The official languages are English, Filipino, and Spanish. Most of the people speak a dialect of English that is very difficult to understand.

The country is composed of more than 7,000 islands, the principal city of **Manila** being located on the island of Luzon. Your tour of the city should include the Ayala Historical Museum; the Cultural Center; the National Museum; the Nayong Filipino, a showcase of the country's six major regions exhibiting typical living quarters and handicrafts; the wealthy residential area of Forbes Park; and the walled city at Intramuros, the site of the first Spanish settlement.

Although shopping in Manila does not compare with shopping in Hong Kong, Singapore, or Bangkok, there are bargains to be found in handicrafts, rattan, sarongs, embroideries, ladies' bags, and rings. The best shopping areas are in the Ermita district, along Roxas Boulevard and the Makati Commercial Center. Those wishing to try their luck at craps, roulette, blackjack, baccarat, and fan tan can be accommodated twenty-four hours a day at a large casino in the Philippine Village Hotel. Most of the major luxury hotels and restaurants are located in the Ermita and "reclaimed area" districts along Manila Bay. The Philippines Plaza Hotel and Shangri-La are large hotels that command impressive views of the bay and offer a wide range of amenities.

Typical Philippine food includes *lechon* (pig on a spit), chicken and pork *adobo* (a spicy dish), *lumpia* (a crêpe-like food combining coconut, pork, shrimp, and vegetables in a tissue-thin wrapping), various fresh local fish, and delicious pineapple, bananas, mango, and papaya. Although the food is not as tasty, colorful, or well-prepared as Chinese food, the local San Miguel beer is one of the richest, most tasty brews I have come across. Western-style foods (Continental, French, Italian, steaks, and so on) and token Filipino fare can be found at restaurants and in all the major hotels, where you will also find nightclubs and discos for dancing.

If your time is not too limited, the real beauty of the islands is to be found outside of the densely populated, dirty cities. A two-hour drive to Pagsanjan Falls will take you past native villages, green-clad mountains, and beautiful palm forests to an interesting river and waterfall. Here you can rent a canoe with two skilled paddlers and "shoot the rapids." The trip up and down the river takes about one-and-a-half to two hours, during which you wind through tall hills covered with giant palms. Parts of the river are calm, with water buffalo lazily bathing in the sun, while other portions contain strong currents and rapids.

The half-day trip to Hidden Valley is one of the most rewarding excursions I have ever experienced in my travels. Here you can hike down a 1-mile trail through a forest of countless varieties of tropical trees, past natural pools to a picturesque waterfall. The first pool you encounter provides one of the most satisfying treats for the senses you could imagine. The setting is that of two blue-green pools separated by a tiny waterfall surrounded by hills laden with tropical trees and vegetation. The water is clear and warm and the area smells of fragrant flowers. Swimming in that pool is an occasion you will never forget and never equal. The price of about $7.50 per person to enter Hidden Valley includes lunch, soft drinks, and full use of the facilities.

The excursion to Hidden Valley can be combined with a trip to Pagsanjan and can be completed in about nine hours. If you rent a car and drive from a hotel it will cost about $100, or you can go by taxi for about $60.

SAMOA

Samoa consists of sixteen islands in the South Pacific, the six most easterly ones being owned by the United States. The 192,000 people are mostly Polynesian. The temperature is hot and humid, getting up to the nineties during the day. There is a great deal of heavy rain in the winter months. Most of the restaurants serve American-style food. You can attend a tribal feast that is called *fia-fia* and is similar to the Hawaiian *luau,* the Tahitian *tamaaroa,* and the Fijian *mangiti,* featuring pig, chicken, or fish steamed over a hot stone oven. American Samoa's main island, **Tutilla,** consists of volcanic formations surrounded by coral reefs, with green tropical forests and small villages.

The main village, Pago Pago (pronounced "Pango Pango"), is adjacent to the harbor, contains a few craft shops, grocery stores, and K-mart-style department stores. The only hotel, the Rainmaker, is a five-minute walk from where your ship docks, and contains two hundred rooms. It is located on a peninsula jutting out into the bay and includes a small pool, an area to swim in the bay, a restaurant, and a souvenir shop. If you take a drive along the South Coast, you will pass a few small villages, the airport, numerous small churches, native huts called *fales,* and eventually arrive at Amanave Beach, which is somewhat picturesque but has no changing facilities and too many rocks to permit serious swimming. The organized tours afford an opportunity to sample typical island food and folklore shows. You may wish you had passed up the food. Golfers can play the nine-hole course near the airport.

SINGAPORE

The island of Singapore is situated at the southern extremity of the Malay Peninsula, only 85 miles north of the equator, with a hot and humid climate varying from seventy-five degrees at night up to ninety degrees during the day. The country is only 26 miles long by 14 miles wide and was a British colony for 140 years. In 1963, it became part of the Federation of Malaysia, but tensions between Malays and ethnic Chinese led to Singapore becoming a separate nation two years later. Its population of 2 1/2 million is 76 percent Chinese, 15 percent Malay, and 9 percent mixed English, Indian, and Pakistani. You will find it to be the cleanest, most modern country in Eastern Asia.

Your sightseeing tour of Singapore should include the lush botanic gardens, an excellent venue for walking or jogging, the golden Hindu temple of Sri Mariamman, China Town, the House of Jade, the Van Kleef Aquarium, the Tiger Balm Gardens, Zoological Gardens, the food stalls in the street markets, the Jarong Bird Park, Raffle's City, and the panoramic cable-car ride from Mt. Faber to Sentosa Island. Sentosa Island lies directly across from the World Trade Center, and those not opting for the cable-car ride can take a five-minute ferryboat or a bus. The best way to obtain a feel for the island is to take the free monorail excursion. The beaches here are beautiful, and a good destination is the Rasa Sentosa Resort, which lies on a palm-lined, white-sand protected beach across from the Underwater World Oceanarium and monorail stop. Other attractions here include Fantasy Island, an enormous water-theme amusement park; Volcanoland Theme Park; Fountain Gardens; the Coralarium; Asian Village; Fort Siloso; and several historical museums.

Although prices are somewhat higher than in Hong Kong, Singapore offers good free port shopping. You will find large varieties of cameras, watches, radios, antiques, leather goods, jewelry, ivory, and carpets. The major shopping areas are Change Alley, Raffle's City, the numerous large shopping centers along and near Orchard Road, Singapore Handicraft Center, Tanglin Shopping Center, Far East Plaza, Shaw Center, Lucky Plaza, Tangs, Scotts, Tong Building, and Wisma Atria.

Singapore boasts numerous restaurants with excellent Western, Chinese, and Indian cuisine. The best French/Continental restaurant is the Latour at the Shangri-La Hotel. There are other Continental restaurants in all the luxury hotels. Fancy (expensive) Chinese restaurants include the Shang Palace at the Shangri-La and Pine Court at the Mandarin. The famous Raffles Hotel has been restored and is the "'in place" for high tea; there you can gorge yourself on dim sum and lavish pastries as well as more typical British high-tea fare. You can inexpensively sample a variety of all the foods of Eastern Asia in the food stalls at Newton Circus and at Rasa Singapura behind the Handicraft Center and on Sentosa Island.

There are Asian cultural shows offered with dinner at many of the larger hotels, as well as at nightclubs, discos, and supper clubs. The luxury hotels offering the most facilities, restaurants, and entertainment are the Shangri-La, Ritz-Carlton, Westin, Oriental, Mandarin, Hilton, Pan Am, and Hyatt hotels.

SOCIETY ISLANDS—FRENCH POLYNESIA
(BORA BORA, MOOREA, AND TAHITI)

French Polynesia, or the Society Islands, is a group of fourteen inhabited islands in the South Pacific, 4,200 miles southwest of San Francisco, that enjoys an ideal climate and trade winds with temperatures ranging from a low of around seventy to the upper eighties. December through April can be humid and rainy.

The islands are administered as an overseas territory of France, and French is the official language. Life is quite informal, and jackets and ties are seldom seen.

I found the Tahitian people working in the hotels, restaurants, and shops to be unhelpful, impatient, and generally rude. This gives one a feeling of annoyance when visiting these otherwise lovely islands.

Although there are numerous French-style restaurants in the hotels and in Papeete (Tahiti), none approach the quality of French restaurants in Europe or in the United States. Shopping is limited to souvenirs, T-shirts, *pareos* (native skirts), and a few French imports. If possible, you will enjoy attending a *tamaaroa,* a native feast similar to a *luau,* at one of the hotels, where a pig or chicken will be roasted over hot stones and served with vegetables, fruits, and coconut.

The largest of the islands, but—contrary to popular belief—not the prettiest, is **Tahiti,** with its main town of Papeete. Here you can stroll down a picturesque waterfront looking out at the island of Moorea, shop for a few French imports, dine at several so-so French restaurants, or take a drive around the island and visit the Gauguin Museum, the blowhole at Arahoko, the Cascade of Vaipahi, the water grotto of Maraa, and the waterfalls and rapid streams that cut into the steep mountains. There are no great beaches on the island of Tahiti; however, there are three "first-class" (not deluxe) hotels that have pools and beaches, and will arrange deep-sea fishing, water-skiing, or a tour of the lagoon. The Tahiti Beachcomber Parkroyal is about 4 miles from Papeete (your best bet). The Maeva Beach is just next door. Tahara'a is located 6 miles from Papeete in the opposite direction, and boasts a very picturesque 3/4-mile strand of black-sand beach with warm waters and a slight surf. You can try the restaurants in the hotels; or La Chaumiere or Belvedere up in the mountains (a short taxi ride away), which offer a good view of the island; or you can try Acajou, Magridone, or Jade Palace in Papeete.

Bora Bora is a small, unspoiled dream island with haunting mountains and some of the most beautiful palm tree-lined, snow-white beaches in the world. The waters surrounding the main island (which is only 20 miles in circumference) are protected by a coral reef that creates miles of a beautiful aqua-colored lagoon containing tiny pristine islets where you can sun on virgin beaches and swim in crystal-clear waters.

The main town of Vaitape is composed of small grocery stores, a hospital, and a few souvenir shops. In the lagoon, across from town, set on its own private island is the Bora Bora Lagoon Resort, where you may wish to make arrangements to have lunch and spend the day. This is as close to paradise in the South Seas as you will find. Other possibilities to spend your day in port include Hotel Bora Bora, 3 miles from town, and Moana Beach Parkroyal Hotel, a mile farther down the road. These hotels are quite posh by Polynesian standards, with excellent restaurants and lovely crescent-shaped, palm-lined white-sand beaches that each extend for a half-mile. There is snorkeling in the waters in front of the hotels. Two new resorts opened on motus (islets) in the lagoons in 1998, Pearl Beach and Le Meridien.

There is only one road that circles 17 miles around the island. You can navigate around this road and explore the island by renting a Jeep "funcar," moped, or bicycle.

Probably the most spectacular experience to be had in Bora Bora is watching the sun set slowly over the lagoon and mountains, followed by the illumination of the sky and sea to a bright orange and purple.

Moorea is another incredibly lovely, lush, tropical island somewhat larger than Bora Bora, only 12 miles from the island of Tahiti, accessible by launch or air taxi. Here there are numerous needle mountain spires (including the fabled Bali Hai), green valleys, and white-sand beaches bordering a protected lagoon. You can take the 37-mile drive around the island by car or motor scooter. The most picturesque spot is Belvedere, about a 15-minute drive west of the airport. Here you proceed up a road through pineapple fields, coconut palms, and numerous varieties of tropical vegetation to a lookout point where you have a magnificent view of Cook's Bay, Papetoai Bay, and Moorea's jagged mountain peaks. You can swim, snorkel, water-ski, take a sailboat ride, play tennis, and have lunch at any of the three largest hotels on the island: Club Med (about a 35-minute drive west of the airport), Club Bali Hai (about a 10-minute drive west of the airport), and Kia Ora (about a 5-minute drive south of the airport). The most upscale resort on the island is the Moorea Beachcomber Parkroyal, an excellent place to spend a few days before or after your cruise. A branch of Dolphin Quest is located at the resort.

There is no special shopping center, only an occasional boutique offering native dresses, *pareos,* T-shirts, and wicker baskets. On the road behind Club Med are shops and small restaurants. The Plantation and L'Aventura located here are excellent choices for a French dinner in charming island settings.

Rangiora in the Tuamotu Archipelago in French Polynesia, located 200 miles northwest of Papeete, is composed of a series of islands and motus surrounding a blue lagoon. The one major hotel, Kia Ora, is composed of beachfront and overwater bungalows, a restaurant and a so-so beach. Unless you opt for snorkeling, diving, or a glass-bottom-boat excursion, the only other choices are a scenic walk along the lagoon on the Pacific side of the island.

Raiatea and **Tahaa.** These two mountainous islands, located immediately to the south of Bora Bora, 125 miles northwest from Tahiti, share a common coral foundation and a protected lagoon filled with small white-sand motus. Mt. Tefateaiti, rising 3,333 feet, dominates Raiatea, and Mt. Ohiri at 1,935 feet is the highest point on Tahaa.

There are no respectable beaches on either island, but snorkeling, scuba-diving, and swimming opportunities are offered on sailing excursions to the motus. A popular way to explore Raiatea is a tour that commences in a motorized outrigger canoe along the perimeter of the island and up the jungle Faaroa River, followed by a Jeep ride back along the single road that stops along the way to explore small coconut and vanilla plantations, waterfalls, and the base of verdant mountains. A boat shuttle operates between Raiatea and Tahaa. The few small hotels have no beaches and are not worth visiting.

THAILAND

Bangkok, the capital of Thailand (known as Siam until 1939), with its six million inhabitants, 94 percent of whom are Buddhists, is a city of contrasts. At first glance, it appears to be a noisy, polluted city with hundreds of hotels, massage parlors, shops, poverty, and horrendous traffic jams. Further exploration reveals a fascinating, well-preserved Oriental culture represented by its beautiful temples, palaces, and the more primitive way of life to which many of its people still cling.

Any visit to Bangkok must start with an early-morning cruise down the Chao Phraya River (River of the Kings) to the "floating markets." The trip will start at the dock next to the Oriental and Shangri-La hotels and will take you past the huts and junks of the "river people," past numerous Buddhist temples (called *wats*), and past the marketplace where the river people come in their dugout canoes to buy and sell their wares. Before you return, your boat will visit one of the most famous and colorful *wats,* The Temple of the Dawn. You can also take an afternoon tour into the adjoining countryside on the "Rice Barge Cruise" to view rural family life along the canals.

In the city, you will want to tour the magnificent Grand Palace housing the chapel of the Emerald Buddha, which is thirty-one inches high, carved out of emerald-colored jasper, and adorned with gold and jewels. You will also want to visit the famous Golden Buddha, which is 5 1/2 tons of solid gold.

An interesting afternoon tour outside the city goes to the Rose Garden, where energetic young Thais entertain you with an excellent cultural show that includes Thai boxing, sword fighting, classical and folk dancing, and elephants at work.

The five most posh hotels with pools, restaurants, entertainment, and other facilities are the Oriental (which is considered by many to be the "best hotel in the world"), the Shangri-La, the Regent, the Peninsula, and the Dusit Thani. The best French-style restaurants are The Normandie, which sits on top of the Oriental Hotel, overlooking the River of the Kings. This ultra-posh, romantic, and expensive dining room features gourmet French cuisine with menus created by acclaimed French chefs. Angelini, the Italian restaurant at the Shangri-La, is also excellent.

You can try authentic spicy Thai food at numerous restaurants throughout the city. It is best to get a recommendation from a local resident. Several tourist Thai restaurants that provide a fixed menu of toned-down Thai dishes, together with Thai dancing. These include the Thai restaurants located on the river at the Oriental and Shangri-La hotels, as well as the Spice Market at the Regent.

The stores offering the best variety of Thai silks, handicrafts, paintings, and jewelry are located in the shopping centers adjacent to the Sheraton Shangri-La and Siam Intercontinental hotels.

Some ships dock near the resort town of **Pattaya,** 85 miles from Bangkok. This is a rather crowded strip of resort hotels, souvenir shops, restaurants, massage parlors, and mediocre beaches. The largest and most secluded hotel with the best beach, pool, tennis courts, and restaurants is the Royal Cliff, which occupies some impressive acreage on a cliff overlooking the Bay of Thailand.

Phuket is a small island south of the mainland in the Andaman Sea. The beaches here are among the best in the world. Amanpuri Resort is situated on a coconut plantation on Surin Beach and is one of the most romantic and exotically beautiful resorts in the world—as well as an excellent choice for lunch and a refreshing swim in warm, crystal-clear waters. The Dusit Laguna, Sheraton Grand Laguna, and the luxurious Banyon Tree resorts are located at the Laguna Phuket Resort complex on Bang Tao Beach. At Banyon Tree there is a full-scale spa facility and 18-hole golf course. A cruise around Phang Nga Bay is a must. Here you will find a labyrinth of forested limestone pillars rearing out of the Andaman Sea. You can explore caves, caverns, mangrove-lined tropical rivers, and the island where the James Bond movie *Man with the Golden Gun* was filmed. Half-day cruises to numerous pristine islands and excellent diving and snorkeling locations are also available, including excursions to the Surin Islands, Similan Islands, Rok Nok, Khai Nok, and Phi Phi Islands. Other sights of interest include the Tone Sai Waterfall in Khao Phra Taew Park, a national preserve; the Marine Station, with its display of more than 100 species of fish; the temple of Wat Chalong; and Phuket Town. Shopping for Thai silk and batik fabrics, precious stones and silver, gold, copies of designer watches, souvenirs, and lacquerware items is best along Patong Beach, a colorful area lined with hotels, restaurants, and shops, which is located across from Phuket's most populated public beach.

VANUATU

This Y-shaped archipelago of 82 islands covering 400 miles in the Melanesia area of the South Pacific, northwest of Fiji, north of New Zealand, and east of Australia, gained its independence from a combined French and English rule in 1980 when it was known as New Hebrides. There are two main islands, Espiritu Santo and Efate.

Luganville, or Santo, as it is locally called, is the only large town on Espiritu Santo, where 100,000 U.S. servicemen were stationed during World War II. Today there is little of interest in town save the open-air farmers' market by the river or a stroll along the paths separating the native homes. Possible tours include snorkeling at Million Dollar Point, an outrigger canoe ride on the Sarakata River, or a tour around the island to see some historic points from World War II.

Port Vila on Efate Island is the administrative, commercial, and tourist center lying on a sleepy lagoon bordered by vibrant tropical jungles. Here you can take a glass-bottom boat ride circumnavigating Port Vila's harbor, snorkel and swim in a secluded bay, spend the day at two of the island's larger resorts—Le Meridien or Le Lagon Parkroyal (which are only 5 minutes from town), or take a helicopter ride and view dense, impenetrable jungles, breathtaking waterfalls, clear rivers, and blue lagoons. The 15-minute drive to Mele Maat is a must. Here you can climb up a jungle mountain path over a succession of charming pools fed by cascading waterfalls.

VIETNAM

Wedged between, China, Laos, Cambodia, and the South China Sea, this historic, war-ravaged country about the size of Norway but with a vastly larger population has become a favorite visit for cruise ships traversing Southeast Asia.

Ho Chi Minh City (formerly Saigon), with its over five million population, is the largest, most dynamic of the Vietnamese cities and the center of culture and commerce. In the middle of the commercial section, not far from the harbor, are Saigon Square and Dong Khoi Street, an area with numerous hotels, shops, art galleries, and restaurants. The Rex Hotel gained public notice during the Vietnam War; however, several more modern hotels have recently been built, including the Sofitel, Hyatt, Marriott, Continental, and Caravelle. Points of interest include Reunification Hall (formerly the Presidential Palace), the Museum of Vietnamese History, the view from the top of the new modern trade center, and Choulan, the bustling Chinese quarter. A don't-miss attraction is the superb water-puppet show, a unique Vietnamese art form. Another enjoyable experience is the performance of traditional Vietnamese musical instruments offered throughout the day at Reunification Hall.

Da Nang, located in the center of the country, is another favorite port of call. Sightseeing should include: visits to the former trade center of the country in Hoi-An, where today you can visit art galleries and silk factories; a climb to the top of Marble Mountain, the sight of many battles during the Vietnam War, and which today offers an excellent panorama of the surroundings; and the modern, five-star Furama Hotel that sits in the middle of famous China Beach. Tours are generally offered to the imperial city of Hue, to the Ho Chi Minh Trail, and the Cham Museum, which houses the world's best collection of art from the Cham civilization. Lunch by the pool at the Furama Hotel is a delightful experience and affords an opportunity to sample a variety of Asian cuisine.

Hanoi, the capital of Vietnam, a two- to three-hour drive from the port of Haiphong (or a one-hour helicopter ride), is less cosmopolitan and less colorful than Ho Chi Minh City. The hordes of bicycles and motorcycles that do not stop at intersections, nor for pedestrians, make it a real challenge to cross streets. (This is also true throughout the country.) The main tourist attractions include the grandiose, Stalinist-style mausoleum of Ho Chi Minh, the country's most revered leader; his former homes with their surrounding gardens and ponds; the Ho Chi Minh Museum; the One Pillar Pagoda; the Temple of Literature, a well-preserved example of Vietnamese architecture housing 82 stone tablet artifacts; and the 36 streets in the old quarter of town, where each street is named after the merchandise offered, i.e., "Fish Street," "Meat Street," "Vegetable Street," "Basket Street," etc.

East Africa and the Indian Ocean

Well-traveled cruisers looking for new and exotic cruise areas are beginning to explore the eastern coast of Africa and the unusual islands in the Indian Ocean that stretch from the southern tip of Africa to India.

For decades, most of the superliners offering world cruises visited the ports of Durban, Madagascar, Mombasa, Zanzibar, and the Seychelle and Maldive group of islands. Recently, several of the more upscale vessels have offered a series of seven- to fourteen-day cruises in this area, usually embarking or terminating at Mombasa, the port for Kenya, allowing passengers a pre- or post-cruise option to enjoy a safari experience to Nairobi and game reserves.

COMORES ISLANDS

Anjouan, Grande Comore, Mayotte, and Moheli—the four islands in the Comores—are located between Madagascar and Mozambique, Africa, in the Indian Ocean. The islands have a long history. During the nineteenth century, they were ruled by sultanates, and the major industries were the export of spices and slaves. Slavery was abolished in 1904, and in 1912 the four islands became French colonies. In 1975, all of the islands except Mayotte became independent. Having wisely voted to retain the French influence, Mayotte is the only island in the Comores with a decent standard of living and not suffering from overpopulation and poverty. The people of the Comores speak French, Arabic, and a native dialect. They are mostly Moslems, and many practice polygamy.

Most cruise ships stop at **Anjouan** because it is the most scenic of the four islands with verdant hills, mountains, and valleys covered with towering palms, banana trees, and tropical forests dotted with waterfalls and streams—all looking down to the blue waters of the Indian Ocean. The port town of Mutsamudu is dirty, crowded, and of little interest. You will want to drive out into the country to the scenic point at Mt. Ntingui to a factory that processes oil from the ylang-ylang flower used in French perfumes or to one of the picturesque beaches. The best beach is at Moya Plage, where there is a nice hotel; however, it takes 90 minutes to drive there. One mile from town is a small, scenic white-sand beach connected to Comotel Al-Amal, where there is also a small pool, bar, and restaurant.

The largest of the Comores is **Grande Comore**. In town, you can stroll through a clutter of homes and narrow alleys reminiscent of Greek island villages (but much dirtier). You can drive out to see the Karthala Volcano, which has the largest crater in the world. The best beach is at Maloudja, also the location of the best hotel. Other choices may include Novotel Ylang-Ylang and Istranda Palace.

Mayotte, the least impoverished of the four islands and still a French colony, is surrounded by a coral reef. Many private yachts anchor at the beach at Soulou to shower and picnic at the waterfall located there. The best beach for swimming and snorkeling is at N'Goudja, where there is also a decent hotel. **Moheli** has little development; however, there are good beaches at Miremani, Sambadjon, Sambia, and Itsamia.

KENYA

Kenya, an independent republic within the British Commonwealth, intersected by the equator, is possibly the destination that offers the greatest variety of attractions for visitors to Africa. You can visit Nairobi, East Africa's most cosmopolitan city, then go on safari through some of the best game reserves in the world, or relax at a beach resort along the clear, blue waters of the Indian Ocean.

One day to explore this country is not nearly sufficient. Therefore, many cruise ships when calling at **Mombasa**, the port city of Kenya, generally arrange overnight or two- to four-day pre- and post-cruise excursions. Because you will want to make the most of your time, I suggest that you make arrangements with a reliable tour organization to plan and conduct your tour. Abercrombie & Kent (A & K) and Micato Safaris are deservingly the favorites of the major cruise lines, including Renaissance and the *Sea Goddesses*. Micato has been owned and operated for more than twenty-five years by the Pinto family. Micato itineraries include a warm, personalized orientation dinner at the home of Felix and Jane Pinto, high atop Lavington Hill overlooking the twinkling lights of Nairobi; excellent professional English-speaking tour guides in modern, air-conditioned safari vehicles; and guaranteed reservations at Kenya's best hotels, lodges, and tent camps. A & K is well known around the world and offer a comparable Safari experience. United Touring is another large operator in the area.

If your cruise commences or ends in Kenya, you will fly in or out of Nairobi's international airport. The best hotels in Nairobi include the venerable Norfolk, Nairobi Safari Club, Hilton, Serena, and Intercontinental. Windsor Hotel and Country Club is situated 30 minutes from Nairobi and 20 minutes from the airport in a suburb surrounded by parks, woodlands, and coffee plantations. This is the most comfortable choice for a few days of rest, relaxation, and possibly a few rounds of golf.

For dining in Nairobi, your best bets are the Grill Room at the Norfolk (Continental), Tamarind (seafood), and Carnivore (unique game). You will want to visit the National Museum and Aviary to view its collection of tribal ornaments, native wildlife, and Dr. Louis Leakey's exhibit on prehistoric man; Karen Estates, former home of Baroness Karen von Blixen, who wrote *Out of Africa* and other literary works under the pseudonym of Isak Dinesen; Giraffe Manor, where you can hand-feed elegant giraffes; and Nairobi National Park with its impressive lion population and animal orphanage.

Of course, the greatest attraction in Kenya is a camera safari to one of the country's magnificent game reserves. If you only have time for one such reserve, the largest concentration of game to be observed is at the Masai Mara Park, which borders the Serengeti in Tanzania. Game that abound here include giraffes, elephants, lions, baboons, zebra, gazelles, impalas, and wildebeests. Mara Sopa Lodge, located near a native Masai village, enjoys an enviable elevated location with breathtaking views of Olooliumutia Valley and the Mara plains. Other lodges in the Masai include Mara Serena and Kakrok. For those wishing to "rough it" at a modern equipped tented camp, the best of the lot are Gouvenor's Camp, Sarova Mara, Siana Springs, and Kichwa Tempo.

Other top safari destinations include mountain lodge Treetop Hotel in Mt. Kenya National Park, where you can view a multitude of animals when they come to drink at a waterhole around which the lodge is built. While in this area, you may want to spend a day or two relaxing at the world-famous Mt. Kenya Safari Club, set in a lovely park in the foothills of snow-capped Mt. Kenya and surrounded by the world's most famous game conservation park. The resort was once owned by the late William Holden, but is now owned by Lonrho Hotels. The private game reserve and animal orphanage adjacent to the resort are owned by actress Stephanie Powers and the renowned conservationists Don and Iris Hunt.

Still other excellent national parks in which to view game include Samburu, Amboseli, Tsavo, and Aberderes.

The port city of **Mombasa,** an old town rich in history, is located largely on an island that connects to the mainland by causeway. The airport is on the mainland, but the port and city are on the island. Of interest is Fort Jesus, built by the Portuguese at the turn of the sixteenth century, which dominates the harbor and the old town itself. The two best hotels are the Castle in the middle of town and the Outrigger Hotel at Ras Liwatoni on the beach. Numerous beach hotels stretch out to the south and north of mainland Mombasa, and there is a national marine park and scuba diving at Malindi. Traditional African dance can be observed at Giriami Villages.

Lamu Island, a small Kenyan island that sits off the coast with an exclusively Muslim population, is a place that appeals to some tourists for an "away-from-it-all" holiday. Several cruise ships make a short visit here after Mombasa. Lamu is often referred to as the Katmandu of Africa and was popular with the hippies in the sixties and early seventies. It is a rather dirty town with not much of interest other than the museum with its display of a traditional Swahili house and models of various types of *dhow,* the unique wood boat that is the major method of transportation (other than donkey) around the island. If you have a few hours, the best bet is to take the 45-minute walk along the coast, or a short *dhow* ride to Shela Village, using Peponis' Hotel as your home base. The beach extending for several miles past Peponis' is a magnificent stretch of light sand, dunes, and small palms lapped by the warm waters of the Indian Ocean. Here you can also wander around the small Islamic Village and have a cold beer or snack at Peponis'.

MADAGASCAR

Madagascar, the fourth-largest island in the world, is thought to have geologically split off from Africa. It was not inhabited until A.D. 500, when it was settled by

Indonesians and Malaysians. In 1500, the Portuguese came to settle and colonize, and they were followed by the Dutch, British, and French. The country was a French colony from 1896 until it gained its independence in 1960. The population of eleven million is Malagasy, a mixture of black Africans, Indonesians, and Arabs. The language is French; however, France and most of the Western world lost interest in Madagascar after its independence, and today it is a poor, overpopulated country that experiences very little tourism.

Most cruise ships visit Nose Be and Nose Komba, two small tropical islands that lie off the northwest coast of the main island. This is a very picturesque area, one where the sea is generally calm and picture-postcard little islands peek out of the water with green peaks surrounded by blue sky and low-hanging, puffy cumulus clouds.

From the dock at **Nose Be,** you can either walk about a half-mile or take the shuttle bus into town. If you walk, you will pass by the large colonial-style homes built by the French in the early 1900s, which are now dilapidated. In town, there is an open marketplace and a few craft and souvenir shops. You can take a 45-minute drive across this verdant island of rolling hills, rivers, towering palms, sugarcane, coffee, and banana and ylang-ylang trees to the Audilana Beach Hotel. Formerly a Holiday Inn (1960s vintage), it lies on a beautiful tan-sand beach covered with tall palm trees where you can bathe in the very warm, clear waters of the Indian Ocean. The hotel also has a small pool, bar, restaurant, and casino.

Nose Komba is a tiny island best known for its rare lemur sanctuary. Your tender will leave you off on a picturesque brown-sand beach with coral reefs for snorkeling, surrounded by hills covered with deep-green tropical flora. You can walk through a secluded, self-sustaining native village to an area where the rare lemur habitates. If you bring bananas, the friendly primates will jump on your shoulder and consume the bananas out of your hand. It's messy, but fun. The natives of the village are very friendly, the children are darling, and if you wish, you can purchase seashells, primitive handicrafts, or linens.

The beach is excellent for snorkeling, but you need to wear plastic sandals if you are venturing out in the water for a swim.

MALDIVE ISLANDS

Referred to by Marco Polo as "the flower of the Indies," the Maldives lie 450 miles southwest of Sri Lanka and consist of 1,190 tiny, palm-decked coral islands in 26 atoll clusters that trail down the Indian Ocean and overlap the equator. Only 220 are inhabited by a population totaling 270,000, which consists of a mixture of Sri Lankans, Indians, Indonesians, Malayans, Arabs, Africans, and Europeans. The Maldives broke away from Great Britain in 1965 as an independent Islamic republic. Twenty-five percent live in Male, the capital, where most of the inhabitants fish for a living. More than 80 islands have opened small hideaway resorts, the nearer ones in the north and south Male atolls being accessible by motorboats or water taxis called "dhoni." The others can be reached by helicopter and seaplane from the airport that sits on a small island near Male.

There is not much of interest in Male other than the Sultan's Park, the National Museum, and a few souvenir shops. The real reason for visiting the Maldives is to witness the beauty of the hundreds of pristine islands and submarine life. The waters are crystal clear—ideal for swimming, snorkeling, and diving.

Most of the resorts offer extensive diving programs and are frequented by scuba-diving enthusiasts. However, in recent years several luxury resorts have opened that feature not only great diving programs, water sports, and incredible fine-white-sand, palm-studded beaches and lagoons, but also sumptuous beach-front and over-water bungalows, good dining, and upscale service. Four Seasons on Kuda Huraa Island and Banyon Tree on Vabbinfaru Island are both in the north Male atoll, only a 25-minute motorboat ride from Male or the airport. Other popular resorts accessible by motorboat include Kurumba Village on Vihhamana Fushi, Full Moon on Furanafushi, Bandos Island Resort, and Paradise Island Resort on Lankanfinolhu Island.

Some ships visit the Maldives because they are directly on the route between Africa and India, as well as to other Asian countries. Be certain that the ship intends to provide a tour of the islands, assist you with your own arrangements to book transportation to an island, or at least hold a beach party on one of the islands; otherwise, stopping here is not very rewarding.

OMAN

Oman is the oldest of all of the established Arab countries. Muscat, known as the "capital region," is made up of three distinct cities, separated geographically by hills and ridges, each with its own particular identity. Muscat is the old port area and the location of most of the places of interest; Matrah, to the northwest, is the main trading district and the country's most important harbor; Ruwi, a few miles inland, is a modern commercial and administrative center. The coastline is dynamic, with jagged rocky cliffs rising above picturesque, whitewashed towns with mosques and minarets.

Visitors will want to tour the old city of Muscat to view the spectacularly beautiful Al-Alam Palace and gardens flanked by two sixteenth-century Portuguese forts, Jalali to the east and Mirani to the west. Another impressive Portuguese sixteenth-century fort sits atop a cliff near the harbor in Matrah and affords a good panorama of the city.

Sightseeing in Oman should also include a visit to the Natural History Museum as well as the Oman Museum, which houses old manuscripts, local arts and crafts, and displays of Omani architecture and design. Bargaining at the souks in Muscat and Matrah are popular tourist priorities. Here you will find antique jewelry, souvenirs, sandals, colorful textiles, gold, silver, spices, and incense.

Dining is best and safest at one of the better hotels such as Al-Bustan Palace Intercontinental, a five-minute drive past Muscat, where you will find a long strand of beach, a pool, tennis courts, numerous restaurants, and a good example of Arabian opulence.

Those wishing to take a long walk or jog will especially appreciate the corniche, the road and path along the gulf extending from the harbor in Matrah to the town of Muscat, a distance of about 2 miles.

SEYCHELLE ISLANDS

These unique, dynamically beautiful tropical islands that encompass a 75-square-mile archipelago are located in the Indian Ocean near the equator, a thousand miles east of Kenya and a thousand miles away from any other land mass. The islands were uninhabited until the mid-eighteenth century, when France took possession. Over the years, the 115 islands (80 of which are still deserted) were settled by Europeans, Africans, and Asians, and today the 70,000 inhabitants speak Creole, French, and English.

These islands are geologically unique in that they are of solid-granite origin rather than volcanic rock, with dramatic cliffs that rise from the sea, carpeted with lush vegetation and interesting boulder formations that are the debris of gigantic movements of the earth's crust thousands of years ago. The Seychelle beaches are the very best in the world, and the warm seas surrounding the islands offer countless opportunities for swimming, water sports, scuba, and snorkeling. Several of the islands are home for rare species of sea birds and plant life found nowhere else in the world. The weather is hot, humid, and sometimes windy during the monsoon seasons. December and January are the worst months, and May through October are the best.

There are several international airplane flights each week into **Mahé**—the largest of the islands. The harbor at Mahé's largest city, Victoria, is the port of call for many cruise ships. Ninety-five percent of the population of the Seychelles is on Mahé. It is here that you will find the major hotels, the best restaurants, and the best shopping, as well as 68 beautiful beaches. The most pristine and picturesque beaches are Anse Royale on the southeast coast and Anse Intendence on the southwest coast; the most popular, but not the most beautiful, is at Baie Beau Vallon, where numerous hotels are located.

The capital town of Victoria, which sits near the harbor, is very clean but not terribly interesting. There are a number of shops and boutiques, as well as several restaurants. The better hotels, resorts, and restaurants are located around the island and not in Victoria.

Presently, the only first-class resort on the island is the Plantation Club at Baie Lazare, which offers lovely grounds, very comfortable accommodations, and many amenities. Other hotels with the same facilities are the Equator at Grande Anse, Meridian at Barbaron, Sunset Beach, Meridian Fisherman's Cove, Berjaya Beau Vallon Bay Beach Resort, Notholme, and Coral Strand, all on Beau Vallon Bay. All of these hotels have beaches, pools, tennis courts, shops, and good restaurants. The best restaurants are Chez Plume at Anse Boileau, La Perle Noire at Beau Vallon, and Le Corsaire and LaScala at Bel Ombre.

To really appreciate this incredibly lush island, you should rent a car or mini-moke or hire a taxi to drive you around Mahé. Nowhere in the world can you witness such incredible beauty.

Praslin lies to the northwest of Mahé, and is a 2 1/2-hour ferryboat ride or 15-minute propeller flight. Here you can enjoy the one-mile walk through the 450-acre Valley-De-Mai, a lovely forest and the home of the botanical rarity, the Coco de Mer Palm, as well as such rare birds as the black parrot, blue pigeon, and bulbul. This 7-mile-long island is surrounded by a coral reef and boasts numerous silver-white-sand beaches. Cote d'Or and Anse Volbert make up a 2 1/2-mile stretch of white-sand beach lined with palm trees only 5 or 6 miles from the pier where your tender docks. Here you can swim, snorkel, and have lunch or a snack at one of the small hotels or restaurants located along the beach, including Berjaya Praslin Beach Hotel, Paradise Hotel, and Acajou.

A few miles farther down the road you will experience one of the most idyllic beaches in the world, the incomparable Anse Lazio. The setting of palms, pines, seagrapes, and flowers is breathtaking; the powder-white sand is firm and excellent for strolling and jogging; and the absolutely crystal-clear warm waters are the very finest for swimming. Adjacent to this extraordinary beach is an equally extraordinary semi-open-air restaurant, Richelieu Verlaque's Bon Bon Plume, which features exceptional fresh fish, seafoods, Creole dishes, French wines, and other beverages and overlooks the panorama of Anse Lazio. Those opting to spend their day ashore at Anse Lazio and Bon Bon Plume will be rewarded with one of the most exquisite island experiences they may ever encounter.

The best resorts on the island are La Reserve, L'Archipel, and Acajou. If you are in Praslin in the evening, the two best restaurants are the charming semi-open-air restaurant sitting on an over-water jetty at La Reserve and the elegant Tante Mimi, situated in a colonial-style building above the casino and serving Continental cuisine.

La Digue, a 30-minute boat ride from Praslin or 3 hours from Mahé, is the most beautiful, pristine, and photographed of the Seychelle Islands. The breathtakingly scenic Anse Source D'Argent, in my opinion, is the most beautiful beach setting in the world. Here, warm turquoise waters with the mildest of currents lap silver-white-sand beaches and tiny private coves interspersed with geometric gray boulder formations, palm trees, and other tropical flora and green hills in the background. This is the scene that appears most often on postcards and brochures depicting the Seychelles. The island is surrounded by a coral reef, and opportunities to snorkel and swim are abundant.

From La Passe, where your boat or tender docks, you can walk or rent a bicycle or oxcart for the two-mile trek through town, past La Digue Lodge (a small hotel) and L'Union Estate, to Anse Source D'Argent. Select any of the private coves to leave your towel and snorkel gear. After you have strolled along the mile or so of sandy paths, rock formations, and coves, and taken some of the most scenic photos imaginable, you will want to settle down and enjoy the sun, soothing warm waters, and picturesque surroundings. This is the perfect romantic hideaway. If you have no one with whom to share romance, it is a great place to sit and reflect.

There are many other spectacular beaches on the island, including Grand Anse and Petite Anse (two magnificent half-mile-long expanses of white sand beach with crystal-clear waters and heavy waves and current), as well as Anse CoCo, Anse

Fourmis, Anse Banane, Anse Patates, and Anse Gaulettes. If time permits, you can ride a bicycle around the island, although there are some places where you will have to proceed by foot. The winds and currents can be rather strong from May through October, and generally the safest place to swim is at Anse Source D'Argent. Places to visit include Black Paradise Flycatcher Reserve, a 37-acre shaded woodland where these rare birds make their home; and L'Union Estate, an old coconut plantation with a traditional colonial house, shipyard, colony of giant tortoises, and horseback riding.

Aride, a nature reserve, is two hours by boat from Mahé. Wardens, who live on the island, will take you on a tour of nature paths to view the beautiful Wright's gardenia, other flora indigenous to the island, and the largest collection of sea birds in the world, including the roseate sooty and bridled tern, the lesser and common noddy, and the white-tailed tropic bird. The pure white-sand beach in front of the wooded area is very beautiful, but swimming and snorkeling can be a bit dangerous when the waves are high.

Curieuse is a small island two miles long that is a half-mile from the north coast of Praslin. Here you can take a rather rugged nature walk across a steep hill to a swamp to view a colony of 100 giant Aldalra tortoises. The long stretch of white-sand beach is picturesque and borders clean, warm waters ideal for swimming and some of the best snorkeling in the Seychelles. Several cruise ships offer barbecues or picnics here.

Cousins is a 70-acre island bird reserve sanctuary for the rare Seychelle ground doves, weaver birds, toc toc, and thousands of other species. There is a half-mile expanse of beach, but the water is generally pretty rough and snorkeling is only fair. **Bird Island, Desroches,** and **Poivre** are three islands offering good game fishing.

UNITED ARAB EMIRATES

Dubai, which lies 100 miles down the coastal road from Abu Dhabi, is really two cities divided by an inlet from the Persian Gulf known as "The Creek." On the north side of The Creek is the village of Deira and on the south, Dubai. Your ship will dock at Port Rashid on the Dubai side, two miles from the center of town. With a half-million inhabitants, it is the second largest of the seven emirates, offering the visitor a distinctive blend of modern city and timeless desert.

A number of Western hotels, such as the Intercontinental, Hyatt Regency, and Sheraton, offer deluxe accommodations, fine dining, shops, panoramic views, and a good home base for your exploration. You will want to sample Arabian specialties such as a *hummus* (a chick pea and sesame seed puree), *taboule* (cracked wheat salad with tomatoes, mint, and parsley), and the variety of spicy lamb dishes, fish, and seafood indigenous to the region. In the small restaurants, the traditional repast is *shawarma,* grilled slivers of lamb or chicken mixed with salad and stuffed inside pita-bread pockets. Several hotels and tour organizations feature "desert safari dinners," where guests enjoy a barbecue dinner under the stars while seated on a carpet under a canopy.

You will want to browse the traditional souks and tiny shops of the old town core and test your skills at bargaining. The famous Gold Souk in Dubai has hundreds of shops and gold is sold by its weight. Persian carpets here are considered the best buys outside of Iran. Also, there are modern multilevel shopping malls at Al Rega Road, Karama, Al Dhiyafa Road, and Bani Yas Square.

Dubai is home to the annual PGA Desert Golf Classic and the only 18-hole golf course in the emirates with real greens. Swimming and water sports are available at Jumeirah Beach Park and Al Mimzer Park, south of the port.

A fun way to cross The Creek is on a shared water taxi called abras. The Creek offers a picturesque glimpse of the city's trading heritage.

Places of interest include: Al Fahide Fort, renovated in 1970 to house an archeological museum; the view from the top of the World Trade Center; Dubai Zoo; the camel racetrack; the shops and restaurants at Holiday Center; the Textile Souk on Al Fahidi Street; the Spice Souk; the Gold Souk; Majlis Gallery; and Juneira Mosque, a spectacular example of modern Islamic architecture.

ZANZIBAR ISLAND, TANZANIA

Known as the "Spice Island," Zanzibar has been ruled at one time or another by Egyptians, Indians, Chinese, Portuguese, Persians, Dutch, Arabs, and English. The island reached prominence during the nineteenth century as the hub of the slave-trading industry and as a major grower and exporter of spices—especially cloves, which are grown on plantations around the island. Ninety percent of the island's inhabitants are Muslims, and Arab influence is present in the architecture, numerous ruins, and customs.

If you do not opt to take an organized tour, you can readily hire an English-speaking taxi driver for about seven to ten dollars an hour. You may wish to explore the labyrinth of narrow winding streets with whitewashed coral houses, shops, restaurants, and public buildings in the "Old Stone Town" area. Attractions here include two former sultans' palaces, a Portuguese fort built in 1700, a mosque, several cathedrals, a museum, the old slave market, and the indoor/outdoor public market, where produce, fish, and meats are sold. The favored restaurant amongst tourists in the Old Stone Town is Fisherman's Restaurant, which features fresh fish, lobster, and other seafood.

To appreciate the tropical splendor of Zanzibar, you must drive out to the beaches, native villages, and spice plantations. Zanzibar is a major producer of cloves. A lovely spot to spend a few hours is Mawimbine Club Village, on the west side of the island where you dock, about a 15-minute drive from town. This is a charming tropical resort with sixty-four thatched bungalows set in lush gardens with a pool, bar, restaurant, and a nice strand of white-sand beach. Water sports and deep-sea fishing can be arranged here. Down the road is a small native village and spice plantation that can be visited in combination with the drive to Mawimbine.

There are a number of fine beaches on the opposite (east) side of the island at Jambiani and Bwejuu, but you probably will not have enough time to get there.

Transatlantic Crossings

When planning your European vacation, why not plan to sail at least one way? Prior to the jet age, cruising to and from Europe was considered by many as "the only way to go." Today, however, the relaxed luxury of sailing abroad has given way to the desires of the typical traveler who wishes to take in as much as he can in as short a time as possible. Those of you who find it difficult to immediately unwind at the beginning of a vacation may find that a five-day ocean crossing is just what the doctor ordered. Others who have been exhausted from the hustle and bustle of a whirlwind European tour may prefer to take a relaxing cruise home to rest up before going back to the demands of everyday life.

As the cruise lines are scheduling a greater number of cruises in the Caribbean and Mediterranean, their ships are making fewer transatlantic crossings. Whereas thirty years ago a traveler leaving for Europe had numerous vessels to choose from, today only a few ships make regularly scheduled trips. However, it is possible to cruise on numerous lines when they are repositioning their vessels between the United States and Europe in late spring and early fall.

Some ships make a few crossings by the southern route. This route takes from five to fifteen days, depending on your point of embarkation and ports of call. Typically, the ships stop at a few of the following ports: Lisbon, Algeciras, Barcelona, Cannes, Genoa, Naples, and Piraeus.

The *QE2* (Cunard Line) has a number of regularly scheduled crossings by the northern route to such ports as Southampton, Le Havre, and Bremerhaven, which take from five to seven days.

For a number of years, the *QE2* has offered an attractive "air-sea" package under which they fly you one way to or from London (including an option on the Concorde) and provide three nights' accommodations at a Cunard Hotel— all for the price of little more than the one-way cruise fare.

As pointed out earlier in the book, when sailing transatlantic, you will find that the seas are rougher than in the Caribbean or Mediterranean, and that the southern route will allow more sunny days on deck than the northern route.

However, don't let these factors discourage you. Sailing on a modern luxury liner is an unforgettable experience. If your vacation plans will not permit a longer cruise and Europe is on your agenda, treat yourself to a transatlantic crossing for at least one leg of your trip.

Length of Cruise

How long a cruise should you take? The answer, of course, depends upon how much time you have available, as well as what length vacation you may prefer. If you are the type that becomes fidgety after having spent a week at a vacation spot, you also probably will become restless should you spend longer than a week at sea. On the other hand, if it takes you a week just to unwind and longer vacations are your preference, a longer cruise will appeal to you.

The duration of a cruise can vary from a one- or two-day journey to "nowhere" to an around-the-world cruise that may take from 90 to 120 days. If you have only a short time to spend afloat, you may wish to consider cruises to "nowhere" from New York, Miami, Fort Lauderdale, Orlando, or Los Angeles, which are offered by a number of the cruise lines. On these outings, the ships merely sail out into the ocean for one or two days, giving the passengers a sample of life aboard a cruise ship at sea. One or two ships of Carnival, Royal Caribbean, Premier, Disney, and Norwegian offer short-duration cruises (three or four days) from Florida to the Bahamas. Ships of the Costa and Royal Olympic lines offer three- and four-day cruises from Piraeus to the Greek islands and Turkish Coast. In addition, there are a few short cruises running from time to time from Los Angeles and between islands in the Caribbean.

If you can spend a week, there are numerous seven-day cruises offered by the major cruise lines. Cruises from New York to Bermuda and the Bahamas are run on a regular basis out of New York by ships of the Holland America, Celebrity, and Royal Caribbean cruise lines. Years ago, the Norwegian Caribbean Line (renamed Norwegian Cruise Line in 1988) pioneered the concept of regular seven-day cruises from Florida to the Caribbean, and today every major cruise line offers regular seven-day Caribbean cruises from Florida. If you prefer a seven-day cruise from Los Angeles to ports in Mexico, you can be obliged by ships of the Carnival and Royal Caribbean lines. Several ships that offer three- and four-day cruises to the Greek islands and Turkish Coast also have seven-day itineraries. Most lines offer regular spring, summer, and early fall cruises in the eastern and western Mediterranean. Many of the lines offering cruises from Florida also make weekly trips from Puerto Rico to a variety of Caribbean islands. Almost all of the other major cruise ships offer a number of seven-day cruises from time to time in various seas of the world, but not on a regular basis. Thus, the traveler with only seven days to spend has a great variety of ships and cruise areas from which to choose.

These seven-day cruises are of three basic types. There are the barnstorming cruises that make as many as six or seven stops in seven days, giving you maximum exposure to a number of different ports for your dollar but affording little time to catch your breath. Then there are certain cruises that hit only a few ports and let you spend most of your time playing and relaxing on ship. The third type of seven-day cruise makes short trips, such as from New York to Bermuda and Nassau. These ships dock in one port several days, acting as your hotel and leaving you plenty of time to explore the island.

There are a number of cruises with eight- to thirteen-day durations, but the ten-day to fourteen-day cruise has become extremely popular because it coincides with many travelers' two-week vacations and offers plenty of time to call on a large number of ports while still leaving several relaxing days at sea. Many of the previously mentioned lines offer regular ten- or fourteen-day itineraries traversing the Panama Canal, or leaving from Florida to the Caribbean, from Los Angeles to Mexico or Alaska, as well as from various Mediterranean ports to other ports on the Mediterranean.

If you wish to cruise to the Hawaiian Islands, the South Pacific, the Far East, South America, or the Northlands, your cruise, by necessity, will be of a longer duration unless you can arrange to fly part of the way and take only a portion of the itinerary. Ships of the Cunard, Renaissance, Radisson Seven Seas, Silverseas, Crystal, Holland America, and Seabourn lines specialize in long cruises that call on ports in several continents and sometimes circumnavigate the globe. Some of the superliners (such as the *QE2, Royal Viking Sun*, and *Vistafjord*) and the Crystal and the Holland America ships make one or more of these "longer" or around-the-world journeys each year. Renaissance, Princess, Radisson Seven Seas, Seabourn, Silversea, Holland America, Crystal, and a number of other cruise lines feature fascinating itineraries for some of their vessels in the Far East, visiting such exotic ports of call as Bali, Singapore, Bangkok, Phuket, Bombay, and Hong Kong. Many of the other cruise lines have indicated they will be entering this market in the near future.

Although it is always dangerous to generalize, one can say that the majority of passengers on the longer cruises are usually over fifty-five, retired, semiretired, or of independent means, since the everyday working man seldom can afford to take so much time off for a vacation. The first-time sailors tend to gravitate toward the seven- to fourteen-day cruises that offer the larger sampling of ports. It would be difficult to make any additional generalizations. Most other categories of cruise vacationers will select cruises with durations and itineraries matching their personal tastes. However, there is often a geographical proximity between the cruiser's hometown and the ports of embarkation.

If you are contemplating a longer cruise, you may wish to avoid too small a vessel, since you will want more space to move around. Although it may be intimate and even cozy to frequent the same public rooms of a small ship on a seven- or even fourteen-day cruise, after a month or so you could be climbing the walls. The larger vessels offer more space, facilities, and public rooms, as well as a greater variety of people to meet.

In conclusion, I feel that however long your vacation, however extensive or limited your budget, wherever it is you prefer to cruise, and whatever your preference in ships, there exists a cruise vacation meeting your requirements—and a cruise vacation is one experience in life that should not be missed.

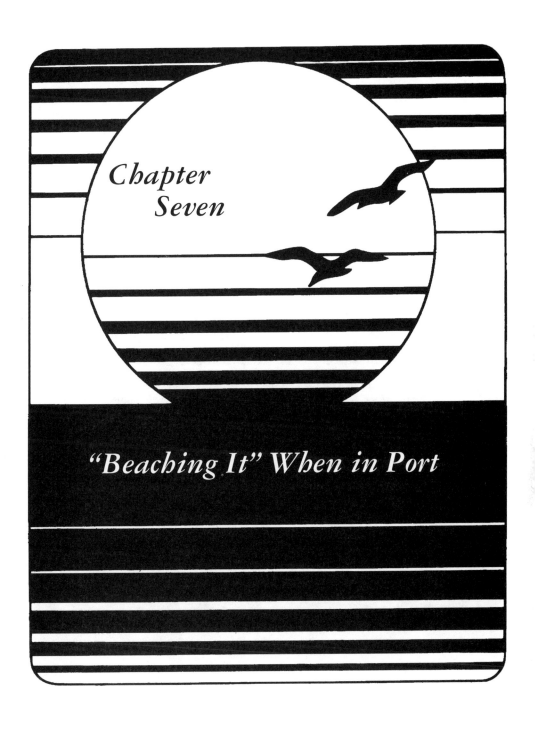

Chapter Seven

"Beaching It" When in Port

Since childhood, I have retained fond memories of romping about on a beautiful beach. I recall the total experience—the smell of the salt water, the tingling of spray from the waves, the hot sand on the bottom of my feet, the warm sun on my shoulders, and the exhilaration of a cool dip. Those who share this nostalgic identity with the sea may feel that a vacation is not complete unless it includes staying at a beach resort. However, it is possible to combine "cruising" and "beaching."

Most every ship cruising the Caribbean, Mexico, and Hawaii spends the majority of days in ports where beach aficionados can dawdle away lazy hours on a variety of lovely beaches. Just pack a small bag with a beach towel, change of clothes, and suntan lotion and head out for your favorite watering hole.

Although there are countless beautiful virgin strands, many are unsafe for swimming and offer no facilities for changing clothes or purchasing a cold drink. Therefore, I generally prefer selecting a beach with facilities adjoining a resort hotel. Often, these are among the most beautiful on the island. The following is an alphabetical list of my favorites:

Africa and Indian Ocean

KENYA

Along Kenya's shoreline, there are long strands of beach with numerous hotels that stretch both to the north and south of Mombasa. In addition, there is also a good sand-dune beach on Lamu Island at Shela Village past Peponis' Hotel.

NOSE BE (MADAGASCAR)

The best beach is at the Audilava Beach Hotel, where there is also a pool, tennis court, and other facilities.

SEYCHELLES

The islands of the Seychelles boast the finest beaches in the world. On Mahé the best beaches are at Anse Royale, Anse Intendence, and Grand Anse, on Praslin at Anse Lazio and Anse Volbert, and on La Digue at Anse Source D'Argent, Grand Anse, and Petite Anse. Actually, every beach in these islands is incredible. The beaches offer the most idyllic settings and warmest water. They are incomparable.

TANZANIA

If your ship stops at Zanzibar Island, a fifteen-minute drive from port will take you to Mawimbine Club Village, where there is a good beach for swimming in the warm Indian Ocean.

Australia

There are numerous large, sandy beaches in the suburbs of Sydney, described earlier in chapter 6. All of the islands around the Great Barrier Reef boast lovely beaches for swimming, including Lizard Island and Hayman Island.

The Caribbean and Atlantic

ANGUILLA

The beach at Malliouhana is the best and least windy on the island. The beaches at Cap Juluca, Shoal Bay, and Sandy Island are also very picturesque and enjoyable.

ANTIGUA

You can't go wrong at any of the alleged 365 beaches. My preference is to spend the day at the beaches at St. James's Club or Halcyon Cove, because of the additional facilities.

ARUBA

Your best bet is the long stretch of white-sand beach fronting the strip of deluxe hotels that includes the Aruba Sheraton, Aruba Caribbean, Americana, Holiday Inn, Concorde, and Hyatt. All of these hotels have swimming pools, tennis courts, and informal poolside dining. The water is usually quiet and warm and without waves or surf. The hotels are located less than ten minutes from the harbor.

BAHAMAS

Abacos—Here you will find miles of virgin beach on Treasure Cay or Guana Cay. These are among the most beautiful unspoiled beaches in the Caribbean.

Grand Bahama (Freeport/Lucaya)—The beach in front of the Holiday Inn Hotel in Lucaya is unquestionably the best on the island; however, it involves an expensive twenty- to thirty-minute taxi ride from the harbor. Most cruisers utilize the beach across from the former Xanadu Princess. The beach is crowded and the sea often too shallow for serious swimming.

Nassau—The best beaches are at Cable Beach and on Paradise Island. The most pristine, unspoiled strand is lined with pine trees and fronts the posh Ocean Club. To get there, cross over the toll bridge to Paradise Island, go straight to the sea, turn right, and walk about three blocks. If you turned left, you would be at a very nice beach in front of what formerly were the Paradise Island and Britannia Beach hotels and now is the Atlantis Hotel complex. All of these hotels have large pools, tennis courts, changing facilities, and informal outdoor restaurants. The public beach near the Paradise Paradise Hotel, which is recommended by most of the cruise ships, is often crowded, although the water is warm, clear, and excellent for swimming.

BARBADOS

One of the more interesting beaches in the Caribbean is at the bottom of the cliff at Marriott's Sam Lord's Castle. This is the Atlantic side of the island, and the surf is high and swimming is sometimes dangerous. The hotel itself is most unusual and has exceptional facilities. Tamer beaches can be found on the Caribbean side at Sandy Lane, Glitter Bay, Royal Pavillion, and Paradise Beach Club. All of these hotels are less than an hour's ride from the harbor. The beach at Sandy Lane is one of the best in the Caribbean.

BERMUDA

One of my personal favorites is the several miles of pink-sand beach directly to the left of the Southampton Princess Hotel. Here you will find little coves, shady hills, and warm, clear water. The Southampton Princess is only a fifteen- to twenty-minute ride from the harbor.

CARACAS (VENEZUELA)

The only beach is at the Macuto Sheraton in La Guaira. It is not very beautiful and not worth the special trip unless you are going to the hotel for other reasons. The pool at the Macuto is much nicer than the beach.

CARTAGENA

Your best bet is the public beach in front of the Hilton. At the Hilton, there are tennis courts, an outdoor bar, and several restaurants.

CAYMAN ISLANDS

Many consider the 7-mile stretch of beach on Grand Cayman Island to be one of the most beautiful in the Caribbean. This is the favorite of scuba divers and snorkelers. A five-minute taxi ride from town will take you to the Hyatt Regency Grand Cayman, the largest and best hotel on the island. Go down to the beach, turn left (or right), and walk for miles on an unspoiled, white-sand beach lined with pines and palms. The Hyatt, Treasure Island, Westin, and Holiday Inn are the only hotels here offering a pool, tennis, restaurant, snorkeling gear, and a large private beach area.

CURAÇAO

There are nice beaches at the Sonesta Beach Hotel, Curacao Caribbean Hotel, and Princess Beach Hotel.

DOMINICAN REPUBLIC

If your ship stops at Santo Domingo, the nearest beach is at Boca Chica. There are hotel pools in town in El Embajador, the Ramada, and the Sheraton. If time allows, go to the beach at Casa de Campo in La Romana. This is one of the best beaches on the island, and Casa de Campo is possibly the most complete resort in the Caribbean. Costa ships stop at their private beach at Serena Cay.

FORTALEZA (BRAZIL)

Within 7 miles of town, there are lovely beaches at Iracema, Meirelles, Mucuripe, de Futuro, and Caca e Pesca.

GRENADA

Grand Anse Beach in front of the Grenada Beach Hotel and Spice Island Inn is convenient because it is only a short taxi ride from town and offers the most facilities. This is a long, fine, white-sand beach with warm, deep-blue waters. However, the constant stream of hawkers and peddlers that aggressively approach you with beads and spices is so annoying that it is difficult to relax. Most of the other hotels with beaches are a great deal farther away, and the taxi rides can be prohibitively expensive.

GUADELOUPE

My favorite is the picturesque beach at the Club Med Caravelle. You will have to make advance arrangements and pay a fee to get through the gates. Sneaking onto the property also is possible if this doesn't make you uncomfortable. There are also nice beaches, pools, and tennis courts at the Frantel, La Creole Beach, and Meridien-Guadeloupe.

HAITI

Port-au-Prince does not have a decent beach. The Club Med at Montrouis is about the best, but it is 1 1/2 hours from town. There are swimming pools at El Rancho, Castel Haiti, Holiday Inn, and the Splendid Hotels.

JAMAICA

Ocho Rios—If your time is limited, you may wish to settle for a beach at the foot of Dunn's Falls after climbing the most important scenic attraction in Jamaica. If you prefer a private beach, pools, tennis courts, and other amenities, you can try any of the larger hotels, such as San Souci and Ciboney. So-so beaches and pools can be found at the Renaissance Hotel, which is located near where your ship docks.

Montego Bay—Most cruisers end up at the public strip known as Doctor's Cave Beach or Cornwall Beach, where there is an underwater marine park. Those wishing a private beach with tennis, pools, restaurants, and other facilities should try Round Hill, Tryall, the Half Moon, or the Holiday Inn.

Negril—The best beaches in Jamaica are at Negril; however, it takes several hours to reach this area from Montego Bay, and this would prevent you from exploring any other part of the island.

MARTINIQUE

The best beach is at Club Med-Buccaneer's Creek. However, this is a several-hour drive from Fort-de-France, and advance arrangements would have to be made here as in Guadeloupe. You may prefer to take a twenty-minute motor launch ride from Fort-de-France to Pointe du Bout, where the Meridian and Bakoua hotels are located adjacent to each other. Both hotels offer mediocre, "partially topless" beaches, tennis courts, a swimming pool, and French-Creole restaurants.

PUERTO RICO

The beaches in Puerto Rico contain darker sand and lack the pristine beauty of the beaches on many of the other islands. If your time is limited, the closest beach with facilities would be at the Caribe Hilton Hotel, which is only five minutes by taxi from the harbor. The beaches at the Sheraton and El San Juan are also nice. If you have an entire day, you may wish to take a long ride out to the Hyatt Dorado or the Hyatt Regency Cerromar. Although the beaches are nothing special, these resorts are in tropical settings containing acres and acres of beautiful grounds, sensational golf courses, good tennis courts, and miles of scenic paths; and Cerromar has one of the most exotic, interesting pool complexes in the world. Another option is the recently renovated El Conquistador Hotel, one hour in the opposite direction, which has its own private island beach with numerous watersport facilities.

RECIFE (BRAZIL)

You can choose from Pina or Boa Viagem beaches in the city, with its 5-mile ocean promenade lined with coconut palms, or from the more pristine beaches at Piedade, Venda Grande, Candeias, or Borra de Jangadar—all a 10- to 20-mile drive away.

RIO DE JANEIRO (BRAZIL)

The city is lined with a long stretch of beach that is most noted for its local color. The most populated beach is Copacabana. Ipanema runs a close second. The only hotel directly on a beach is the Sheraton, which is at the juncture of Ipanema and Gavea.

ST. LUCIA

There are good beaches with full facilities at either La Toc, the Club Med, or Jalousie Plantation.

ST. MAARTEN

The beach near the airport in front of Mullet Bay Resort is the best. There is a little surf here, which makes swimming more interesting. Planes on a landing approach right overhead can become annoying. The beach at La Samana is also magnificent; however, you would have to make special arrangements with the hotel. Orient Beach, about a fifteen-minute ride from Philipsburg, is reminiscent of Tahiti Beach in St. Tropez, France, with topless and nude bathing and numerous small beach restaurants and boutiques.

TRINIDAD

The nearest beach is 14 miles from the capital at Maracas Bay. There are no facilities here. You may be better off settling for the pool at the Trinidad Hilton.

VIRGIN ISLANDS

St. Croix—There are nice beaches, tennis courts, and informal restaurants at the Carambola and the Buccaneer Beach Hotel. Buck Island would be the best choice.

St. John—The several horseshoe-shaped, private beaches at Caneel Bay Resort are possibly the loveliest in the Caribbean. A day in port at this resort is a "must" whenever possible. The tennis courts are excellent and usually empty; and the paths running through the acres of vegetation are a jogger's dream. The Westin is also exquisite; however, the beach is not as desirable as those at Caneel. Trunk Bay is the best choice for snorkelers.

St. Thomas—Magen's Bay is deservingly reputed to be one of the top beaches in the world. I personally prefer spending the day at the Virgin Grand Resort and taking my dip at "nearby" Coki Beach. There is also good swimming at Marriott's Frenchman's Reef on Morningstar Beach, only a five-minute taxi ride from the harbor.

Europe

Because there are not many "great beaches" in Europe, I will mention just a few that make up in local color what they lack in pristine beauty. Some of the best strands can be found on the island of Ibizia and at Hotel Formentor on the Spanish island of Majorca. Other sandy beaches include Lido Beach near Venice, the numerous beaches in Mykonos and Skiathos, Tahiti Beach in St. Tropez, the beach resorts in Kusadasi and Marmaris (Turkey), and the main beach in Tel Aviv. Some colorful beach resort areas with little sand include the beaches of Capri, Cannes, Nice, Corfu, Rhodes, Costa del Sol, and the Italian Riviera.

On the island of Calvi, there is a long strand of beach surrounded by a pine forest to the left of the main part of town. In Cannes, the beach club in front of the Majestic Hotel is the best place to spend the day; however, voyeurs will want to walk in either direction to take advantage of the exotic human scenery. The beaches in Marbella are widely frequented, but you will probably prefer the pools at the various hotels.

Far East

There are a few great beaches in the Far East. The best "resort beach" areas can be found at Phuket and Pataya in Thailand; Penang, Langawi, and Sabah in Malaysia; and Bali in Indonesia. Repulse Bay in Hong Kong is just so-so. The small uninhabited islets a short boat ride from the Tanjung Aru Beach Resort in Sabah and those in Phuket and its neighboring islands offer some of the most beautiful beaches and best swimming in the world.

Mexico

ACAPULCO

Although none of the beaches in Acapulco compare with those in the Caribbean or Cancún, the best of the lot is in front of the Princess and Pierre Marques hotels. The myriad of pools at the Princess is interesting and exciting.

CABO SAN LUCAS

The best beach for swimming is in front of the Hacienda Hotel, five minutes from where you disembark from your tender. The beach fronting the Solmar and Finistera hotels is more picturesque, but too dangerous for swimming.

CANCUN

There are 10 miles of beautiful white-sand beach stretching in front of the all of the hotels in the hotel area. Here the water is clear but the waves can be too strong for safe swimming.

COZUMEL

Playa del Sol, about a twenty-minute drive from town, offers the best sand, swimming, and facilities.

MANZANILLO

The beaches at Las Hadas and Grand Bay Resorts are very nice, as are the picturesque pools.

PUERTO VALLARTA

The beaches in Puerto Vallarta, as in Acapulco, are not exceptional. The hotels with beaches closest to the harbor are the Posada Vallarta, Fiesta Americana, and the Holiday Inn.

ZIHUATANEJO-IXTAPA

The beach that runs along the stretch of high-rise hotels in Ixtapa or the more private beach at the Camino Real are the best.

Middle East

Sandy beaches can be found in Herzelia, Elat, and Tel Aviv in Israel; Kusadasi and Marmaris in Turkey; and in Cyprus; however, they are nothing to write home about. For those cruising the Greek islands, the beaches are best at Mykonos and Skiathos. The beaches at Lindos in Rhodes, Corfu, Kos, and Crete are decent.

Pacific

FIJI

The best beach on the big island of Viti Levu is found at The Fijian Resort. There are lovely, pristine beaches in the Yasawa Islands group and on Mana Island, Beachcomber Island, Plantation Island, Treasure Island, and Turtle Island. These also are among the best in the world.

HAWAII

For those cruising the Hawaiian Islands, you will want to consider the following beaches:

Oahu—The best strand is in front of the Kahala Mandarin Oriental, fifteen minutes from Waikiki, and at Ihilani. The beaches in Waikiki are too crowded with tourists; however, the beach in front of the Hilton Hawaiian Village is the best of the lot.

Maui—The beach in Kaanapali fronting all the hotels, the beaches at Wailea, or the beach at Kapalua Bay resort are your best bets.

Kauai—One of my favorite beaches in the world is Lumaha Beach, where *South Pacific* was filmed. Although this involves an hour-and-a-half drive, you will be rewarded with witnessing as much as Mother Nature can provide. There are no facilities here, and swimming is dangerous in the winter months. If you do not have time to visit Lumaha, then bodysurfers will want to go to Poipu, between the Sheraton and Hyatt resorts, and nonsurfers will prefer the facilities at the beach fronting the Kauai Marriott at Kauai Lagoons. The Hyatt Regency Kauai, with its pool complex and protected beach, is your most exotic locale.

Hawaii—If your ship docks at Hilo, you will enjoy the scenic black-sand beach at Kaimu. This may be too dangerous for swimming. At Kona, the best beach belongs to the Mauna Kea Beach Hapuna and Mauna Lani. Nearby at Hilton Waikoloa is one of the most extensive and imaginative pool complexes in the world.

NEW CALEDONIA

Ile des Pins is a lovely pine-studded island with numerous chalk-white beaches ideal for swimmers, divers, and sun worshipers.

TAHITI

Bora Bora—In Bora Bora, there are numerous little islets with nothing but palms, sandy beaches, and crystal-clear waters sitting in a very large protected lagoon. The lovely little Motu Tapu, a private island about a half-mile in circumference, is pristine. The half-mile of crescent-shaped beach at the Bora Bora Hotel on the mainland offers some good snorkeling close to the shore. Romantics may prefer the setting at Bora Bora Lagoon Resort on Motu Toopua, which can be reached by the resort's private launch.

Moorea—In Moorea, the best beach with facilities is at the Club Med, where there is snorkeling and countless watersports. There is also a beach with watersport facilities at the Bali Hai, Kia Ora Hotels, and Moorea Beachcomber Parkroyal.

Tahiti—On the big island of Tahiti, the black-sand beach at Hotel Tahara'a and the Strand at the Tahiti Beachcomber Parkroyal are the best places to swim and sun.

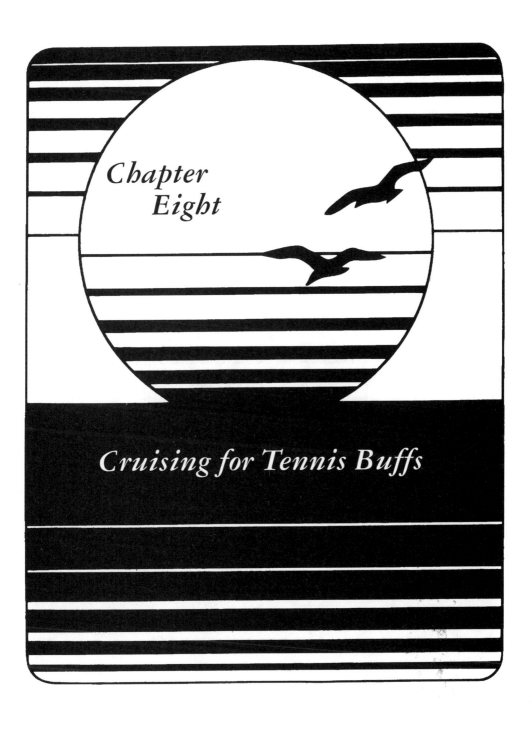

Chapter
Eight

Cruising for Tennis Buffs

Many of my friends who are ardent tennis buffs have avoided cruising because they could not conceive of taking a vacation without playing tennis. Being somewhat of a tennis aficionado myself, I have always managed to include tennis with my cruises. Because it is possible to play tennis in almost every Caribbean, Mexican, and South American port of call, I merely select ships with multiport itineraries. Ships offering three ports in four days, six ports in seven days, or eleven ports in fourteen days will permit ample opportunity to keep your game from getting rusty.

From experience, I would not recommend public tennis courts or tennis clubs. It is far easier and less time-consuming to play at the courts in the various hotels, which are also usually maintained in better condition. Because many hotels do not permit nonresidents to use their facilities, it is often necessary to represent yourself as a guest. If this slight bit of deception offends you, the alternatives are to make arrangements with the management or offer the person in charge of the courts a fee.

The following list contains those tennis facilities I have found to be the most desirable and most accessible from where your ship may dock:

Acapulco: Acapulco Princess Hotel or the Pierre Marques (a twenty-minute ride from port), or the Acapulco Plaza (a five-minute ride from port).

Anguilla: Malliouhana Hotel and Cap Juluca.

Antigua: St. James's Club, Halcyon Beach Resort, Curtain Bluff.

Aruba: Hyatt, Holiday Inn, Sheraton, Americana, Aruba Caribbean, or Concorde.

Barbados: Sam Lord's Castle (a thirty-minute ride from port, but a lovely place to spend the day), Sandy Lane, Glitter Bay, or Royal Pavillion.

Bermuda: Southampton Princess.

Cabo San Lucas: Las Ventanas.

Cancun: All hotels on the strip.

Caracas: Macuto Sheraton Hotel in La Guaira.

Curaçao: Sonesta or Curaçao Caribbean.

Eastern Mediterranean: On Corfu, at the Corfu Holiday Palace; in Limassol (Cyprus) at the Amathus Beach Hotel, Four Seasons, or Le Meridien; in Tel Aviv (Israel) at the Hilton; in Jerusalem (Israel) at the Hyatt or King David; in Kusadasi (Turkey) at the Fantasia and Onur; in Athens at Astir Palace complex in Vouliagmeni; in Rhodes at The Rhodos Palace or Dionysos; and in Skiathos at the Skiathos Palace.

Fiji: The Sheratons, the Fijian Resort, or the Hyatt.

Grand Cayman Island: Holiday Inn or Hyatt Regency Grand Cayman.

Great Barrier Reef: Hayman Island.

Grenada: Grenada Beach Hotel.

Guadeloupe: Club Med Caravelle (you have to "sneak" in) or Le Meridien.

Haiti: At Port-au-Prince, the Club Med, Holiday Inn, or El Rancho.

Hawaii: In Oahu, the public courts at the foot of Diamond Head, the hotel courts at the Kahala Mandarin Oriental, or the Ihilani; in Maui, Kapalua Bay, Four Seasons, Grand Wailea, the Maui Hyatt, or the country club at Wailea; in Kauai, the Hyatt; in Kona, Mauna Kea, Mauna Lani, or Hilton Waikoloa.

Jamaica: In Montego Bay, Round Hill, the Half Moon, Holiday Inn, or Intercontinental; in Ocho Rios, the Renaissance, San Souci, or Syboney.

Kenya: Windsor Hotel and Country Club near Nairobi and Mt. Kenya Safari Club.

Malaysia: In Penang, at the Rasa Sayang; in Sabah, at the Tanjung Aru Beach Resort; in Langkawi, at the Radisson, Sheraton, or Datai.

Martinique: Bakoua Beach, the Meridien, or Club Med.

Nassau: Holiday Inn, Radisson Grand, Atlantis, or Ocean Club (all located on Paradise Island) or Cable Beach near the harbor.

Peter Island: Peter Island Resort.

Puerto Rico: In San Juan, the Caribe Hilton, Holiday Inn, Sheraton, or El San Juan; or drive out to the lovely Hyatt Dorado or Hyatt Regency Cerromar hotels (a forty-five-minute to one-hour drive from port) or the El Conquistador (a 40-mile drive from port).

Puerto Vallarta: Melia Posada Vallarta, Fiesta Americana, or Holiday Inn.

Rio de Janeiro: Sheraton or Intercontinental hotels.

Santo Domingo: El Embajador, the Sheraton, or Casa de Campo (a two-hour drive).

St. Barts: Guanahani.

St. Croix: at Carambola or Buccaneer.

St. John: Caneel Bay or Hyatt Regency St. John.

St. Lucia: Latoc or Club Med.

St. Maarten: Mullet Bay, La Samanna, or Little Bay Beach.

St. Thomas: The Frenchmen's Reef, Virgin Grand, Lime Tree, or Ritz-Carlton.

Seychelle Islands: On Mahé, at the Sheraton Plantation, and other resorts.

Singapore: Shangri-La and Rasa Sentosa.

Tahiti: On the big island, the courts at Maeva Beach Hotel, the Hyatt, or the Tahiti Beachcomber Parkroyal; in Bora Bora, at Bora Bora Lagoons or the Hotel Bora Bora; and in Moorea, at the Club Med, Moorea Beachcomber Parkroyal, or the Kia Ora Moorea Hotel.

Thailand: In Pataya, at the Royal Cliff, in Bangkok at the Oriental, or in Phuket at Amanpuri or Banyon Tree.

Virgin Gorda: Little Dix Bay Resort or Bitter End.

Western Mediterranean: On Capri, at the Luna or Grand Quisisana; in Cannes, at Montfleury; in Cap Antibes at Hotel du Cap; in Majorca, at Formentor, Arbella, or Son Vida; in Marbella, at Puente Romano or Los Monteros; in Portfino, at the Splendido; in San Remo, at the Grand; in Lake Como at Villa d' Este; in Taormina, at the Holiday Inn; in Venice, at Grand Hotel des Bains, the Excelsior Palace, or Cipriani.

Several cruise lines have introduced tennis programs on many of their cruises. Well-known tennis pros give group lessons aboard ship, then organize tennis matches while in port. These programs have met with enthusiastic approval by tennis-oriented cruisers. Hopefully, more of these tennis programs will be offered on cruise lines in the future.

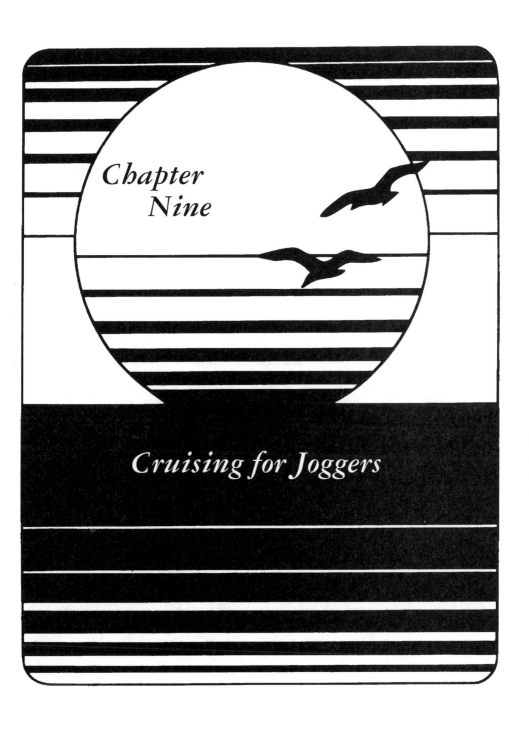

Chapter
Nine

Cruising for Joggers

Like so many health-oriented travelers, during the past decade I have become addicted to the sport of jogging as a program for staying fit and trim. The widely held notion that on a cruise one pigs out and adds a quick ten pounds has frightened away many weight-conscious joggers. If you are one of this dedicated breed, allay your fears. It is possible to run (or take a long walk) every day on the vast majority of cruises.

Just as the inveterate gambler will choose a ship that either has its own casino or visits ports that offer gambling, so a dedicated jogger (or walker) will want to select a ship that provides a jogging track or one that makes sufficient stops to afford him or her ample opportunity to follow the regular program.

In recent years, most of the large- and middle-size ships have provided special areas for jogging. Often this involves romping around the circumference of an outside deck, or running back and forth in a horseshoe path. Although the giant vessels of Royal Caribbean, Princess, Carnival, Costa, and Crystal Cruises, and the *Norway* and *QE2* offer the longest, uninterrupted expanse, most of the others have designated deck space to accommodate those wishing to walk off meals or jog. The dimensions for most ships sailing can be found in chapter 11.

Whenever possible, most seasoned joggers (and walkers) prefer a straight open path in sufficiently beautiful or interesting surroundings to break up the innate boredom of their daily routine. In those ports where there is insufficient time to seek out an ideal stretch of ground, I have settled for running through the main commercial areas, using this as an opportunity to sight-see and obtain the lay of the land. Although it is feasible to jog in almost every port, some offer more desirable options than others. (Forrest Gump may have jogged across the U.S., but sometimes I feel like I have jogged around the world.) The following are some of my personal recommendations in alphabetical order:

Acapulco (Mexico): The beach that fronts the Acapulco Princess, Pierre Marques, and Mayan Palace hotels is ideal. If you wish to remain closer to port, your only choice is to run along the sidewalks that border the main hotels on Acapulco Bay. The beach itself is too congested for jogging.

Alaska: On most stops in the inland passage, you can jog from the dock into town.

Amsterdam (Holland): If you walk out from the Marriott Hotel (in the center of town), turn right, and proceed for one block, you will find the entrance to a lovely park. You can run for several miles around this park, or you can exit at the opposite end. Several blocks from this exit (to your right) is a long stretch of park that leads to the zoo. A map of the city will help you find the exact locations.

Anguilla: Wherever you spend the day, there are roads and trails along which you can jog and enjoy the scenery, which includes goats and sheep. Those who prefer running on the beach will enjoy the stretch between Malliouhana and Cocolobo or in front of the villas at Cap Juluca. Another good area is the private sand road to the left of Cap Juluca.

Antigua: Jogging along the beach at any of the major resorts is a treat. If you start at Halcyon Cove, you can head toward town and go for miles.

Aruba: You can run for several miles along the beach or the road bordering the Sheraton, Aruba Caribbean, Concorde, Americana, Hyatt, and Holiday Inn hotels.

Athens: The botanical gardens in the middle of town is the most desirable locale; however, along the waterfront in Piraeus or at Vouliagmeni is also picturesque.

Bahamas: In Nassau, I prefer starting at the base of the pine-studded path in front of Paradise Paradise Hotel (to the left of the Holiday Inn on Paradise Island), proceeding straight up to Club Med, taking a left turn, and then continuing past the bridge to the Ocean Club and around the golf course to return by the beach. Because this involves several zig-zags, a map of Paradise Island would prove helpful. Other options include the 5-mile, round-trip jaunt from the harbor across two bridges to Coral Island, where Coral World is located; and jogging along the sidewalks emanating from Cable Beach. In Freeport, there are numerous quiet beach roads that front the hotels. In the Abacos, you can enjoy an uninterrupted, several-mile run on the beaches.

Bali (Indonesia): If you are in the Nusa Dua area, there are numerous sidewalks between the various resorts, and you can either run along these sidewalks that border the main road or along the beach.

Bangkok (Thailand): Since this is such a polluted city, your best bet is the 2-mile run around colorful Lumpini Park, in front of the Dusit Thani Hotel.

Barbados: If you spend the day at Sam Lord's Castle, you are relegated to the roads that run in front of the hotel. If you spend the day at Sandy Lane, there are numerous roads starting from behind the tennis courts near the golf course.

Barcelona (Spain): From where your ship docks in the main harbor, you can turn right and run for several miles on the walk that surrounds the sea. The more scenic areas are too far away.

Bermuda: The doorman at the Southhampton Princess will give you directions for a 3- to 5-mile romp that takes you behind the golf courses and lighthouse (to the right of the hotel) and permits you to return on the cliff road overlooking the sea. As an alternative, you can run in the opposite direction along the various beaches, starting at Horseshoe Beach.

Bora Bora (French Polynesia): The main island is 20 miles in circumference and has only one road that encircles the island in clear view of the lagoon. You can run for as many miles as you wish on the road from any point, or you can go the entire 20-mile distance around. If you start from the center of town at Vaitape, it is about 3 1/2 miles to Hotel Bora Bora. A more scenic run would start at Hotel Bora Bora and extend in the opposite direction from town past the new Club Med.

Buenos Aires (Argentina): If time permits, the botanical gardens and surrounding parks offer the best scenery and least congestion.

Cabo San Lucas: You can jog along the road where the tenders disembark for about a mile and a half to the Hacienda Hotel.

Cancún (Mexico): Because the sand is really too soft to permit running along the beach, you are better off jogging along the sidewalks that abut the road that connects all the major hotels.

Cannes (France): For the most local color, you will want to jog down the long stretch of walk known as "The Croissette," which is adjacent to the beach across from all the hotels.

Capri: Alas, this lovely island is so broken up with villas, walks, and hills that there is no level stretch of road that lends itself to jogging. The best I could do was to take the path that is located to the right as you walk out of the Grand Quisisana Hotel. It extends for a mile or so to the Punta Tragara Hotel. (Watch out for dog droppings.)

Caracas (Venezuela): If you spend part of the day at the Macuto Sheraton Hotel in La Guaira, you can run along the roads that line the sea (to your right as you walk out of the hotel). Otherwise, you will be relegated to the seedy harbor area next to your ship, where it is possible to run along a sidewalk for several miles (to your right as you leave the dock).

Cartagena: You can run along the sidewalk along the waterfront all the way from the old town to the Hilton. As an alternative, you can jog from your ship to town or to the ancient fortress, both being about a mile from the harbor.

Cayman Islands: Unquestionably, one of the best runs I have experienced is along Seven-Mile Beach. You can run for several miles in either direction if you start at the Holiday Inn or Hyatt.

Copenhagen: It is possible to run from the middle of town west on Sonder

Boulevard and N.Y. Carlsberg Vej to the zoo, past the Carlsberg Beer Factory. Another interesting itinerary would be to head out from the middle of town north on Vester Farimagsgade and Norre Farimagsgade to the botanical gardens and nearby Rosenborg Castle and continue north along Oster Volgade to the Langelinie Pavilion, the site of the *Little Mermaid* statue. Locals seem to prefer to jog along the canal that starts behind the Sheraton Hotel and extends for about 2 miles toward Langeline.

Corfu: Although you can easily jog through the town that is in front of the harbor, you may prefer the dirt roads and countryside commencing at the Holiday Palace, or the beach at Paleokastritsa.

Cozumel (Mexico): You can run along the side of the main road that follows the sea commencing in the middle of town and extending out past all the hotels and villas. If you go out to the Playa del Sol, you can run for several miles in either direction along this picturesque strand of beach.

Curaçao: Starting at the hotel complex near the Sonesta, you can run for several miles on a road next to the sea that goes into Willemsted.

Cyprus: The 10-mile stretch of walkways along the beach between the harbor and Le Meridien Hotel offers numerous possibilities.

Dominican Republic: From Santo Domingo, there is a path running for miles along the sea in the direction of the airport. The best jogging trails are at Casa de Campo or the Club Med at Punta Cana.

Dubrovnik: The downhill jog from the President Hotel to the harbor is easy and picturesque.

Fiji: The jogging track along the golf course overlooking the ocean at The Fijian Resort is your most picturesque choice. You can also jog along the beach at the Sheratons for several miles in either direction.

Great Barrier Reef: Many ships offer passengers the opportunity to spend the day at Hayman Island, where there are picturesque trails behind the resort.

Grenada: Starting at the Grenada Beach Hotel, you can run for several miles in either direction along the beach road. There are also roads leading from the harbor toward Grand Anse Beach.

Guadeloupe: Starting at the Club Med Caravelle, you can run along the main road in either direction.

Hawaii: In Oahu, the best stretch for jogging is around the park at the foot of Diamond Head or the paths along the beaches at Ihilani; in Maui, it is along the golf course and stretch of hotels and condos in the Kanapaali area or along the sea at Wailea; in Kauai, it is on the road from Breneke Beach to the Sheraton or the Hyatt, or around the golf course and lagoons at the Marriott Kauai.

Helsinki: The route from the harbor to the Esplanade is a colorful one.

Hong Kong: There is no ideal place to jog in this crowded city. The only open stretch extends on the harbor walk between the railroad station and the *Star Ferry* on the Kowloon side.

Ibizia: You can run for several miles on the walks that surround the harbor where your ship docks.

Ile des Pins, New Caledonia: This island is ideal for jogging on expansive beaches.

Israel: In Tel Aviv, you can proceed for miles down the scenic beach path behind the Hilton, Sheraton, and Dan hotels, or run through the resort area of Herzelia. In Jerusalem, you will enjoy running anywhere, taking in the exotic sights. A scenic run would start at the Hyatt past the University to the Intercontinental.

Istanbul (Turkey): This city is so crowded, that there is really no good place to run. You just do the best you can on the streets. It is possible to follow the path along the harbor from where your ship docks. As you exit the terminal, turn right and continue toward Ciragan Palace and Casino.

Ixtapa: You can jog along the sidewalk that runs in front of the string of high-rise hotels.

Jamaica: In Montego Bay, you may enjoy running from the harbor along the main road toward the airport past the main hotels; and in Ocho Rios you can run from the harbor toward Dunn's Falls.

Kota Kinabala: From Tanjung Aru Beach Resort, proceed along the beach or beach road toward the airport.

Kuangchow (People's Republic of China): I preferred jogging in Luihua and Yuexiu parks adjacent to the Dong Fang Hotel or the paths inside the Canton Zoo. For a different experience, you can run alongside the people cycling on special paths to and from work.

Kusadasi (Turkey): As you exit the harbor facing the town, you can turn left and run along the coast for several miles past the Koru-Mar Hotel.

Lisbon: Although you can follow the walk adjoining the harbor, a more desirable area is Estoril.

London: The best place for jogging is either around Hyde Park or through Green Park and St. James Park, where you can take in Buckingham Palace, Westminster Abbey, and Parliament.

Majorca: The best jogging is along the pine-studded paths leading out from Hotel Formentor, on the far tip of the island. You can also run along the waterfront near the harbor or along the road that encircles the Son Vida property.

Manila (Philippines): Starting at the Philippine Plaza Hotel, you can proceed for miles along Manila Bay on a clear path without venturing into the crowded city.

Manzanillo: There are good jogging paths at Las Hadas and Grand Bay Resort.

Marbella: You can run along the beach from the Punta Romano Resort into town.

Marmaris, Turkey: From port you can proceed indefinitely along the harbor past scenic hotels and resorts until it is time to turn around.

Martinique: The best path is on the road behind the Meridien and Bakoua Beach hotels.

Mazatlan: You can run for miles on the road that extends along the waterfront from town past the various hotels.

Moorea (French Polynesia): You can jog in any direction along the road that runs 37 miles around the island; it has a beautiful blue lagoon on one side, and palm trees and green-clad mountain spires on the other.

Moselle and Rhine Rivers (Germany): You will have a truly unique experience if you jump off your riverboat while it is going through a lock and meet it when it pulls into the next town. Anyone who runs a ten-minute mile or better should arrive before the boat. If this does not appeal, you can run along the riverbank at almost every port of call.

Mykonos: You can jog on the road leading out to the beach, San Stefanos, to the right of the main square (as you face the sea).

Nairobi: The paths extending along the golf course and entrance to Windsor Golf & Country Club are the best.

Nice: Running from the harbor along the walk adjacent to the beach, across the road from the hotels and apartment buildings is the most colorful, but it also very crowded.

Oman: The road along the Corniche from the harbor to Al-Bustan Palace is very picturesque.

Palermo (Sicily): If you don't make it out to Citta del Mare or the beaches at Mondelo, your best bet is running along the "smelly" waterfront for several miles to the right (facing the sea) of where your ship docks.

Paris: Running down any street of the city is colorful, but the most picturesque expanse would be adjacent to the River Seine on the Left Bank. I also enjoyed running around the Tuileries Gardens early in the morning (about three-quarters of a mile around) or along the paths in the Bois de Boulogne.

Penang (Malaysia): Starting at the Rasa Sayang Hotel, you can jog along the beach up to the Casuarina Beach Hotel.

Phuket: You can jog along any of the beaches or the roads behind the beaches.

Portofino: Although somewhat dangerous due to traffic, you can run from the town of Portofino to Santa Margarita and back.

Puerto Rico: From the harbor, near the old town where your ship docks, it is possible to jog along the waterfront to the Caribe Hilton Hotel for about 3 miles. Should you spend the day at the Hyatt Dorado or Cerromar Beach hotels, the road connecting these resorts offers some picturesque jogging, as do the golf courses.

Puerto Vallarta (Mexico): You can run down the main road from the harbor past the Posada Vallarta, Holiday Inn, and Fiesta Americana hotels (with considerable pollution), or along the beach.

Rhône and Saône Rivers (France): Here again you can run along the riverbank at almost every port of call.

Rhodes: You can run along the expansive harbor into Rhodes Town or on walks anywhere in the city.

Rio de Janeiro (Brazil): You can run for miles along the black-and-white mosaic walks that border Copacabana and Ipanema beaches, commencing at the Meridien Hotel and continuing as far as the Sheraton.

Rome: The most charming area in which to jog is the Borghese Gardens; however, it is possible to jog around the entire city. Those wishing to combine their sightseeing with exercise can jog from the Forum and Coliseum along the Tiber River to the Vatican.

St. Barthelemy: You can run along the road where the cruise ships dock in a semicircle, or in the direction of Shell Beach, or along the beach and beach road at Baie de St. Jean.

St. Croix: There are picturesque trails along the sea at Carambola Resort or at Buccaneer.

St. John: On the grounds at Caneel Bay Resort are numerous paths that will take you past lovely trees, flowers, and tropical plants.

St. Lucia: You can jog along any of the beaches or country roads. Latoc Resort is a good starting point.

St. Martin: Try jogging along the golf course and beach at Mullet Bay Resort.

St. Petersburg, Russia: You can proceed for miles along the harbor, or venture out into Nevsky Prospekt.

St. Thomas: You can jog along the road by the Virgin Grand Hotel, Magens Bay Hotel, or Lime Tree Beach Hotel. If time is a factor, you can jog from the harbor where the ship docks into the main part of town along the waterfront.

Seychelle Islands: Jogging on any of the silver-white-sand beaches is excellent. Generally, the sand is firm. My favorites for jogging were Anse Lazio and Anse Volbert on Praslin, Grand Anse on Mahé, and Grand Anse on La Digue (or jogging from town to Source D'Argent).

Singapore: The botanical gardens offer the most picturesque possibility in this lovely city. The paths on Sentosa Island are also ideal for joggers.

Stockholm: You can run from the harbor into town and follow the sea to the amusement park area.

Sydney (Australia): Hyde Park, which runs through the center of the city, and the Botanical Gardens near the Sydney Opera House are the best areas for jogging here.

Tortola: The beach at Cane Garden Bay offers the most desirable jogging possibility. Otherwise, the roads along the harbor will accommodate.

Vancouver, B.C.: Running through Stanley Park is an extraordinary experience.

Venice: The walk bordering the Adriatic in the Lido Beach area is the most picturesque and least-interrupted jogging area in Venice. You can start at the Grand Hotel de Bains and proceed for several miles past the Excelsior. An alternative is along the Grand Canal, past the parks about 1 mile to the left of San Marco, near where the cruise ships dock.

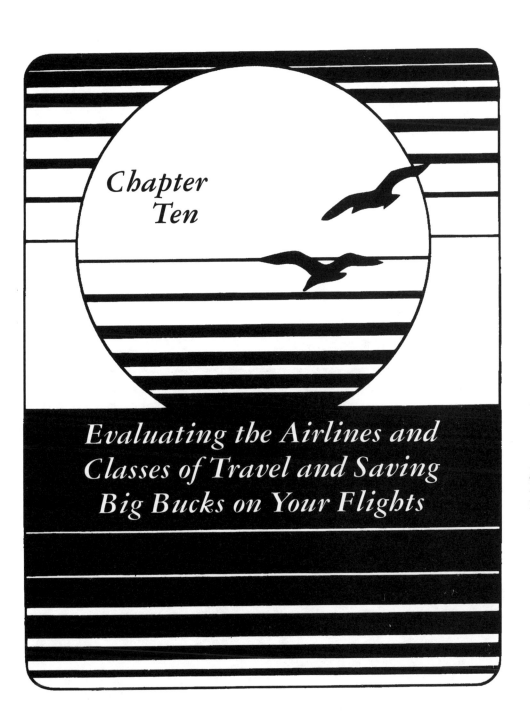

Chapter Ten

Evaluating the Airlines and Classes of Travel and Saving Big Bucks on Your Flights

For most of us, the vacation commences when we arrive at the airport and board the plane. The hassle and drudgery of planning, packing, and preparing for the trip are forgotten; the routine of our day-to-day lives is left behind; and our focus shifts to the upcoming vacation—which can get off to a good or bad start depending upon our experience during the flight. Arriving at our destination rested, well fed, and well attended to without any glitches can set a positive tone; whereas, the reverse can leave us in an ugly state of mind.

Some cruise lines are superior to others and ships of the same line and cabins at the same ship may differ in size, comfort, and amenities. Similarly, the same differences can be found on the various airlines.

When planning your trip, you may be limited to those airlines and flights servicing your destination. However, since the airlines frequently announce over the loudspeaker at the conclusion of your flight, "we know you have a choice of air carriers," the purpose of this chapter is to assist you in making that choice. We will explore the differences in equipment (model of aircraft) and the differences among the major airlines between first, business, and coach classes. We will compare comfort, services, dining, amenities, and entertainment and what each offers in its frequent-flyer program.

When selecting a particular flight, the criteria that I would recommend considering includes the type of aircraft utilized (747, 767, 727, DC-10, etc.); the width of the seats, to what degree they recline, and the leg and storage space;

the ratio of flight attendants to passengers being serviced; the number of wash-rooms for a given number of passengers and their cleanliness; the quality of meals and beverages; the personal amenities furnished passengers, such as eye masks, socks or slippers, and travel sundry kits; the caliber of in-flight entertainment including number of movies and short subjects, musical programs, and utilization of personal video machines; the air safety record; whether or not there are special airport lounge facilities for business- and first-class travelers; the policy concerning carry-on and check-in baggage; and the frequent flyer programs, including which other airline programs are honored by the line in question and which other airlines credit miles earned on the airline in question.

An important consideration when planning a flight is whether to spend the additional amount necessary (or to use up your frequent-flyer miles) to fly in first class or business class. The difference in price is very significant; business class frequently costs twice the price of a regular coach ticket and first class costs three to four times more than a coach ticket. If you compare discounted or super-saver fares, the difference is even greater.

Personally, I have found that flying first class on domestic flights in the United States and even within Europe was not very special on any of the air carriers. Other than wider seats and more leg room, there is little else to write home about. Dining and service are not comparable to what you will experience on a trans-ocean crossing and food and wine selections are generally only a small cut above coach. On flights that do not take place at meal time, snacks are very limited and the only perk is free alcoholic beverages. In addition, airlines generally use their smaller, less desirable craft and less-experienced flight attendants for domestic runs. There-fore, those contemplating a big economic splurge or saving up frequent-flyer miles may prefer waiting for a trans-ocean flight in order to get more value for their money or miles, as the case may be.

On trans-ocean flights, class upgrades deserve a higher degree of consideration. However, the higher-priced experience varies greatly among airlines. First class on a widebodied jet can be highly rewarding and relaxing, especially in the front cabin of 747s on carriers that have provided sufficient space for seats to recline to simulate the sleeping position. These aircraft also afford very generous storage space for carry-ons, including closets to hang garment bags. Air France's "L'Espace," which is gradually being introduced on its Airbus A-340, Boeing 747-400, and Boeing 767, is an innovative design for seat conversion. The width between arm rests is 21 inches and the seat reclines 180 degrees to a horizontal position; all of which is embellished with down pillows, quilted slippers, and sleeping suits. The seat is equipped with an in-seat telephone and individual video. On British Airways 747-100, 747-200, 747-400, and 747s, the first-class cabins also have revolution-ary accommodations where the seats not only gradually recline to a total horizon-tal position with a lumbar support, but also have retractable dividers with private reading lamps so that one passenger can stay up and read while a companion goes to bed. The seats are equipped with individual TV and radios operated by personal remote controls; and at the end of the allotted passenger space, there is a wood partition with a retractable "buddy" (jump) seat to permit traveling companions to chat, play board games or dine tête-à-tête. Singapore, Lufthansa and many of the other major airlines are gradually adopting similar innovations on some of their craft. However, where non-widebodied jets are employed, the comfort level does not come close and space limitations do not permit the same degree of comfort. Therefore, you would be well advised to obtain all pertinent details about the type of plane and composition of the first-class cabin before booking your flight.

Similarly, business class also varies among aircraft, and the most spacious accommodations again are found on the 747s. Where the airline has split the business-class section between the main cabin and the upper level, the upper level area tends to be more comfortable and quieter and frequently enjoys better service. The distance between your seat and the one in front of you can vary as much as a foot on different aircraft, which represents a significant difference in how far you can stretch your legs and tilt back your seat. Smaller planes generally do not offer a business-class section and many airlines are dispensing with first-class altogether and have combined first and business and assigned a new "class" designation for its more desirable cabin areas. Where there is no first class section, business class tends to be more upscale.

Here again, on British Airways and Air France's 747s, the seats recline almost 130 degrees with a lower leg cushion and include built-in, remote-control TVs and radios; however, the seats on these companies' Concorde flights are quite close together, providing only a bit more space than in the average coach.

United and American are following the lead of British Airways and Air France and introducing 180 degree reclining seats, 6'6" in length in first class, and improved business-class seats with adjustable seat cushions, lumbar supports, winged headrests, and individual reading lights.

Food, service, and amenities generally will be better in business class than coach and will be even better in first class. However, "better" is a relative term, and the caliber of these items varies on the different airlines.

One of the best first-class flights I experienced was six years ago on United between Chicago and Singapore. The first-class cabin was only half full and I was rewarded with extremely attentive service. Dinner featured Beluga-Malossol caviar expertly served with the appropriate accouterments; Swedish Gravlax, a salad of expensive greens mixed at your table (seat); and lobster raviolis and filet mignon carved from a cart. Alcoholic beverages included Dom Perignon Champagne, VSOP Courvoisier Cognac, a premier cru Puiligny Montrachet, a Nuit St. George, and several classified French Bordeauxs. Four recently released full-length movies were presented and the complimentary overnight survival kits contained a bevy of designer-brand sundries and cosmetics. A more recent first-class flight on United between Hong Kong and Los Angeles, where the first-class cabin had a larger capacity, exhibited similar food and service but was not as good as the prior experience. First class on Singapore Airlines was also quite impressive. On Northwest Airlines 747 flights across the Pacific and Southeast Asia, the first-class section accommodates eight to ten passengers on the second level of the aircraft, which allows maximum space and comfort and gives one the feeling of being on a private jet.

On the flip side, first-class flights on numerous other airlines, as well as other routes on the aforementioned carriers, did not include the same quality of cuisine, the variety of expensive wines, nor the impeccable service. Business class on all of the airlines does not measure up to the special treatment you receive in first class. Seats are almost as comfortable but are closer together and do not extend to the same horizontal position. On-board amenities are a bit scaled down. Service is not as attentive and dining and beverages are not close to that served in the front of the plane. In fact, on some flights food and service were only a smidge better than that found in coach. However, on a number of airlines where first and business classes have been combined, I found food, service, and amenities approaching the first-class level. This was especially true on Cathay Pacific. British food critic Egon Ronay rated Air France number one in the food department, followed by KLM.

For those considering a transatlantic Concorde flight offered by British Airways and Air France, remember that the flights are offered only between London and Paris and New York and Washington, D.C. Although transatlantic flying time is cut in half, for those that must change aircraft (and possibly airports) to complete their trip, the total time savings may not be significant. As indicated earlier, seats on the Concorde are very close together. Food and beverages are first class, but, by necessity, served poorly due to lack of time and space. These flights seem best suited to passengers who do not need to change planes and who feel that saving a few hours is worth thousands of dollars and foregoing the creature comforts of first class on other aircraft.

"Coach" is pretty much "coach" on most airlines (the original "Greyhound" of the skies), where the comfort level depends chiefly on the type of aircraft and the number of passengers on any given flight. Up until the deregulation in the late 1980s, the average coach seat offered a 34-inch pitch, providing adequate leg room. Today the average pitch is an uncomfortable 31 inches, and often even less. Boeing 737s and 757s, with rows of three seats on each side of a single aisle, offer the least space, whereas the A-320 Airbus and Boeing 777 offer the most. Several of the European and Asian airlines provide better service and better food; however, I have yet to experience excellence or any degree of comfort on a "coach" flight. Helpful hints would include reserving an aisle and window seat for two and hoping no one will book the middle, opting for a bulkhead or emergency exit seat to obtain more leg room, and sitting at the front of the plane in order to exit earlier. Avoid seats in the last row or in front of an emergency exit, which may not recline. Where movies are to be shown, you will want to be certain your seat has a clear view to the screen. If you cannot abide airplane food or the advanced special-request options (for those on special diets or ordering children's meals), then I recommend packing your own repast or picking something up at the airport. A survey conducted in 1998 indicated that U.S. airlines spent $3.17 on food for each domestic passenger. When describing his overall opinion of the coach flights he experienced, Egon Ronay commented that the seats were "kneecrunching, the food disgusting and the lavatories inadequate." I am afraid that I have to agree. In fact food and service on domestic U.S. flights (if available at all) has recently reached new lows.

There is a rising tide of consumer dissatisfaction with airline practices. In 1999, six consumer-rights bills were introduced in the U.S. House and Senate. These bills are designed to protect passengers from arbitrary airline practices and poor treatment. It was further proposed that the airlines' liability for losing luggage and bumping passengers be doubled. According to the University of Michigan's "American Customer Satisfaction Index," the airline industry ranked 32nd in customer satisfaction, just ahead of the Internal Revenue Service.

The major world airlines are beginning to adopt sophisticated systems that feature a video screen at each seat with a choice of movies, video games, shopping, and even gambling. These cost millions of dollars to install in an aircraft and will first appear on trans-oceanic flights in first and business classes on the larger carriers. Japan Airlines introduced special eyeglasses fitted with tiny video screens to its first class passengers in June 1998. At the cost of $500 per pair, the glasses simulate the experience of watching a 62-inch movie screen.

A survey of publications that rate airlines in 1999 indicated that Singapore Airlines was *Conde Nast, Zagat,* and *Business Traveller International*'s choice for the best overall airline. Midwest Express was the choice for the best of the U.S. airlines.

Travel and Leisure's Readers' Survey rated Singapore, Qantas, Swissair, Cathay Pacific, and Thai as their choices for the top five airlines; and Midwest Express, Alaska, United, Delta, and American as their five favorite U.S. carriers. The 1999 *Conde Nast Readers' Survey* ratings for international routes had Singapore at the top, followed by Swissair, Quantas, Japan, and Virgin Atlantic; and for domestic, Midwest took the honors, followed by Alaska, United, American, and Horizon. Personally, I do not agree with all of these selections and believe that "readers' surveys" must be discounted somewhat due to the fact that many of the parties casting a vote have limited flying experience and have not flown on a fair sampling of the various airlines.

For those concerned with safety records, *Conde Nast* conducted an in-depth statistical study. Their article included the following data: in an average year, 200 Americans die in airplanes, 42,000 in auto accidents, 13,000 in falls; 6,500 are poisoned and 2,900 choke on food. The most fatal crashes occurred on Boeing 727s (which is also the aircraft longest in service); the airports with the most accidents since 1955 are JFK (New York), O'Hare (Chicago), LAX (Los Angeles), and Heathrow (London). U.S. airlines have one fatality for every 7.5 million passengers, whereas the overall fatality rate is a little less than one per million. Airlines never experiencing a fatality included Southwest, Ansett, KLM, America West, Hawaiian, Sabena, Singapore, and Quantas; whereas those with the most fatalities were Vietnam, China, Egypt Air, Philippine, Air India, Korean Air, and Midwest Express.

Certainly obtaining the best price for your ticket is a major consideration. Because air fares change constantly, there is no substitute for checking out the price of the various carriers. I have found that when exploring the price of a ticket with an airline, a travel agent, and over the Internet, prices can vary from day to day and even from hour to hour depending upon cancellations and the airline making additional low-cost fares available. Therefore, when time permits, it may be prudent not to be rushed into purchasing your ticket, but rather to check on the lowest fare over several days or weeks with different sources.

At best, airline pricing is complicated and on any given flight, passengers in the same area of the plane are paying widely divergent fares. Business travelers and others who book flights on short notice generally end up paying the highest fares, whereas those that have the luxury of booking several months in advance and who are willing to travel mid-week, on off-hours, or from less popular airports have first crack at the lower super-saver tariffs. Recently, I found that off-season fares offered for round-trip flights to Europe for a weekend were lower than those from Chicago to New York.

The International Air Transport Association is a cartel of most of the world's major airlines and attempts to control prices; however, most airlines have sources to unload unsold seats at discounted prices through third parties such as consolidators and discount travel agents.

For those of you interested in accomplishing big savings on your next flight, two books devoted to this topic are Michael William McColl's *The Worldwide Guide to Cheap Airfares,* and Wunder and Leach's *Airfare Secrets Exposed.* In addition, there is *Consumer Report,* travel newsletters, and numerous web sites that have sprung up that list the best fares available on different dates for the various routes. Some travel web sites allow you to tell the airlines what you want to pay for a ticket to a particular destination at a specific time. If an airline chooses to accept your offer, it will e-mail back an acceptance, or it may make a counteroffer.

McColl suggests three major sources of "cheap tickets": consolidators, charter flights, and air-courier services. He describes consolidators as akin to factory-outlet stores that are used by most airlines to unload empty seats, especially as the date of the flight approaches. I have found that the Sunday travel section of most big-city newspapers carries numerous consolidator ads with sample prices. Rarely do the consolidators come through with the prices advertised; however, savings from 1/3 to 2/3 off of regular coach fares are readily available. Generally, consolidator tickets are non-refundable, only available in coach, cannot be upgraded with frequent-flyer miles, and are the best value in off-seasons. However, there are exceptions to all of the above. Different airlines use different consolidators and some receive bigger discounts from airlines with whom they do the most business. Therefore, it is best to price-shop several before booking any particular flight. As further precautions, it is best to use a consolidator with a local office and to verify the reservation that is made on your behalf with the airline. Wunder and Leach also list consolidators located in the various U.S. cities, as well as "bucket shops" (as consolidators are known in London and Germany).

Many companies offer charter airplane flights with nonstop service to popular destinations during busy seasons. Although these planes tend to be packed and uncomfortable, budget-minded travelers can often save 15 to 50 percent off of regular coach fares. Most travel agents can book these flights for you, as well as Group Inclusive Tour (G.I.T.) Fares and Tour Operator Packages, all of which offer fares generally lower than the airlines. You can take advantage of these packages and not utilize the land arrangements.

An air courier is someone who delivers packages for companies in the international overnight shipping business such as Federal Express or DHL. There are air-courier companies (listed in both of the above guides) who broker tickets for these shipping companies. Typically the passenger gives up his checked-baggage allowance to make space for the courier's packages, agrees to travel on a specific flight at a specific time, helps the courier clear customs with the merchandise, and in return receives a discount of 50 percent or more on his air ticket. Thus, those who are interested in pursuing this route must be able to carry on all of the luggage they personally require and have a certain amount of flexibility in their time for travel. Unfortunately, the courier company dictates the dates and destinations for travel and provides very limited opportunities to bring a companion.

Other price-saving approaches would be to use discount travel agents (who kick back a portion of their commission); to fly on a "low-fare" airline such as Midway Airlines, Midwest Express, Kiwi, American Trans Air, Frontier, Airtran, Delta Express, Pro Air, Reno Air, Southwest, or National Air in the U.S. and Air Europa, Virgin Express, Ryanair, and City Bird on international flights; or to book space on flights bound to popular destinations at busy seasons and volunteer to get bumped at the airport in exchange for free travel on the next available flight.

The low-fare/no-frills air carriers fly the same type of planes as the majors and are subject to the same regulatory safety standards. However, they often operate from less-central or less-popular airports, offer no meals, even on longer flights (which may be a blessing), and will not make advance seating assignments. The Internet weekend specials offered by major carriers afford attractive deals (try www.webflyer.com). Also airlines offer "Senior Savings' coupon books" (for those over 62), "air-pass" multi-flight coupon books of discount tickets for travelers who reside in a different country (similar to a Eurail Pass); and some, such as American and TWA, offer special student fares.

An airline's policy regarding check-in and carry-on baggage is another concern for passengers. Ideally we would all prefer to travel light and not have to worry about heavy suitcases and the inconvenience of maneuvering suit bags and parcels through the aisles of the plane. However, recreational travel on cruise ships and to fine resorts often requires us to include a variety of workout and sports equipment, a number of diverse outfits for evening wear, and a full complement of sundry items. Those who prefer to have a different outfit daily are doubly cursed. Therefore, information on the number and weight of suitcases allowed to be checked in and dimensions of those to be carried onto the plane is a necessity. Often, I witness passengers at international airports feverishly attempting to eliminate a prohibited suitcase by stuffing clothes into other pieces of luggage or their coat pockets to avoid expensive surcharges. All of this can be avoided by calling the airline in advance for their policies on the flight you have booked. Baggage allowances do vary among the airlines and are uniformly more liberal in first class.

Rercently airlines have adopted a far more restrictive policy regarding "carry-ons," which is strictly enforced. Therefore, if you expect to be allowed to retain your carry-ons, it is best to comply with the airline's quoted limits. While on the subject of carry-ons, it should be noted that airlines frequently lose luggage temporarily due to placing it on the wrong flight. However, until it is returned, you must survive with what you are wearing or what you placed in your carry-on. Therefore, I recommend treating your carry-on as a survival kit that affords you at least 48 hours worth of clothes and sundries. Of course, valuables should always be kept on your person.

Passengers traveling first class and business class are often entitled to admittance to a private lounge that provides special amenities ranging from comfortable chairs, telephones, coffee, tea, soft drinks, pretzels, and newspapers to free alcoholic beverages, Continental breakfasts, small sandwiches, sophisticated business equipment, meeting rooms, and even showers and changing rooms. The availability of these facilities varies among the airlines and the airport involved. Often airlines with no lounge in a particular airport may offer reciprocity to selected other carriers. The private lounges located in the major airports around the world tend to be better and more plentiful than in the less-traveled locations. Possibly, the best-equipped, most amiable lounges offering the most amenities are the First Class and Club World Class lounges of British Airways, especially at Heathrow.

Many airlines have membership clubs where an annual fee ranging from $100 to $300 entitles you to the use of all of that airline's and its affiliates' private lounges around the world, regardless of what airline you are flying or the type of ticket you hold. Some of these even permit a one-day membership that generally runs from $25 to $50. Those considering joining an airline's private club should investigate which airports have branches, the facilities available, and whether there are any affiliated airline clubs that offer reciprocity.

Acquiring mileage awards on frequent-flyer programs has become as popular a pastime as the lottery and clipping grocery coupons. Today you can earn points not only by flying but also by using a particular credit card, renting a car, or staying at a hotel. I once read an article that indicated American Airlines was launching a program that will award one mile for each dollar in interest you pay on your mortgage. However, as the airlines create more and more ways to earn miles, they end up with more and more miles waiting to be redeemed. To counteract this potential problem, the airlines periodically increase the number of miles required for a particular reward, as well as create earlier expiration dates that often fall due before the holder can arrange for a trip.

Those of us who have attempted to cash in our air miles have often experienced the reality that the hype is a lot more appealing then the actuality. Unfortunately, the most desirable dates for travel, such as holidays, are usually blocked out; and at other times, only a limited number of seats on any given flight are available. Therefore, those wishing to use their frequent-flyer miles must book early and often be willing to travel on a day or at a time other than is optimum for their travel plans.

In order to maximize your frequent-flyer mileage awards, it is often advantageous to give your free award ticket to a traveling companion, pay for your own ticket, and thereby earn additional miles. Also, if you pay for a discounted coach ticket and use miles to upgrade, you still earn frequent-flyer miles for the flight; whereas if you used the miles to purchase the entire ticket, you would receive no future frequent-flyer miles for the flight. This may be especially valuable on longer flights. However, many airlines will not permit upgrades when using consolidator or discounted tickets.

The various airlines have different policies with regard to the number of miles they require for any given award, as well as with which other airlines they give or receive reciprocity. Because the programs offered by the various airlines are constantly changing, it is necessary to obtain their latest frequent-flyer brochures at least annually. You will then wish to compare the number of miles each requires for a free coach-, business-, or first-class ticket to various destinations; how many miles for an upgrade; how long a period you have to cash in your miles; which other airlines honor their miles; and whether they honor miles earned on other airlines.

For most of us, it is preferable to decide upon one or two favorite airlines in order to accumulate enough miles to earn an award. If you are constantly flying on different airlines, it is difficult to build up a meaningful balance. Further, building up miles on any given airline often results in being able to acquire various levels of "Elite Status" that entitles you to preferential check-in, use of special lounge facilities, easier access to bookings, last-minute upgrades when space is available, and other perks. The mileage necessary to reach Elite Status varies among the airlines, but generally requires 15,000 to 25,000 miles per year. Once attained the status extends through the following 12- to 14-month period.

Hopefully the above has provided you with some food for thought, and you will be able to make future flight arrangements more wisely and economically.

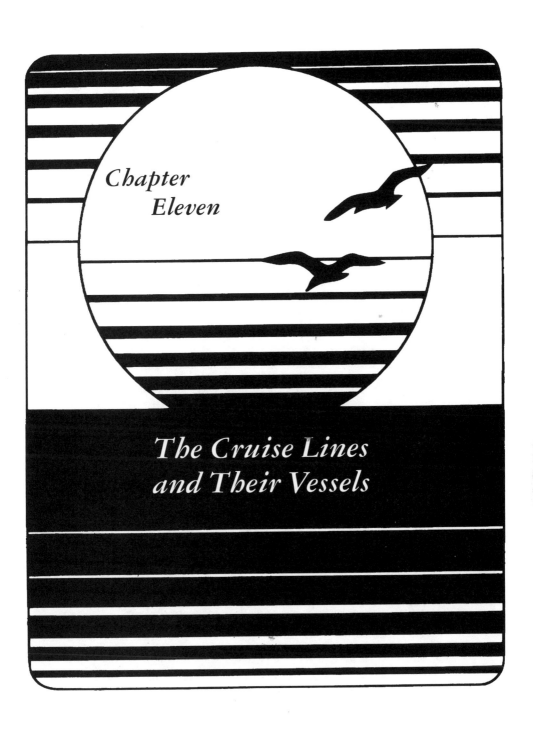

Chapter Eleven

The Cruise Lines and Their Vessels

In this chapter, you will find a section describing every major cruise line, including photographs for those we were able to obtain them from, a dinner menu, and a daily program for most of the ships of each line. The synopsis at the beginning of each section lists the vessels currently sailing, their former names, the date they entered service, the date they were refurbished, gross tonnage, length and width, maximum passenger capacity, number of cabins, nationality of officers and crew, usual itineraries, and my overall ratings, i.e., Ribbon Awards. (An explanation of the significance of the Ribbon Awards is given in chapter 12.) Briefly, the ships are divided into four market categories based on per diem prices for average cabins, on-board costs, and the economic class of passengers the cruise line seeks to attract:

Category A   (black ribbons) being the most expensive—Deluxe.
Category B   (crisscrossed ribbons) being the next most expensive—Premium.
Category C   (diagonal ribbons) being the middle-priced market—Standard.
Category D   (white ribbons) being the least expensive—Economy.

The ships are then rated on a six-point system, six+ ribbons being the highest. Only oceangoing cruise ships are rated. No ratings are given for riverboats.

In the text of each section, you will find a brief history of the cruise line, a description of the physical makeup of each ship, including cabins, inside and outside public areas, dining, service, pricing, usual itineraries, and my opinion of the strongest points.

Note: Commencing with the prior (1999) edition we changed our ribbon award system from a five-point system to a six-point system in order to conform with rating systems used in other cruise guides and to avoid confusion for our readers.

The intent of this chapter is to provide readers with as much information as possible in a succinct, organized fashion, so as to enable them to make their own intelligent selections for their cruise vacation.

THE CRUISE LINES
AND THEIR VESSELS

ABERCROMBIE & KENT
AMERICAN CANADIAN CARIBBEAN LINE, INC.
AMERICAN HAWAII CRUISES
AQUA VIVA CRUISE LINES
CARNIVAL CRUISE LINES
CELEBRITY CRUISES
CLIPPER CRUISE LINE
CLUB MED CRUISES
COMMODORE CRUISE LINE
COSTA CRUISE LINES
CRYSTAL CRUISES
CUNARD LINE (CUNARD BRAND AND SEABOURN BRAND)
PETER DEILMANN EUROPAMERICA CRUISES
THE DELTA QUEEN STEAMBOAT COMPANY
DISNEY CRUISE LINE
EUROPE CRUISE LINE/1ST CLASS HOLIDAYS
EUROPEAN WATERWAYS
FRENCH COUNTRY WATERWAYS
HAPAG-LLOYD
HOLLAND AMERICA LINE
K D RIVER CRUISES OF EUROPE
MEDITERRANEAN SHIPPING CRUISES
METROPOLITAN TOURING'S GALAPAGOS CRUISES
NORWEGIAN CRUISE LINE
ORIENT LINES
P & O CRUISES
PREMIER CRUISE LINE
PRINCESS CRUISES
RADISSON SEVEN SEAS CRUISES

RENAISSANCE CRUISES, INC.
RIVERS OF EUROPE/DANUBE CRUISES AUSTRIA
ROYAL CARIBBEAN CRUISE LINE
ROYAL OLYMPIC CRUISES
SEA AIR HOLIDAYS, LTD.
SEABOURN CRUISE LINE (SEE CUNARD LINE, ABOVE)
SHERATON NILE CRUISES
SILJA LINE
SILVERSEA CRUISES, LTD.
SONESTA HOTELS AND NILE CRUISES
STAR CLIPPERS, INC.
STAR CRUISES
WINDJAMMER BAREFOOT CRUISES
WINDSTAR CRUISES
WORLD EXPLORER CRUISES

ABERCROMBIE & KENT
1520 Kensington Road
Oak Brook, Illinois 60521
(800) 323-7308

ACTIEF: entered service 1980; reconstructed 1989; 100' x 16.5'; 11-passenger capacity; 6 cabins; British officers and crew; cruises on River Thames, Great Britain.

ALOUETTE: entered service 1986; 98' x 16'; 6-passenger capacity; 3 cabins; cruises to Burgundy and Franche Comté in France.

ANACOLUTHE: 210' x 24'; 51-passenger capacity; 26 cabins; cruises on Seine and Yonne rivers in France.

CAPRICE: 128' x 17'; 22-passenger capacity; 11 cabins; cruises on Franche Comté and eastern Burgundy.

CHANTERELLE: refurbished 1994; 128' x 16'; 24-passenger capacity; 14 cabins; cruises in upper Loire, France.

EXPLORER: (formerly *Lindblad Explorer* and *Society Explorer*); entered service 1969; renovated 1992; 2,398 G.R.T.; 238' x 46'; 100-passenger capacity; 50 cabins; European officers and Filipino crew; transatlantic cruises and cruises in Antarctica, the Amazon, and the North Atlantic, including Reykjavik, Iceland, and Spitsbergen, and Norway.
(Medical Facilities: P-1; EM, CLS, MS; N-0; CM; PD; EKG; TC; EPC; OX; WC; OR; CCP; TM; LJ.)

FLEUR de LYS: entered service 1986; 129' x 16.5'; 7-passenger capacity; 4 cabins; British officers and mixed crew; cruises in the Burgundy and Franche Comté regions of France.

HALAS: entered service 1911 (subsequently rebuilt as a yacht in the eighties and refurbished); 160' x 28'; 30-passenger capacity; 15 cabins; Turkish crew; cruises along Turkish Coast.

HIRONDELLE: entered service 1994; 128' x 16'; 8-passenger capacity; 4 cabins; cruises Burgundy and Franche Comté in France.

L'ABERCROMBIE: entered service 1982; refurbished 1991; 128' x 16'; 22-passenger capacity; 11 cabins; British officers and British and French crew; cruises in central Burgundy.

LAFAYETTE: entered service 1983; refurbished 1991; 128' x 16'; 22-passenger capacity; 12 cabins; British officers and British and French crew; cruises in lower Burgundy, France.

LIBELLULE: entered service 1996; 128' x 16'; 20-passenger capacity; 10 cabins; French and British officers and crew; cruises in Champagne region of France.

LITOTE: entered service 1979; refurbished 1991; 128' x 16'; 20-passenger capacity; 10 cabins; French officers and French and British crew; cruises on canals of northern Burgundy, France.

LORRAINE: 128' x 17'; 22-passenger capacity; 11 cabins; cruises in Alaska.

MARJORIE II: entered service 1998; 128' x 16.5'; 12-passenger capacity; 6 cabins; cruises on the Seine and Yonne rivers between Paris and Auxerre; and in Holland during Tulip season.

NAPOLEON: entered service 1991; 129' x 16.5'; 12-passenger capacity; 6 cabins; cruises on Rhône River in Provence, France, and Saône in Burgundy.

REMBRANDT: 133' x 16'; 18-passenger capacity; 10 cabins; cruises in Belgium and Holland.

RIVER CLOUD: entered service 1996; 360' x 37'; 90-passenger capacity; 45 cabins; European officers; Danube River cruises.

ROAD TO MANDALAY: 126-passenger capacity; 330' long; 66 cabins; cruises the Ayeyarwady River in Myanmar.

SEA CLOUD: entered service 1931; renovated 1979 and 1993; 360' x 50'; 69-passenger capacity; 34 cabins; international officers and crew; Mediterranean and Caribbean cruises. (**Category A—Not Rated**)

SUN BOAT II: 64-passenger capacity; 32 cabins; Nile River cruises.

SUN BOAT III: 40-passenger capacity; 20 cabins; Nile River cruises.

SUN BOAT IV: 84-passenger capacity; 42 cabins; Nile River cruises.

VINCENT VAN GOGH: entered service 1997; 217' x 23'; 32-passenger capacity; 16 cabins; Dutch officers and crew; cruises in Holland and Belgium.

Abercrombie & Kent is one of the largest tour operators in the world, specializing in the upscale travel market. Many of its tours include sailing on cruise ships, riverboats, and barges. Although the various vessels (other than the *Sun Boat*s and

Explorer) are independently owned and operated by several companies, A & K markets them and, in many situations, has chartered the entire ship or boat for its tours.

A & K has offered barge and river cruises since the sixties. Today, it offers 14 barges with itineraries in the Burgundy, Provence, Champagne, Alsace, and Loire Valley regions of France; on the Thames in Great Britain; plus river cruises through the canals and rivers of France, Austria, Germany, Hungary, Holland, and Belgium and on the rivers of Egypt and Myanmar. Most of the barges have a dining room, lounge, and outdoor observation area. These are small, intimate vessels offering a unique experience, with the emphasis on the scenic regions visited and good food and wine.

The boats are marketed as deluxe, with per diem prices ranging from $200 to $700 per night. Prices usually include all meals, wine, open bar, transportation, transfers, and sightseeing.

A & K is also marketing Antarctic, North Atlantic, and Amazon expedition cruises on the *Explorer,* formerly of Society Expeditions. The *Explorer* carries 100 passengers in 50 outside 160-square-foot cabins, two of which are suites with queen-size beds. At the top of the ship, on Bridge Deck, is a health club, sauna, hospital, and radio room. Below, on Boat Deck, are sunning space, a swimming pool, a lecture hall, a hair salon, and ten cabins. Next are a library and the *Explorer* lounge. The remaining cabins are on the two lower decks. Prices range from $128 per person per night for the lowest category cabin on the transatlantic cruise, up to $964 per person for a suite on an Antarctica sailing. Prices do not include international airfare. The ship was built to sail in Antarctica and has Zodiacs for in-depth explorations.

The 160-foot *M.Y. Halas* was built in Scotland in 1911 as a coastal cruiser and was converted to a yacht-like cruise vessel in the 1980s. Its fifteen deluxe cabins and suites accommodate thirty passengerse for a unique cruise experience from Istanbul along the Turkish Coast, including visits to Kusadasi, Ephesus, Ankara, and Antalya. Turkish cuisine is featured. Prices range from $300 to $525 per day.

The *Sea Cloud* was originally built as a private yacht for E. F. Hutton and Marjorie Merriweather Post in 1931. This luxurious four-masted barque sailing ship was renovated in 1979 and 1993 and now offers luxury sailing cruises to private groups and as part of A & K itineraries in the Mediterranean and Caribbean.

The *Road to Mandalay* is owned by London-based Venice Simplon-Orient Express, Ltd., which put this 330-foot-long river cruiser into service in 1996 to ply the waters of the Ayeyarwady River. The northbound itinerary departs from Pagan and goes upstream to Mandalay, and the southbound does the reverse. Only portions of two days are spent sailing, and the riverboat spends most of its time as a riverfront hotel at either end of the line, permitting passengers easy access to the points of interest in Myanmar (formerly Burma), including the famous Shwedagon Pagoda in Yangon (formerly Rangoon). The vessel has 66 cabins accommodating 126 passengers and includes a swimming pool, lounge, observation deck with a bar, a dining room, piano bar, and a main-deck observation lounge. Breakfast and lunch are served buffet style, and an open-seating, four-course, set-menu dinner is offered nightly.

Strong Points:

Intimate, elegant, scenic as well as educational experience, with good food and beverages on the various barges, riverboats, and small cruise ships, and with packaged land and air arrangements by one of the most successful tour operators.

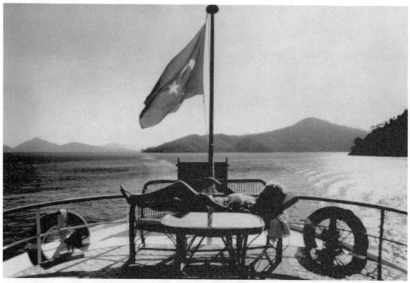

Courtesy Abercrombie & Kent

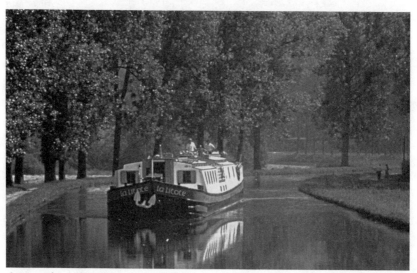

Courtesy Abercrombie & Kent

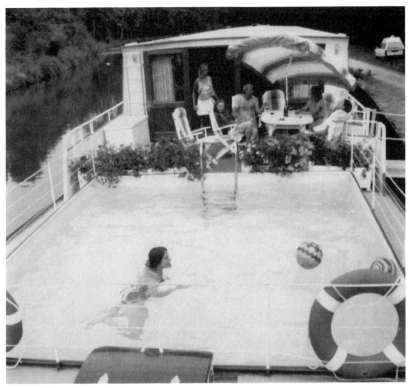

Courtesy Abercrombie & Kent

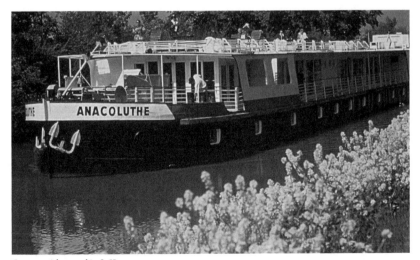

Courtesy Abercrombie & Kent

AMERICAN CANADIAN CARIBBEAN LINE, INC.
461 Water St.
P.O. Box 368
Warren, Rhode Island 02885
(800) 556-7450
(401) 247-2350 FAX

GRANDE CARIBE: entered service 1997; 98 G.R.T.; 183' x 40'; 100-passenger capacity; 50 cabins; U.S. officers and crew; cruises through Panama Canal, Belize, Guatemala, Erie Canal/Sanguenay River, Nova Scotia, Maine, and Canada. **(Category D—Not Rated)**

GRANDE MARINER: entered service 1998; 98 G.R.T.; 183' x 40'; 100-passenger capacity; 50 cabins; U.S. crew; cruises to Bahamas, Caribbean islands, Central America, Erie Canal/Sanguenay River, and Newfoundland/Labrador Canada. **(Category D—Not Rated)**

MAYAN PRINCE: entered service 1992; 98 G.R.T.; 175' x 38'; 92-passenger capacity; 46 cabins; U.S. crew; cruises in Caribbean, New England, and Newfoundland/Labrador Canada. **(Category D—Not Rated)**

NIAGARA PRINCE: entered service 1994; 98 G.R.T.; 175' x 40'; 84-passenger capacity; 42 cabins; U.S. crew; cruises in Caribbean, West Palm Beach to New Orleans, New England, Great Lakes, and Newfoundland/Labrador Canada. **(Category D—Not Rated)**
(Medical Facilities: There are no health care or handicap facilities aboard these vessels.)

The owner, president, and designer of the ships of ACCL, Luther H. Blount, founded the cruise line in 1966. These uniquely designed smaller ships specialize in destination cruises to out-of-the-way ports of call which larger vessels cannot navigate, throughout the Caribbean, Newfoundland/Labrador, New England, and Panama Canal/Central America.

Public areas include one dining room that accommodates all passengers in a single seating and one lounge used for receptions and lectures. Some staterooms have upper and lower berths, while others have two lower berths and some can be made into a double bed. All have small private facilities and limited storage.

The line advertises itself as "the original small ship cruise line . . . no-frills, informal, unpretentious, casual and friendly . . . with an emphasis on the destination, not the ship . . . no room service, no glitz and 'bring-your-own-bottle bar policy' . . . we offer unpretentious adventure for the mature, experienced traveler. . . ." Prices range from $150 to $200 per person per night, with most itineraries averaging about 12 days.

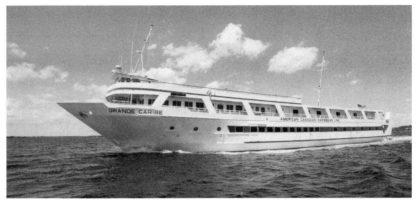

Courtesy American Canadian Caribbean Line, Inc.

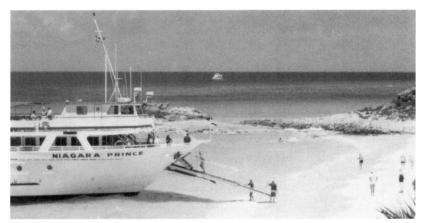

Courtesy American Canadian Caribbean Line, Inc.

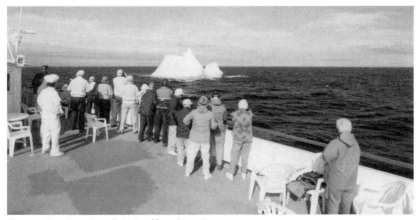

Courtesy American Canadian Caribbean Line, Inc.

AMERICAN HAWAII CRUISES
Robin St. Wharf
1380 Port of New Orleans Place
New Orleans, Louisiana 70130
(800) 765-7000
(504) 599-5579 FAX

SS *INDEPENDENCE:* (formerly *Oceanic Independence*); entered service 1951; refurbished 1980, 1989, 1991, 1994, and 1999; 20,221 G.R.T.; 682' x 89'; 1,021-passenger capacity; 446 cabins; American officers and crew; one-week cruises around the Hawaiian islands.

 +

(Medical Facilities: C-O; P-1; N-1; CM; PD; EKG; TC; PO; OX; WC; ICU; TM.)

American Hawaii Cruises was formed by an investment company that introduced the refurbished *Independence* to seven-night Hawaiian cruises in 1980. In 1993, the line was acquired by The Delta Queen Steamboat Company, and thereafter the parent company's name was changed to American Classic Voyages Company. The *Independence* was the first ship sailing under a U.S. flag with a U.S. crew since the demise of the United States, Matson, and American President lines. The *Constitution* was added in 1982, but due to the high cost associated with refurbishing the *Constitution,* the ship was taken out of service. The *Independence* embarks from Honolulu and calls at the ports of Kona and Hilo on the big island of Hawaii, as well as at the islands of Kauai and Maui. With the exception of one day at sea, the other days are spent in port, which maximizes your opportunity to explore the Hawaiian islands. Brochure rates start at about $175 per day per person, with most cabins averaging $280 and suites costing from $354 to $468. On most cruises children under 18 sharing cabins with two full-fare adults cruise free except for taxes and port charges. It is possible to take three- or four-day segments. The three-day cruise sets sail from Honolulu and stops at Kauai to let cruisers disembark in Maui, where the four-day itinerary begins, calling at both Hilo and Kona on the big island and terminating in Honolulu.

The *Independence,* originally built in the fifties, retains some of the original design of ships of that era. In the 1990s, over $78 million was spent on her renovation; however, little of this is visible, and the ship appears to have enjoyed better days. Most cabins are on the lower decks, and there are more inside accommodations than outside. Those wishing for luxury are best off opting for one of the suites located on the three upper decks. There are more than a hundred cabins that can accommodate a third or fourth passenger.

Public facilities include an exercise room, pool, theater, show lounges, lounges for drinking, a conference center, a children's playroom, a youth recreation center, a jogging track, and many of the usual facilities found on cruise ships. There is no casino because Hawaiian law does not permit gambling. In 1996, the line introduced a "Floating Greens of Hawaii" golf program where passengers can choose among 18 golf courses on four different islands, with tee times arranged by the ship's shore excursion staff.

The young, all-American crew unfortunately is not as efficient at service as European crews on other ships, and the food is plentiful and quite good for a ship in this price range, but not gourmet. The buffet breakfasts near the pool are especially plentiful and complimentary; soft drinks and juices are served around the clock. These are cruises that appeal to older couples and families wishing to see the Hawaiian islands in comfort without the inconvenience of flying from island to island and seeking out resorts and restaurants. The mood is nostalgic and Polynesian, and there are good programs for the children.

Strong Points:

Magnificent itinerary for those wishing to visit all of the major Hawaiian islands with minimum effort. Good appeal for families and older couples.

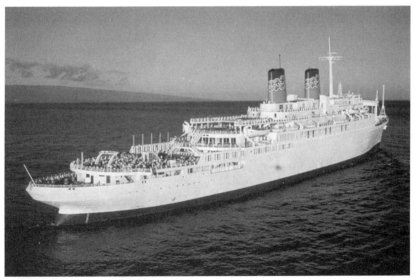

Courtesy American Hawaii Cruises

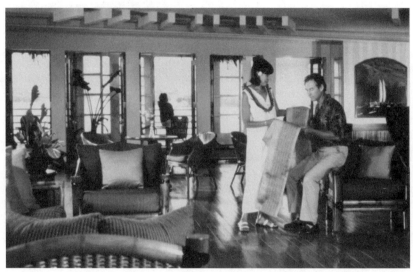

American Hawaii Cruises and the Bishop Museum of Honolulu have created a permanent shipboard interactive exhibit—the first of its kind—aboard the SS Independence *in its Kama'aina Lounge. The exhibit teaches about the customs and way of life of the Hawaiian people. It focuses on navigation and voyaging, geography and geology, arts and crafts, costumes, religion, gods and legends, food, and plants and animals. The Kama'aina Lounge is like a typical Hawaiian living room. On both sides of the room, doors open onto open-air lanais with comfortable rattan furniture. The hardwood floor is covered with area rugs featuring brightly colored Hawaiian lei borders.*

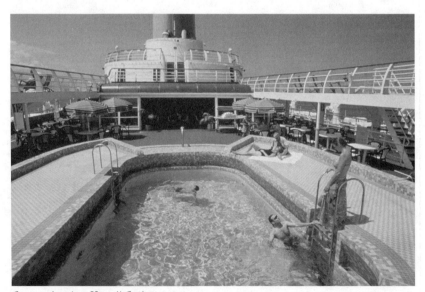

Courtesy American Hawaii Cruises

YOUR·DAILY GUIDE TO PARADISE

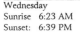

SS INDEPENDENCE
AMERICAN HAWAII CRUISES
VOYAGE 823

CAPTAIN MARK ZARYNOFF
MASTER

March 27, 1996

Wednesday		Kahului, Maui
Sunrise 6:23 AM		Dock: 8:00 AM
Sunset: 6:39 PM	Word of the Day: **Haleakala: House of the Sun**	Sail: 6:00 PM

TOUR DEPARTURE INFORMATION

M1	Haleakala Crater	Departs from the pier at 8:30 AM
M2	Iao Valley/Tropical Plantation	Departs from the pier at 8:30 AM
M3	Hana Adventure	Departs from the pier at 8:30 AM
M4	Lahaina Spree	Departs from the pier at 10:00 AM
M5	Haleakala/Hana by Helicopter	Individually Scheduled/Check Tickets
M6	West Maui Mountains/Molokai by Helicopter	Check Tickets
M8	Bicycle Haleakala (Day Trip))	Departs from the pier at 8:30 AM
M9	Atlantis Submarine (Transportation not provided)	10:30 AM check-in, Lahaina
M12	Molokini Snorkeling/Fourwinds	Cancelled
M13	Club Lanai	Cancelled
M14, 15 & 16	Whale Watching (Transportation not provided)	Check Tickets
M17	Coastal Kayak	Departs from the pier at 8:30 AM
M18	Lahaina Shuttle	Departs from the pier at 9:00 AM
M19	Horseback Riding (Transportation not provided)	Check in at ranch at 12:30 PM
M20	Hana Rainforest Walk	Departs from the pier at 9:00 AM

INDIVIDUALLY SCHEDULED TOURS depart from the pier. Please check tickets for times.
OTHER TOURS please be on the pier five minutes before your scheduled time.
The Shore Excursion Office will be open today from 7:00 AM - 12:00 PM, and 3:00 - 8:00 PM.

REMINDER: PLEASE BOOK TOURS FOR THURSDAY BY 10:00 AM TODAY. MAHALO!

AVIS RENT- A- CAR will shuttle passengers with advanced reservations to and from their office every 15 minutes from 8:00 AM until 5:00 PM.

Gangway: Aloha Deck/Purser's Foyer & Hawaii Deck/Aft

6:00	**AM**	RISE AND SHINE AEROBICS: JILL starts the day the healthy way.	**Conference Center**
6:45	**AM**	EXERCISE: Easy stretch out with JILL before Walk-A-Mile.	**Sun Deck**
7:00	**AM**	EXERCISE. WALK-A-MILE. JILL has the lap log available. It is not to late to get started and earn a "Ship Shape" certificate for walking 5 miles.	**Boat Deck**

9:15 AM	**CRAFT CLASS** **Hoi Hoi Showplace**

CRAFT CLASS
LEARN TO MAKE HAIR BARETTES with SEA SHELLS
with AUNTIE KAUI. Makes a great souvenir.
Also join KAUI for her EARRING CLASS at 10:30 today.

10:00	**AM**	HAWAIIAN ARTS and CRAFTS: On *display until sailing*.	**Ohana Deck Pool Side**
10:30	**AM**	**SHELL EARRING CLASS with KAUI.** Here is another opportunity to make a terrific souvenir for yourself or a loved one.	**Hoi Hoi Showplace** **Kama`aina Deck**
2:30	**PM**	FABRIC FLOWER CLASS with KAUI.	**Hoi Hoi Showplace**
3:00	**PM**	**UKULELE CLASS:** Join GLENN to learn an easy song.	**Kumu Study**
3:00	**PM**	**HULA LESSONS:** Learn the "Hukilau Hula". with KAUI. It's not too late to join in and graduate a "Hula Master" Friday night.	**Hoi Hoi Showplace** **Kama`aina Deck**
4:00	**PM**	**TEA TIME:** LANEY entertains, while you curb your appetite.	**Commodore's Terrace**

4:00	PM	TALENT SHOW sign-up and rehearsal	Hoi Hoi Showplace 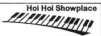

4:00 PM — TALENT SHOW sign-up and rehearsal — Hoi Hoi Showplace

Calling all passengers! Join KYM, EUGENE, ROB and CHRIS for a rehearsal for Friday night's great show.
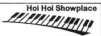

4:00 PM — HAWAIIAN IMPLEMENT CLASS — Kumu Study / Kama`aina Deck
Kumu, HAUNANI teaches the art of playing ancient Hawaiian Instruments. This class will also have a graduation on Friday.

4:30 PM — BROADWAY ON THE PACIFIC — Kama`aina Lounge / Kama`aina Deck
Join DOUG and LANEY for a "Celebration" of the music of Irving Berlin as you enjoy a light snack.

4:30 PM — LINE DANCING: Join JILL for another terrific class. She will be reviewing some of the old dances as well as teaching new ones. — Ohana Lounge / Ohana Deck

4:45 PM — $$ CASH JACKPOT BINGO $$ — Hoi Hoi Showplace

Here is our second session. Is today your lucky day? Join KEITH, KYM, and KAUI to find out.

5:00 PM — HAWAIIAN SAIL-AWAY MUSIC with ISLAND SERENADE. — Ohana Deck

5:30 PM — PORT TALK ON HILO, HAWAII WITH KYM. This talk is for those passengers not going on a guided tour. — Hoi Hoi Showplace / Kama`aina Deck

6:30 PM — "LET THE GOOD TIMES ROLL" — Hoi Hoi Showplace / Kama`aina Deck

starring
THE RAY KENNEDY ENTERTAINERS

This is for our second seating Passengers
Tonight BREK, MEENA, JENNIFER, WAYNE, LORI and KELLIE take you back to the time when dancin' was HOT and the world was in love with "Rock & Roll".

7:00 PM — BEACH BLANKET BINGO PARTY. Join BRIAN your bartender for some lively fun and special drinks until closing. — Surfrider Bar / Sun Deck

7:30 PM — DANCE TO THE SOUNDS OF THE SS INDEPENDENCE ORCHESTRA. — Hoi Hoi Showplace / Kama`aina Deck

7:30 PM — TV THEME SONG TRIVIA WITH LANIKAI — Ohana Lounge / Ohana Deck
Calling all couch potatoes! See how well you know TV themes.

8:15 PM — "LET THE GOOD TIMES ROLL" — Hoi Hoi Showplace / Kama`aina Deck

starring
THE RAY KENNEDY ENTERTAINERS

This is for our First seating Passengers
Tonight BREK, MEENA, JENNIFER, WAYNE, LORI and KELLIE take you back to the time when dancin' was HOT and the world was in love with "Rock & Roll".

9:15 PM — Dance to the 50's beat of the SS INDEPENDENCE ORCHESTRA. EUGENE LEBEAUX sets the tempo to dance, dance, dance. — Hoi Hoi Showplace / Kama`aina Deck

9:30 PM — KARAOKE — Ohana Lounge / Ohana Deck
Join the RAY KENNEDY ENTERTAINERS to be the star of our trendy sing-a-long party.

9:30 PM — BROADWAY ON THE PACIFIC — Kama`aina Lounge / Kama`aina Deck
Headliner DOUGLAS DUNNELL and LANEY BURKE will share with you "YESTERDAY'S TODAY". Enjoy the music of Broadway revivals such as "Showboat" and "Guys and Dolls" LANEY will start you off with some favorites at 9:15 PM.

| 10:00 | PM | FRIEND'S OF BILL W. MEETING | Boat Deck Lounge |

| 10:30 | PM | | Ohana Lounge
Ohana Deck |

50's/60's SOCK HOP

Tonight, slick back your hair, put on those bobby socks and join your crazy & wild Cruise Staff, KYM, LANIKAI, & THE RAY KENNEDY ENTERTAINERS for an evening of laughs and prizes. Be ready for the ever popular "ELVIS HUNT."

| 11:15 | PM | LATE NIGHT DANCING with LANIKAI YOUR D.J. | Ohana Lounge |

DINING AND LOUNGES

BREAKFAST SERVICE:

CONTINENTAL (Danish & Coffee)	5:30 AM	to	10:00 AM	SURFRIDER BAR
ALI'I BREAKFAST	6:00 AM	to	9:00 AM	OHANA BUFFET
BREAKFAST (Open seating)	7:30 AM	to	9:30 AM	HIBISCUS DINING ROOM

LUNCHEON SERVICE:

HAUOLI LUNCHEON	11:30 AM	to	1:30 PM	OHANA BUFFET
LUNCH (open seating)	12:00 PM	to	1:30 PM	HIBISCUS DINING ROOM
HAUOLI HOT-DOGS & HAMBURGERS	2:30 PM	to	4:00 PM	OHANA BUFFET

DINNER SERVICE: ATTIRE: CASUAL EVENING WEAR

	FIRST SEATING	A. 5:45 PM	DINING ROOMS
		B. 6:00 PM	
	SECOND SEATING	C. 8:00 PM	
		D. 8:15 PM	

MOON LIGHT SNACK: | 10:30 PM | to | 12:00 AM | OHANA BUFFET |

LOUNGE HOURS:

OHANA LOUNGE	9:00 AM	to	2:00 AM	OHANA DECK/AFT
HAPA HAOLE	2:30 PM	to	12:00 AM	KAMA`AINA DECK/AFT
SURFRIDER BAR	10:00 AM	to	10:00 PM	SUN DECK/AFT

DRINK SPECIALS

DRINK OF THE DAY: LAHAINA LEMONADE - $3.00
DRINKS OF THE WEEK: BIG KAHUNA OR LAVA FLOW - $4.75
SMOOTHIE OF THE DAY: (NON-ALCOHOLIC) - PINEAPPLE $3.00
Hot coffee, tea, & soda are available around the clock in the Ohana Buffet.

*** SPECIAL "BEACH BLANKET BINGO" PARTY IN THE SURFRIDER BAR ***
GET A "TIDAL WAVE" DRINK SPECIAL WITH A COMPLIMENTARY BAMBOO CUP FOR ONLY $2.50 FROM 7:00 PM UNTIL CLOSING. OR GET A LOWENBRAU FOR $1.50, OR A WARSTEINER FOR $1.50 'TIL THEIR GONE. AT 9:00 JOIN BRIAN YOUR BARTENDER TO TRY TO WIN PRIZES.

HAPPY HOUR IN THE SURFRIDER AND OHANA BAR - ALL WELL DRINKS $2.50 FROM 5:00 pm TO 7:00 pm
****

BEACH TOWELS are available at the Bell Stand for those guests spending the day on shore. Please return beach towels to the hampers located at the gangway.

YOUR OPINION COUNTS! You will receive a COMMENT CARD! Please drop your completed form at the Purser's Office by 8:00 PM on Friday. A random comment card will be drawn for a $50.00 prize.

PHOTO SALES: All photos are on display in the Photo Gallery on Aloha Deck/Aft or Starboard Lanai Ohana Deck. Try a special souvenir such as a key chain or postcard.

TODAY'S MOVIES IN THE KAUAI THEATER				
THE INDIAN IN THE CUPBOARD	ADVENTURE	(PG)	96 MINUTES	10:00 AM
NOW AND THEN	COMEDY	(PG-13)	102 MINUTES	2:00 PM
AN AFFAIR TO REMEMBER	ROMANCE	(NR)	114 MINUTES	5:00 PM
JUMANGI	ADVENTURE	(PG)	104 MINUTES	7:45 PM
AN AMERICAN QUILT	DRAMA	(PG-13)	117 MINUTES	9:45 PM

Courtesy American Hawaii Cruises

AQUA VIVA CRUISE LINES
(formerly known as French Cruise Lines)
c/o K D River Cruises of Europe
2500 Westchester Avenue
Purchase, New York 10577
(914) 696-3600
(800) 346-6525—Eastern U.S.
(800) 858-8587—Western U.S.

M.S. *ARLENE:* entered service 1986; 1,375 G.R.T.; 300' x 35'; 104-passenger capacity; 53 cabins; French officers and crew; cruises on the Rhône and Saône rivers in France.

M.S. *NORMANDIE:* entered service 1989; 1,375 G.R.T.; 300' x 35'; 104-passenger capacity; 53 cabins; French officers and crew; cruises on the Seine River in France.

(Medical Facilities: No medical facilities aboard ship—medical facilities available ashore only.)

Aqua Viva Cruise Lines (formerly known as French Cruise Lines) commenced operations in 1990, offering seven-night Provence and Burgundy cruises on the Rhône and Saône rivers between Chalon and Avignon on the M.S. *Arlene,* and seven-night Normandy cruises on the Seine River between Honfleur and Paris on the M.S. *Normandie.*

The line is represented in the United States by K D River Cruises of Europe. The *Arlene* and *Normandie* are the first larger vessels to offer itineraries down the aforementioned rivers. Previously only small river barges offered trips through the waterways of France. Although advertised by the company as cruise ships, a more appropriate description would be large, modern riverboats.

Both vessels carry approximately one hundred cruisers on two passenger decks, with cabins toward the stern and public areas forward. On the top deck are the reception desk, bar, and lounge, with the restaurant immediately below, not unlike the layout of K D's riverboats. Cabins, though small and simple, are adequate and include large picture windows, limited storage space, color TVs with in-house movies, three-channel music systems, hair dryers, individual climate controls, telephones, and private, tiled bathrooms with toilet, sink, and shower. Atop the ship are the sun deck and observation area.

The *Normandie* features seven-night cruises up and down the Seine River between Honfleur, where the Seine flows into the English Channel, and Paris. The ship visits the quaint Norman town of Caudebec; Rouen, known for its spires, bell towers, and Gothic architecture; Les Andelys, where you can visit the famous twelfth-century Chateau Gaillard, a castle built by Richard the Lionhearted; the medieval town of Vernon; and Giverny, with its Claude Monet house and gardens.

The *Arlene* offers seven-night cruises between Chalon and Avignon that pass through the picturesque Burgundy, Rhône, and Provence areas, thus affording passengers an opportunity to visit the vineyards where French Burgundy and Rhône wines are made, as well as some of Provençal France's most renowned (*Michelin Guide*) two- and three-star restaurants. Stops include Mâcon, in the heart of the Burgundy wine country; Lyon, gastronomic capital and one of the largest cities in France; Tournon, where you can take an old steam train in the photogenic region of Ardeche; and the historic villages of Viviers, Arles, and Avignon.

There is a limited number of service staff, with one person taking on the combined jobs of hotel manager, purser, and social director. Some crew members speak English, but some familiarity with French will prove helpful. However, the cuisine is extraordinary French fare, with some of the best breads, cheeses, and desserts to be found on any vessel in service. The executive chefs are members of the Confrerie de la Chaine des Rotisseurs.

Prices for the ships range from $214 per night per person on the lower deck to $241 per person on the top deck. (Prices can vary with relative value of currencies.)

Strong Points:

Comfortable, relaxing experience enabling passengers to visit some of the most picturesque and charming areas of France while enjoying sensational French cuisine.

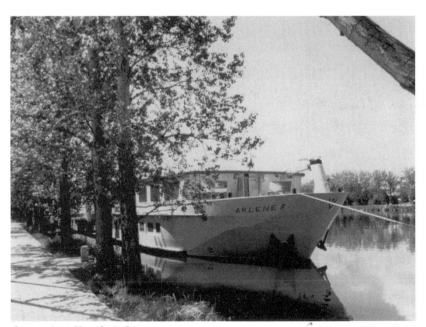

Courtesy Aqua Viva Cruise Lines

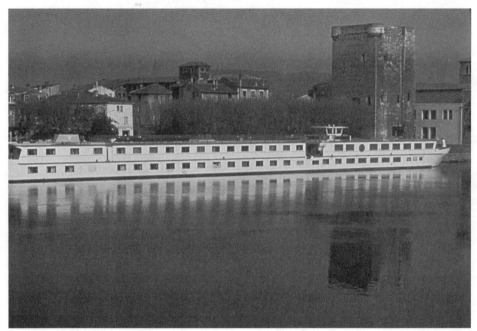

Courtesy Aqua Viva Cruise Lines

Dinner

Dîner d'Au Revoir et Cocktail
Farewell Dinner and Cocktail

~ ~

Velouté de volaille aux cèpes et son croûton
Cream of Chicken Soup with Mushrooms and Crouton

~ ~

Coussinet de Sole et Saumon à la Crème d'Oursin sur
son lit de Tagliatelles de Légumes
Fresh Sole and Salmon with Cream Sauce
on a bed of Fresh Pasta

~ ~

Crépinette de Médaillon
de Veau forestière sauce Paprika
Stuffed Medallions of Veal with Paprika Sauce

Tête de Champignons farcie,
Mousseline de Celeris, Croquette de Maïs
Stuffed Mushroom Cap, Celery Mousse,
Corn Croquettes

~ ~

Bouquet de cresson aux dés de chèvre
et pignons de pin
Watercress Salad with cubed Goat Cheese and Pine Nuts

~ ~

Gratin de Fraises au cointreau et son coulis
Fresh Strawberries with Cointreau Sauce

AQUA VIVA CRUISE LINES

Preliminary Sailing Schedule

M/S NORMANDIE

HONFLEUR - PARIS

DAY 1:   HONFLEUR

  6:30 p.m.   Embark the M/S NORMANDIE

DAY 2:   HONFLEUR

(Full-day tour to Caen Peace Museum and Normandy Landing Beaches)

  Evening   Depart Honfleur

DAY 3:   CAUDEBEC/ROUEN

  Morning   Arrive Caudebec
  Lunch   Depart Caudebec
  Evening   Arrive Rouen

DAY 4:   ROUEN/LES ANDELYS

  Lunch   Depart Rouen
  Evening   Arrive Les Andelys

DAY 5:   LES ANDELYS/VERNON

  Lunch   Depart Les Andelys
  Afternoon   Arrive Vernon

DAY 6:   VERNON/PARIS

  Early Morning   Depart Vernon
  Evening   Arrive Paris

DAY 7:   PARIS

                    Farewell Party & Illumination Cruise

DAY 8:

  8:00 a.m.   Disembark the M/S NORMANDIE

Schedule is subject to slight variations.

Courtesy Aqua Viva Cruise Lines

CARNIVAL CRUISE LINES
3655 N.W. 87th Avenue
Miami, Florida 33178
(800) 372-9501

CARNIVAL DESTINY: entered service 1996; 101,353 G.R.T.; 893' x 116'; 2,642-passenger capacity; 1,321 cabins; Italian officers and international crew; alternate seven-day cruises in eastern and western Caribbean.

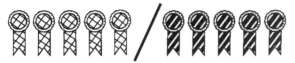

CARNIVAL TRIUMPH and *CARNIVAL VICTORY:* entered service 1999 and 2000 respectively; 102,060 G.R.T.; 893' x 116'; 2,758-passenger capacity; 1,379 cabins; Italian officers and international crew; itineraries to be determined.
(Medical Facilities for *Destiny, Victory,* and *Triumph:* C-27 (except *Destiny,* C-25); P-1; EM, CLS, MS; N-4; CM; PD; BC; EKG; TC; PO; EPC; OX; WC; ICU; X; M; LJ.)

CELEBRATION: entered service 1987; 47,262 G.R.T.; 733' x 92'; 1,486-passenger capacity; 743 cabins; Italian officers and international crew; seven-day cruises from New Orleans to the western Caribbean.

(Medical Facilities: C-14; P-1; N-3; CM; PD; BC; EKG; TC; PO; EPC; OX; WC; OR; ICU; M; LJ.)

ECSTASY and *FANTASY:* entered service 1991 and 1990 respectively; 70,367 G.R.T.; 855' x 103'; 2,040 and 2,044-passenger capacity; 1,022 cabins; Italian officers and international crew; three- and four-day cruises from Port Canaveral to the Bahamas on *Fantasy* and from Miami to the Bahamas, Key West, and Cozumel on *Ecstasy.*

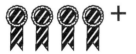

(Medical Facilities: C-20; P-1; EM, CLS, MS; N-3; CM; PD; BC; EKG; TC; PO; EPC; OX; WC; ICU; M; LJ.)

HOLIDAY: entered service 1985; 46,052 G.R.T.; 727' x 92'; 1,452-passenger capacity; 726 cabins; Italian officers and international crew; three- and four-day cruises from Los Angeles to Ensenada and Catalina.

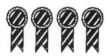

(Medical Facilities: C-15; P-1; EM, CLS, MS; N-2; CM; PD; CB; EKG; TC; PO; EPC; OX; WC; ICU; M; LJ.)

JUBILEE: entered service 1986; 47,262 G.R.T.; 733' x 92'; 1,486-passenger capacity; 743 cabins; Italian officers and international crew; seven-day Alaska cruises and 11- and 12-day Hawaii cruises; 10-day southern Caribbean cruises; 11-, 12-, 13-, 14-, and 16-day Panama Canal cruises.

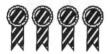

(Medical Facilities: C-14; P-1; N-3; CM; PD; BC; EKG; TC; PO; EPC; OX; WC; OR; ICU; M; LJ.)

SENSATION, FASCINATION, IMAGINATION, INSPIRATION, ELATION, and *PARADISE:* entered service 1993, 1994, 1995, 1996, 1998, and 1998, respectively; 70,367 G.R.T.; 855' x 103'; 2,040-passenger capacity; 1,020 cabins; Italian officers and international crew; seven-day Caribbean cruises and Mexican Riviera cruises.

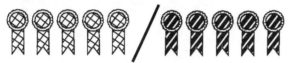

(Medical Facilities: C-20; P-1; EM, CLS, MS; N-3; CM; PD; BC; EKG; TC; PO; EPC; OX; WC; ICU; X; M; LJ.)

TROPICALE: entered service 1982; 36,674 G.R.T.; 660' x 85'; 1,022-passenger capacity; 511 cabins; Italian officers and international crew; four- and five-day cruises from Tampa to Key West, Grand Cayman, and Cozumel.

(Medical Facilities: C-11; P-1; N-3; CM; PD; BC; EKG; TC; PO; EPC; OX; WC; OR; ICU; M; LJ.)

Note: Passenger capacities listed are based on double occupancy.

Carnival Corporation's major owner, the Arison family, started the company in the early seventies with the purchase of the *Empress of Canada* from the Canadian Pacific Line. After a refurbishing, it entered the Caribbean market in 1972 as the *Mardi Gras.* This was followed by the purchase and refurbishing of the sister ship, *Empress of Britain,* which commenced service in 1976 as the *Carnivale.* The former *S.A. Vaal* of the Union Castle Line, refurbished for more than $30 million and renamed the *Festivale,* was added in 1978. Major advertising and promotion of these vessels as the "Fun Ships," together with attractive air-sea packaging, quickly brought Carnival to the top of the heap as one of the most financially successful cruise lines in the industry.

This led to the construction of the *Tropicale* for more than $100 million, designed to be the forerunner of the cruise line's updated, full-capacity "Fun Ships" of the eighties. It entered service in 1982 with Mexican Riviera cruises from Los Angeles. Continued financial success and belief in the future of the American cruise market led to the construction of three new vessels in the 46,000–48,000-ton category. The *Holiday* entered Caribbean service in 1985, followed by the *Jubilee* in 1986 and the *Celebration* in 1987. With the addition of these newer ships with expanded passenger capacity doing seven-day Caribbean itineraries, the aging *Mardi Gras* and *Carnivale* were relegated to three- and four-day runs from Florida to the Bahamas. Subsequently, the *Mardi Gras* and *Carnivale* were sold to Epirotiki Lines and the *Festivale* to Dolphin Cruise Line.

Today, Carnival is one of the leading cruise lines in the middle to upscale cruise market, with ships that have the capacity to put 24,554 passengers afloat each week. If you add passengers sailing on Holland America, Windstar, Costa, Cunard, and Seabourn, its subsidiaries, its passenger capacity is further increased. The casual, amusement-park environment, plethora of activities and entertainment, round-the-clock partying, and attractive packaging have attracted a new generation of younger cruisers—singles, couples, and families. This is one of the few major cruise lines where 70 percent of passengers are under fifty-five years old, with 30 percent under age thirty-five. Carnival offers discounts ranging from $50 to $200 to members of the American Association of Retired Persons.

The *Tropicale, Holiday, Jubilee,* and *Celebration,* although garish, are quite modern. The spacious rooms include closed-circuit color TVs with current movies and music, built-in safes, very generous dresser and closet space, telephones, large bathrooms, and twin beds that convert to king-size. About 65 percent of the cabins are outside with large picture windows, and each ship features from ten to twelve suites with outside verandas and bathtub Jacuzzis. In my opinion the biggest negatives with the three over –46,000-ton ships are the larger number of passengers and the lack of public facilities to accommodate them when the ships are filled. Seven-day cruises (without airfare) on all the ships range from $1,129 per person for the least expensive accommodations up to $2,679 (high season) for the veranda suites.

Carnival contracted to build eight 70,000+-ton sister cruise ships with $225 million-plus price tags in the 1990s: the *Fantasy* commenced service in March 1990, the *Ecstasy* in June 1991, the *Sensation* in late 1993, the *Fascination* in 1994, the *Imagination* in 1995, the *Inspiration* in 1996, and the *Elation* and *Paradise* in 1998. The 101,353-ton *Carnival Destiny,* with more than 1,300 cabins, entered service in 1996. Sister ships to the *Carnival Destiny,* the *Carnival Triumph* and *Carnival Victory* entered service in 1999 and 2000; and an 82,000+-ton ship is scheduled for delivery in late 2000. Two additional sister ships to the *Carnival Destiny,* to be named *Carnival Conquest* and *Carnival Glory,* are scheduled to enter service in 2002 and 2003 respectively.

The *Fantasy, Ecstasy, Sensation, Fascination, Imagination, Inspiration, Elation,* and *Paradise* are very similar in layout and design; however, they differ in decor, and with each new ship there have been innovations and improvements. Joe Farcus, interior architect for all of the Carnival ships, attempts to create a "fantasy vacation environment." The later entries have less dazzle, are a bit more traditional in decor, and, in my opinion, are more tasteful. The *Paradise* is a smoke-free ship, and violators will be expelled from the ship and fined.

Each of these ships measures a little over 70,000+ tons, extends approximately 855 feet in length, has 1,020 cabins that accommodate 2,040 double and 2,594 if all of the upper berths are filled. Standard cabins measure 183 to 190 square feet and are quite spacious, featuring twin beds that convert to king-size, closed-circuit color TVs, private safes, telephones, generous closet and drawer space, and bathrooms that are larger and with greater storage than found on most ships in its market category. Forty percent of the cabins are inside; however, they are very similar to the outside accommodations except that they have no windows or portholes and are about 10 to 20 percent smaller. The 28 most expensive suites have verandas, refrigerators, a small sitting area, a small walk-in closet, and a combination Jacuzzi tub and shower. The 26 demi-suites are a bit larger than the standard cabins and include a very small sitting area and veranda. The full suites measure 350 square feet with 71-square-foot balconies, and they only cost about 20 percent more than a deluxe outside cabin.

The focal point of each ship is a spectacular grand atrium rising seven decks to an immense skylight, with two glass birdcage elevators traversing between top and bottom. The majority of the cabins except the demi- and veranda-suites are located on the four lower decks, with the public rooms and two dining rooms on the upper levels of the ship.

Public rooms include a multilevel, state-of-the-art show lounge with a turntable stage and rising orchestra pit, and several more intimate lounges that feature a variety of nightly entertainment ranging from disco with mirrored dance floors, neon arcs, and copper lightning bolts to variety acts, comedians, and semi-well-known entertainers. Extending into the wee hours, there is something nightly for everyone.

The casinos are among the largest afloat, with numerous blackjack, roulette, craps and Caribbean poker tables, and more than 200 slots. The library and cardrooms are more traditional and offer a quiet respite. The boutiques at the Galleria Mall feature jewelry, logo items, T-shirts, men and women's cruise and formal wear, liquor, and sundries.

Sport and health enthusiasts will appreciate the rubberized jogging tracks, the vast pool deck areas, and the fabulous Nautica Health Spas, which include an aerobics room, an immense gymnasium with weights, cardiovascular and exercise equipment looking out to the sea, men and women's locker rooms with sauna steam and Swiss showers, a hairdressing salon, and an area featuring numerous beauty and massage treatments normally found only at fancy spas.

Dining standards on the Carnival ships have significantly improved over the years, and they now offer an impressive variety of dining possibilities with varied menus. The two main dining rooms serve all three meals in two sittings. Seven-course dinners are featured, which include a variety of appetizers, soups, salads, pasta entrees, and desserts, with steak, chicken, and health options always available. The large indoor-outdoor lido restaurants referred to as the Seaview Bistros offer a full-scale breakfast buffet and a lunch buffet that includes a salad bar, frozen yogurt, and freshly made pasta as well as hamburgers, hot dogs, and various warm dishes. One section of these restaurants, which provides a casual, alternative dining venue, offers pizza hot from the oven around the clock.

The line features an extensive organized children's program on all ships known as "Camp Carnival." Additionally, the ships offer children's menus, young counselors, and video game rooms. Activities and entertainment seem designed to appeal to single and married young adults (under forty-five); and on my most recent cruise, my impression was that the line is moving even further toward attracting this market. Of course many of the activities will also appeal to older cruisers as well.

The *Carnival Destiny* was the first cruise ship to measure over 100,000 tons. She carries a crew of 1,070 that can service 1,321 staterooms with a potential passenger capacity of 3,400; however, the normal passenger count with two to a stateroom is 2,642. Upon entering the ship, you will be overwhelmed by the humongous central atrium with its birdcage elevators traversing the numerous decks of the ship. No less impressive are the three-level, 1,500-passenger-capacity Palladium show lounge; the two bi-level elegant dining rooms featuring numerous intimate booths; the full-facility spa/fitness center; the giant outdoor lido area with four pools, the longest water-slide at sea, Jacuzzis, a swim-up bar, and magradome; a plethora of bars, lounges, shops, and facilities for children of all ages; and the alternative-dining restaurant on Lido Deck with eclectic offerings, including numerous food stations featuring pizza, pasta, and Chinese and Mexican specialties. The stateroom accommodations are also innovative, with larger-than-average cabins all with direct-dial telephones, remote-control televisions, private room safes, generous storage, large showers, and hair dryers. Four hundred thirty-two accommodations have balconies, and there are 40 suites, and 8 penthouse suites. About 30 percent of the cabins are inside. For passenger convenience, there are soda and ice machines on each deck, and most also have laundromats. For cruisers who enjoy the extra facilities and options found on megaships, the *Carnival Destiny* will surely fill the bill.

Carnival Cruise Lines features a new golf program, headed by professionals from the PGA, which includes lessons both aboard ship and during golf excursions at top courses in the Bahamas, Mexico, and Caribbean islands.

Seasoned cruisers indoctrinated with ships offering understated elegance, impeccable service, gourmet dining, and a relaxed atmosphere may find Carnival's "Fun Ship" environment a little unsettling. However, those who are young at heart; not terribly fussy; who seek a ship with a lively environment, very comfortable accommodations, round-the-clock activities, and filled to the brim with fellow passengers of similar persuasion will be Elated, Fascinated, Inspired, Jubilant, or in Paradise (depending on their choice of vessels).

Carnival Corporation is a publicly owned company that also owns the Holland America Line, Windstar Cruises, and Seabourn Cruise Line, all of which are operated and promoted as separate products. In 1997 Carnival and Airtours initiated a joint tender and purchased Costa Crociere. In 1998 Carnival Corporation acquired Cunard and merged the line with Seabourn. Currently it is in discussions with shipyards to design a vessel that would be the world's longest luxury ocean liner, as a companion to the *QE2*.

Strong Points:

Spacious cabins on glamorous newer ships, a plethora of daytime and evening activities and entertainment, a casual lively atmosphere, good food, and plenty of fellow passengers from twenty to fifty-five years old.

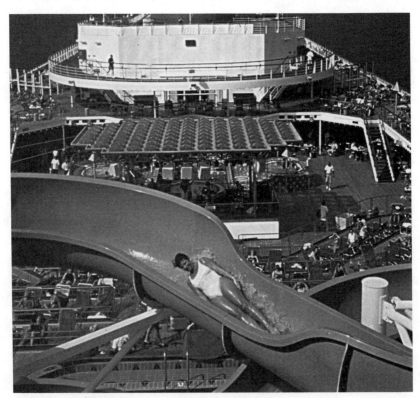

Courtesy Carnival Cruise Lines

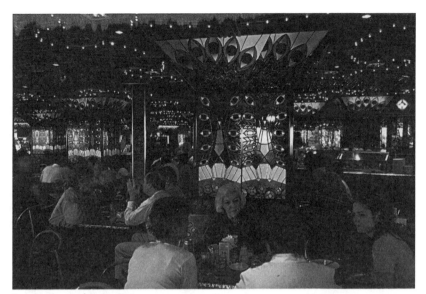

Courtesy Carnival Cruise Lines

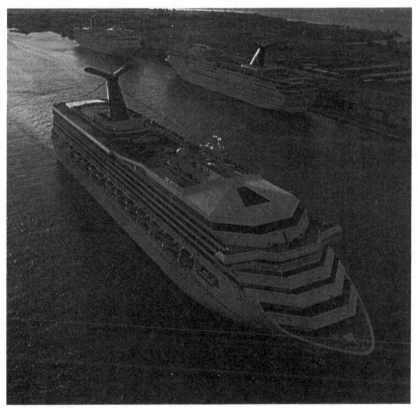

Courtesy Carnival Cruise Lines

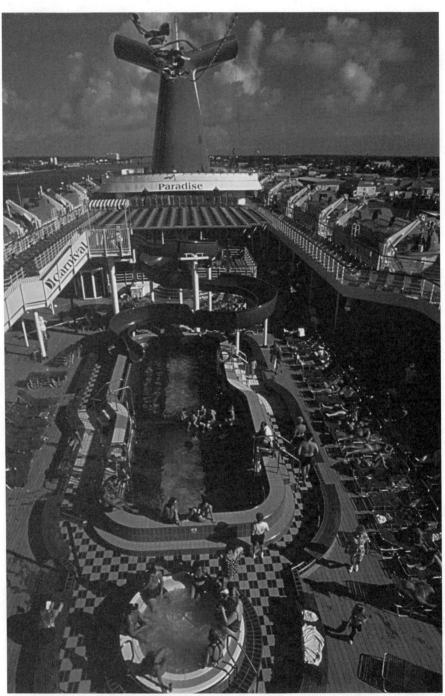

Courtesy Carnival Cruise Lines

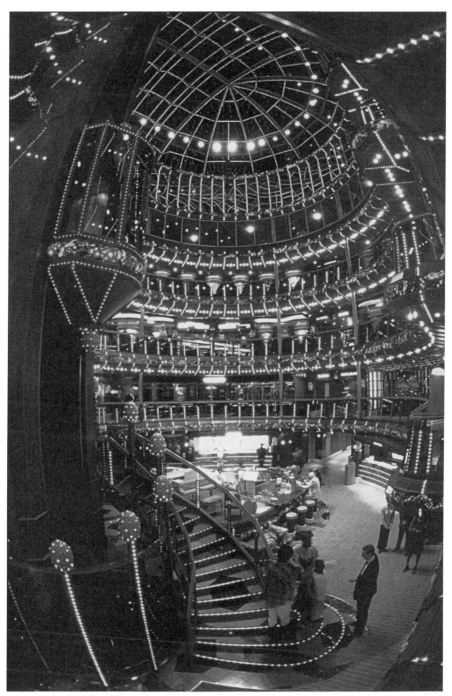

Courtesy Carnival Cruise Lines

Sunrise 7:12 am

Tuesday, January 30, 1996

Sunset 6:26 pm

Captain: Gianpaulo Casula

Hotel Manager: Dennis Dearborn

Cruise Director: John Heald

Fun Ship Sea Day!

Walk through the Bridge
See the largest enclosed bridge aboard any cruise ship.
9:30am .... Meets in the Dynasty Lounge

Snorkel Rental Desk Opens
10:00am .... Empress Deck

"Trivia Quiz"
10:00am .... Dynasty Lounge

Horse Racing
Crazy Fun, bring $3.00 and your Horse could be a WINNER
2.00pm .... Dynasty Lounge

Friends Of Bill W
1:00 pm .... Library

Nautica Spa Demo's
10:00am Glamor Hair Demo .... Aerobics Studio
3:30pm - Learn The Art Of Massage .... Aerobics Studio

Free Blood Pressure Clinic
4:00-5:00pm .... Empress Deck Lobby

Art Auction # 2
Win a valuable Art Masterpiece! Simply by attending our new and exciting art auction. Original oil paintings, watercolors, popular limited editions lithographs and serigraphs will be available. Don't Miss It!
4:45pm Auction ....Xanadu Lounge
(Viewing For Auction #3 7.30, 8.30, 9.30 & 11.15pm in the Curiosity Library)

Galley Tour
See the Galley in Operation
4:00pm ....Meets in the Dynasty Lounge

Guacamole and Salsa Party
5:15 - 6:00pm and 7:15 - 8:15pm
Join your new friends for happy hour bar prices, live music and complimentary chips and salsa................................. Promenade Deck

---

2:30PM   DYNASTY LOUNGE
The Hilarious

THE
MARRIAGE SHOW

With your Cruise Director JOHN
Don't miss one of the funniest events of
the cruise

Cayman & Jamaica
Adventure
INFORMATION

Join your Cruise Director, JOHN
for this important meeting about:

- Beautiful Cayman Beaches
- What to do and not to do
  while in these two ports of call.
- The Exciting Dunn's River Falls Tour

11:00am
Dynasty Lounge
Atlantic and Promenade Deck, Forward

Today At A Glance

Time	Event	Location
6:30 am	Continental Breakfast	Horizon Bar & Grill
7:00 am	Spa & Gym open	Sports Deck
	Walk-a-Mile	Sun Deck
7:45am	Main Sitting Breakfast	Pride & Spirit Dining Rooms
8:00am	Lido Breakfast	By Pool Lido Deck
	Breakfast Buffet	Horizon Bar & Grill
	Slots Open	Casino
	Pools and Whirlpools Open	Lido Deck
	Step Basics	Aerobic Studio
9:00am	Late Sitting Breakfast	Pride and Spirit Dining Rooms
	Gift Shops open	Atlantic Deck
	Body Sculpting	Aerobic Studio
9:30am	Bridge Tour	Meets in the Dynasty Lounge
10:00am	Video Diary & Snorkel Desk Opens	Empress Deck
	Photo Gallery Opens	Empress Deck
	Trivia Time	Dynasty Lounge
	Glamor Hair Demonstration	Aerobics Studio
10:30am	Bingo	Dynasty Lounge
11:00am	Cayman & Jamaica Adventure Talk	Dynasty Lounge
	Library Opens	Atlantic Deck
11:30am	Tour Sales Begin	Dynasty Lounge
11:50am	Message from the Captain	Bridge
12:00 noon	Full Casino opens	Casino
	Sun Lovers Lunch	Horizon Bar & Grill
	Main Sitting Menu Lunch	Pride& Spirit Dining Rooms
1:00pm	Take A Picture With One Of Coreys Birds	Open Decks
1:00pm	Slot Tournament Starts	Casino
1:30pm	Late Sitting Menu Lunch	Pride & Spirit Dining Rooms
2:00pm	Horse Racing	Dynasty Lounge
	Library Opens	Atlantic Deck
2:30pm	Marriage Show	Dynasty
3:30pm	Learn The Art Of Massage	Aerobics Studio
3:30pm	Ice Cream & Treats	Horizon Bar & Grill
	Bingo	Dynasty Lounge
4:00pm	Galley Tour	Dytnasty Lounge
	Afternoon Tea	Pinnacle Club
4:15pm	Step 2 The Beat	Aerobic Studio
4:45pm	Art Auction #2	Xanadu Lounge
5.15pm	Guacamole and Salsa Party	Promenade Deck
5.30pm	Pre-Dinner Cocktail Music	Mirage & Pinnacle
6:00pm	Main Sitting" Oriental Dinner"	Both Dining Rooms
7:15pm	Guacamole and Salsa Party	Promenade Deck
7.15pm	Big Band Dance Music	Dynasty Lounge
8:00pm	Bingo	Dynasty Lounge
8:15pm	Late Sitting "Oriental Dinner"	Both Dining Rooms
8:30pm	Showtime (Main)	Dynasty Lounge
9.15pm	Calypso Sounds	Xanadu Lounge
9:30pm	Sing Along Time	Mirage Bar
	Piano Music	Dream Bar
10:00pm	Party Music	Shangri-La Lounge
10:00pm	Disco Opens	Illusions Disco
10:30pm	Showtime (Late)	Dynasty Lounge
12:15am	Late Show	Xanadu Lounge
12:30am	Dessert & Pastry Buffet	Pride Dining Room
1:30am	Mini Buffet	Horizon Bar and Grill
24 Hours	Pizzeria	Horizon Bar and Grill

Courtesy Carnival Cruise Lines

Gift Shops

Galleria Shopping Mall

They offer a full range of items including souvenirs, perfumes, jewelry liquor,Imagination t-shirts only $11.95 and a convenience section. Also .
GOLD BY THE INCH - ORDER TODAY
Open 9:00am - 10:00pm ....Atlantic Deck

Information Desk

The Purser's Information Desk is located on the Empress Deck, Midship. Here you will find our Pursers who will answer your questions, assist you with lost & found items The desk is open 24 hours for your convenience.
Open 24 hours.. Purser's Lobby

Miscellaneous

Wake- up Call

You can use your cabin telephone to program wake -up calls! Simply lift the handset, and dial "37" then the **Hour** and **Minutes** of your wake-up call. (Example: To set the call time to **7:45am**, dial 37. then dial **07** for the hour then **45** for minutes.) and (To set the call time to **3:30pm**, dial **37** , then dial **15** for the hour then **30** for minutes. To clear a wake-up call just dial *37 and hang up.   All previously programmed calls will be erased.

Phoning Home

You can call anywhere in the world direct from your cabin.

Infirmary

Located Deck 3 Forward.   Doctor's consulting hours are 9am-11am & 3pm-5pm. In Case of an emergency please call the Information Desk on 7777

SWIMMING POOLS

The swimming pools are open from 8:00am - 7:00pm. The Jacuzzis will open from 8:00am - 10:00pm

Looking Ahead

We arrive tomorrow in Grand Cayman at approximately 7:30am. Get ready for a fantastic day ashore to just sit back and relax or shop till you

Laundry Service Note:

Due to enviornmental laws, all laundry service & laundry rooms must be closed while in Cayman waters. This will be from Wednesday 1:00am until Wednesday 6:00pm. We apologize for any inconvenience.

M.S. IMAGINATION

CAPTAIN'S GALA DINNER

The Master Summons All Who Sail with Him to Dine as Royal Guests in a Spectacular Celebration of the Seagoing Life. All Aboard are to Heed the Captain's Wishes of Making Merry on this Special Occasion. The Captain has Ordered the Very Best of Everything for His Guests, For on His Night, He Salutes Each of You.

APPETIZERS

TOMATO AND FRESH MOZZARELLA
Marinated in Basil and Olive Oil

ALASKAN SMOKED SALMON
With Condiments

PANFRIED FROG LEGS
Garlic and White Wine

STUFFED BLUE CRAB

SOUPS

MEDITERRANEAN SEAFOOD   **CREAM OF BROCCOLI**

CHILLED STRAWBERRY

SALADS

Mixed Garden Greens with Herb Infused Vinaigrette

CAESAR SALAD
Romaine Lettuce with Croutons, Parmesan Cheese and Caesar Dressing

PASTA

PENNE SICILIANA
With Eggplant, Zucchini and Tomato Cream Sauce

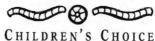

CHILDREN'S CHOICE

SEA DOG   **QUARTER DECK CHICKEN BURGER**

MACARONI AND CHEESE   **RIBS ON THE BARBIE**

FRENCH FRIES   **ICE CREAM CAKE**

A Complete Wine List, Your Preferred Beer, Water, Soft Drink and Cocktail is Also Available.
Guests on Special Diets are Requested to Advise the Restaurant Manager of their Requirements.

ENTREES

SPA BROILED SWORDFISH STEAK
Garlic Aioli, with Sugar Snap Peas and Cauliflower

GRILLED JUMBO SHRIMP
Served over Mushroom Risotto

OAK-SMOKED PORK LOIN
Champagne Cabbage and Mashed Potatoes

TOURNEDOS OF BEEF TENDERLOIN
Red Wine Mushroom Sauce, Sugar Snap Peas and Lorette Potatoes

BAKED VEGETABLE PRINCESS
*Vegetarian Entrée: Seasonal Vegetables Baked in a
Cheese Sauce and Topped with Asparagus*

AVAILABLE ON REQUEST
Grilled Chicken Breast, Sirloin Steak, Pasta with Tomato Sauce and Baked Potato

❱❱

CHEESES

PORT SALUT   BRIE   GOUDA   IMPORTED SWISS   DANISH BLEU

❱❱

DESSERTS

SPA CHOCOLATE BAVAROIS   **FRUIT TRANCHE**

BLACK FOREST GATEAU   **BAKED ALASKA**

ICE CREAM
Vanilla, Chocolate, Strawberry, Butter Pecan

SHERBET
Orange, Pineapple, Lime

❱❱

BEVERAGES

FRESHLY BREWED COFFEE: REGULAR OR DECAFFEINATED

ESPRESSO   CAPPUCCINO

ICED, HOT AND HERBAL TEAS

MILK   SKIMMED MILK   HOT CHOCOLATE

SPA NAUTICA SPA FARE
*These Items are Lower in Calories, Sodium, Cholesterol and Fat.
Salads Prepared with Diet Dressing; Desserts Prepared with a Sugar Substitute.*

Courtesy Carnival Cruise Lines

CELEBRITY CRUISES
1050 Caribbean Way
Miami, Florida 33132
(305) 539-6000
(800) 437-3111
(800) 437-9111 FAX

CENTURY: entered service 1995; 70,606 G.R.T.; 858' x 105'; 1,750-passenger capacity; 875 cabins; Greek officers and international crew; offering seven-night cruises from Ft. Lauderdale to the east and west Caribbean. Itineraries to be determined.

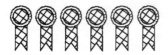

GALAXY: entered service 1996; 77,713 G.R.T.; 858' x 105'; 1,870-passenger capacity; 935 cabins; Greek officers and international crew; cruises from Los Angeles and Vancouver to Alaska, and from San Juan to the southern Caribbean and Transcanal.

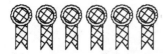

HORIZON: entered service 1990; refurbished and renovated 1998; 46,811 G.R.T.; 682' x 95'; 1,354-passenger capacity; 677 cabins; Greek officers and international crew; cruises from Ft. Lauderdale to the southern Caribbean and Transcanal, and cruises from New York, Baltimore, Charleston, Norfolk, Philadelphia, and Wilmington to Bermuda.

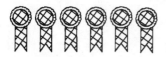

MERCURY: entered service 1997; 77,713 G.R.T.; 858' x 105'; 1,870-passenger capacity; 935 cabins; Greek officers and international crew; cruises to the west Caribbean, Transcanal, and the Pacific Coast, and from Vancouver to Alaska.

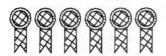

ZENITH: entered service 1992; refurbished and renovated 1999; 47,225 G.R.T.; 682' x 95'; 1,374-passenger capacity; 687 cabins; Greek officers and international crew; cruises from San Juan and Acapulco, Transcanal cruises between San Juan and Acapulco, Transcanal and South America cruises, and cruises from New York to Bermuda.

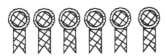

(Medical Facilities: Celebrity's parent company, RCI, advises that all ships have full medical facilities and equipment and are staffed with highly qualified physicians and nurses trained in trauma, emergency medicine, and general practice; however the cruise line has a policy of not providing specifics and suggests passengers concerned contact the medical department of the cruise lines prior to sailing.)

Note: Six ribbons is the highest rating given in this edition to ships in the premium market category.

In 1990 Chandris created a new Celebrity Cruises division to compete in the middle to upscale cruise market, while also continuing its Fantasy Cruises division at the budget end of the cruise market. For its new Celebrity Cruises division, Chandris rebuilt, lengthened, redesigned, and refurbished the former *Galileo* in 1989, renaming her *Meridian,* and built *Horizon,* which entered service in 1990, and *Zenith,* which entered service in 1992. The two divisions promoted their ships like separate companies and did not advertise the "Chandris" name. In 1994 the name of the U.S. company was changed to Celebrity Cruises, Inc. In 1995, 1996, and 1997 Celebrity introduced three 70,000+-ton innovative hi-tech vessels, *Century, Galaxy,* and *Mercury.* In 1997 *Meridian* was sold.

In the summer of 1997, Royal Caribbean Cruise Ltd. acquired Celebrity and now operates Celebrity Cruises as a separate brand.

The *Horizon* and *Zenith* were cleverly conceived ships for the nineties, recently updated for the new millenium. Although each carries more than 1,300 passengers, you never feel crowded, a result of the careful design in public areas. All the staterooms are similar in size, layout, and amenities—being among the roomiest "average" staterooms afloat. Each has two twin beds or one double bed, ample closet and dresser space, a three-channel radio, an interactive television with remote control, telephones with ship-to-shore capacities, electronic safes, dressing tables, and large bathrooms with hair dryers and plush bathrobes. The regular suites have a small sitting area, mini-bars, butler service, and a few additional features, but they are not much larger than the average staterooms. Those requiring a suite will prefer the Presidential Suites, at 340 square feet on *Horizon,* or the 500-square-foot Royal Suites on *Zenith.* These suites include separate sitting rooms, walk-in closets, numerous additional amenities, and marble baths with whirlpool jets in the tubs (as do the suites on the other Celebrity ships).

On top of the ships is the new AquaSpa^{SM} facility that houses a beauty salon, treatment rooms, fitness area and changing rooms with steam and sauna for men and women, saunas, jogging tracks, and an upper level of deck chairs overlooking the pool. The next deck below features two swimming pools surrounded by lounge chairs, a bar, and a music bandstand, as well as the lido restaurant, outdoor grill, and panoramic observation lounge. Casual alternative dinners are offered atop ship in the lido restaurants.

The next two decks contain the higher-priced staterooms, with remaining accommodations being toward the bottom of the ship, below the two main public deck areas. The main public deck areas include the large two-level theater/show lounges; several other smaller show and cocktail lounges; a disco; a large casino with slots, roulette, blackjack, and craps; an electronic game room; and an attractive dining room. When the *Horizon* received a major refurbishment and renovation in 1998, and the *Zenith* in 1999, the AquaSpa^{SM} facilities were added along with intimate Martini Bars, Michael's Clubs, trendy cigar bars, and Cova Café's featuring coffees, liqueurs, chocolates, and other innovative features.

There is a high ratio of service staff to passengers (1:2). Service in the dining rooms, staterooms, and various lounges is the best in the premium market and among the best in the industry, and the ships carry a large number of social and entertainment staff. The diversity and presentation of food offerings at all meals as well as buffets are amazing. Entertainment is also exceptional.

In December 1995 Celebrity entered the megaship market, introducing the innovative $320 million, 70,000+-ton, 815-foot, 1,750-passenger *Century,* followed by the 77,713-ton, 852-foot, 1,870-passenger *Galaxy* in December 1996, and its sister ship, *Mercury,* in November 1997, giving Celebrity 8,206 lower guest berths at sea. In collaboration with Sony Corporation, the vessels are equipped with the most sophisticated array of entertainment options and interactive audio, video, and in-cabin entertainment systems presently available on any cruise ship. These hi-tech amenities include a fully equipped, state-of-the art conference center, with electronic voting chairpads and broadcast capabilities; a 921-seat multilevel, amphitheater-style show lounge designed to accommodate Broadway-scale productions with its revolving stage, hydraulic orchestra pit, and sophisticated special-effects capability; a revolutionary hi-tech-equipped lounge and disco; and in-cabin interactive televisions featuring the Celebrity Network, an innovation that permits guests to order room service, select their dinner wine, purchase shore excursions, gamble at casino games charged to their personal accounts, review their shipboard account, and purchase pay-for-view movies. *Galaxy* and *Mercury* are very similar in physical layout to *Century* but with different decors and various innovations, including martini bars, magradomes that slide over the rear pool areas when the weather is inclement, family staterooms that hold up to five persons, Sony Wonder computer equipment with free classes, and larger verandas in the Sky Suites.

All of the 875 staterooms on *Century* and the 935 on *Galaxy* and *Mercury* include very ample closet and drawer space, convertible twin beds, dressing table and mirror, direct-dial telephones, mini-bar-refrigerators, electronic safes, hair dryers, terry-cloth robes, interactive television systems, and nice-size bathrooms with showers, sinks, and storage more generous than on most ships. The eight 637-square-foot spacious Royal Suites with 131-square-foot verandas and the 20 Sky Suites with even larger verandas include video systems, marble baths with whirlpool jets, champagne, personalized stationery and business cards, afternoon tea and snacks, nightly hors d'oeuvres, and 24-hour butler service. Eleven additional deluxe cabins also have verandas. The two 1,219-square-foot Penthouse Suites include a master bedroom with its own bathroom, living room, dining room, kitchen pantry, powder room, large balcony with an outdoor Jacuzzi, and sophisticated security system that can be combined with the adjoining suite to accommodate two additional guests. Comfort and service in the suites emulate that found on more expensive ships that compete in the deluxe-category cruise market. Cruisers who demand luxurious suites, personalized butler service, and gourmet cuisine but who also require ships offering an abundance of activities and entertainment will find the "suite life" on all Celebrity vessels viable alternatives to many of the more expensive deluxe cruise ships. There are also a number of wheelchair-accessible staterooms on the three larger ships, and the design of these vessels is especially well adapted for the handicapped.

The ships are attractively furbished in contemporary/Art Deco designs with out-standing, multimillion-dollar art collections assembled by Christina Chandris. The two-tiered Grand Restaurants feature majestic staircases; a piano balcony, where soft dinner music is played by a quartet; two-story picture windows looking out to the sea; and Continental menus and wine lists developed by renowned chef Michel Roux. In the dining rooms, the gourmet-quality meals are imaginatively presented and are served European style. The overall dining experience is the best in the premium market and one of the reasons Celebrity has gained high praise throughout the travel industry. Complimentary room service is available around the clock; casual buffet-style breakfasts and lunches are offered atop ship at the Lido Cafés, which feature four separate buffet areas; casual dinners are also offered in this area on most evenings; and for additional variety there are hamburger/hot-dog grills and pizza ovens by the pool, wine and espresso bars, caviar and champagne bars, and English men's-club-style lounges featuring fine hand-rolled cigars, premium liqueurs, spirits, and cognacs.

The ships also offer AquaSpa^{SM}, the most complete health spas at sea, operated by Steiner Transocean, Ltd. In addition to a large, fully equipped exercise and aerobics room with dozens of cardiovascular machines, a hair salon, his and hers dressing rooms with showers, steam, and saunas, there also is a marvelous thalassotherapy pool and a bevy of beauty, health, relaxation, and massage treatments available. AquaSpa^{SM} packages may be booked in advance and range in price from $200 to $699.

Other public facilities on each of these three ships include 7,500-foot casinos; impressive observation lounges which convert to discos at night; cabaret-style nightclubs; advanced technology, supervised children's playrooms and numerous electronic-game facilities; three-story Grand Foyers that rise from the marble main lobbies with extensive shopping galleries; lido decks with two attached swimming pools, four whirlpools, designated sport areas, small jogging tracks, and several bars; golf simulators, where for a fee guests can play a full round of golf on one of three courses; and libraries and cardrooms. These are truly three of the most full-facility resorts at sea, and passengers may have difficulty pulling themselves away in order to allot time for visiting ports.

Commencing in 1999, all of the Celebrity vessels will feature an option for casual dining on most nights of every cruise. The menu will initially include a fresh fruit cocktail, Caesar or lettuce salad, lasagna al forno, broiled salmon steak, spit-roasted chicken, grilled sirloin steak, a variety of pizzas, key lime pie, and black forest cake.

Celebrity frequently changes itineraries, and it is best to obtain their most recent brochures before making your travel plans. Celebrity presently is focusing on the Caribbean, Bermuda, Alaska, Transcanal, and South American markets. However, seasonal Mediterranean and European cruises are also offered. Two new vessels will join the Celebrity fleet in the next millennium.

Strong Points:

Celebrity Cruise's ships have been well received by their guests, travel writers, and travel agents. The spacious, full-amenity staterooms and suites, superior dining, excellent service and total dedication to passenger satisfaction, innovative entertainment options, and vast array of facilities make Celebrity one of the best buys and the top contender in the premium cruise market. The 70,000+-ton ships offer an exceptional experience on the most state-of-the-art, high-tech vessels afloat, with the option to purchase accommodations as sumptuous as those offered on the more expensive luxury-category cruise ships. The Celebrity fleet tries harder, has exceeded our expectations, and has received our highest rating in the premium-cruise market category.

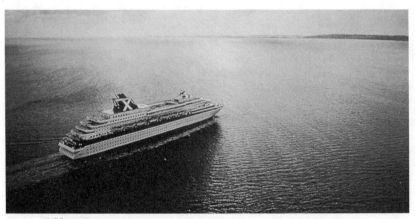

Courtesy Celebrity Cruises

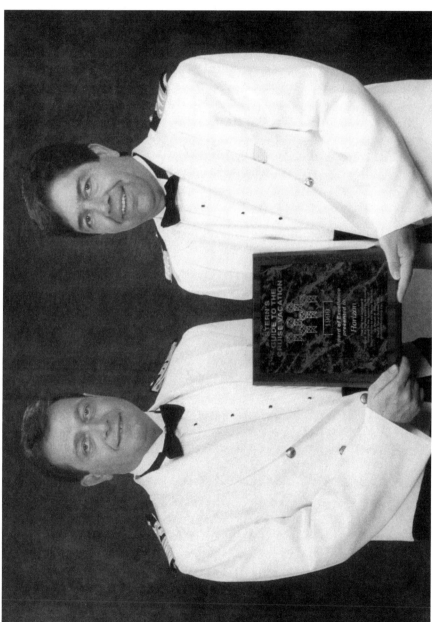

Courtesy Celebrity Cruises

AQUASPA^{SM}

Celebrity Cruises features its own custom-brand AquaSpa^{SM} program to provide guests with an exclusive spa resort vacation at sea. The AquaSpa^{SM} programs are the most comprehensive and sophisticated spa programs in the cruise vacation market.

AquaSpa^{SM} offers guests an architecturally unique spa facility at sea that features exclusive treatments. Whether it uses the serenity of a Japanese bathhouse or images from the Moorish and Ottoman worlds, AquaSpa^{SM} creates a warm and natural retreat in which guests can cleanse and purify the body, mind, and spirit. Incorporating the ancient traditions found in the mineral springs of Turkey and the therapeutic lure of the Dead Sea, AquaSpa^{SM} provides an exotic and serene environment for the complete range of beauty and health treatments offered within the program.

Celebrity Cruises' *Mercury* evokes tranquil and natural images that embody the essence of ancient Middle Eastern therapeutic traditions. Screens detailed with teakwood, echoing lattice windows, and marble walls banded with contrasting colors create an atmosphere of protection and privacy reminiscent of the Alhambra, the epitome of Moorish palaces. Arched walls clad in ceramic mosaics adorn the thalassotherapy pool area, while grid patterns shaped to resemble arches echo throughout the salon and therapy areas. Special heating and insulation in the Rasul treatment area and steam room heat the walls and floors to enhance comfort for guests even further.

Custom-designed for Celebrity Cruises by the prestigious Steiner Leisure Ltd. of London, the AquaSpa^{SM} programs have been created in response to a growing

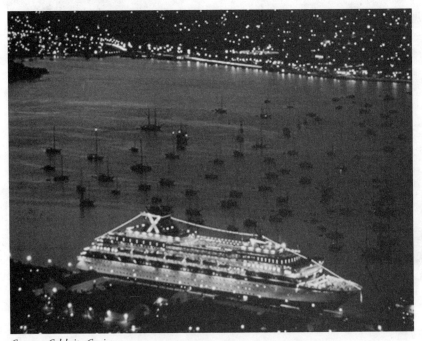

Courtesy Celebrity Cruises

demand among sophisticated consumers for luxury spa services that not only pamper but also help address the stress caused by contemporary pressures. Recognizing the therapeutic link between cruising and body and mind rejuvenation, Celebrity and the Steiner organization have created spa treatment programs that integrate the spa experience with a premium cruise environment.

The AquaSpa^{SM} programs, which can be booked prior to cruising on any Celebrity ship, offer both male and female guests a choice of three different levels to provide a balance of treatments, classes, and consultations at select price points ranging from \$200 to \$699. The basic entry-level (Silver), intermediate-level (Gold), and the top-level (Platinum) packages appeal to guests seeking a comprehensive spa vacation. Both the Silver and the Gold levels provide packages with either a fitness or a pampering focus, while the Platinum-level package provides both fitness and pampering services.

AquaSpa^{SM} programs are offered on all the Celebrity Cruises vessels and, combined with Celebrity's award-winning cuisine and on-board service, signal the cruise line's emergence as a world-class, premium spa destination. (Courtesy Celebrity Cruises)

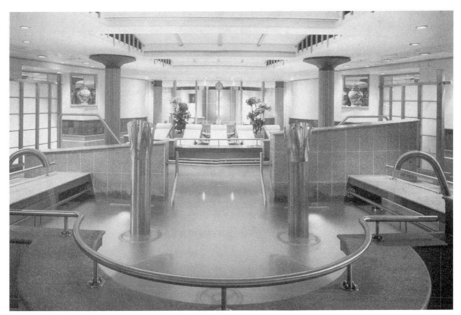

Aqua Spa^{SM} Courtesy Celebrity Cruises

MICHEL ROUX

Internationally acclaimed Master Chef Michel Roux continues Celebrity's award-winning heritage of serving the finest cuisine available at sea. Elevating the art of fine cuisine to an intimate and elegant dining experience is simple and easy to achieve with the talents of Mr. Roux. The Celebrity Fleet, comprised of *Century, Galaxy, Horizon, Mercury,* and *Zenith,* has been awarded numerous top industry honors for spectacular cuisine since the cruise line's inception in 1990.

In his role as consultant for Celebrity Cruises, Mr. Roux has been actively involved in the design of the new ships' galleys, created the award-winning ship menus, developed the wine list, and assisted with the training of the executive restaurant staff. Without compromising quality or quantity, Roux took on the task of creating menus that are easily workable on board the ships. For Roux, the presentation must be kept simple. It should look like food—unpretentious and fresh as possible. All food is prepared from scratch using only the finest produce, fresh herbs, aged beef, and fresh fish, provisioned weekly. Mr. Roux also revises and updates the menus approximately every six months. Alternating with Mr. Roux's inspections, his sous chefs review the ships to ensure that the quality and presentation of the cuisine uphold Celebrity's highest standards.

Onboard Services recognized Celebrity Cruises' cuisine and service in its first year of operation with the magazine's highest honors. In 1992, 1993, 1994, and 1995, *Ocean and Cruise News* lauded Celebrity Cruises for serving the best cuisine in the industry. America Online's Cruise Critic User Poll ranked all of Celebrity Cruises' ships among the "top ten best" in cuisine for 1997 and 1998. *Mercury* was the only cruise ship in the world in 1999 to be awarded a membership into the Epicurean International Associates.

Michel Roux is one of Britain's most famous French chefs and the recipient of three Michelin stars for his restaurant, the Waterside Inn at Bray in Berkshire, England. The Waterside Inn was recognized twice as the "Restaurant of the Year" and is the recipient of three stars in the *Egon Ronay Guide.*

Mr. Roux has won a number of medals, prizes, and honors from the world's most noted culinary institutions. He has served as a consultant in the establishment of currently top-rated restaurants in France, the United Kingdom, and the United States. The author of several cookbooks, Mr. Roux is a member of L'Academie Culinaire de France, the Association Relais et Desserts, and the Benedicts Club, and he is the vice president of the Board of the Association Relais et Chateaux. (Courtesy Celebrity Cruises)

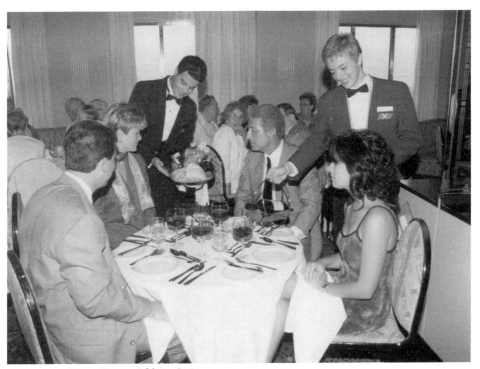

Dining Room. Courtesy Celebrity Cruises

Celebrity Cruises excels in the attention its staff devotes to passenger satisfaction. A testament to the philosophy of the staff is best exemplified by the words of one of its more popular captains.

CAPTAIN IOANNIS PAPANIKOLAU

The cruise industry has become most competitive, and I feel that all of us working on board cruise ships, or in the industry in general, have a responsibility toward our guests to fulfill their cruising expectations.

Because approximately 40 percent of our guests on each cruise are first-time cruisers, it is up to us on board to ensure that they enjoy their anticipated experience. Of course, all our guests on board are treated to the same service; however, if a first-time cruiser is subjected to a bad experience and their expectations not fulfilled, they may never want to cruise again—on any cruise line. Therefore, I personally make it my goal and responsibility, as well as instilling the philosophy in my crew, to ensure that all our guests are given the very best service.

I feel it very important for a captain to know his guests personally and to spend time socializing with them, listening to suggestions or improvements they may have, and acting on those suggestions. In this way I also set an example to my crew to be friendly and helpful to our guests, giving them the best possible service, rendered with a ready smile.

Ioannis Papanikolau

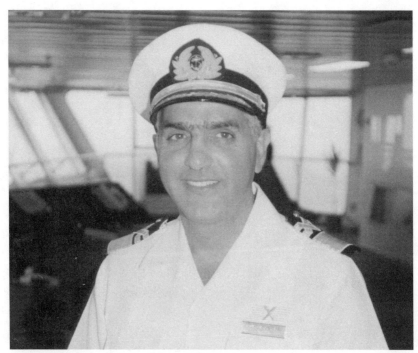

Captain Papanikolau. Courtesy Celebrity Cruises

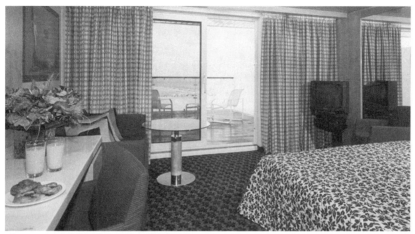

Sky Suite. Courtesy Celebrity Cruises

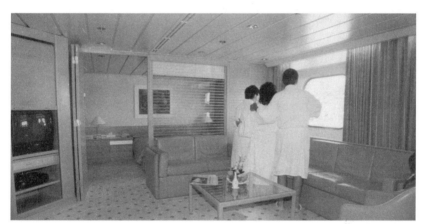

Royal Suite. Courtesy Celebrity Cruises

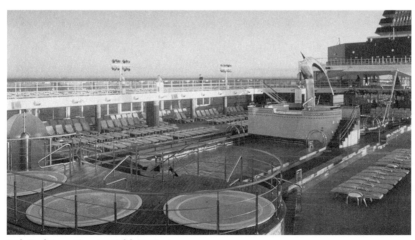

Lido Pool Area. Courtesy Celebrity Cruises

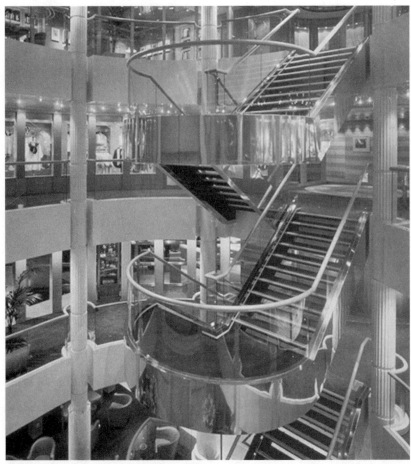

Atrium—Grand Foyer. Courtesy Celebrity Cruises

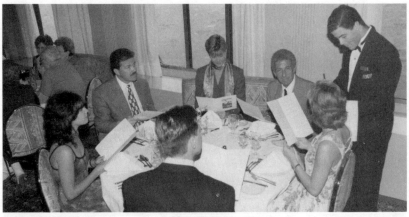

Dining Room on the Zenith. *Courtesy Celebrity Cruises*

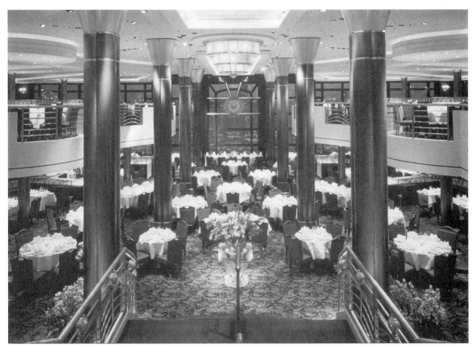

Main Dining Room. Courtesy Celebrity Cruises

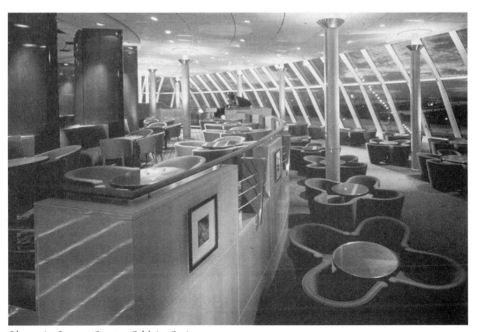

Observation Lounge. Courtesy Celebrity Cruises

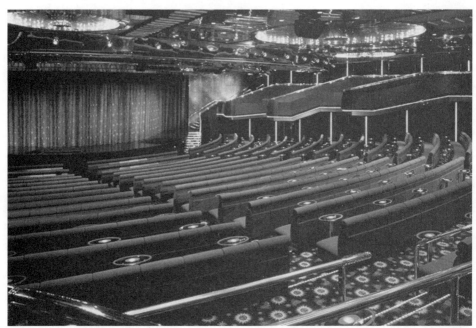

Main Show Lounge. Courtesy Celebrity Cruises

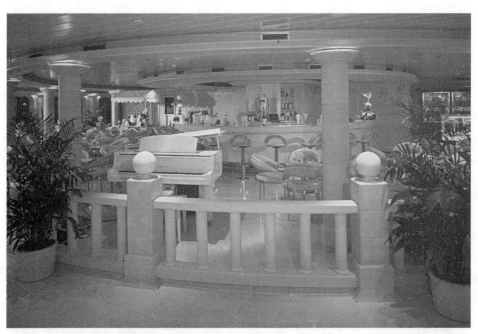

Cova Café on Horizon. *Courtesy Celebrity Cruises*

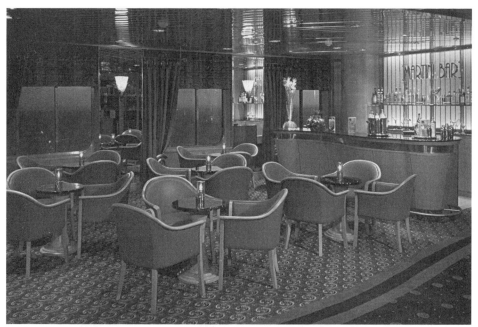

Martini Bar on Horizon. *Courtesy Celebrity Cruises*

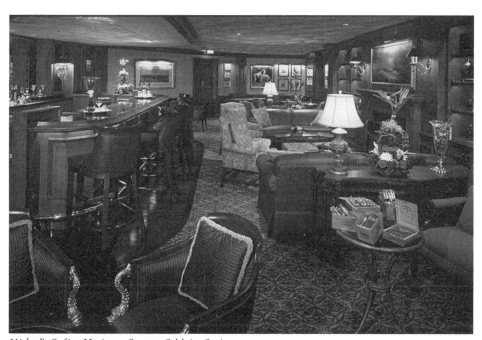

Michael's Café on Horizon. *Courtesy Celebrity Cruises*

GOOD MORNING

7:00am (approx.)	**Enjoy our arrival at Georgetown, Grand Cayman Island.** Anchorage at approximately 7:00am. Tender service begins shortly thereafter, please listen for announcements. (See Tender Service information, page 2.)		
8:00am	Be sure to pick up your **Shopping Map.** Available all day.	Gangway	3
8:30am	Catholic Mass with Father Wagner.	Cinema/Conference Cnt.	6
★ 8:30am	Walk A Mile with your Entertainment Staff.	Sky Deck	12
9:00am	The Pools are open. Have a morning swim to start your day.	Poolside, Resort Deck	11
10:00am	Daily Quiz available in the Library. Answers available after 3:00pm.	Library	8
10:00am – 11:30am	The Library Bookcase is open.	Library	8
10:30am	Staying Aboard? The Entertainment Staff organizes indoor games.	Card Room	6
10:30am	**Goldwyn Movie Time:** "The Bishop's Wife." 113 mins.	Cinema/Conference Cnt.	6
11:00am	Celebrity Social Hour. Chat with the Entertainment Staff.	Tastings	6
11:00am – 2:00pm	Suntan to today's selection of Music.	Poolside, Resort Deck	11
11:30am – 12:30pm	**Special Cruise Consultation.** Drop by for a chat with **Cynthia** and get all the details on Celebrity's vacation choices, and itineraries.	Grand Foyer	5 Port

GOOD AFTERNOON

1:30pm	**Movie Time:** "Shine." 105 mins.	Cinema/Conference Cnt.	6
★ 2:30pm	Pool Volleyball Challenge with the Entertainment Staff.	Poolside, Resort Deck	11
2:30pm – 4:00pm	The Library Bookcase is open.	Library	8
3:30pm	Looking for Bridge players? Meet with your fellow guests.	Card Room	6
3:30pm – 5:00pm	**Concert** at the poolside amphitheater, starring **Onyx.**	Poolside, Resort Deck	11
3:45pm – 4:15pm	**(Preview) Park West Art Auction At Sea.**	Rendez-Vous Square	6
4:15pm – 5:15pm	**(Auction)** All fine art is duty-exempt, shipped worldwide, and offered to all at great prices! Art expert **Jon** hosts.	Rendez-Vous Square	6
4:00pm	Tea Time. The Verossa Strings bring you a relaxed mood.	Oasis Café	11
4:00pm	**Celebrity Enrichment Series.** Geology Lecturer **Gilles Allard** presents "Geological mapping techniques and adventures throughout the world."	Cinema/Conference Cnt.	6
4:15pm	**Snowball Jackpot Bingo.** Join the **Entertainment Staff** for fun. Advance purchase of bingo cards from 3:45pm – 4:15pm Deck 7 Aft.	Savoy Night Club	7
4:30pm	**Last tender leaves the shore. All aboard please.** **The GALAXY is scheduled to sail for Port Everglades, Florida.**		
4:30pm	Friends of Bill W. meet in the ...	Meeting Room	6
5:15pm	**The GALAXY TV Program.** With **Don, Doug Cameron** and special guests. *(Rebroadcast tonight on Channel 68).*	Celebrity Theater	6, 7
5:15pm	**Jewish Sabbath Service.** Conducted by one of your fellow guests.	Cinema/Conference Cnt.	6

GOOD EVENING
This Evening's Dress throughout the ship (after 6:00pm): **Formal.**
Ladies: *A dressy outfit.* **Gentlemen:** *Dark suit & tie, tuxedo, or dinner jacket.*
(Please maintain Formal dress code throughout the evening).

5:00pm – 8:30pm	Happy Hour. Enjoy a selection of cocktails at only $2.95 each.	Savoy Night Club	7
5:00pm – 1:00am	**Tasty Cigars** and conversation plus a cigar rolling demonstration.	Michael's Club	6
5:15pm – 6:00pm	**The Martini Bar.** Savoy Night Club and	Savoy Night Club	7
& 7:45pm – 8:45pm	Savoy Melody Makers.		
5:15pm – 6:00pm	**Musical Pre-Dinner** cocktails, music and dancing with **Casanova.**	Rendez-Vous Square	6
6:00pm & 9:00pm	**Goldwyn Movie Time:** "An American in Paris." 114 mins.	Cinema/Conference Cnt.	6
7pm, 9pm, 11pm	**Blue Seas Lotto.** A chance to win $50,000.00.	Fortunes Casino	7
7:15pm – 8:30pm	**Casanova's** musical rendezvous.	Rendez-Vous Square	6
9:45pm – 1:00am	Our Musical Duo **Casanova** entertains around Karaoke.	Rendez-Vous Square	6
10:00pm – 11:00pm	**Disco Music Hour** with **D.J. Doug.** *(Minimum age 18 years.)*	Stratosphere Lounge	12

Courtesy Celebrity Cruises

$\mathcal{T}$HE $\mathcal{C}$HEF $\mathcal{P}$RESENTS

We take pride in presenting Chef Michel Roux's recommendation
for this evening's meal, foods especially designed
to complement each other and provide a fine dining experience.

SHRIMP COCKTAIL
*Served with Gulf Sauce flavored with Cognac
or a zesty Cocktail Sauce*

CREAM OF BROCCOLI
A classical American Creamy Soup

CAESAR SALAD
*A culinary classic; crisp Romaine Lettuce tossed with Croutons,
freshly grated Parmesan Cheese and distinctive Caesar Dressing*

PRIME RIB OF BEEF
*America's favorite; the finest cut of Roasted Beef
presented with natural Pan Juices and our own fresh creamed Horseradish*

BAKED ALASKA
*A blazingly spectacular Dessert
with layers of Sponge Cake, Ice Cream and Meringue*

$\mathcal{T}$HE $\mathcal{W}$INE $\mathcal{S}$TEWARD $\mathcal{S}$UGGESTS

The following Wines are recommended to complement the Chef's Selection
Chardonnay, Régnard et Fils, Petit Chablis
Cabernet Sauvignon, Jordan, Alexander Valley, Estate Bottled

WINES BY THE GLASS

White: Chardonnay, Raymond Vineyards, Napa Valley

Red: Cuvée Georges, Duboeuf, nv

$\mathcal{B}$EVERAGES

Freshly Brewed Regular or Decaffeinated Coffee   Iced Coffee

Tea, Herbal and Iced Tea   Hot Chocolate   Milk

1:30am – .....   **D.J. Doug** blasts off to a new musical universe! *(Minimum age 18 years.)*   Stratosphere Lounge   *12*

He is unrivalled in Europe as one of the most innovative
and exceptional of restaurateurs.

$\mathcal{A}$PPETIZERS

Seasonal Fruit with Rum and Black Currant Syrup

* Shrimp Cocktail   Supreme of Chicken Terrine

Sweetbreads with Crisp Potato Pancake

$\mathcal{S}$OUPS

Cream of Broccoli   Mussel Veloute

* Chilled Gin and Tomato Consomme with Straw Mushrooms

$\mathcal{S}$ALADS

Caesar
Romaine Lettuce, Parmesan Cheese and Croutons

Iceberg Lettuce, Zucchini, Yellow Squash, Celery, Scallions

Roquefort   Red Wine Vinaigrette   Caesar   * Spicy Tomato

$\mathcal{E}$NTREES

Halibut Steak
*Broiled Alaskan Halibut complemented by a Beurre Blanc,
enhanced with preserved Black Beans*

Broiled Lobster Tail
*Topped with green Asparagus Tip,
presented with melted Drawn Butter*

Canard à l'Ananas
*Crisply roast Long Island Duckling complemented by
grilled Pineapple and a Duck flavored Cinnamon Sauce*

* Scaloppine di Vitello al Limone
*Thin slices of milk-fed Veal enhanced by a natural Sauce
with the delicate essence of Lemon*

Prime Rib of Beef
*The finest cut of Prime Rib presented with baked Idaho Potato,
natural juice and creamed Horseradish*

$\mathcal{D}$ESSERTS

Baked Alaska   * Frozen Lemon Yogurt with Dark Cherries

An array of Petits Fours, with the Chef's compliments

Coffee, Vanilla, Piña Colada or * Sugar-free Ice Cream   Today's Sherbet

Fruit and Cheese

An assortment of fresh seasonal Fruit complemented by fine Cheese

Roquefort   Camemebert   Gruyere   Cheddar

Courtesy Celebrity Cruises

CLIPPER CRUISE LINE
7711 Bonhomme Avenue
St. Louis, Missouri 63105
(800) 325-0010
(314) 727-6576 FAX

CLIPPER ADVENTURER: (formerly *Alla Taravosa*) entered service 1975 and converted 1998; 4,364 G.R.T.; 330' x 53.5'; 122-passenger capacity; 61 cabins; international officers and crew; cruises around Western Europe, Baltic, British Isles, Scandinavia, Greenland, the Canadian Arctic, the East Coast of North America, South America, and Antarctica. **(Category C—Not Rated)**

CLIPPER ODYSSEY: (formerly *Oceanic Odyssey*) entered service 1989; 5,200 G.R.T.; 340' X 51'; 120-passenger capacity; 60 cabins; international officers and crew; cruises in North and South Pacific and Indian Ocean. **(Category C—Not Rated)**

NANTUCKET CLIPPER: entered service 1984; 95 G.R.T.; 207' x 37'; 102-passenger capacity; 51 cabins; American officers and crew; cruises to eastern seaboard of the U.S., Canada, the Great Lakes, and the Virgin Islands. **(Category C—Not Rated)**

YORKTOWN CLIPPER: entered service 1988; 97 G.R.T.; 257' x 43'; 138-passenger capacity; 69 cabins; cruises the western seaboard of U.S., Grenadines, Mexico's Sea of Cortez, Costa Rica, Panama, British Columbia, and Alaska's Inside Passage. **(Category C—Not Rated)**
(Medical Facilities: There is a physician on *Clipper Adventurer* and on other ships when ships are not within sight of U.S. or Canada.)

Clipper Cruise Line was started in 1982 by Barney Ebsworth. In December 1996 INTRAV, a deluxe-tour operator, acquired Clipper Cruise Line, with Paul H. Duynhouwer acting as president and CEO of both companies.

The *Newport Clipper,* the line's first ship, which set sail on its first voyage in 1982, is no longer part of the fleet. The *Nantucket Clipper* joined the line in 1984, and the *Yorktown Clipper* in 1988. The *Nantucket Clipper* and *Yorktown Clipper* are shallow-draft ships designed to operate in coastal waters. Because of their size, these ships are able to explore areas and ports inaccessible to larger cruise ships. They carry fewer than 140 passengers, and the on-board ambiance is intimate and unregimented.

The line acquired a Russian passenger vessel, renamed it the *Clipper Adventurer,* and refitted and renovated her for an April 1998 inauguration. She boasts an ice-strengthened hull, which enables her to sail to Greenland, the Canadian Arctic, and in Antarctica. There are four decks with 61 outside cabins, a dining room, lounge, beauty shop, gift shop, and library. Itineraries planned for 1998 included the Iberian Peninsula, the western Mediterranean, western Europe, the British Isles, Greenland, Hudson Bay, Arctic Canada, the eastern coasts of North and South America, the jungle rivers of South America, Antarctica, and the Falkland Islands.

In addition to those listed above, the line offers a casual, intimate cruise experience with specialized itineraries that include the St. Lawrence Seaway, the Thousand Islands, the Maine coast and Bay of Fundy, New England's coastal islands, Chesapeake Bay, the Great Lakes, the Intracoastal Waterway, the antebellum South, the Caribbean, Costa Rica, the Panama Canal, the lower Caribbean and Orinoco River, the Grenadines, the Sea of Cortez, San Francisco and the Sacramento River Delta, the Pacific Northwest, British Columbia, and Alaska's Inside Passage.

Cruise rates range between $1,250 per person for six-day cruise itineraries to $16,690 per person double occupancy for a suite on a 23-day Antarctica cruise. For single occupancy, add approximately 50 percent. All cabins are outside, are small with large picture windows, and have twin beds and private bathroom facilities. There are no tubs, telephones, TVs, private room safes, or special bathroom amenities. There are hair dryers on the *Clipper Adventurer.* All vessels have attractive public areas, including window-lined observation lounges.

Open-seating dining is offered in a simply but pleasantly furnished dining room with windows looking out to the sea. The mood and dress are casual. There are no formal nights. The restaurants emphasize American and Continental cuisine.

There is neither a casino nor the usual shipboard activities and entertainment. Emphasis is on the destination and sights, and the ships carry several motorized landing craft that permit landings inaccessible to most ships and tenders. Naturalists and historians are on hand to lend substance to the enjoyment of places visited. The ships frequently cruise during the day with one or more destination visits and are often docked at night to permit evenings ashore.

In late 1998, the line purchased the 5,200-ton *Oceanic Odyssey* from Spice Islands Cruises, renamed her *Clipper Odyssey,* and will commence operating her as a Clipper Cruise Line vessel in late 1999, with itineraries in the North and South Pacific, Australia, New Zealand, and Southeast Asia. The 60 staterooms each have a small tub and shower, a hair dryer, mini-bar, and television with VCR attachment and music channels. Dining is single seating, featuring American and Continental cuisine as well as regional specialties. Public areas include a main lounge and bar, a library, swimming pool, Jacuzzi, sauna, jogging track, gymnasium, boutique, and beauty salon.

Strong Points:
Unusual itineraries on casual, more intimate vessels.

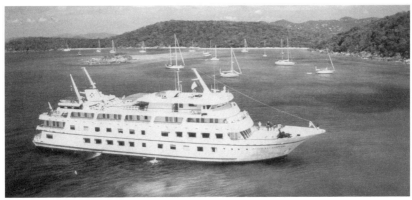

Courtesy Clipper Cruise Line

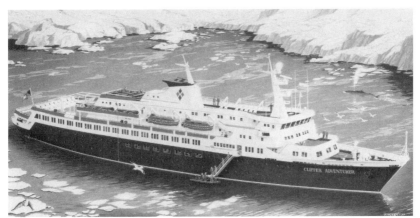

Courtesy Clipper Cruise Line

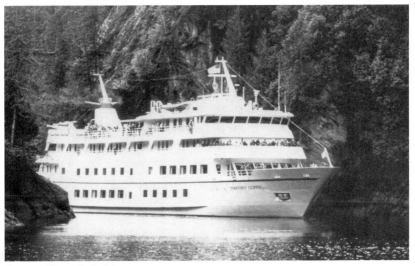

Courtesy Clipper Cruise Line

APPETIZER
Blackened Sirloin of Beef
Thinly Sliced Cajun Style Beef
Served Chilled with Red Onion, Tangy Mustard Sauce,
And Fresh Baked Melba Toast

SOUP
Navy Bean

SALAD
Spinach Salad
Fresh Picked Spinach Garnished with
Chopped Egg, Diced Bacon, and Sliced Mushrooms
Served with Our Own Hot Bacon Dressing

Tossed Crisp Green Salad * Choice of Dressing
Fresh Fruit Salad

SEAFOOD
Grilled Swordfish
Fresh Swordfish Steak Broiled to Perfection
Served with a Light Lemon Sauce

ENTREE
Roasted Duckling
A Boneless Breast of Long Island Duckling
Roasted Slowly Until Fork Tender
Accompanied with A Lingonberry Sauce

PASTA
Fresh Pasta Noodles Tossed with a
Pesto Cream Sauce
Garnished with Grated Romano Cheese

VEGETARIAN ENTREE
Stuffed Bell Pepper
Fresh Peppers filled with Seasonal Fresh Vegetables and Rice
Bound with a Zesty Tomato Sauce

VEGETABLE AND STARCH
Steamed Cauliflower
Wild Rice Pilaf

DESSERT
Fresh Berry Shortcake

New York Style Cheesecake with a Fresh Berry Sauce

A Variety of Ice Creams, Toppings and Jello

Courtesy Clipper Cruise Line

NANTUCKET CLIPPER

EXPLORING THE YACHTSMAN'S CARIBBEAN
ABOARD THE *NANTUCKET CLIPPER*

Tuesday, January 28, 1997
Sopers Hole, Tortola and
Roadtown, Tortola

Roadtown is the capital of the British Virgin Islands. This portion of the Virgin Islands includes 40 islands, islets and cays (points of land too small to be called islands). At 1,715 feet, Sage Mountain is the highest point on Tortola and is the focal point for a 92-acre park protecting remnants of a natural rain forest. This preserve provides an area for reforestation of native West Indian Mahogany.

6:00 a.m.   **DEPARTURE** of the *NANTUCKET CLIPPER* en route to Roadtown, Tortola.

7:00 a.m.   **WAKE-UP CALL** can be heard on CHANNEL "C" of your stateroom radio.

7:00 a.m.   **EARLY BIRD BREAKFAST** is available in the Observation Lounge until 9:00 a.m.

7:30 a.m.   **APPROXIMATE ARRIVAL** of the *NANTUCKET CLIPPER* in Roadtown, Tortola.

7:45 a.m.   **BREAKFAST** is served in the Dining Room until 8:15 a.m.

8:00 a.m.   **SAGE MOUNTAIN PARK HIKE:**
             If you are interested in taking a hike of Sage Mountain please meet Matthew
             on the dock at this time. Your return to the ship will be approximately 12:00 p.m.
             Please wear sturdy, comfortable walking shoes and loose clothing.

8:30 a.m.   **Departure of the PETER ISLAND SNORKEL EXCURSION:**
             Passengers signed-up for this snorkeling excursion should meet Matthew at the
             Main Deck transverse at this time. The snorkel tender will pull up to the Main Deck
             hatch. Your return to the ship will be approximately 11:00 a.m.

9:00 a.m.   **Departure of the CANE GARDEN BAY BEACH BUS:**
             Passengers signed-up for this excursion are asked to meet Matthew on the dock at this
             time. Your return to the ship will be approximately 12:00 p.m.

9:30 a.m.   **Departure of the TORTOLA ISLAND TOUR:**
             Passengers signed-up for this excursion are asked to meet Matthew on the dock at this
             time. Your approximate time of return to the ship is 12:00 p.m.

9:30 a.m.   **Departure of the PETER ISLAND SNORKEL EXCURSION:**
             Passengers signed-up for this snorkeling excursion should meet Matthew at the
             Main Deck transverse at this time. The snorkel tender will pull up to the Main Deck
             hatch. Your return to the ship will be approximately 12:00 p.m.

12:30 p.m.   **LUNCH** is served in the Dining Room. A soup and sandwich buffet is also available
             in the Observation Lounge.

1:45 p.m.   **Departure of the third PETER ISLAND SNORKEL EXCURSION:**
             Passengers signed-up for the third snorkeling excursion should meet Matthew at the
             Main Deck transverse at this time. Towels and swim belts will be available for you.
             Your return to the ship will be approximately 4:15 p.m.

2:00 p.m.	**Departure of the CANE GARDEN BAY BEACH BUS:** Passengers sign-up for this excursion are asked to meet Matthew on the dock at this time. Your return to the ship will be approximately 5:00 p.m.
2:15 p.m.	**Departure of the second TORTOLA ISLAND TOUR:** Please meet Matthew on the dock at this time if you have signed-up for the Tortola Island Tour. Your return to the ship will be approximately 5:00 p.m.
2:45 p.m.	**Departure of the fourth PETER ISLAND SNORKEL EXCURSION:** Passengers signed-up for this snorkeling excursion should meet Matthew at the Main Deck transverse at this time. Your return to the ship will be approximately 5:15 p.m.
5:45 p.m.	**LECTURE PRESENTATION:** All passengers are invited to join your on-board naturalist, AJ Lippson, for an informative presentation entitled, "THE BLOOMS OF THE CARIBBEAN", in the Observation Lounge.
7:15 p.m.	**DINNER** is served in the Dining Room.
9:00 p.m.	**AFTER DINNER ENTERTAINMENT** in the Observation Lounge. Enjoy music of the Caribbean performed by the local band, *SPLASH*.
········	**FEATURE PRESENTATION:** Once the Dining Room has been cleared and cleaned, we will begin this evening's feature presentation...

EXTREME MEASURES
Starring Hugh Grant and Gene Hackman

F.Y.I.	**FOR YOUR INFORMATION** *The *NANTUCKET CLIPPER* will depart Roadtown Tortola at 5:30 a.m. en route to Leverick Bay, Virgin Gorda. *TOUR SIGN-UP DEADLINES* If you would like to participate in the following tours please sign-up at the Hospitality Desk today: **WRECK OF THE RHONE SNORKEL - offered *THURSDAY MORNING* THE INDIANS SNORKEL - offered *THURSDAY AFTERNOON* HIGHLIGHTS OF THE BVI SNORKEL - (All Day) *THURSDAY***

Courtesy Clipper Cruise Line

CLUB MED CRUISES

40 West 57th Street

New York, New York 10019

(800) CLUB MED

(212) 315-5392 FAX

CLUB MED II: entered service 1992; 14,000 G.R.T.; 617' x 66'; 392-passenger capacity; 196 cabins; European officers, international crew, and international Club Med social staff; cruises in Caribbean and Mediterranean.

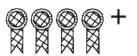 +

Club Med's first cruise venture, *Club Med I,* initiated service in February 1990. *Club Med II* followed in 1992. At 617 feet, these two graceful ladies currently represent the cruise industry's largest sailing vessels, carrying five masts and seven computer-controlled sails. *Club Med I* was sold to Windstar Cruises in 1997 and now sails as the *Wind Surf.* During the fall, winter, and early spring, *Club Med II* sales in the Caribbean, but in the late spring and summer she shifts to the Mediterranean, offering cruises that vary in length between 3 and 12 days to islands and ports around the Mediterranean.

Prices range from $250 to $335 per day per person double occupancy, and 30 percent more for single occupancy. Reasonable air-sea packages that include land options at Club Med Villages are available.

All of the spacious cabins measure 188 square feet and are located on the bottom three decks. There are also five suites. Thirty-five of the cabins can accommodate three passengers and six can accommodate four. All cabins have twin beds that can be converted to king-size, and every stateroom includes a telephone, four-channel TV, radio, refrigerator, mini-bar, private safe, large mirrors on the walls, an unusually generous amount of wardrobe and storage space, and bathrooms with showers, large sinks and vanities, separate toilet compartment, and numerous shelves.

The ship carries its own sailboats, scuba gear, windsurf boards, water skis, launches, and sports platform. There are two saltwater swimming pools, and the ships feature golf programs in many of the ports. Massages, saunas, and facials are offered, and a well-equipped fitness center is located atop the ship.

Two open-seating restaurants provide a variety of dining options, from lavish Club Med-style breakfast and lunch buffets, with both indoor and outdoor seating available in the top-deck restaurant, to more formal waiter service in the mid-deck. On a recent Mediterranean cruise, I found the freshly baked breads, rolls, and fresh fruits and cheeses especially outstanding. There are very acceptable French house wines provided *gratis* at lunch and dinner, as well as an à la carte wine list. A no-tipping policy prevails, as at other Club Meds. Room service is available.

Other public facilities include a piano bar and lounge, several additional bars by the pools, a boutique, hairdresser/beauty salon, and a gambling casino offering black-jack, roulette, and slot machines. After dinner, the G.O.'s (genteel organizers/social staff) provide you with typical Club Med-style entertainment, followed by late-night dance music in the disco at the bottom of the ship. Club Med provides a very good cruising experience; however, I found that activities, entertainment, and shore excursions are not as well developed as those found on more conventional cruise ships. It is possible that this ship will be sold by the line to Windstar.

Strong Points:

An upscale Club Med experience at sea offering comfortable cabins and great watersports, French food, and the opportunity to visit tropical islands and great beaches in the Caribbean or some unusual ports in the Mediterranean.

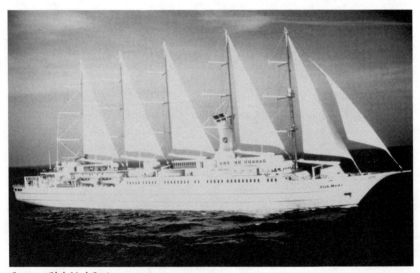

Courtesy Club Med Cruises

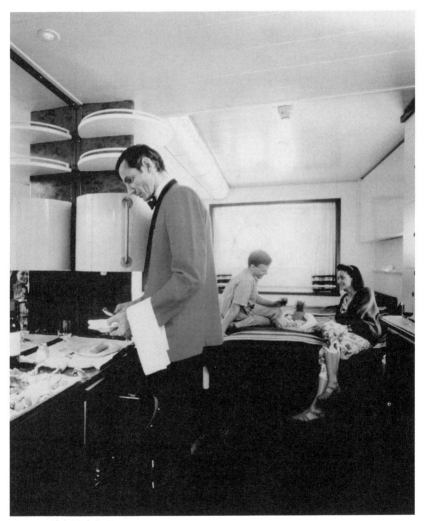

Courtesy Club Med Cruises

Club Med 1

SAMPLE DINNER MENU

PARISIAN CREAM SOUP

or

CHILLED CUCUMBER YOGURT GAZPACHO

****

SMOKED SALMON WITH WHIPPED CREAM

or

BEEF CARPACCIO

****

RACK OF LAMB IN GARLIC SAUCE

or

BROILED ENTRECOTE STEAK IN BORDELAISE SAUCE

or

VEAL ROAST WITH MUSHROOMS

****

CHEESE BOARD

****

DESSERT

Club Med 1

Menu

"SAINT GERMAIN" SOUP (Pea Soup)
or
ICED CAROTTS CREAM SOUP WITH ORANGES

★★★★

SMOKED SALMON WITH GRAPEFRUITS
or

SHRIMPS AND FRESH MUSHROOMS SALAD WITH COGNAC

★★★★

FROG LEGS IN "PROVENCALE" STYLE
WITH PUREE OF TOMATOES WITH BASIL
or
SWEETBREADS IN "PERIGOURDINE"STYLE

★★★★

GRILLED BEEF RIBEYE WITH "BORDELAISE" SAUCE
or
DUCK FILLET WTIH SHERRIES
or
BROCHETTE OF LEG OF LAMB WITH HERBS

★★★★

CHEESE BOARD

★★★★

SABAGLIONE WITH CHAMPAGNE

or

FRUITS WITH THE 2 SHERBETS

COMMODORE CRUISE LINE
4000 Hollywood Boulevard, Suite 385 South Tower

Hollywood, Florida 33021

(800) 237-5361

(954) 967-2100

(954) 967-2147 **FAX**

ENCHANTED CAPRI: (formerly *Island Holiday, Arkadya,* and *Azerbajian*); entered service 1976; refurbished 1997; 15,410 G.R.T.; 515' x 71'; 488-passenger capacity; 244 cabins; international officers and crew; 2-night cruises from New Orleans to Mexico. **(Category D—Not Rated)**

ENCHANTED ISLE: (formerly *Argentina, Veendam, Monarch Star,* and *Bermuda Star*); entered service 1958; refurbished 1972, 1985, 1990, 1994, and 1997; 23,395 G.R.T.; 617' x 84'; 725-passenger capacity, double occupancy; 361 cabins; European and American officers and international crew; seven-night cruises from New Orleans to the western Caribbean and Mexico.

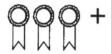

(Medical Facilities for *Enchanted Isle* and *Enchanted Capri:* C-2; P-1; CLS, MS; N-1; CM; PD; BC; EKG; TC; PO; EPC; OX; WC; ICU.)

UNIVERSE EXPLORER: (formerly *Brasil, Monarch Sun, Volendam,* SS *Canada Star, Liberte, Queen of Bermuda,* and *Enchanted Seas*); entered service 1958; refurbished 1972, 1985, 1990, 1994, and 1995; 23,500 G.R.T.; 617' x 80'; 736-passenger capacity, double occupancy; 369 cabins; European and American officers and international crew; on lease to the Institute of Shipboard Education and World Explorer Cruises. **(Category D—Not Rated)**
(Medical Facilities: Information not provided for this ship.)

Commodore Cruise Line was founded in 1966 by Sanford Chobol, a Miami hotel owner, who sold the line to a Finnish group in 1981. Today it is owned by a Florida financial group. The former vessels of the fleet were the M/S *Caribe* and the M/S *Boheme,* which were sold in 1981 and 1986, respectively. The *Caribe,* which started life in 1953 as the *Olympia* of the former Greek Line and was purchased by Commodore in 1983, was sold in 1993. The *Enchanted Isle* and *Enchanted Seas,* sister ships that commenced service in 1958 as the *Argentina* and *Brasil,* spent many years as Holland America vessels *Veendam* and *Volendam* and were frequently refurbished. Subsequently, they were operated as the *Bermuda Star* and *Queen of Bermuda* for Bermuda Star Line (BSL Cruises), which was absorbed by Commodore in 1990. The ships were then renamed the *Enchanted Isle* and the *Enchanted Seas,* respectively. The *Enchanted Seas* is now known as the *Universe Explorer.* In 1998, Commodore Cruise Line, in partnership with Isle of Capri Casinos, Inc., introduced two- and five-night sailings from New Orleans on the *Enchanted Capri.*

Commodore specializes in value-oriented cruises with per diem rates starting as low as $70 and escalating to $207 for a suite. Third and fourth passengers in the cabin pay less, and there are also attractive air-sea packages from 90 U.S. gateways.

The *Enchanted Isle,* at 23,395 tons, and *Universe Explorer,* at 23,500 tons, are medium-size sister ships with spacious cabins and plenty of open deck space. Eighty percent of the cabins are outside. They offer the usual facilities, including several public lounges, large dining rooms, lido buffet restaurants, pools, gyms, saunas, casinos, libraries, bars, shops, and more. Most public rooms are on the Promenade Deck, except for the dining room, which is two decks below, on the Main Deck. Forty cabins recently were fitted with double beds, and nine suites were added, two with balconies. Bargain fares and a plethora of activities make this one of the best buys in the cruise industry.

The *Enchanted Isle* offers seven-night itineraries departing from New Orleans and sailing to the western Caribbean and Mexico.

The *Universe Explorer* is under lease to the Institute for Shipboard Education as the 100-day Semester at Sea student program and to World Explorer Cruises for summer Alaska sailings.

Eighty percent of the cabins on the *Enchanted Capri* are outside. The ship features an Isle of Capri Casino, one of the largest onboard casinos in the Caribbean. It also has a large dining room, pool, bars, shops, theater, and a disco. Most public rooms are located on the Capri Deck. Sand Dollar Lounge is located on the Sky Deck and the Theater and Hideaway Disco on the Fiesta Deck. She alternates two and five-night cruises from New Orleans. The two-night cruise to nowhere sails down the Mississippi and out into the Gulf of Mexico before returning to New Orleans. On five-night sailings, the ship sails to Mexico.

Strong Points:

Commodore historically offers some of the most value-oriented seven-night cruises available, making it possible for low-budget cruise enthusiasts or first-time cruise passengers to partake of the entire cruise experience.

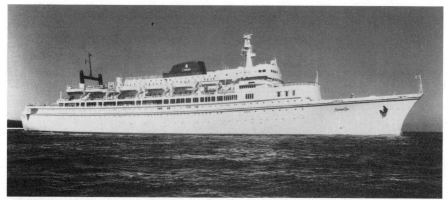

Universe Explorer, *courtesy Commodore Cruise Line*

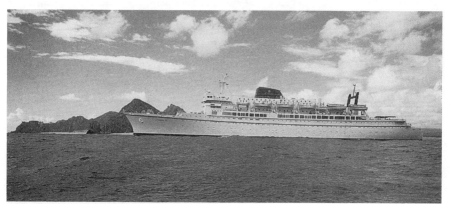

Enchanted Isle, *courtesy Commodore Cruise Line*

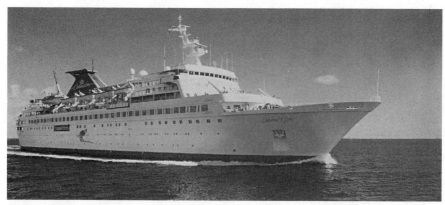

Enchanted Capri, *courtesy Commodore Cruise Line*

Welcome Dinner

Appetizers

SMOKED NORWEGIAN SALMON
Served with capers and lemon twist.

ESCARGOT BOURGUIGNON
Snails sautéed in shallots, parsley, lemon juice, red wine and sweet butter.

Soups

LOBSTER BISQUE
Pieces of lobster simmered in a cream soup and laced with old brandy.

FRENCH ONION SOUP AU GRATIN
Classic French onion and beef bouillon soup served with cheese croutons and oven baked.

Salads

CAESAR SALAD
Romaine lettuce tossed in caesar dressing sprinkled with grated parmesan cheese and croutons.

SLICED TOMATO AND RED ONION

Dressings

GREEN GODDESS - FLORIDA - ITALIAN

Entrees

GULF OF MEXICO SHRIMPS, JAMBALAYA
Jumbo shrimps simmered in diced tomatoes and garlic, spiced with southern herbs and served with dirty rice.

GRILLED CORNISH GAME HEN
Half a cornish hen seasoned with fresh herbs, Dijon mustard and garlic, served with dirty rice.

ROAST RACK OF LAMB, MINT JELLY
Tender spring lamb served with rissole potatoes.

ROASTED TENDERLOIN OF BEEF, MUSHROOM SAUCE
The heart of beef tenderloin served with red wine mushroom sauce.

Vegetables

BUTTERED GREEN BEANS - SUCCOTASH
DIRTY RICE

Desserts

FLORIDA KEY LIME PIE
A classic Key West dessert revealing a unique flavor of the Sunshine State.

TIRAMISU
Mascarpone cheese and Italian lady fingers flavored with espresso coffee.

BANANA FOSTER
Sliced island bananas simmered in a sweet butter, natural sugar and banana liqueur.

Ice Creams & Sherbets

SELECTION OF ICE CREAMS & SHERBETS

Dessert Sauces

CHOCOLATE - STRAWBERRY

Fruits & Cheeses

An Assortment of Domestic and International Cheeses accompanied by a selection of Fresh Fruits from the Cart.

Courtesy Commodore Cruise Line

WHAT'S UP

SCHEDULE OF DAILY ACTIVITIES

S/S Enchanted Isle

VOYAGE #281

AT SEA

8:00	CATHOLIC MASS is celebrated with Father Tamburello	Spyglass Lounge
8:00	Sign up sheets for WHEEL HOUSE TOUR are available.	Main Deck Fwd.
9:00	Brain Teasers and Crossword Puzzles. (Available at the Main Deck Fwd. Lobby)	
9:00-1:00pm	PHOTOGRAPHERS AVAILABLE FOR QUESTIONS	Photo Gallery

CRUISE FIT WORKOUT

9:30		Stretch and Tone. (Bring a towel & meet in the Neptune's Lounge)	C-Deck Aft.
10:00		Walk-A-Mile. Meet at . . .	Life Boat #1 - Boat Deck

9:45	***The Art of Napkin Folding*** *Dress up your table with a little help from our Dining Room Staff*	Grand Lounge

10:00	## ART AUCTION AT SEA No taxes, no duty, prices 30-70% off gallery prices!!	Bistro

10:00	Informal gathering of Horse Racing Fans. Hosted by David Pascale, join fellow racing enthusiasts, discuss and share your love & stories of events and triumphs "at the track".	Library

10:15	## IT'S BLOODY MARY BINGO! **WIN $$$ PLUS A BLOODY MARY**	Grand Lounge

11:00	## 'YOUR LIPS ARE MOVING' **The Edgar Bergen, Charlie McCarthy & Montimer Snerd Story** <small>A Multi-Media Presentation by foremost Bergen authority Teddy Davis. Bring your own cameras and meet Charlie McCarthy</small>	Neptune's Lounge
11:00-12:00	OUR SHORE EXCURSION MANAGERS and PORT LECTURER are available for inquiries.	Lobby Main Deck Fwd.

11:15	## TEAM TRIVIA CHALLENGE **With Dan and the Cruise Staff** Join us for more Laughs as we Explore the World of Completely Useless Information.	Grand Lounge
11:30-2:00	**Our Deck D.J. Danny Plays some of your favorite music.**	Poolside

-AFTERNOON-

1:00	SPECIAL HONDURAS TOUR BRIEFING FOR THOSE GUESTS WISHING TO LEARN ABOUT OUR OTHER ITINERARY.	Disco
1:00	ICE CARVING DEMONSTRATION	Poolside
1:00	TRAPSHOOTING gets underway. (Nominal charge)	Upper Deck Aft.
1:30	POOL GAMES! Fun in the sun with the Cruise Staff. (Weather Permitting)	Poolside
2:00	ZYDECO MUSIC ON DECK	Poolside

2:00	## STAR SEARCH TALENT SHOW SIGN UP If you can dance, sing, or tell a clean joke, come sign up with **George** for Friday's show. **We will register the First Ten Acts Only!**	Spyglass Lounge

2:15	# HIGH SEAS HORSERACING **WIN $$$$ AS THE FUN CONTINUES!!** Bet a Hunch and Win a Bunch at Commodore's Ups and Downs!	Grand Lounge

2:15	GOLF PUTTING & GOLF CHIPPING CONTEST! Win a prize!!!	Grand Lounge
3:00	FRIENDS OF DR. BOB & BILL AND LOIS W., meet in the . . .	Spyglass Lounge

3:15 Approx.	Join your Cruise Director, **Dan**, for ## THE NEWLYWED/NOT SO NEWLYWED GAME **A Re-creation of the Popular T.V. Game Show.** **JOIN US FOR MORE LAUGHS!**	Grand Lounge

4:30 - 5:00 pm	### Reef Roamer Farewell Get - Together For all passengers who took part in the Reef Roamer tours...	Grand Lounge

4:45	All couples wishing to renew their wedding vows, please sign up at this time. Registration will finish at 4:55 pm.	Spyglass Lounge
5:00	RENEWAL OF WEDDING VOWS Join us for a ceremony to renew your vows of marriage.	Spyglass Lounge
5:00	KIDS - HAVE YOUR PHOTO TAKEN WITH "COMMODORE CUDLEY"	Main Deck Fwd.

5:15- 6:00	**Nothing But Love Songs with ALAN LEE at the piano** *Piano Man Special: "Cuba Libre" only $2.50 (Bacardi, Cola and Lime)*	Spyglass Lounge

¤ *EVENING* ¤

PLEASE REMEMBER TONIGHT'S DRESS.... JACKET & TIE, THANK YOU.

| 7:15-8:15 | **ART AUCTION FINAL PREVIEW** with Matthew | Main Deck Fwd. Lobby |

| 7:30 ☺ | **CLUB COMMODORE PAST PASSENGERS PARTY** (Please bring your invitation) Please enter via the Photo Gallery. | Grand Lounge |

| 7:30-8:15 & 9:30-Close | *JOIN US FOR THE PIANO MELODIES OF ALAN LEE* Piano Man Special: "Cuba Libre" only $2.50 (Bacardi, Cola and Lime) | Spyglass Lounge |

Guests are requested to refrain from smoking during tonight's performances. Due to copyright laws video taping is not permitted, and please, do not reserve seats. Thank you.

| 8:30 1st Sitting 10:30 2nd Sitting | **GALA SHOWTIME** | Grand Lounge |

DON'T MISS THIS SHOW!

BACK BY POPULAR DEMAND...
COMEDIAN

STEVE ZIMMERMAN
and MORE MAGIC with
DAN STAPLETON

Music by: The Enchanted Isle Orchestra   *Musical Director: George Schneider*

9:15-10:15	THE ENCHANTED ISLE ORCHESTRA Plays for your dancing pleasure.	Grand Lounge
10:00	**KARAOKE TIME!** YOU MAY BE THE NEXT STAR!	Neptune's Lounge
11:00- Close	**Player's Special: all drinks $2.50 (except premiums)** Jackpot Special "Three Sevens" $2.50 (Scotch, Blended Whisky and Bourbon served with Grenadine & Orange Juice)	Casino
11:15-12:00	Great Music to dance to by THE ENCHANTED ISLE QUARTET	Grand Lounge
11:30 - Close	**MUSIC UNDER THE STARS** with Deck DJ Danny	Poolside
12:00	**GALA BUFFET** A DISPLAY OF CULINARY DELIGHTS. (Doors open for Picture-taking only -11:30 p.m.)	Riviera Dining Room
12:30MN-Close	**"THE BEAT GOES ON"** in our Disco	Neptune's Lounge

DINING HOURS FOR TODAY

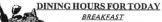

BREAKFAST

| 7:30- 9:30 | OPEN SITTING BREAKFAST | Riviera Dining Room |
| 7:00-10:00 | BUFFET BREAKFAST | The Bistro |

LUNCH

	12:00 - First Sitting - Second Sitting - 1:30	Riviera Dining Room
12:00- 2:00	LITE BUFFET LUNCH	The Bistro
12:00- 1:45	ENJOY HAMBURGERS & HOTDOGS	Poolside
4:00- 4:45	AFTERNOON SNACKS	The Bistro

CAPTAIN'S FAREWELL DINNER

| | 6:00 - First Sitting - Second Sitting - 8:15 | Riviera Dining Room |

Formal pictures will be taken outside the Dining Room (Doors will be closed 15 minutes after posted sitting time.)

(Passengers are advised that tank-tops or caps are not to be worn in the Dining Room at any time and shorts are not to be worn after 6:00 p.m.)

| 12:00 m.n.- 12:45 a.m. | **GALA BUFFET** (11:30 p.m., Picture-taking) | Riviera Dining Room |

🕐 BAR HOURS FOR TODAY

THE BISTRO- Tel. 15	8:00 AM - CLOSE	**MONTE CARLO CASINO BAR-** Tel. 3935	12:00 NN - CLOSE
GRAND LOUNGE- Tel. 3923	9:30 AM - 12:30 AM	**NEPTUNE'S LOUNGE -** Tel. 3930	9:30 PM - CLOSE
SPYGLASS LOUNGE- Tel. 3929	4:00 PM - CLOSE		

DRINK SPECIALS OF THE DAY

Eye Opener from 9:00 a.m.-12:00 n.n. - **BLOODY MARY & SCREW DRIVER - $2.75**

Drink Special of the Day: **"MAI-TAI"** - $2.75 (Rum; Creme de Almond liquor; Orange; Pineapple & Lemon Juices)

Non Alcoholic Special: **ORANGE COOLER -** $1.75 (Orange and Cranberry Juices)

Special Coffee- HAVANA COFFEE $2.75 (Bacardi Rum; Frangelico & Whipped cream)

All Cocktails in Souvenir Glass - $4.95   Refill price - $3.95

Draft Beer Special - Murphys Stout

☎ AT YOUR SERVICE

🛈 PURSER'S OFFICE/INFORMATION DESK (Main Deck Fwd.,Tel. 0)	OPEN 24 HOURS
⊕ INFIRMARY Located on D-Deck Forward. (Service Fee Charged)	9:00 AM -10:00 AM
(For Emergencies, Call The Purser's Office, Available 24 Hrs., Tel. 0)	4:00 PM - 5:00 PM
🎧 RADIO ROOM (Tel. 3983)	8:00 AM -12:00 MN
🏋 GYMNASIUM (Upper Deck Midship)	6:00 AM -10:00 PM
🛶 SHORE EXCURSIONS (Main Deck Forward)	11:00 AM -12:00 NN
(Tour Order Form drop box available after 11:00 AM)	
🎁 GIFT SHOP (Promenade Deck Midship) (Watches $69.95!, Make Up 50% off))	9:00 AM - 9:00 PM
💈 BEAUTY SALON & MASSAGE THERAPY	
C-Deck Midship (Tel. 3951)	9:00 AM -12:00 NN & 2:00 PM - 7:00 PM
🎰 CASINO SLOT MACHINES (Promenade Deck Fwd.)	10:00 AM - CLOSE
TABLES-	2:00 PM - 6:00 PM & 7:30 PM - CLOSE
(Children under the age of 18 are NOT allowed in the Casino.)	
PING PONG TABLES	9:00 AM - 8:00 PM
📷 PHOTO GALLERY (Inquiries , Tel. 3961) Photographers in Attendance,	9:00 AM - 1:00 PM

Courtesy Commodore Cruise Line

COSTA CRUISE LINES
80 S.W. 8th Avenue
Miami, Florida 33130
(800) 462-6782
(305) 375-0676 FAX

COSTA ALLEGRA: (formerly *Alexandra*); entered service 1969; totally rebuilt 1992; 30,000 G.R.T.; 615' x 84'; 820-passenger capacity; 410 cabins; Italian officers and international crew; cruises in South America, Mediterranean, and Northern Europe.

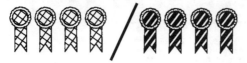

COSTA ATLANTICA: entered service 2000; 84,000 G.R.T.; 957' x 106'; 2,112-passenger capacity; 1,056 cabins; Italian officers and international crew; itinerary to be determined.

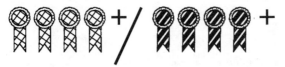

COSTA CLASSICA: entered service 1991; 53,000 G.R.T.; 718' x 98'; 1,308-passenger capacity; 654 cabins; Italian officers and international crew; Caribbean cruises; cruises to the Greek Isles from Venice in the summer.

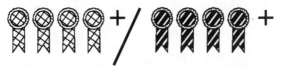

COSTA MARINA: (formerly *Italia*); entered service 1969; rebuilt 1990; 25,000 G.R.T.; 572' x 84'; 776-passenger capacity; 388 cabins; Italian officers and international crew; Northern Europe and South America cruises.

COSTA RIVIERA: (formerly *Guglielmo Marconi*); entered service 1963; rebuilt 1985; refurbished 1990, 1994, 1996, and 1998; 31,500 G.R.T.; 700' x 94'; 972-passenger capacity; 487 cabins; Italian officers and international crew; Mediterranean cruises, the Canary Islands, Egypt, and Israel.

COSTA ROMANTICA: entered service 1993; 54,000 G.R.T.; 722' x 102'; 1,356-passenger capacity; 678 cabins; Italian officers and international crew; Caribbean cruises in winter and Mediterranean summer cruises.

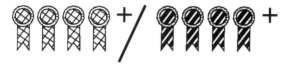

COSTA VICTORIA: entered service 1996; 76,000 G.R.T.; 824' x 105'; 1,928-passenger capacity; 964 cabins; Italian officers and international crew; Caribbean cruises in the winter and Mediterranean cruises in the summer.

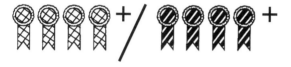

[Medical Facilities: Cruise line indicated there were one physician and two nurses aboard each ship but furnished no additional information.]

Note: Passenger capacity reflects double occupancy. Ships are capable of carrying more passengers.

Up until 1997, when it was acquired by Carnival Corporation and Airtours, the controlling owners of Costa Cruises were the Costa family, whose business ventures date back to 1860. Costa made its entrance into the cruise industry in 1948, when it introduced Italy's first air-conditioned passenger ship, the *Anna C,* which carried clients between Italy and South America. During the fifties, sixties, and seventies, the company added eight more vessels, some named after the grandchildren of its president, the *Federico C, Franca C, Carla C, Andrea C, Enrico C, Eugenio C, Giovanni C,* and *Flavia.* From time to time, it chartered other ships, including the *Leonardo da Vinci* and *Amerikanis,* as well as the *Daphne* and *Danae.* The latter two vessels were originally converted for cruising by the Carras line, a large Greek shipping enterprise, and subsequently leased and sold to Costa. Costa has sold off its older ships (including the *Enrico Costa, Eugenio Costa, Carla Costa, Daphne,* and *Danae*), renovated others, and streamlined down to the present six vessels listed above, offering cruises in the Caribbean, Northern Europe, South America, in the Mediterranean, and trans-Atlantic. In January 1998 Costa announced an agreement for the delivery of an 84,000-ton vessel in 2000, to be named *Costa Atlantica.*

The keynote for Costa is Italian ambiance and spirit. On all the ships you will find friendly Italian officers, romantic Italian orchestras, and helpful cruise directors and social staff. The officers and others holding important positions are Italian; however, the waiters, cabin attendants, and remainder of the crew are recruited from India, Goa, South America, and other areas around the world and have varying cruise experience. Generally, you do not find big-name entertainers, and the food, although ample, is not gourmet. The wine list offers an excellent selection of Italian wines at reasonable prices.

The ships doing Caribbean itineraries pretty much follow the pattern of other cruise ships in the Caribbean mass market and carry many Spanish-speaking passengers, as well as Italian and European families who have crossed the sea to enjoy a warm Caribbean winter cruise. When sailing in the Mediterranean, you will have mostly Italian and a smattering of other European shipmates, and you'll hear announcements in Italian, French, English, German, Spanish, and other languages. The food, entertainment, and activities are somewhat more geared to the European clientele. However, for those of you wanting a totally cosmopolitan and different experience, these cruises offer a unique opportunity to sail "Italian style" with Italians and passengers from around the world on a more intimate basis. During Christmas holidays and the summer months, you will find many young adults and also families traveling with children, as well as on-board activities to accommodate them. A less elegant and more party-oriented atmosphere pervades.

Recently, the *Costa Classica* has been marketed primarily to the European market year-round, and on *Costa Allegra* and *Costa Marina,* South American clientele predominates on cruises in their indigenous areas.

Prices vary from ship to ship and depend upon the season and cruise grounds. Costa quotes cruise-only cabins from $110 to $200 per person per day, with suites as high as $550 per person per day in the Mediterranean. An average outside cabin on a seven-night Caribbean cruise costs about $1,000 per person, including port charges but not airfare. On all ships third and fourth passengers sharing a room pay less than the regular fare. This is one of the least expensive, full facility/activity cruise experiences, with special appeal to Spanish- and Italian-speaking travelers.

The Costa Riviera received a $37 million renovation after its purchase in 1983. It originally entered service as the *Guglielmo Marconi* with the Italian Lloyd Triestino Line. All staterooms were refurbished during the renovation, with 285 located outside, 202 inside, and 52 with queen-size beds. The public rooms include several show lounges, a disco, a large casino, a special pizzeria, a cinema, a large dining room, and numerous more intimate nooks and bars. Outside, in addition to the pool and sun deck, are three Jacuzzis that have proven popular with the guests. Additional renovations took place in 1996 and 1998.

In the summer of 1990, Costa introduced the *Costa Marina,* a 25,000-ton rebuilt container ship that accommodates 776 passengers in 388 cabins for seven-night Northern European cruises from Copenhagen. South American cruises are scheduled for the winter, usually carrying a predominately South American clientele.

In early 1991 the *Costa Classica* entered service, the first totally new ship built by Costa since the *Eugenio Costa.* At 53,000 tons, with a capacity to accommodate 1,600 passengers (1,308 double occupancy) at a cost of $325 million, it is one of Costa's larger vessels. Two-thirds of the cabins are outside, and 20 percent have double or queen beds. All cabins and the ten veranda suites include radio, cable TV, phone, private safes, hair dryers, and good storage space. In addition to the main restaurant, there is a pizzeria, a pastry and coffee shop, and an indoor/outdoor lido restaurant. There is also a health spa with a few exercise machines, sauna, steam, whirlpools, massage, and other body treatment facilities; a gambling casino; and a 1,500-square-foot conference center for business meetings. She offers seven-night cruises to the Greek Isles during summer months and Caribbean cruises during the winter. The ship is marketed year-round primarily in Italy. An almost identical sister ship, *Costa Romantica,* entered service in November 1993. All cabins are large compared to other Costa ships, and the suites offer additional space, comfort, amenities, and privacy. The clientele is mostly Italian in the Mediterranean and predominately American in the Caribbean. In 2000 she will offer summer cruises in Northern Europe.

In December 1992, *Costa Allegra* was added to the fleet after a multimillion-dollar rebuilding at the Mariotti Shipyard in Genoa. At 30,000 tons, the ship can accommodate 820 passengers in 410 cabins, more than half of which are outside. The interior design is composed of skylights, transparent tiles, glass-roofed atriums, greenhouse domes, bold colors, flowing waterfalls and streams, and art and murals by some of Europe's leading artists. Public facilities include a meeting center; imaginative lounges, bars, and showrooms; a circle of shops; a casino; a large restaurant; a disco; a pool; an indoor/outdoor café; and a Romanesque spa featuring exercise equipment, aerobics, free weights, whirlpools, steam/sauna, massage, and a beauty parlor. A special low-calorie spa menu is also offered in the dining room. From May through October, she offers Mediterranean and Northern Europe cruises. During the winter months, she sails in South America, catering to a South American clientele.

The 76,000-ton, 1,928-passenger ship *Costa Victoria* entered service in the summer of 1996. She offers Mediterranean itineraries during the summer and Caribbean cruises the remainder of the year. The ship features a grand atrium spanning seven decks, extending to a crystal dome at the top. Public facilities include an Italian-style spa and fitness center that houses an indoor pool, sauna, steam room, whirlpool, and an exercise room with a limited number of cardiovascular machines and other equipment; a walking/jogging track around Deck 6; a lido area with two outside pools, four whirlpools, basketball, shuffleboard, and one miniature tennis court; two main dining rooms, a four-station buffet restaurant with an outdoor area overlooking the sea, a pizzeria, ice-cream bar, and poolside grill; a two-deck show lounge, a tri-level lounge for dancing and other entertainment, a disco, a large fully stocked casino, and several lounges and bars. The decor of the ship is austere compared to most large ships built in the nineties and does not include the expensive art found on Celebrity, Princess, Royal Caribbean, and Holland America vessels, nor the glitz and spectacle of the Carnival line. Cabins—though functional, with adequate storage, private safes, mini-bars, hair dryers, and remote-control televisions—are relatively small, having no sitting areas or balconies. The limited number of suites and mini-suites is not as large or as posh as those on many of Costa's competitors; however, the availability of two extra beds in the large walk-in closet areas makes them a viable alternative for families.

Strong Points:

Friendly service and spirit with an Italian theme; an opportunity to travel with numerous Italian and international passengers; special appeal for Spanish- and Italian-speaking passengers; an abundance of families and children's activities during holidays and summer months; full-facility ships with a lot happening for reasonable tariffs.

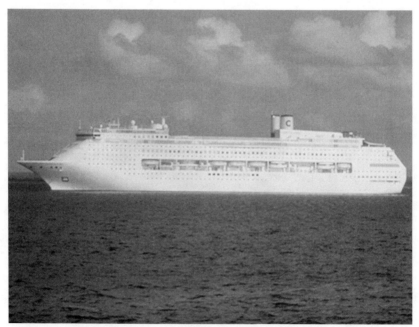

Courtesy Costa Cruise Lines

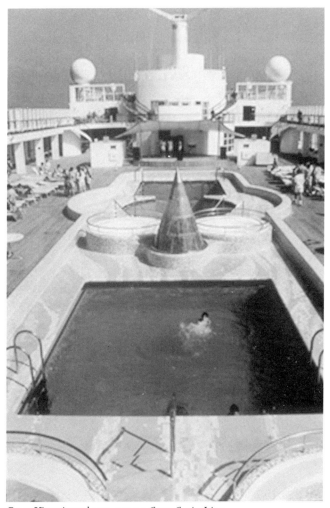

Costa Victoria *pool area, courtesy Costa Cruise Lines*

at sea

Time	Today on Board	Place & Deck
8.00am	**Morning Walkathon**	*Jogging Track, 6*
9.00am	**Aerobics, Abs, Butts & Tighs** with your Gym Instructor	*Pompei Spa, 6*
9.30am	Good Morning from the Navigational Bridge	
9.30am	**Bridge Players** meet our directors Alan and Mary Jane	*Jolly Cardroom, 7*
9.30am-5.30pm	**Private individual golf lessons** available from our resident PGA Golf Professional. Golf practice area. Nominal fee required.	*Deck 12, forward*
10.00am	**Aquagym** with the Costa Victoria Dancers	*Poolside, 11*
10.30am	**Wacky Putting contest, round #1.** Bring your favourite putter and your putting skills. Golf practice area. Nominal fee required.	*Deck 12, forward*
10.30am	*Cooking Italian Style* : with your Maître D' team	*Orpheus Grand Bar, 6*
11.00am	**Poolgames** with your cruise staff	*Poolside, 11*
11.00am	*A Morning at the Opera. Today: Otello*	*Concorde Plaza, 7*
11.00am	**Wine Tasting Demonstration.** (Nominal fee: US $5.00)	*Capriccio Bar, 7*
11.00am	**Bad Hair Demonstration.** Join the Salon Team! Learn helpful and styling techniques	*Orpheus Grand Bar, 6*
11.00am	**Jackpot Bingo!!!** Cover your card in 48 numbers or less and you'll win US$ 1200 guaranteed!	*Festival Theater, 6*
11.15am	**Doubles ping pong tournament** - Prizes for the winners	*Poolside, 11*
11.30am	**Anti-cellulite seminar.** Join the spa therapist to see how to smooth away cellulite and lose inches permanently	*Orpheus Grand Bar, 6*
noon-2.00pm	**Unity** plays caribbean music	*Poolside, 11*
12.30-1.45pm	**Kuba** plays classical piano	*Orpheus Grand Bar, 6*
2.00pm	**Art Auction Preview:** Join Carey, your onboard Art Consultant for a personal viewing of our fine woeks of art	*Concorde Plaza, 7*
2.00pm	**Seaweed Secrets.** Are you on it? Boost your health and lifestyle with this amazing seminar	*Orpheus Grand Bar, 6*
2.00-4.00pm	Our **Port Lecturer Robert** is available to answer all your island shopping questions	*Planetarium Hall, 5*
2.15pm	**History of Astrology:** lecture by Luise and John Hounihan	*Conference Center, 7*
2.15pm	**Darts Tournament** with your Cruise Staff	*Poolside, 11*
2.30pm	**Arts and Crafts** with our directors Olga and Jennifer	*Tavernetta, 12*
2.30pm	**Bridge players** meet Alan and Mary Jane	*Jolly Cardroom, 7*
2.30pm	**Superquiz** with the Cruise Staff	*Orpheus Grand Bar, 6*
2.45-4.30pm	Listen to the tropical melodies by *Unity*	*Poolside, 11*
3.00pm	**Park West Gallery Art Auctions at Sea:** Save for 50%- 80% off gallery prices on masters of Rembrandt, Picasso, Dali to contemporary artists Max & Tarkay. Opening bids as low as 25$! **Free raffle** - work of art valued at US$1,000! Cruise Special - free champagne for every 5 works purchased!	*Concorde Plaza, 7*
3.00pm	**Reflexology.** Bring a partner and experience this unique therapy of the footpressure points	*Capriccio, 7*
3.00pm	**Bill W. Meeting**	*Meeting room #2, 7*
3.00pm	**Complimentary gaming lessons** with your casino staff	*Montecarlo Casino, 7*
3.00pm	**Circuit Training** with your Gym instructor	*Pompei Spa, 6*
3.00pm	**Super Poolgames** with your cruise staff - Let's have fun!!	*Poolside, 11*
3.15pm	Cinema Time! *My best friend's wedding* (105 min.)	*Conference Center, 7*
3.15pm	Horseracing! Meet Orlando and the Cruise Staff and place your bets	*Festival Theater, 6*
3.15-4.00pm	**Musical Quiz** with Richard Raphael	*Orpheus Grand Bar, 6*
3.30pm	**Italian lesson** with Paola	*Tavernetta, 12*
3.30pm	**Scrabble Competition** with your Cruise Staff	*Capriccio Bar, 7*
3.30pm	**Wacky Putting contest, round #2.** Bring your favourite putter and your putting skills. Golf practice area. Nominal fee required.	*Deck 12, forward*
4.00pm	**Jackpot Bingo!!!** If you cover your card in 49 numbers or less you could win US$ 1400!	*Festival Theater, 6 & 7*
4.00pm	**The Sanctuary:** stretch, relax, aromatherapy, music...Wonderful to de-stress! Join your fitness directors	*Tavernetta, 12*
4.00pm	**Dance class** with our instructors Richard and Carol	*Orpheus Grand Bar, 6*

9.15pm
1st sitting

SHOWTIME

11.00pm
2nd sitting

Micki Spoon, John Ciotta & Colin Charles
and featuring the *Costa Victoria Dancers*
with music by Mark Mac Gregor and the Costa Victori Orchestra

---

Tonight at 8.30pm in the Orpheus Grand Bar, deck 6

Richard Raphael Entertains!
A Tribute to Andrew Lloyd Webber
(this show is 30 minutes in duration)

Music for everyone!

Orpheus Grand Bar
5.30-7.00pm	Karena and Michelangelo
7.30-8.30pm	Karena and Michelangelo
8.30-9.00pm	Richard Raphael entertains

Planetarium Martini Bar
5.30-6.30pm	Music with Kuba
8.00-9.00pm	Music with Kuba
9.00pm-midnight	Mr. X plays piano

Orpheus Grand Bar
9.15pm-1.30am	Let's dance with Jackpot Duo

Concorde Plaza
8.30pm-1.30am	Music with "Fausto's Band"

Capriccio Piano Bar
5.30-6.30pm	Piano entertainment with Richard Raphael
7.45-8.45pm	Music by Kuba
9.30-11.30pm	Wonderful melodies by Karena and Michelangelo
11.30pm-12.30am	Music by Kuba
12.30-1.30am	Music by Richard Raphael

The Tavernetta
10.00pm-2.00am	Music with Art Mathews and his "pocket orchestra"

Rock Star Disco
from 11.30pm disco music with our DJ Giorgio

---

your hotel

Breakfast

Coffee and croissants for early risers,
Bolero Buffet, deck 11 ....6.30am
Breakfast in your cabin................................7.30-10.00am
Sinfonia Restaurant, deck 5
first sitting (no table reservation)...............................7.30am
second sitting (no table reservation).........................8.30am
Fantasia Restaurant, deck 5
first sitting (no table reservation)...............................7.30am
second sitting (no table reservation 8.30am
Self Service, Bolero Buffet, deck 11.................7.30-10.00am
Croissants, La Terrazza, deck 11 ....10.30-11.30am

Lunch

Fantasia Restaurant, deck 5 (from table 1 to 100)
first sitting 12.00pm
second sitting 1.30pm
Sinfonia Restaurant , deck 5 (from table 101 to 231)
first sitting 12.00pm
second sitting 1.30pm
Self Service, Bolero Buffet, deck 11 ....12.30-2.30pm
Grill
Grill Nettuno, deck 11 ....12.30-2.30pm

For those passengers who enjoy relaxing in the sun, you may enjoy a limited selection luncheon, at the Buffet, deck 11. For those, who prefer a complete lunch, the Restaurant is available at opening hours listed in the "Today".

Afternoon Tea

Bolero Buffet, deck 11 ....4.00-5.00pm
served with pizza, sandwiches and pastries

Pizzeria

Pizzeria, deck 12 ....2.30-8.30pm & 9.30pm-1.00am

Ice Cream

Pizzeria, deck 12 ....10.00pm-midnight

Captain's Gala Dinner

Fantasia Restaurant , deck 5 (from table 1 to 100)
first sitting...6.15pm
second sitting..8.45pm
Sinfonia Restaurant, deck 5 (from table 101 to 231)
first sitting...6.15pm
second sitting..8.45pm
In order to guarantee the best service, guests are kindly asked to respect meal hours. If you are more than 15 minutes late, please contact the Maitre D'.

Late Night Buffet

Galley Buffet
Fantasia Restaurant, deck 5.....................................12.15am

Bar

Planetarium Hall Bar, Bohème deck 9.00am-midnight
Grand Bar Orpheus, Traviata deck 8.00am-1.30am
Rock Star Disco Bar, Traviata deck ....11.00pm-........
Festival Bar, Traviata deck 5.00pm-1.00am
Concorde Bar, Carmen deck 5.00pm-1.30am
Capriccio Bar, Carmen deck 11.00am-3.00am
Bellavista Bar, Carmen deck 7.00pm-12.30am
Sirena Bar, Rigoletto deck 8.00am-6.00pm
Terrazza Caffè Bar, Rigoletto deck 10.30am-6.00pm
Tavernetta Bar, deck Butterfly 5.00pm-2.00am
Neptuno Bar, Rigoletto deck noon-2.30am

Today's cocktail : **Screwdriver**
(Vodka - Orange Juice)

Italian Dinner

Appetizers

Prosciutto e Melone
Parma Ham with Melon

Coppa di Arance e Kiwi al Maraschino
Iced Orange and Kiwi Cocktail with Maraschino

Mozzarella in Carrozza
Mozzarella on Toast dipped in golden Butter, served with Tomato Coulis

Soups

Consommé Milanese
Consomme with Rice and Tomato Strips

Pasta e Fagioli alla Napoletana
Pasta and Bean Soup Neapolitan Style

Salad

Primavera
Garden Greens with sliced Cucumbers, Spring Onions and Radish Rose
Choice of Dressing

Pasta

Lasagne al forno Emiliana
Layers of freshly made Pasta, filled with a creamy ground Beef Sauce and
Enhanced with Cheese

Entrées

Zuppa di Pesce Cioppino
Rockfish, Lobster, Clams and Mussels, simmered in a light Tomato Sauce
garnished with Vegetables and Garlic Croutons

Carré d'Agnello ai Profumi del Tigullio
Roast Rack of Lamb wih Herb Crust, served with Gratinated Potatoes

Scaloppina alla Parmigiana
Breaded Tender Escalope of Turkey, topped with Ham, Cheese and Tomato
served with Chateau Potatoes

Vegetables

Selection of the Day

Cheese

Parmigiano, Bel Paese, Gorgonzola

Desserts

Tiramisù Veneziano
Babà Tarantella
Watermelon Sherbet
Tri-flavoured Ice Cream
Fresh Fruit in Season

Beverages

Freshly brewed regular or decaffeinated Coffee
English or Herbal Tea

CRYSTAL CRUISES

2049 Century Park East, Suite 1400

Los Angeles, California 90067

(310) 785-9300

CRYSTAL HARMONY: entered service 1990; 49,400 G.R.T.; 791' x 105'; 940-passenger capacity; 480 staterooms; Norwegian and Japanese officers, European hotel and dining staff; international crew; Transcanal, Mexico, Caribbean, South America, Pacific, Southeast Asia, Australia/New Zealand, South Pacific, Orient, and Alaska/Canada cruises.

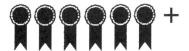 +

CRYSTAL SYMPHONY: entered service 1995; 50,200 G.R.T.; 781' x 99'; 940-passenger capacity; 480 staterooms; Norwegian and Japanese officers, European hotel and dining staff, international crew; Middle East, China/Orient, Southeast Asia, Mexican Riviera, Transcanal, South Pacific, Australia/New Zealand, Europe, Mediterranean, Baltic, and Black Sea.

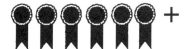 +

(Medical Facilities: P-1; EM, CLS, MS; N-2; CM; PD; BC; EKG; TC, PO; OX; WC; ICU; X; M; TM; LJ; and 4 wheelchair accessible cabins on *Harmony* and 7 on *Symphony*.)

Note: **Six+ black ribbons is the highest rating given in this edition to ships in the deluxe market category.**

Crystal Cruises, a subsidiary owned by Nippon Yusen Kaisha (NYK) of Japan and based in Los Angeles, launched its first luxury-class ship, the *Crystal Harmony,* in the summer of 1990, followed by *Crystal Symphony* in 1995. With construction costs of $200 million and $250 million respectively, these are two of the largest, most spacious ships competing in the luxury cruise market. These sleek vessels boast some of the largest luxury penthouses afloat, with outdoor verandas in all penthouses as well as in more than 50 percent of the staterooms.

The 480 staterooms on *Harmony* and *Symphony* are composed of the four Crystal Penthouses on *Harmony* and the two on *Symphony,* measuring 948 and 982 square feet respectively (one can really spread out here); 26 additional penthouse suites on *Harmony* and 18 on *Symphony,* measuring 492 square feet; 32 penthouses on

Harmony and 44 on *Symphony* at 360 square feet; 198 outside deluxe staterooms with verandas on *Harmony* and 214 on *Symphony;* 201 additional outside staterooms on *Harmony* and 202 on *Symphony;* and 19 inside staterooms only on *Harmony.* All penthouses and staterooms have twin beds that convert to queen- or king-size beds, mini-refrigerators, hair dryers, robes, makeup mirrors, private safes, showers and bathtubs, large closets, writing-makeup desks, voice mail, 14-channel color TV and radio systems that include CNN and videocassette players, and 24-hour room service. All non-veranda cabins on *Symphony* have large picture windows. The Crystal Penthouses feature oversized Jacuzzis, Jacuzzi-tub-showers, an additional enclosed shower stall, and walk-in closets. Describing the accommodations on these ships is more akin to describing the accommodations at a luxury resort rather than on oceangoing vessels.

The central focus of both ships is the magnificent Crystal Plaza atrium lobby. Leading off this area are a casino; a disco; a piano bar; a 277-seat Hollywood Theater; a bistro offering an assortment of international coffees, wines, pastries, and snacks; and a 3,000-square-foot shopping area. A number of lounges, bars, and showrooms (including the observation lounges) afford 270-degree views. The Caesars Palace at Sea Casinos, operated by the famed Las Vegas gaming operation, are designed to look like Roman forums, each with blackjack tables, slot machines, a craps table, baccarat, and a roulette table. Elaborate Broadway-style productions are offered throughout the cruise, in addition to cabaret entertainers, classical concerts, and several dance bands.

The Crystal Spas offer aerobics and jazzercise instruction coordinated by a full-time fitness director, and also an assortment of exercise equipment, saunas, and steam rooms. Featured at the Crystal Salons are facials, massages, makeup instruction, manicures, and hairstyling. There are two swimming pools: the Seahorse pool, with two adjacent Jacuzzis; and the Neptune indoor/outdoor pool, with a swim-up bar serving all beverages, hotdogs, hamburgers, pizza, ice-cream creations, and deli sandwiches. Additionally, the ship has a full promenade deck plus an outdoor track above the pool for jogging or walking, a paddle-tennis court, skeet shooting, and shuffleboard facilities.

Crystal was the first cruise line to offer alternative dinner restaurants at no extra charge. In addition to luxurious main dining rooms, passengers can opt for Japanese specialties at the intimate Kyoto Restaurant on *Harmony* or Asian specialties at Jade Garden on *Symphony,* as well as superb Italian cuisine in the romantic Prego Restaurants on both vessels. Casual breakfast and lunch buffets are offered both indoors and alfresco at the Lido Cafés near the pools. All meals, as well as snacks, are available around the clock through extensive room-service menus. Smoked salmon and other expensive delicacies are offered at the buffets, and hot and cold hors d'oeuvres are served each evening in the lounges. The breakfast buffet includes freshly made omelets and Belgian waffles, delicious pastries, fresh fruits, and other standard items, while the luncheon buffets offer numerous eclectic dishes, freshly made pasta and Caesar salad, and a variety of delectable desserts. Special theme buffets are also offered on each cruise. Passengers ensconced in the penthouses enjoy complimentary liquors, nightly hors d'oeuvres and/or caviar trays in their rooms, free pressing, shoe shines, personalized stationery, and personal butler services.

Other special features available to all passengers include 24-hour front-desk service, two European-trained concierges to assist you with travel and land arrangements, a Crystal Ambassador (gentleman) host program for the mature ladies, self-service launderettes throughout the ship, satellite telephone service, descriptive videos of all shore excursions, and access to private business offices equipped with computers, telefaxes, and secretarial services on request. The ships often feature on-board enrichment programs.

Before the *Crystal Harmony* commenced service, the owners and operation staff wisely researched all of the other major cruise vessels to determine which facilities, activities, and amenities would be most desired by knowledgeable and sophisticated cruise enthusiasts. The result is a uniquely excellent cruise experience that combines the impeccable service, gourmet dining, and spacious accommodations found on the small, luxury, yacht-like vessels with the state-of-the-art facilities and high-caliber entertainment and activities offered on the major ships of today's most popular cruise lines.

Prices average about $425 per day, per person, for a deluxe outside stateroom. Crystal Penthouses run over $1,000.

Strong Points:

Excellent dining and service; spacious and comfortable accommodations in all categories; special pampering for Crystal Penthouse occupants; and the ultimate in luxury on large, full-facility ships; considered by most to be the best of the large luxury ships afloat.

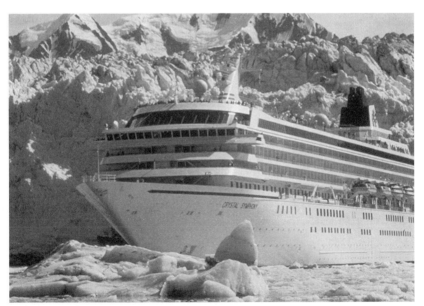

Courtesy Crystal Cruises

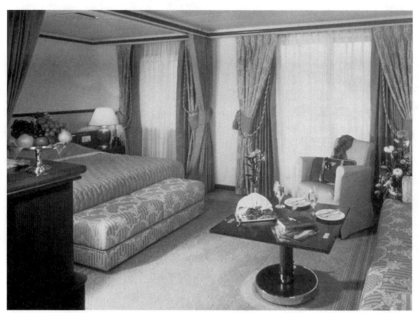

Courtesy Crystal Cruises

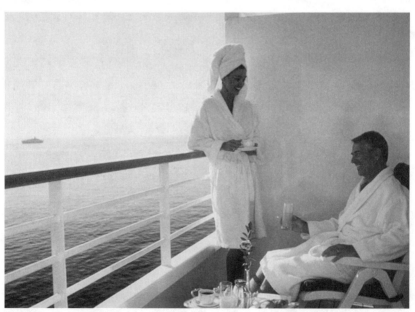

Courtesy Crystal Cruises

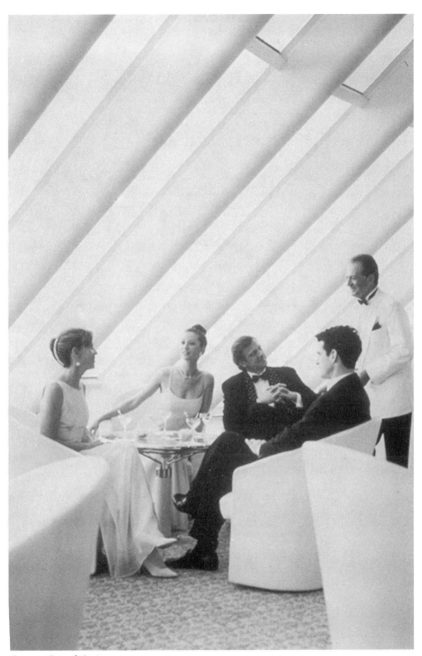

Courtesy Crystal Cruises

CRYSTAL SYMPHONY

MONDAY, JANUARY 12, 1998
"LATIN INTERLUDE" CRUISE
AT SEA, EN ROUTE TO LOS ANGELES

Maître d'Hôtel **Leo Assmair**   *Executive Chef* **Josef Lumetsberger**

CAPTAIN'S GALA DINNER

ON BEHALF OF THE OFFICERS, STAFF, AND CREW OF CRYSTAL SYMPHONY,
I WOULD LIKE TO BID ALL GUESTS LEAVING US
"PA GJENSYN," "AU REVOIR," BUT NOT "GOOD-BYE."

I SINCERELY HOPE YOU HAVE ENJOYED YOUR STAY ON BOARD WITH US,
AND THAT WE SHALL BE SHIPMATES AGAIN IN THE VERY NEAR FUTURE.

CAPTAIN HELGE BRUDVIK, COMMANDER

CHEF'S SUGGESTIONS

Iced Russian Sevruga Caviar with Traditional Condiments, Blinis and Melba Toast

Cream of Asparagus "Argenteuil"

Roasted, Herb-Marinated Quail
*On Braised Summer Cabbage with Apples,
Potato Coins, and Cassis Flavored Gravy*

The American Institution – Baked Alaska Flambe en Parade

FOR OUR VEGETARIANS

Papaya Boat Filled with Tropical Fruit, Sprinkled with Grand Marnier

Irish Cobbler Potato Strudel
With Caramelized Onions, Early Morels, on Port Wine Reduction Sauce

Blackberry Mousse with Cassis Mirror

CELLAR MASTER SUGGESTIONS

CHAMPAGNE
By the Bottle: *Mumm Cordon Rouge, Reims NV* – $42.00
By the Glass: *Louis Roederer Brut Premier, Reims NV* – $8.50
By the Glass: *Moët & Chandon, Cuvée Dom Pérignon, Epernay 1990* – $19.00

WHITE WINE
By the Bottle: *Babcock Vineyard Grand Cuvée Chardonnay, Santa Ynez Valley 1995* – $48.00
By the Glass: *Cuvaison Chardonnay, Carneros 1996* – $7.00

RED WINE
By the Bottle: *Jordan Cabernet Sauvignon, Alexander Valley 1993* – $45.00
By the Glass: *Chimney Rock Cabernet Sauvignon, Napa Valley 1994* – $7.50

CRYSTAL SYMPHONY

APPETIZERS

Iced Russian Sevruga Caviar with Traditional Condiments, Blinis, and Melba Toast

Pâté de Foie Gras of Duck with Warm Brioche

Alaskan Halibut Carpaccio with Vegetable Vinaigrette

Papaya Boat Filled with Tropical Fruit, Sprinkled with Grand Marnier

SOUPS

Beef Consommé with Truffle and Goose Liver Croutons

Cream of Asparagus "Argenteuil"

SALAD

The Commander's Salad
Selected Salad Bouquet with Tomatoes, Cucumbers, Carrots,
Endive, and Daikon Julienne, Served with Balsamic Vinaigrette

Traditional favorite dressings available, plus today's specials:
Fat-Free Tomato Basil and Low-Calorie Creamy Caesar Dressing

SHERBET

Refreshing Kir Royal Sherbet

MAIN COURSES

Broiled King Crab Legs
Served with Melted Lemon Butter or Sauce Hollandaise,
Steamed Fresh Garden Vegetables, and Saffron Pilaf Rice

Roasted, Herb-Marinated Quail
On Braised Summer Cabbage with Apples,
Potato Coins, and Cassis Flavored Gravy

Filet of Beef Wellington
Pink Roasted Tenderloin of Beef in Flaky Puff Pastry,
With Sauce Perigourdine, Assorted Fresh Young Vegetables, and Château Potatoes

Grilled Wisconsin Veal Medallions
On Creamy Morel Sauce, Fresh Vegetable Bouquet, and Angel Hair Pasta

SIDE ORDERS

Fresh Vegetable Bouquet   Braised Summer Cabbage   Saffron Pilaf Rice

Potato Coins   Château Potatoes   Angel Hair Pasta with Tomato Sauce

Upon request, dishes are available without sauce. Vegetables are also available steamed, without butter or salt.

CRYSTAL SYMPHONY

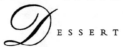

MONDAY, JANUARY 12, 1998
"LATIN INTERLUDE" CRUISE
AT SEA, EN ROUTE TO LOS ANGELES

Maître d'Hôtel **Leo Assmair** *Executive Chef* **Josef Lumetsberger**
Executive Pastry Chef **Harald Neufang**

SWEET FINALE

The American Institution – Baked Alaska Flambe en Parade

Blackberry Mousse with Cassis Mirror

Sugar-Free Chocolate Cake

*Vanilla, Spumoni, Black Walnut, and Chocolate Ice Cream
With Your Choice of Assorted Toppings*

Freshly Frozen Non-Fat Peanut Butter or Chocolate Yogurt

Refreshing Kir Royal Sherbet

Tropical Fruits in Season

Plantation Pralines, Truffles, and Petits Fours

SELECTIONS FROM THE CHEESE TROLLEY

St. Loupe   Tilsiter   Bel Paese   Monterey Jack   Dana Blue

Served with Crackers and Biscuits

BEVERAGES

Freshly Brewed Coffee   Decaffeinated Coffee   Cafe Latté   Cappuccino

Espresso   Selection of International Teas

AFTER DINNER DRINKS

As a Digestif, we would like to recommend:

Tia Maria – $3.75   Late Bottled Vintage Port – $5.75

Grand Marnier – $4.00   Remy Martin Cognac V.S.O.P. – $5.00

or your favorite classic after dinner liqueur, available from your bar waiter

Courtesy Crystal Cruises

── CRYSTAL SYMPHONY ──

GOOD MORNING

6:00am – 8:00am	**The Crystal Spa and Fitness Center** is open for your workout enjoyment.	Crystal Spa	12

7:00am	**Crystal Symphony is scheduled to anchor off Cabo San Lucas.** Please make yourself comfortable in one of the ship's public areas as you await the announcement that the ship has been cleared, and you are free to proceed to the tender area.

7:30am	**Walk-a-thon.** The clipboard is set up for you to log in your laps.	Promenade Deck	7
9:00am	**Jigsaw Puzzle "in Progress"** in the Bridge Lounge. Add a piece!	Bridge Lounge	6
9:00am – Noon	**The Library is open** to check out books, videos, and today's quiz. Christina the Librarian is there to assist you.	Library	6
9:00am – 6:00pm	**Table Tennis, Shuffleboard, and Paddle Tennis** are available for in-port, open play.		

11:30am	**All guests back aboard the last tender, please.**
Noon	**Crystal Symphony is scheduled to sail for Los Angeles.**

GOOD AFTERNOON

12:15pm	**Trivia.** Join in the fun with Social Hostess Teri Ralston.	Avenue Saloon	
1:30pm	**Crystal Visions Enrichment Lecture.** Health and Fitness Expert Richard Helfrich tells you how to "Slow the Aging Process."	Galaxy Lounge	6
2:00pm – 4:00pm	**Duplicate and Rubber Bridge Games** with Roberta Salob.	Bridge Lounge	6
2:30pm	**Movie:** *George of the Jungle.* Brendan Fraser stars. Rated PG-13, 1:37.	Hollywood Theatre	6
2:30pm	**Shuffleboard Tournament** with Sports Director Kim Walters.	Promenade Deck *Aft*	7
2:30pm	**Complimentary Dance Class.** Join Dance Instructors Tony & Margaret Long.	Galaxy Lounge	6
2:30pm	**Golf Lessons and Tips** with Golf Pro Sam Randolph at the golf net.	Sun Deck	12
3:00pm	**Fitness Class:** *Total Body Conditioning* with your Fitness Director Hazel.	Crystal Spa	12
3:30pm	**Auction The Premier Collection.** Today we feature the most exclusive works in our collection by the renowned masters such as Miro, Erté, Picasso, and more. Join Tommy Varzos for a look at these exclusive works. *Complimentary mimosas.* Art Auction preview at 2:30pm.	Starlite Club	6
3:30pm	**Paddle Tennis** with Sports Director Kim Walters.	Wimbledon Court	12
3:30pm – 4:30pm	**Crystal Afternoon Tea Time** serenaded by the Manila Trio.	Palm Court	11
4:00pm	**Fitness Class:** *Stretch and Relax* with your Fitness Director Hazel.	Crystal Spa	12
4:30pm	**Friends of Bill W.** meet in the private room of…	Jade Garden	6
5:30pm	**Catholic Mass** celebrated by Reverend Thomas Kiefer.	Hollywood Theatre	6

GOOD EVENING

5:30pm *(Main Seating)* & 7:45pm *(Late Seating)*	**All guests are cordially invited to the Farewell Cocktail Party.** The Commander of Crystal Symphony, **Captain Helge Brudvik**, personally greets you at the entrance.	Starlite Club	6
5:30pm – 6:15pm & 7:45pm – 8:30pm	**Jeff Walters** plays the Crystal Piano during the pre-dinner cocktail hours.	Crystal Cove	5
6:45pm – 7:30pm & 7:45pm – 8:30pm	**Tommy Dodson** entertains at the piano bar. Join him for a great evening of music.	Avenue Saloon	6
8:00pm and 10:30pm	**Movie:** *The Game* starring Michael Douglas. Rated R, 2:08.	Hollywood Theatre	6
9:30pm – 10:30pm	**Jeff Walters** entertains at the Crystal Piano.	Crystal Cove	5
9:30pm – 12:30am	**The Manila Diamonds** play for your dancing and listening pleasure.	Palm Court	11
10:30pm – 12:30am	**Tommy Dodson** entertains.	Avenue Saloon	6
11:30pm – 12:15am	**The Manila Trio** serenade for the Late Night Snack (buffet to 12:30am).	Crystal Plaza	5

Monday's Dining Hours

Formal Night

THE LIDO CAFE AND GARDENS, LIDO DECK 11
Early Bird Coffee (port side) .... 5:00am – 5:30am
Early Risers Buffet (Continental) .... 5:30am – 6:30am
Breakfast Buffet .... 6:30am – 10:00am
Bouillon .... 11:00am – 11:30am
Asian Cafe *(Around Neptune Pool)* .... **Noon – 1:30pm**

THE BISTRO, TIFFANY DECK 6
Late Risers Coffee with Danish Pastries .... 9:30am – 11:30am
Bistro Snacks, Tarts, and Pastries..................... 11:30am – 6:00pm

THE TRIDENT SNACK BAR, LIDO DECK 11 ...... 11:00am – 6:00pm

THE ICE CREAM BAR, LIDO DECK 11 .... 11:00am – 6:00pm

THE PALM COURT, LIDO DECK 11
Crystal Afternoon Tea Time.............................. 3:30pm – 4:30pm

THE CRYSTAL DINING ROOM, CRYSTAL DECK 5
Breakfast (open seating) .... 7:00am – 9:00am
Luncheon (open seating) .... Noon – 1:30pm
Gala Farewell Dinner (Main Seating) 6:15pm
Gala Farewell Dinner (Late Seating) 8:30pm

CRYSTAL PLAZA, CRYSTAL DECK 5
Late Night Snack .... 11:30pm – 12:30am

JADE GARDEN, TIFFANY DECK 6 (Offering Asian Cuisine)
Dinner .... 6:00pm – 10:00pm

PREGO, TIFFANY DECK 6 (Offering Italian Cuisine)
Dinner .... 6:00pm – 10:00pm

Reservations for Jade Garden and Prego Restaurants: For these alternative dining areas, we ask you to please come by and make reservations in person with Mario, our Maître d', in the Prego Restaurant from 10:30 to 11:30am, and from 5:00pm to 6:00pm. Please note that both Jade Garden and Prego Restaurants are non-smoking areas.

Avenue of the Stars Shops
Open today from sailing to 9:00pm.

Caesars Palace at Sea Casino
Open today: **Slots:** 1:00pm to 2:00am. **Table Games:** 1:00pm to 6:00pm and 9:00pm to 2:00am.

Library, Tiffany Deck 6
The Library is open today from 9:00am to Noon, 2:00pm to 6:00pm, and 8:00pm to 11:00pm.

Crystal Hair Salon and Spa Treatments, Sun Deck 12
Open daily: 8:00am to 8:00pm. For salon & massage appointments, call 3875.

Crystal Spa Fitness Center, Sun Deck 12 Aft
Open daily: 6:00am to 8:00pm. Fitness Instructor Hazel on Duty: Days in Port: By Appointment.

Cruise Sales Consultant
Cruise Sales Consultant Nikki is available to assist you with booking a new Crystal Cruises sailing. *Start your booking on board and make great savings.* The desk is open today from 3:00pm to 6:00pm.

Concierge Desk
Open daily from 7:30am to 7:30pm.

Monday's Bar Hours
Avenue Saloon .... 5:00pm – 1:30am
Bistro .... 9:30am – 7:00pm
Caesars Casino Bar ... 1:00pm – 5:00pm
                          9:00pm – 2:00am
Crystal Cove .... 10:00am – 12:30am
Galaxy Lounge .... 7:15pm – 11:45pm
Palm Court .... 11:00am – 12:30am
Starlite Club .... 9:00pm – Late
Trident Bar .... 10:00am – 6:00pm

TODAY'S SPECIAL DRINK
EUROPEAN CHAMPAGNE COCKTAIL
This one is as elegant as the evening...a mix of Cognac, Grand Marnier, and Champagne. *Price $6.00*

SPECIAL
Late Vintage Port – $3.75
Founders Reserve Port – $2.75

BLOODY MARY HOUR
Crystal Cove • 10:30am to 12:30pm
Palm Court • 11:00am to 12:30pm
Featuring a special menu of Bloody Mary drinks prepared by our barkeepers. Special price: $3.25

Shore Excursion Desk
Open today from 2:00pm to 6:00pm.

Medical Center, Crystal Deck 5
Located on Crystal Deck 5 (starboard corridor, just forward of Front Desk). **Open:** 8:00am to Noon and 2:00pm to 6:00pm. **Doctor's Consultation Hours:** 9:00am to 10:00am and 5:00pm to 6:00pm. **Medical attention (24 hours) call 9911** *(let ring 5 times to page a nurse).* **In an extreme emergency call 3333.**

Photo Shop
Our shop is open today from 1:00pm – 4:00pm. Please order your cruise photos as the "Latin Interlude" cruise is drawing to a close.

Port/Shopping Lecturer
Katy Brodish is at the gangway today from 7:00am to 9:00am to answer your questions on Cabo San Lucas.

Crystal Symphony • Monday, January 12, 1998

Courtesy Crystal Cruises

CUNARD LINE LIMITED
CUNARD LINE BRAND
SEABOURN CRUISE LINE BRAND

6100 Blue Lagoon Drive, Suite 400

Miami, Florida 33126

(800) 528-6273

(305) 463-3000

(305) 463-3010 FAX

CUNARD LINE BRAND

CARONIA: (formerly *Vistafjord*); entered service 1973; refurbished periodically, including 1997 and 1999; 24,492 G.R.T.; 627' x 82'; 675-passenger capacity; 373 cabins; Norwegian officers and European crew; cruises to different areas around the world, including Europe (Northern Europe, and the Mediterranean, Baltic, and Black Seas), the Caribbean, Transcanal, Hawaii, Tahiti, Amazon, and South America.

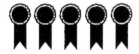

(Medical Facilities:C-6; P-1; EM, CLS, MS; N-1; CM; PD; BC; EKG; TC; PO; EPC; OX; WC; OR; ICU; X; M.)

QUEEN ELIZABETH 2: entered service 1969; refurbished periodically, including 1996; 70,327 G.R.T.; 963' x 105'; 1,500-passenger capacity; 910 cabins; British officers and crew; Caribbean cruises, transatlantic crossings, world cruises, party cruises; cruises to Bermuda, Europe, the Mediterranean, New England, and Canada.

Grill Rooms   **Caronia**

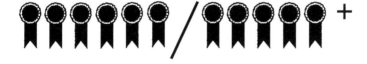

Mauretania

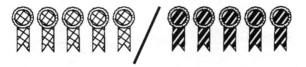

(Medical Facilities: C-4; P-2; EM, CLS, MS; N-2; CM; PD; BC; EKG; TC; PO; EPC; OX; WC; OR; ICU; X; M.)

SEABOURN CRUISE LINE BRAND

SEABOURN GODDESS I and II: (formerly *Sea Goddesses I and II*); entered service 1984 and 1985, respectively; 4,250 G.R.T.; 344' x 48'; 116-passenger capacity; 58 cabins; Norwegian officers and international crew; cruises various areas around the world, including Europe, the Orient, and the Caribbean.

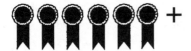

(Medical Facilities: C-0; P-1; EM, CLS, MS; N-1; CM; PD; EKG; TC; PO; EPC; OX; WC; ICU; X; M.)

SEABOURN LEGEND: (formerly *Royal Viking Queen* and *Queen Odyssey*); entered service 1992; 10,000 G.R.T.; 439' x 63'; 204-passenger capacity; 102 suites; Norwegian officers, European staff and crew; cruises Bermuda, the Caribbean, the Mediterranean, Europe, Scandinavia, Panama Canal, and other destinations around the world.

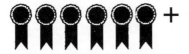

SEABOURN PRIDE: entered service 1988; 10,000 G.R.T.; 439' x 63'; 204-passenger capacity; 102 suites; Norwegian officers, European staff and crew; cruises in Northern Europe, Mediterranean, the Caribbean, South America, Mexico, U.S. East Coast, Canada, and Panama Canal.

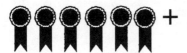

SEABOURN SPIRIT: entered service 1989; 10,000 G.R.T.; 439' x 63'; 204-passenger capacity; 102 suites; European staff and crew; cruises in Mediterranean, Europe, Southeast Asia, East Africa, China, Far East, and Africa.

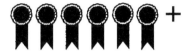

(Medical Facilities for *Legend, Pride,* and *Spirit:* C-4; P-1; EM, CLS, MS; N-1; CM; PD; EKG; TC; PO; OX; WC; ICU; X; M.)

SEABOURN SUN: (formerly *Royal Viking Sun*); entered service 1988; 37,845 G.R.T.; 669' x 95'; 758-passenger capacity; 380 cabins; Norwegian officers and international crew; itineraries around the world.

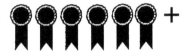

(Medical Facilities: C-4; P-1; EM, CLS, MS; N-1; CM; PD; BC; EKG; TC; PO; EPC; OX; WC; OR; ICU; X; M.)

Note: **Six+ black ribbons is the highest rating given in this edition to ships in the deluxe market category.**

Cunard Line was founded back in 1840 by Samuel Cunard, a merchant from Nova Scotia. His original plan was to provide transatlantic mail service while carrying a few passengers at the same time. The first ship, the *Britannia,* was a 1,150-ton paddlewheel steamer that made the crossing between continents in fourteen days.

Over the years, the Cunard flag has flown on such well-known vessels as the *Aquitania, Mauretania, Lusitania, Franconia, Queen Mary,* and the original *Queen Elizabeth.* Ironically, the Cunard Line not only originated transatlantic passenger service 160 years ago but presently, via the *Queen Elizabeth 2,* is the last major cruise line offering regular transatlantic crossings.

Cunard, as a wholly owned subsidiary of the British conglomerate Trafalgar House, was acquired by the Norwegian construction and engineering firm of Kvaerner in 1996 and was resold to Carnival Corporation in May 1998. Carnival Corporation then merged Cunard with Seabourn Cruise Line (a company organized in 1987). Sixty-eight percent of the new company, Cunard Line Limited, is owned by Carnival Corporation, and 32 percent is owned by Atle Brynestad and a group of Norwegian investors. Seabourn continues to operate as a separate brand. Several of the "Cunard Line" ships were transferred to the "Seabourn Line brand," namely the two *Sea Goddesses* and the *Royal Viking Sun.* They have been renamed *Seabourn Goddess I, Seabourn Goddess II,* and *Seabourn Sun.*

In the mid-1970s, Cunard built the *Princess* and *Countess,* two 17,000-ton ships designed to accommodate the then-emerging mass market of first-time and more economy-minded cruisers. Both of these ships were sold off in the 1990s. In 1983 it acquired the *Sagafjord* and *Vistafjord* from the now-defunct Norwegian America Cruises. The *Sagafjord* ceased operating for Cunard in 1996.

In the summer of 1986, Cunard surprised many observers when it purchased the unique *Sea Goddess I* and *Sea Goddess II,* two yacht-like, superdeluxe ships. In 1994, Cunard acquired the *Royal Viking Sun* and all rights to the Royal Viking logo. This gave Cunard six luxury-class vessels, making it the biggest in the luxury cruise market.

In the early nineties Cunard acquired the ships of Crown Cruise Line, *Crown Monarch, Crown Dynasty,* and *Crown Jewel;* however, all of these vessels were subsequently transferred to other cruise lines.

The original Seabourn ships, the *Pride* and *Spirit,* entered service in 1988 and 1989, respectively, and were heralded throughout the industry as the most magnificent and luxurious smaller vessels ever built. Seabourn ordered a third ship built in 1991 but exercised its option not to buy it. The shipyard, in turn, sold it to Royal Viking Line, where it entered service in 1992 as the *Royal Viking Queen.* When the Royal Viking Line was dismantled by its owners, the ship was transferred to the Royal Cruise Line and renamed *Queen Odyssey.* Royal also ceased operating in 1996, at which time the ship was repurchased by Seabourn and now is known as the *Seabourn Legend.*

The *Queen Elizabeth 2* is a unique ship both in her size (one of the larger ships sailing) and in her continuation of a system whereby passengers paying more for their cabins are entitled to an escalating scale of cabin facilities and frequent different dining rooms, all offering a higher caliber of service and gourmet options. Thus, it is possible to travel less expensively in a small cabin and dine in the Mauretania Dining Room, pay a bit more for a more spacious stateroom and dine in the Caronia Restaurant, or cruise in luxury in a deluxe cabin or suite and enjoy meals in one of the elegant Grill Rooms. Irrespective of which category you book, you will have access to the same ship facilities and participate in the same activities and entertainments.

Queen Elizabeth 2 entered service in 1969 and is still considered one of the most elegant of the floating giants presently sailing. During the late fall and early spring, she offers Caribbean cruises; in January she departs for her annual around-the-world cruise; and in late spring, summer, and early fall makes 17 regular transatlantic crossings. The unique air-sea package that permits you to sail one way to or from Europe and fly the other, with a three-day London holiday, offers a very attractive short vacation.

The 910 cabins and suites are divided into no less than twenty cabin categories. The less expensive cabins on the lower decks on the average sell for $325 per person per day. A standard outside cabin will cost from $350 to $400 per person. These passengers (the majority on the ship) all eat in the 530-seat Mauretania Restaurant (formerly known as Tables of the World and Britannia) in one or two seatings depending on the passenger occupancy of the sailing. A superior outside first-class cabin costing about $500 to $550 per person per day entitles its occupants to eat in the more elegant Caronia Restaurant. Passengers popping for one of the 107 ultra-deluxe cabins for about $650 per person per day enjoy one of the two charming, romantic Princess and Britannia grillrooms, with their dramatic floor-to-ceiling picture windows and posh, red velvet upholstery. Passengers occupying the 121 luxury staterooms and penthouse suites (including 30 with large outside balconies) that cost from $700 per person per day up to $2,000 for the Queen Mary and Queen Elizabeth suites enjoy the exclusive, exquisitely elegant Queens Grill. This dining room has its own private lounge area and private staircase leading to the luxury suites, so its devotees need not mingle with the other passengers should they desire seclusion or anonymity. Because many dignitaries and well-known personalities sail on the *Queen*, this affords them a degree of privacy not available on most other vessels.

The daily menu is similar in all dining rooms, and special orders for such items as caviar, smoked salmon, soufflés, chateaubriand, rack of lamb, lobster, etc., are honored throughout the ship. However, in the three grillrooms special orders are expected, service is even more attentive, and the feel is that of a super-elegant intimate restaurant rather than a dining room on a ship. In addition, the lovely Lido Restaurant offers a casual three-meal-a-day dining option featuring an impressive selection of international offerings attractively served buffet style.

The facilities and activities on the *Queen* are mind-boggling. There are thirteen decks; thirteen elevators; one small indoor and one small outdoor swimming pool with two adjoining Jacuzzis; seven dining venues; a hospital with complete medical services; eight lounges and bars; more than a dozen shops; an expertly managed bookstore and library, the most complete at sea; a fully stocked casino; a 590-seat, two-tier theater; a children's playroom and cartoon cinema; animal kennels; a thirteen-car garage; the "QE2 Spa at Sea" with a thalassotherapy pool, sauna, steam room, massage, therapy, and beauty treatments; a fitness center with an aerobics room and aerobics classes, free weights, exercise and cardiovascular machine, and the indoor pool; a launderette; an Epson computer center; and a separate synagogue. There are also outside sport decks, which include a 1/5-mile jogging track, skeet shooting, paddle tennis, a golf driving range, a putting green, shuffleboard, Ping-Pong, and activities around the clock ranging from bingo, bridge, and backgammon tournaments to wine tastings, financial lectures, pool games, deck horse racing, children's facilities, and just about anything else you can do on a ship. In late 1994, the ship underwent a major $45-million refurbishment, including a modernization of all bathrooms, and in 1996 the refurbishment included extensive work in the dining rooms and other public areas. A major refit and refurbishment is scheduled for 1999 and early 2000.

The *Sagafjord,* which entered service in 1965, and the *Vistafjord,* which entered service in 1973, were built by Norwegian America Cruises (NAC) and acquired by Cunard in 1983. I have always had a warm spot in my heart for NAC, having sailed as a student on the *Stavangafjord* and *Bergensfjord* back in the sixties ($425 round-trip between New York and Copenhagen). The *Sagafjord* and *Vistafjord,* as well as the *Oslofjord,* were built to replace their other vessels and designed as luxury ships, competing in their day with the *Kungsholm* and *Gripsholm* of the Swedish America Line for the well-heeled older cruise market that could afford longer itineraries at higher prices. With the demise of the Swedish America Line in the seventies, the NAC ships had a lock-in of this particular clientele, with Royal Viking Line and the *Queen Elizabeth 2* as their only competition. However, rising fuel, food, and labor costs became prohibitive and NAC—like the Swedish America, Italian, and French Lines before it—finally bit the dust.

In 1994, the *Vistafjord* received a major refurbishment including the addition of two 880-square-foot, bi-level suites and Tivoli, a 40-seat alternative Italian restaurant. In late 1999 she received a major refit and additional refurbishing and her name was changed to *Caronia.* In 1996 the *Sagafjord* was chartered to Transocean Tours after the line made a decision not to make the investment in her future that had been made for the *Vistafjord.* The median age of the passengers historically has been over sixty-five, and the passenger mix includes many Germans and Scandinavians. The *Vistafjord* seems most ideal for mature cruisers who seek concerned service, excellent food, and comfortable accommodations, but are willing to sacrifice some of the spirit, activities, facilities, and glamour found in some of the newer luxury vessels.

This is not to say that the *Vistafjord* does not have activities and many facilities. The ship has nightly entertainment, a small casino, movies, the usual bridge lessons, lectures, and entertainment programs, as well as a health spa, indoor and outdoor pools, and several lounges. She has fascinating and varying itineraries that can take her almost anywhere in the world. Extended cruises with various optional segments are offered regularly. Because prices differ depending upon the cruise area, it is difficult to describe the numerous categories. Food and service are top-notch in the dining room (but not as good at the buffet restaurant near the lido), and the cabin stewardesses are very professional and anxious to please. Cabins in every category tend to be larger than on other ships; 90 percent have bathtubs and some of the luxury cabins and suites have outside verandas. All cabins were recently redecorated and have mini-refrigerators, TVs, VCRs, and new telephone systems.

Since the entrance into the luxury cruise market of the *Sea Goddess I* and *Sea Goddess II* in the mid-eighties, these two beauties have offered cruisers a unique, more intimate, yacht-like cruise experience. There are no cabins, only fifty-seven identical 205-square-foot outside suite rooms, elegantly furnished, with sitting rooms, twin beds convertible to queen-size with down comforters, tub and showers, remote-control color TV, telephone with worldwide direct dial, three-channel music systems, VCRs, safes, terry-cloth robes and slippers, wooden hangers in the closets, large mirrors, large windows looking out to the sea, and around-the-clock room service. There are also fresh plants, flowers, and fruit; a mini-bar; and a refrigerator stocked with complimentary soft drinks, liquors and wines of your choice, and any other snacks requested, including caviar. One larger double suite is available on each ship for those who want more spacious accommodations. The suites on

Decks Three, Four, and Five have large picture windows that look out to the sea; those on Deck Two have portholes. The staterooms do not have verandas and are smaller than those on many of her luxury-class competitors.

The tariff is around $850 to $950 per person per day ($1,400 for a double stateroom/suite) and includes everything from the usual meals, activities, and transportation to some shore excursions, all liquors and soft drinks, all but the most expensive wines, tipping, and special orders. This seems like a lot of money; however, it is not out of line with the cost for suites on other luxury ships. There are a few sailings during the year when the ship is repositioning where the tariff may vary from $400 to $600 per person per day.

Although the atmosphere is more subdued and private, there is nightly entertainment, music and dancing, a small casino with two blackjack tables and slot machines, a main lounge and intimate club with piano bar, a library, a hospital, a hair salon, an outdoor café, an outdoor pool and whirlpool, and a lovely dining room without pre-assigned seating. This is probably the most sophisticated and best dining experience at sea. In addition to the regular menu, guests can order just about anything they desire, including unlimited caviar and champagne. If you desire a romantic, intimate dinner, you can make arrangements to have your table prepared in your cabin or out on the deck. To help ensure outstanding service, a personal preference form is mailed to all guests before their cruise, requesting information on favorite beverages, foods, and activities.

Because the ships are small, they can negotiate cruise areas and shallower ports where some of the larger ships cannot drop anchor. Thus, their itineraries in the Mediterranean, Caribbean, and Orient include some seldom-visited spots, affording passengers opportunities not available except by chartering a private yacht. The *Sea Goddesses* combine the personal attention and elegance of a private yacht with all the amenities and services of a grand ocean liner. The ship carries watersports equipment such as water skis, personal watercraft, windsurfers, and snorkeling gear—all of which can be utilized from a special platform at the stern of the ship. There is also a small gymnasium with exercise equipment (including treadmills, exercycles, and free weights), and a sauna and shower. Exercise classes and a heart-healthy diet menu are offered daily.

These ships offer impeccable service, the finest cuisine, and unparalleled personal attention and elegance. They are for the sophisticated, discerning cruiser and not for Middle America or those seeking a more active cruise program. Following the merger with Seabourn, these ships were renamed *Seabourn Goddess I* and *II.*

In 1994, Cunard acquired the *Royal Viking Sun* and certain Royal Viking trademarks for $170 million. The *Royal Viking Sun,* at 37,845 tons, is the largest vessel to have been built by the Royal Viking Line. Thirty-eight percent of the staterooms (including the eighteen penthouse suites) feature private verandas. All include three-channel radios, TVs, VCRs, mini-bars and refrigerators, security lock drawers, showers, hair dryers, terry-cloth robes, and slippers, and most also have tubs.

For those not wishing to pay the top tariff for the ultra-luxurious penthouse suites, the deluxe-A-grade cabins (junior suites) on Discovery Deck are a desirable option, being very roomy with large closets, additional storage and makeup areas, a separate sitting area, a separate toilet compartment with its own sink and vanity, and an oversized veranda. The suites and some rooms can accommodate a third passenger. The 25 inside cabins are quite small and are best suited for passengers traveling alone.

The elegant main dining room serves all passengers at one sitting, featuring varied culinary offerings. Dress tends to be more formal, and gala balls, as well as private entertainment and cocktail parties, are more prevalent than on other cruise lines. Less formal and simpler fare is offered daily at lunch on the outdoor decks and at the charming, airy Garden Café, which is several notches above casual, poolside restaurants found on other vessels. Actually, the luncheon buffet in the Garden Café was the most imaginative to be found on any cruise ship, with endless varieties of ethnic gourmet offerings, as well as salads, smoked salmon, pastas, seafood, imported cheeses, and mouth-watering desserts and pastries. The midnight buffets and theme buffets tend to be lavish, and room service is available around the clock. Recently, an alternative-dining, Italian-style restaurant, Venezia, was added.

Facilities include two outdoor swimming pools; a gym with state-of-the-art equipment, a spa and sauna, whirlpool, and massage; a beauty salon; golf-putting greens and driving nets; a croquet court; a paddle tennis court; a small casino offering roulette, blackjack, and slots; numerous show and cocktail lounges as well as a lovely observation lounge atop ship; cardrooms; and a plethora of expensive artwork, plants, and elegant Scandinavian furnishings. Among the activities aboard are enrichment lectures on cruise destinations, trap shooting, golf and tennis instructions, card tournaments, production shows, movies, dance lessons, nightly entertainment, religious services, and other typical cruise ship events. Many well-known celebrity entertainers are featured, especially on longer cruises.

Fares vary with the length and location of the cruise and include airfare. Minimum fares average about $450 per person per day. Middle-priced outside doubles run from $650 to $750, deluxe-A-grade cabins (junior suites) go from $900 to 1,100 per person per day, and penthouse suites can cost as much as $1,400 per person. Most passengers are repeaters who would consider no ship other than the *Seabourn Sun* (formerly *Royal Viking Sun*) and adore the staff and officers, many of whom have been with the ship since its inception.

The three all-suite vessels of Seabourn are positioned at the top of the luxury cruise market and are designed to offer the most elegant, luxurious cruise experience afloat, with spacious suite accommodations, open-seating dining with top-of-the-line service and gourmet cuisine, tasteful and elegantly appointed public rooms, excellent watersport and spa facilities, and some of the most desired destinations. Although dress during the day is casual, in the evening gentlemen are expected to wear jackets in the dining room (even on "casual nights"), and the atmosphere is more formal and sophisticated than on other ships. However, guests may opt to have dinner at the Veranda Café, where the dress code is somewhat more casual.

Cruise-only prices average about $761 per person per day (double occupancy), depending upon location of cabin and cruise area. A no-tipping policy is enforced, and there is no charge for soft drinks, wines, or alcoholic beverages (except for certain premium wines, liquors, and brandies). The line offers past passengers discounts on longer segments purchased in advance in certain cabin categories. Any passenger accruing 140 days on board receives a complimentary 14-day cruise on any Seabourn ship.

Itineraries include Northern Europe and the Mediterranean in the spring, summer, and early fall, and the Pacific Rim, Asia, Africa, the Caribbean, South America, and Mexican Riviera the remainder of the year, with several transatlantic positioning cruises. In addition, Seabourn has recently introduced its "As You Like It" program, which permits passengers to select from a variety of air and pre- and post-cruise land arrangements tailored to each passenger's individual tastes and budget. Seabourn's comprehensive air program features competitively priced, negotiated tariffs with major carriers in economy, business, and first class and on the Concorde, as well as on luxurious private jets. Land packages include most prestigious hotels and custom-designed "Signature Series" shore excursions.

Most suites are approximately 277 square feet, with a large, 3-by 5-foot picture window looking out to the sea; twin beds that convert to a queen; color TV with VCR attachment; richly appointed armchairs, sofa, and coffee table; a refrigerator and mini-bar (fully stocked upon embarkation free of charge); a hair dryer; a large walk-in closet with a private safe; and a marble bathroom with twin-sink vanities (except the *Legend,* which has single sink vanities); a shower or shower/tub combination; and ample storage space. There are also larger suites that range in size from 400 to 575 square feet; several have small private verandas.

The health spa on each vessel includes an exercise room, a gym for dance and aerobics classes, steam, sauna, massage, herbal body wraps, two outdoor whirlpools, and an outdoor swimming pool. At the "fold-out marina" off the rear of the ship, passengers can swim, windsurf, water-ski, banana boat, and sail. There is also an underwater observatory in the Nautilus Room of the *Pride* and *Spirit.*

The observation lounges at the top of each ship are glass enclosed and afford a panoramic view for passengers enjoying coffee, tea, or drinks. The club has a piano bar and is the location for evening cocktails and hors d'oeuvres, as well as late-night dancing. There also is a large showroom that can accommodate all passengers; an indoor/outdoor café where imaginative buffet breakfasts, lunches, and dinners are served; a casino; a hospital; a boutique; a self-service launderette; and laundry and dry-cleaning service.

One of the highlights of the Seabourn experience is the elegant, open-seating dining room featuring some of the best Continental cuisine at sea, as well as an extensive wine list priced lower than at most liquor stores back home. A typical dinner may include carefully prepared escargot Bourgouignonne, quail eggs with two caviars and dill cream, broiled Maine lobster in a champagne butter sauce, loin of lamb with eggplant and prosciutto in baked phyllo pastry, bananas flambé à la Foster, crêpes suzette, and raspberry soufflé in a Drambuie sauce. Service is also impeccable. This may be the ultimate cruise experience for a well-heeled, sophisticated cruise aficionado.

Strong Points:

Caronia, formerly *Vistafjord:* Subdued elegance, excellent food and service, and good accommodations; ideal for Northern Europeans and experienced mature cruisers.

Queen Elizabeth 2: A grand ship that exudes class and tradition with great facilities, loads of entertainment, and fine dining at all levels. For those who can pay the price for the Grill Rooms, greater stateroom comfort, more pampering, and an especially elegant sophisticated experience.

Seabourn Goddess I and *II,* formerly *Sea Goddesses I* and *II:* A unique, elegant, intimate, yacht-like experience in luxury cruising. The very best cuisine and the most impeccable service, and the most personal attention of any cruise ship afloat, comfortable accommodations, and interesting, seldom-visited ports for those who can pay the freight.

Seabourn Legend, Pride, and *Spirit:* Top-of-the-line luxury (at top-of-the-line prices), superb food, service, and accommodations, as well as the most desired itineraries. The most spacious and comfortable of the yacht-like cruise ships. For many, these are the best ships in service today.

Seabourn Sun, formerly *Royal Viking Sun:* One of the most elegant of the larger cruise ships in service, offering exceptional food, service, and accommodations with fascinating itineraries and a high ratio of loyal repeat passengers.

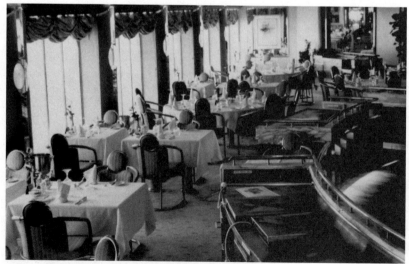

Princess Grill-QE2, courtesy Cunard Line

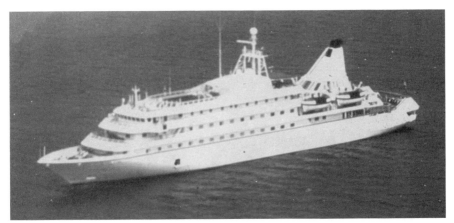

Seabourn Goddess, *courtesy Cunard Line*

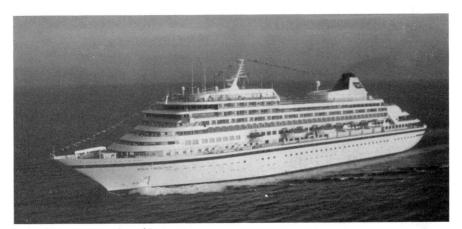

Seabourn Sun, *courtesy Cunard Line*

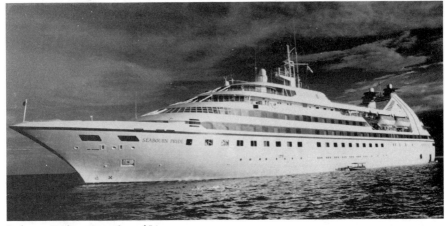

Seabourn Pride, *courtesy Cunard Line*

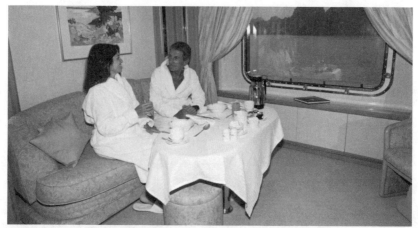

Breakfast in cabin. Seabourn Spirit, *courtesy Cunard Line*

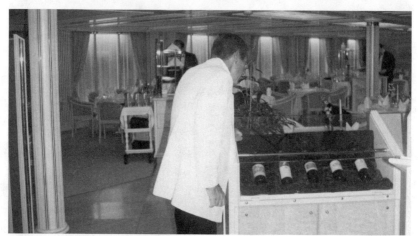

Main Dining Room. Seabourn Spirit, *courtesy Cunard Line*

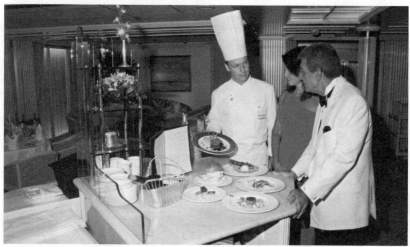

Chef presentation Tasting Menu. Seabourn Spirit, *courtesy Cunard Line*

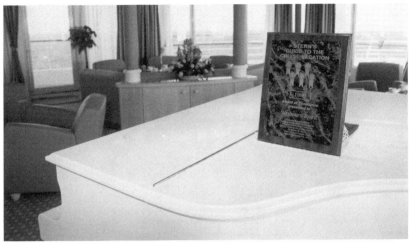

Award Plaque in Lounge. Seabourn Spirit, *courtesy Cunard Line*

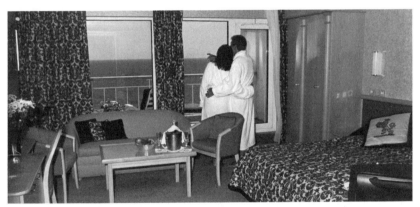

QE2, *courtesy Cunard Line*

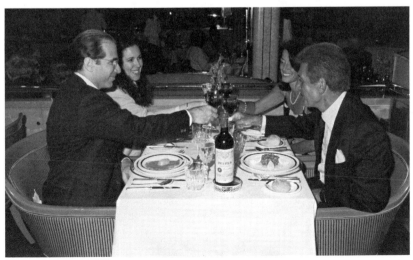

QE2, *courtesy Cunard Line*

DAILY PROGRAMME

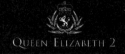

QUEEN ELIZABETH 2

HOTEL MANAGER JOHN DUFFY   MASTER: CAPTAIN WARWICK   CRUISE DIRECTOR SCOTT PETERSON

SUNRISE: 6.21AM   **SATURDAY 21ST MARCH 1998**   SUNSET: 6.43PM

MORNING ACTIVITIES

PLANNING YOUR DAY? UNLESS OTHERWISE INDICATED, MOST ACTIVITIES LAST ABOUT 45 MINUTES

8.00am   **Sabbath Morning Service** with Rabbi Harry Roth in the Synagogue .... 3 Deck A Stairway

At the Fitness Centre Hi-Lo Aerobics *(please wear appropriate footwear)* .... 7 Deck C Stairway

Walk-A-Mile Meet a member of the Steiner staff *(please wear appropriate footwear)* .... Boat Deck Aft

8.15am   **Good Morning QE2** Your Cruise Director Scott presents today's weather report and
informational update until 11.00am .... TV Channel 14

9.00am   **Daily Crossword Puzzle** is available throughout the day .... Library

10.00am   **Bridge Lecture** with Bridge Director Simon Frome .... Yacht Club

QE2 Mid-Ocean Golf Tournament continues. Come and support your fellow passengers .... Sports Area Boat Deck

Computer Lecture Introduction to Windows & Windows 95. An informal lecture by
Computer Expert Harry Barkan *(repeated at 11.00am)* .... Computer Centre

Today's Brain Teaser Quiz is available. All quiz forms must be handed in by 4.00pm .... Library

Morning Games All Scrabble, Backgammon, Canasta, Chess and other game players
- meet in the .... Crystal Bar Starboard Side

Casino Change is available for the slot machines, the tables are open and gaming lessons
with available Casino Staff .... Casino

10.30am   **Crew Boat and Raft Drill** While this in no way affects guests directly, some ship's services and activities are curtailed.
Thank you for your understanding.

11.00am   **Reform Economics - Asian Style** International Relations Lecturer Gloria Wyeth Neumeier talks about
wide open markets, authoritarian politics and a rising middle class produced by Asian economic miracles.
Also the Asian tiger has gone into decline - will it recover - and what are the consequences? .... Theatre

Renewal of Wedding Vows Join Archdeacon Willing and Father Nee and once again
repeat those meaningful words .... Yacht Club

At the Fitness Centre Fabulous Abdominals *(please wear appropriate footwear)* .... 7 Deck C Stairway

Ladies' Table Tennis Open Play Meet a member of the Cruise Staff at the tables .... Upper Deck Aft Port Side

Ship's Daily Total Guess our mileage from sailing time yesterday to noon today.
Cash prizes to be won! ($2.00 per bet.)Last guess is at 11.55am.
(The mileage will be posted on the Navigator's Chart, Quarter Deck by 2.00pm) .... Golden Lion Pub

12.00noon   **Mahe and the Seychelles** An illustrated presentation about this Indian Ocean paradise by
World Cruise Port Lecturer Peter Longley
(to be repeated on TV Channel 14 running continuously from 3.00pm throughout the rest of the day) .... Theatre

Team Trivial Pursuit Combine brain power in teams to play our version of this popular pastime .... Grand Lounge

Complimentary Dance Class with Dance Champions Warren and Daniella Smith .... Queen's Room

Lunchtime cocktails with Jon Courtenay at the keyboard .... Golden Lion Pub

Pianist Peter Campbell Thornton entertains you before lunch .... Chart Room

12.30pm   **Pianist Bryant Olender** plays for your listening pleasure .... Crystal Bar

---

DINING TIMES

QUEEN'S GRILL, PRINCESS GRILL & BRITANNIA GRILL
Breakfast: 8.00am to 9.30am
Lunch: 1.00pm to 2.30pm
Dinner: 7.30pm to 9.00pm

CARONIA & MAURETANIA RESTAURANT
Breakfast: 8.00am to 9.30am
Lunch: 12.30pm to 2.00pm
Dinner: 7.00pm to 9.00pm

THE LIDO
Breakfast Buffet: 8.00am to 10.00am
Luncheon Buffet: 1.00pm to 2.30pm
Afternoon Tea: 4.00pm to 5.00pm
Children's Tea: 5.30pm
Dinner Buffet: 7.30pm to 9.00pm
Midnight Snack: 11.30pm to 12.30am

*Gentlemen are required to wear a jacket
and tie for dinner.
We kindly ask you to refrain from pipe and
cigar smoking in the dining rooms.*

THE PAVILION
Continental Breakfast: 6.00am to 8.00am
Light Grill Dishes: 11.00am to 4.00pm

QUEEN'S ROOM
Afternoon Tea: 4.00pm to 5.00pm

OPEN DECKS
Afternoon Tea: 4.00pm to 5.00pm
(weather permitting)

AFTERNOON ACTIVITIES

2.30pm **Crimson Tide - The Writing of a Techno Thriller** Best-selling writer **Richard Henrick**, author of the original story *Crimson Tide*, gives an illustrated presentation .... Grand Lounge

Matinee Movie: Sling Blade A drama starring Billy Bob Thornton & John Ritter *Running Time: 2 hours 16 minutes. Cert: R (contains violence, profanity and/or adult situations)* .... Theatre

Line Dancing Join Warren & Daniella and learn how to do the latest craze. *No partners needed!* .... Queen's Room

A Different Way to look at food choices and nutrition - designed especially for you at your time of life. A hands-on session with fellow passenger Adeline Shell, PhD. R.D. .... Yacht Club

Duplicate and Party Bridge with Bridge Directors Simon and Carole *(expected duration: approximately 2 hours)* .... Crystal Bar Port Side

Back Care Class Do you suffer with back pain, arthritis or osteoporosis? Join the Steiners' experts and learn how to prevent these problems .... Golden Lion Pub

Computer Workshop Improve your computer skills with Computer Expert Harry Barkan .... Computer Centre

Paddle Tennis Come play in a doubles tournament *(please wear appropriate footwear)* .... Sports Area Boat Deck

Afternoon Games All Scrabble, Backgammon, Whist, Chess and other game players - meet in the .... Crystal Bar Starboard Side

3.30pm **The Royal Promenade Shops on Board** present a fashion show featuring the designs of *Mondi, Frank Usher of London,* and more. Hosted by Social Director Elaine MacKay .... Grand Lounge

Screened Concert *Les Miserables.* A cast of over 250 performers appear in this Royal Albert Hall performance. Presented on a large screen TV via laser disc. Disc 3 of 3 .... Yacht Club

Rubber Stamping Create your own designs using rubber stamps with Arts & Crafts Instructor Joyce Pinfield *(please bring a small pair of scissors)* .... Outside the Crystal Bar Starboard Side

Richard Henrick, best-selling author, is available to sign copies of his book. *Crimson Tide* .... Outside the Library

At the Fitness Centre Body Blitz *(please wear appropriate footwear)* .... 7 Deck C Stairway

Men's Table Tennis Open Play Meet a member of the Cruise Staff at the tables .... Upper Deck Aft Port Side

4.30pm **$$$ Snowball Bonanza Bingo with the Cruise Staff $$$** Cash prizes to be won! The snowball continues with a minimum jackpot of $500!!! *(cards purchased for US dollars only and are available from 4.15pm)* .... Grand Lounge

At the Fitness Centre Step to the Beat *(please wear appropriate footwear)* .... 7 Deck C Stairway

5.30pm **Catholic Holy Mass** is celebrated with Father Eugene Nee .... Theatre

At the Fitness Centre S-T-R-E-T-C-H & Relax *(please wear appropriate footwear)* .... Deck C Stairway

---

THE QE2 WORLD CRUISE OFFICE
Upper Deck Aft, Starboard Side
Open today for tour reservations
from 9.00am to 12.00noon
and from 2.30pm to 5.00pm.

CRUISE SALES MANAGER
Quarter Deck D Stairway
Kent and Tracey will be at their desk from
10.00am to 1.00pmand 3.00pm to 6.00pm
Ask about the additional 5% discount!

BAR HOURS

DRINK OF THE DAY

"BLUE LAGOON"

Vodka, Blue Curacao & Lemonade
$4.00

CRYSTAL BAR
11.00am to 2.00pm and 5.30pm to 12.30am

GOLDEN LION PUB
11.00am to 1.00am

CHART ROOM
11.00am to 1.00am

PRINCESS GRILL LOUNGE
6.30pm to 9.00pm

YACHT CLUB
11.00am to the wee small hours
❀ WINE DESK ❀

AFTER DINNER DRINK

"BONNIE PRINCE"

with
Drambuie
$4.75

SOMMELIER THOMAS GALLAGHER IS AVAILABLE OUTSIDE THE LIBRARY FROM 10.00AM TO 12.00NOON TO GIVE ADVICE ON WINES AND TO TAKE PRE-ORDERS SHOULD YOU WISH.

Courtesy Cunard Line

Queen's Grill Dinner Menu

Hors d'oeuvres Froids

Terrine de Foie Gras Truffée
with a red wine Onion Confit and warm Brioche

Carpaccio of Beef,
Shaved Parmesan Reggianno and Watercress Oil

Iced Sevruga Caviar Malassol
with traditional Condiments and Toast Fingers

Jumbo Prawns Cocktail
with Brandied Horseradish Dressing

Tartar of Salmon and Tuna,
Mesclun Salad and Caper seasoning

Seasonal Fruits and Berries,
topped with Lemongrass Sorbet

Butterfly of Scottish Smoked Salmon
topped with Malassol Caviar and Sour Cream

Le Choix de Viandes

Double Veal Cutlet, Panfried with a Ragôut of Forest Mushrooms

Filet of Beef "Wellington", Sauce Periguord,
Fricassée of Vegetables

Suprême de Faisan a L'Etuve, Façon du Chef

Peppered Filet Steak,
Seasoned with a blend of Five Peppers, Flamed in Cognac
and finished with a Café au Lait Sauce

Mélange de Ris, Foie et Rognon de Veau
Cooked in a Mustard Grain Sauce

Les Rotis

Poulet de Bresse Rôti a l'Anglaise
served with Pan Gravy, Bread Sauce, Chipolatas and Onion Parsley Stuffing

Oven Roast Quail filled with Foie Gras,
on a bed of Lentils

Crispy roast Duck a L'Orange
with Braised red Cabbage, Orange Sauce and Pommes Croquettes

Whole Rack of Lamb "Côtes de Provences"
Served with Lyonnaise Potatoes, Petite Green Beans and Thyme Jus

Courtesy Cunard Line

Les Grillades

Prime Filet of Beef Chateaubriand Béarnaise
Pommes Paille, grilled Tomato and Watercress (for Two)

Grilled Prime Beef - Sirloin - Filet or T-bone,
with Béarnaise sauce and choice of Potato and Vegetables

Paillard of Milk fed Veal with Choron Sauce

To Accompany...

New Potatoes
Gratin Dauphinois
Creamed Potatoes
French Fries
Lyonnaise Potatoes

Steamed Green Asparagus
Puréed Spinach
Crisp Market Vegetables
English Baby Peas
Ratatouille Nicoise

Les Fromages Affinés d'ici et la

Selection of International Cheeses
Bartholivers - Digestives Walnut and Raisin Bread

Courtesy Cunard Line

SEA GODDESS

Monday, January 4th, 1999
At Sea

" The Cunard Spa Menu "
An Ocean of Well Being

Red Oak Leaf Salad with Tomato Vinaigrette
*

Poached Salmon on Leek Julienne and Cilantro Nage
*

Festive Fruit Cake

Vegetarian Dish of the Night

Lasagne of Zucchini, Tomato and Mozzarella

Our Wine Suggestion

Chablis Premier Cru 1993, Burgundy
Clos du Bois 1993, Alexander Valley

Renato Chizzola   *Anton Probst*
Maître d'Hôtel   *Chef de Cuisine*

Appetizers

Bouquet of Baby Lettuce Topped with Pink Roasted Barbarie Duck Breast

Homemade Feta Cheese Terrine with Avocado Tartare

Crispy Fried Spring Rolls with Crab Meat and Thai Chili Dip

Soups

Beef Consommé "Diablotin"

Creamy Vegetable Soup

Chilled Pear Flip

Sherbet

Nectarine

Entrées

Lobster Thermidor

Oven Roast Rack of Lamb "Dijonnaise" with Potato Gratin

Mignon of Buffalo Tenderloin Served with Asparagus Pancakes

Oven Roast Stuffed Woodland Quail on Shoestring Potatoes and Pink Lentils

Salads

Caesar Salad

Marinated Black Eye Bean Salad

Desserts

Banana Chocolate Crêpe

Chocolate Mousse with Almond Tulip

Kahlua Cream with Amarena Cherries

Fruit Sherbets

Selection of Ice Cream

Petits Fours

Assorted International Cheeses and Fresh Fruit

We Proudly Serve 100% Colombian Coffee

Courtesy Cunard Line

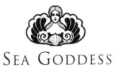

SEA GODDESS

ST. TROPEZ, FRANCE
Friday, July 3, 1998

Sunrise: 05:58   **Sunset: 21:17**

07:00 - 08:00	Early Risers' Coffee	- Outdoor Café
08:00 - 10:00	A la carte Breakfast is served	- Dining Salon
08:00 - 11:00	Breakfast is served	- Outdoor Café

08:00   **Sea Goddess I anchors off St. Tropez, France.**
A continuous tender service will operate throughout the day.

09:00   **"Ramatuelle, Gassin and Grimaud"** tour departs from the gangway.

10:00 - 16:30   **Shuttle bus transfer service to Pampelone Beach will operate on a scheduled
basis. Schedule details are available at the Reception desk.**
(Beach towels are available for collection at the gangway.)

11:00   **Crew Lifeboat Drill.** For the duration of this drill, ship's services may be
curtailed. We apologise for any inconvenience caused.

12:30 - 14:00	A la carte luncheon is served	- Dining Salon
12:30 - 14:00	Luncheon is served	- Outdoor Café

17:00 - 18:00   Afternoon tea is served in the Club Salon.

19:00   The Main Salon is open for cocktails and dancing with 'Two's Company'.
19:30   **The Captain's Farewell Reception in the Main Salon, followed by a brief
review on tomorrow's disembarkation procedures at Monte Carlo, Monaco.**
(This may be heard on radio channel two in your suite approximately 19:45.)

20:00 - 22:00   Dinner is served in the Dining Salon.

22:00   The Piano Bar is open.
22:00   Join *"Two's Company"* for coffee, after-dinner drinks and dancing
in the Main Salon.
22:30   Live music in the Piano Bar with *Vlado.*

23:00   **Last tender departs from shore.**
24:00   **Sea Goddess I sails for Monte Carlo, Monaco.**

00:30(July 4)   The Casino is open for blackjack and slotmachines.

Fitness Schedule	08:00	Awesome Abdominals	- Deck 6
	17:00	Pump it Up	- Deck 6

Beauty Salon / Massages   - 08:00 - 20:00
Telephones   - 24 hour direct telephone service is available from all suites.

JACKET AND TIE IS REQUESTED IN THE PUBLIC ROOMS AFTER 19:00

SEABOURN
HERALD

SUNRISE: 6:39 AM
TUESDAY, DECEMBER 29, 1998
VOL. 3901, NO 11

GUSTAVIA, ST. BARTHÉLEMY

SUNSET: 5:46 PM
EDITOR: JILL GALT
DRESS THIS EVENING: RESORT CASUAL

═══ Good Morning ═══

8:00 am	Today's Quiz is available. The answers will be posted at Afternoon Tea and in the Library after 4:00 pm.	Library
8:00 am	Wake Up and Stretch session with Fitness Director, Lianne.	The Spa
8:30 am	Fitness Class in the Aerobics Studio. Low Impact Aerobics and Body Conditioning.	The Spa
10:00 am	Walk your way back to Ft. Lauderdale! (only 16 rounds to 1 mile).	Sky Bar
10:00 am	The Seabourn Legend is scheduled to anchor off Gustavia, St. Barthélemy. *Please listen for announcements regarding the clearance of the ship by local authorities and commencement of tender service ashore.*	

> We wish our Guests a very enjoyable day in St. Barthélemy. Please remember that if you are staying aboard, books, and videos are available in the Library and that additional indoor games can be found in the Midnight Sun Lounge and in the Boardroom. The Spa, including beauty services, is operating as usual and the Sky Bar and Midnight Sun Lounge are open for your pleasure.

10:15 am	**Tour Departure:** *Catamaran Sail to Rockefeller Beach*	King Olav Lounge

═══ Good Afternoon ═══

2:00 pm	Board Games are available throughout the day for your enjoyment.	Midnight Sun Lounge
4:00 pm	**Afternoon Tea** is served in an elegant surrounding.	Midnight Sun Lounge
4:15 pm	**Tour Departure:** *St. Barts Sunset Sail by Catamaran*	King Olav Lounge

═══ Good Evening ═══

Dress this evening is Resort Casual after 6:00 pm
Jackets are required for Gentlemen in the Restaurant only.

6:45 pm	**The 5th Avenue Quartet** play for your enjoyment during pre-dinner cocktails.	The Club
9:30 pm	**The Seabourn Legend Quartet** invite you to take to the dance floor. *Requests are always welcome!*	The Club
10:00 pm	IMPORTANT! The last tender from shore will depart at this time.	
10:15 pm	**SHOWTIME!** Tonight we invite you to a foot stomping, knee slapping good time as *SEABOURN GOES COUNTRY!* Join the gang as Shane, Johnny, Julien and Jill sing and play some of your favorite Country tunes. Yee Hah!	The Club
10:30 pm	The Seabourn Legend will sail for Virgin Gorda, British Virgin Islands.	

After the show and until the wee small hours enjoy the music of

The 5th Avenue
Duo

At The Club ... "It's The Late Night Place To Be!"

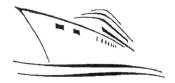

SIMPLICITY

With today's changing lifestyles and the quest for healthier living
through increased nutritional awareness, we at Seabourn, bring you
a daily selection of dishes, that reflect these needs. These dishes,
although low in cholesterol, salt and fat, are high in flavor.

Teriyaki Chicken Salad on Glass Noodles
*

Beef Consommé
*

Garden Lettuce Salad with Your Choice of Low Calorie Dressing
*

Grilled Fresh Swordfish with Lemon on Baked Zucchini
Sautéed Pheasant Breast on Pineapple Cabbage with Whipped Potatoes

A Selection of Steamed Vegetables and Baked Potatoes are always available

A LA CARTE

Caesar Salad Served with Croutons and Shaved Parmesan Cheese
Angel Hair Pasta with Chunks of Fresh Plum Tomatoes, Garlic, Olive Oil and Basil
Baked Fillet of Norwegian Salmon
Crisp Chicken Breast with Rosemary
Grilled New York Cut Striploin Steak with Herb Butter
Grilled Beef Fillet Steak, Madagascar Pepper Sauce
Broiled Double Lamb Chops

All dishes may be ordered with your choice of French Fries, Boiled Potatoes,
Baked Potatoes, Mashed Potatoes, Rice and Vegetables of the Day

The United States Public Health Service had determined that eating uncooked or partially
cooked meat, poultry, fish, seafood or eggs may present a health risk to the consumer.

Chef de Cuisine
Bernd Kessler

Maitre d'Hôtel
Franz Blaskowitz

DINNER

En Route to Limassol, Cyprus, Sunday, October 18, 1998

APPETIZERS

Teriyaki Chicken Salad on Glass Noodles
Californian Sushi Rolls with Wasabi
Fresh Forest Mushroom Ragout Served in a Puff Pastry Case

SOUPS

Lobster Bisque with Cognac
Guinea Fowl Consommé, Vegetable Concasse
Chilled Soup of Exotic Fruits

SALADS

Garden Lettuce with Crispy Bacon Bits and Sunflower Seeds
Jalapeño Caesar Salad with Crisp Chorizo

A TASTE OF THE MEDITERRANEAN

Deep Fried Squid with Garlic Mayonnaise

ENTRÉES

Grilled Fresh Swordfish, Warmed Potatoes, Caper and Citrus Vinaigrette
Glazed Scallops on Whipped Celeriac Mousseline, Lemon Beurre Blanc
Grilled Striploin Steak "Café de Paris," Green Beans and Stuffed Baked Potato
Roast Pheasant Breast, Creamy Juniper Berry Sauce, Champagne Cabbage

VEGETARIAN

Six Onion Risotto with Red Wine and Black Olive Sauce

DESSERT

En Route to Limassol, Cyprus, Sunday, October 18, 1998

SWEET INDULGENCE
Cherry Jubilee
Pumpkin Pie a la Mode
Barlett Pear Poached in Red Wine, Cassis Sauce

ICE CREAM
Vanilla
Maple Walnut
Rum Raisin

SORBET
Pear
Mango-Papaya

FROZEN YOGURT
Vanilla

Chocolate Fudge Sauce
Butterscotch Sauce
Vanilla Pod and Pistachio Sauce

SUGAR FREE / LOW FAT
Fresh Fruit Tart, Fruit Sorbet

ASSORTED INTERNATIONAL CHEESE
From the Cart, Walnut Baguette

SEABOURN'S SELECTION OF
Exotic Teas
Espresso, Cappuccino
Regular and Decaffeinated Coffee

PETITS FOURS

Pastry Chef
Ernst Keinberger

SEA NEWS

Friday, June 12, 1998   Evening Dress: Informal/Jacket & Tie   Sunrise: 6:18 a.m.   Sunset: 9:23 p.m.

Good Morning

8:00	**M/S Vistafjord is due to dock at Vigo, Spain**	
8:00	"Walk A Mile" with our Fitness Instructor	Veranda Deck, aft
8:30	"Morning Stretch" - Morning Stretch with Emma	Veranda Deck, aft

For those passengers remaining on board:

Good Afternoon

2:30	Chess, Back Gammon and Card players meet	Cardroom
2:30	Movie Matinee: *Good Will Hunting;* starring Matt Damon and Robin Williams; Drama; Rated R; 2 hours and 2 minutes	Theater
3:00- 6:00	Cruise Sales Manager Tracey will help you book your next cruise	Purser's Square
4:00	Teatime Melodies with Jon Courtenay at the piano	Ballroom
5:30	Holy Mass with Fr. Waldemar Molinski	Theater
5:30	**All passengers on board! *M/S Vistafjord* prepares to sail!**	
5:30	Friends of Bill W. meet	Library

Good Evening - Tonight's Dress Code is Informal/ Jacket & Tie

6:00	*M/S Vistafjord* **sails for La Pallice (La Rochelle), France** **Enjoy the recorded music on Veranda Deck, aft as we sail away from Vigo**	
6:00 - 7:30	Dance to the music of the Vistafjord Trio; Our Gentlemen Hosts invite you on to the dance floor	Ballroom
6:00 - 8:00	Jon Courtenay awaits you with his collection of Cocktail and Dance Music	Club Viking
7:00	**Early Showtime presents:** **The Classical Quintessence** **"Figaro Plus ...."**	Garden Lounge
8:30	Try your luck in the Casino! You may charge U$ 500 to your cabin daily!	Casino

9:00	The Vistafjord Trio plays music for your entertainment; our Gentleman Hosts will dance with our ladies traveling independently	Ballroom
9:30	Card and Chess players meet for informal games	Card Room
9:30	Late Night Movie: *Great Expectations*; starring Ethan Hawke and Gwyneth Paltrow, Classic; Rated R; 1 hr. and 51 mins.	Theater
9:30	Dance to the Big Band Sound of Toni's Orchestra	Ballroom
10:00 - 11:30	Jon Courtenay plays piano melodies for your listening pleasure	Club Viking
10:00	Listen and Dance to the music of our Vistafjord Trio	Garden Lounge

10:15   **Showtime tonight presents:**   Ballroom

"Spanish Love Songs & More ...."

with international Song Stylist

Peter Fernandez

Accompanied by Toni's Orchestra; followed by dance music

| 11:30 | D.J. Paul plays your requests until the early morning hours | Club Viking |

Late-Night-Thought:

"Our destination is never a place but rather a new way of looking at things".

— Sleep Well —

Cruise Director Carleton Freese

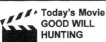
IN THE LIMELIGHT

Social Director Anita Pabst

Social Director Anita Pabst has been traveling around the world by air and by sea throughout most of her life. Originally from Europe, Anita attended school in three different countries, thus she is fluent in English, German and French as well as some Spanish and Italian.

As a young woman, Anita had a thirst for travel and a passion for learning about different cultures, their history and art. She began her career as a flight attendant for TWA traveling international routes. Eventually she moved into the cruise industry after sailing many times as a passenger. She began working aboard Cunard's Vistafjord as a Social Director in 1993 and aboard the Royal Viking Sun. A New York resident for more than 22 years, Anita's second passion is in the field of arts and antiques, on which she also lectures. After leaving the airline business, she attended New York University where she earned a degree as an appraiser in fine and decorative arts. She spent two years as an antique dealer and personally is an avid collector. Another hobby of Anita's is landscape photography. Although antiques and photography will always hold her interest, Anita says that a wanderlust keeps her in the travel industry doing what she loves best - meeting fascinating people, sharing her joie de vivre with them and seeing the world.

Courtesy Cunard Line

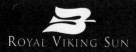

SEA NEWS

Royal Viking Sun

Saturday, April 18, 1998   **Evening Dress: Informal**   **Sunrise: 6:46 a.m.**   **Sunset: 7:50 p.m.**

GOOD MORNING

7:30	Wake Up and Stretch with Fitness Instructor Colin	Norway Deck, aft (Deck 8)
8:00	*Royal Viking Sun* **is scheduled to dock at Hamilton, Bermuda**	
	For those passengers remaining on board:	
8:00	The Daily Crossword is available	Reception Desk
9:00	Indoor games and books are available	Dicken's Library
9:00	Deck Sports Equipment is available to our a.m. athletes	Sports Area
9:00 - 6:00 p.m.	Golf Simulator open for self use (unsupervised) everyday, except during scheduled supervised play	Pebble Beach

GOOD AFTERNOON

12:00	Easy listening cocktail music	Midnight Sun Lounge
2:00	Matinee Movie: *Gone Fishin';* Starring Joe Pesci and Danny Glover; Comedy; Rated PG; 1 hr. 34 mins.	Starlight Theatre
4:00	Afternoon Teatime; finger sandwiches & sweets are served Teatime today with Pianist David Taljaard	Norway Lounge
5:00	Legs, Buns and Tums with Fitness Instructor Colin	Fitness Center
5:15	Holy Catholic Mass is celebrated with Msgr. Joseph Topping, K.H.S., the Rosary will be recited 15 minutes prior to Mass	Starlight Theatre
5:30	**All aboard!** *Royal Viking Sun* **prepares to sail!**	
5:30	Bottom Line with Fitness Instructor Colin	Fitness Center
5:45	Dixieland Sailaway Music with the Tom Haberman Orchestra as we leave beautiful Bermuda	Promenade Deck 7

GOOD EVENING - TONIGHT·S DRESS CODE IS INFORMAL

6:00	*Royal Viking Sun* **sails for Miami, Florida**	
6:00	Hold That Stretch with Fitness Instructor Colin	Fitness Center
6:45	Dancing to the David Ramm Trio; the Guest Hosts will be available for our ladies traveling independently	Midnight Sun Lounge

TODAY·S HOURS
The Shore Excursion Office will be
closed today during our stay in

FOR HAMILTON, BERMUDA
Royal Viking Sun is scheduled to be docked at Front Street, Berth No. 1 at Hamilton,
Bermuda at 8 a.m. today, Saturday, April 18.

6:45	Harpist Toni plays for your cocktail hour pleasure	Stella Polaris Room

7:00

Pre-Dinner Classical Concert
with
Pianist
Nana Mukhadze

Norway Lounge

8:00	Luck be a lady tonight! The Casino is open for your gaming pleasure!	Casino
9:00	Dancing to the David Ramm Trio; the Guest Hosts will be available for our ladies traveling independently	Norway Lounge
9:30	Evening Movie: My Best Friend's Wedding; Starring Julia Roberts and Cameron Diaz; Romantic Comedy; Rated PG-13; 1 hr. 45 mins.	Starlight Theatre

9:45

Showtime tonight presents:
Comic Impressionist
James Stephens III
plus
"The Rhythm is Going to Get You"
an opening number with
The Morag Singers and Dancers
Accompanied by the Tom Haberman Orchestra

Norway Lounge

10:15	Dancing to the David Ramm Trio; the Guest Hosts will be available for our ladies traveling independently	Norway Lounge
10:15	Harpist Toni plays for your late night listening pleasure	Stella Polaris Room
10:30	Dancing to the Tom Haberman Orchestra; the Guest Hosts will be available for our ladies traveling independently.	Norway Lounge
11:00	**Dancing to the David Ramm Trio**	Norway Lounge
11:30	Late Night Snack is served	Garden Cafe
12:00	Dancing continues with the David Ramm Trio	Midnight Sun Lounge

Late Night Thought:
What we need are more people
who specialize in the impossible.
- Theodore Roosevelt
Sleep Well — Cruise Director Bob Haines

Courtesy Cunard Line

PETER DEILMANN EUROPAMERICA CRUISES
1800 Diagonal Road, Suite 170

Alexandria, Virginia 22314

(800) 348-8287

(703) 549-1741

(703) 549-7924 **FAX**

M.S. *BERLIN:* (formerly *Princess Mahsuri*); entered service 1980; 9,570 G.R.T.; 139.3 meters x 17.5 meters; 420-passenger capacity; 210 cabins; German officers and crew; various itineraries around the world.

M.V. *DANUBE PRINCESS:* entered service 1983; refurbished 1997; 200-passenger capacity; 95 cabins; cruises on Danube River and to the Black Sea.

DEUTSCHLAND: entered service 1998; 22,400 G.R.T.; 513' x 75'; 650-passenger capacity; 288 cabins; German officers and crew; various itineraries all over the world.

M.V. *DRESDEN:* entered service 1991; refurbished 1996; 110-passenger capacity; 55 cabins; cruises on Elbe River.

M.V. *KONIGSTEIN:* entered service 1992; refurbished 1998; 58-passenger capacity; 29 cabins; cruises on Elbe, Moldav, and Havel.

S.Y. *LILI MARLEEN:* entered service 1994; 750 G.R.T.; 250' x 32'; 50-passenger capacity; 25 cabins; German officers and crew; sails in the Canary Islands and eastern and western Mediterranean. **(Category B—Not Rated)**

M/S *MOZART:* entered service 1987; refurbished 1997; 2,680 G.R.T.; 396' x 75'; 207-passenger capacity; 99 cabins; international officers and crew; cruises on Danube River and to Romania on the Black Sea.

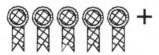

M.V. *PRINCESS DE PROVENCE:* entered service 1991; refurbished 1996; 146-passenger capacity; 71 cabins; cruises on Rhône and Saône rivers.

M.V. *PRUSSIAN PRINCESS:* entered service 1991; refurbished 1996; 142-passenger capacity; 69 cabins; Rhine, Moselle, and Main-Danube Canal cruises, cruises on Dutch and Belgium canals and cruises between Amsterdam and Budapest.

Peter Deilmann Reederei is the owner of the S.Y. *Lili Marleen* sailing ship, the *Berlin* and *Deutschland* cruise ships, and various riverboats, including M/S *Mozart*, *Danube Princess, Prussian Princess, Princess de Provence, Dresden,* and *Konigstein.* The clientele is predominantly from Germany; however, the riverboats typically attract numerous passengers from the U.S., Britain, and other parts of the world.

The M/S *Mozart* presently is the largest and most luxurious riverboat afloat. She offers many of the facilities and entertainment formerly only found on oceangoing vessels.

The 207 passengers are serviced by a complement of eighty crewmembers, sixty of whom are hotel staff. The public areas include an attractive 170-seat lounge, the location for evening dancing, performances, and lectures; a Viennese coffeehouse; a library; an indoor swimming pool, whirlpool, sauna, and solarium center; a beauty salon; a gift boutique; a large, comfortable sun deck area atop the ship; and single-seating dining.

Breakfasts include a cold buffet of juices, fruits, pastries, rolls, cereals, meats, and cheese, as well as eggs and other warm items served from the kitchen. Lunch and dinner feature numerous courses of top-notch Austrian and European cuisine, a step above the level of most other riverboats. At 11:00 P.M., cold cuts, salads, and desserts are offered in the coffeehouse area. There is a band for nightly dancing, and on many evenings, professional entertainers perform.

Cabins are 205 square feet in size, the largest of any riverboat and far more spacious than the average cabin on most cruise ships. Accommodations are air-conditioned and tastefully furnished with picture windows, very generous closet and dresser space, color TV, lock drawers, mini-bars, twin- or queen-size bed, with down comforters, and a large bathroom with toilet, shower, sink, abundant storage, and hair dryers. The ship is also equipped to service small conferences and business groups.

Itineraries include seven-night cruises on the Danube between Passau, Germany, and Budapest, Hungary, with visits to cities and villages in Austria, Hungary, and Slovakia. Prices range in high season from $214 per person per night for an inside cabin on the lower deck to $421 per person for an outside cabin on the higher deck. One hundred of the 104 accommodations are located outside, thus affording panoramic views.

The Danube is possibly the most picturesque river for cruising (see descriptions of ports of call in chapter 6) and a must for aficionados of the riverboat experience. The *Danube Princess* also offers cruises on the Danube between Passau and Budapest, with similar itineraries at prices that run a bit lower than on the *Mozart.*

The S.Y. *Lili Marleen* is a three-masted sailing vessel with Barquentine rigging, measures 250 feet in length, and accommodates 50 passengers with 25 outside cabins. Cabins are decorated with burled wall finishes and pastel upholstery and carpeting and include luxurious tiled bathrooms, hair dryers, lock drawers, and international direct-dial telephones. The restaurant accommodates all passengers at one sitting. Other public areas include an outdoor bar, a lounge and bar, and a small library with an additional bar. Itineraries feature seven-night sailings during the winter months from the Canary Islands, from Nice, Athens, and Turkey during the spring and summer, and from Majorca in the fall. Fares range from about $325 per person per day up to $465.

In addition, the line operates the *Prussian Princess,* offering Rhine/Moselle cruises and selected itineraries on the Dutch and Belgian canals; the *Dresden* and *Konigstein,* which visit ports on the Elbe River in Germany and the Czech Republic; and the *Princess de Provence,* which cruises from Lyon on the Rhône and Saône rivers between Arles and Chalon-sur-Saône.

The *Berlin,* which entered service in 1980, and the new, more luxurious *Deutschland,* which entered service in 1998, are traditional, oceangoing cruise vessels offering exotic itineraries around the world that can be purchased in segments. Cabins on the *Deutschland* include radios, telephones, bathrobes, hair dryers, mini-bars, and safes, and vary in size from 142 square feet for an inside cabin and 210 square feet for a deluxe outside cabin up to 400 square feet for the most expensive suite. Only the two owner's suites have private balconies, and three-quarters of the cabins are outside. Public areas encompass, numerous lounges and bars, three restaurants (the two-seating main dining room, the informal Lido restaurant, and a more intimate à la carte restaurant), a business center, children's playroom, indoor and outdoor pools, boutiques, and a fitness center offering sauna, steam, massage, exercise equipment, and thalassotherapy.

Strong Points:

The *Mozart* is the largest, most elegant, and comfortable riverboat in service, offering itineraries on the Danube, one of the world's most lovely and interesting rivers. The *Lili Marleen* offers a unique/comfortable sailing experience to diverse ports of call. The river vessels afford opportunities to visit some of Europe's more charming villages via Europe's most picturesque rivers.

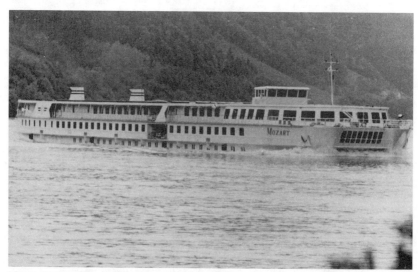

Mozart, *courtesy Peter Deilmann EuropAmerica Cruises*

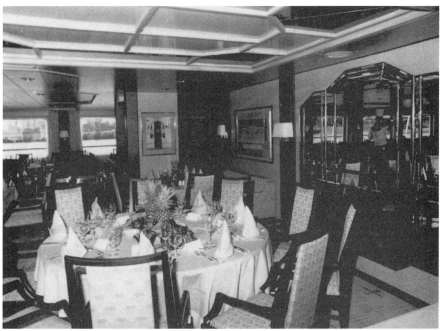

Mozart, *courtesy Peter Deilmann EuropAmerica Cruises*

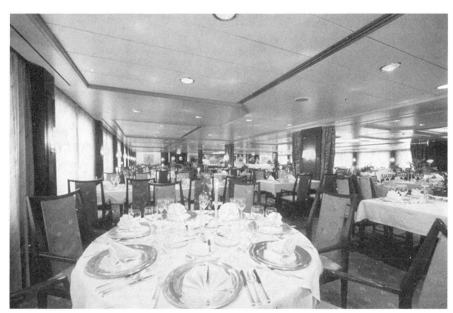

Mozart, *courtesy Peter Deilmann EuropAmerica Cruises*

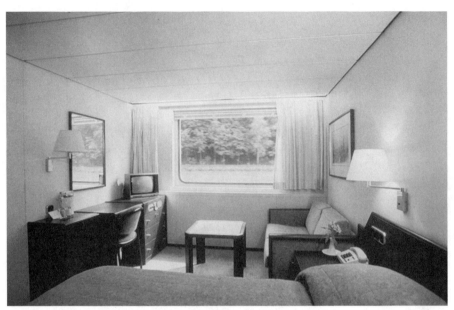

Mozart, *courtesy Peter Deilmann EuropAmerica Cruises*

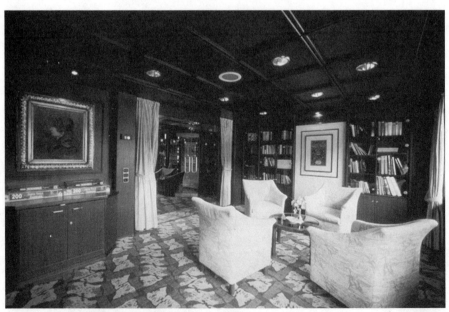

Mozart, *courtesy Peter Deilmann EuropAmerica Cruises*

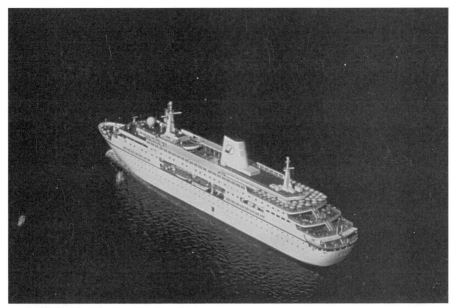

Courtesy Peter Deilmann EuropAmerica Cruises

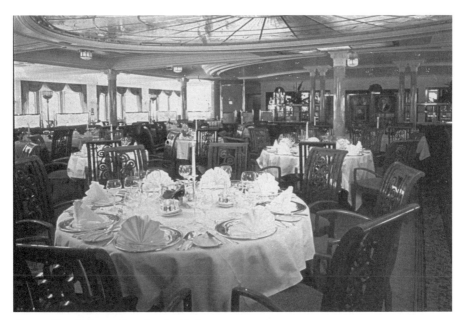

Courtesy Peter Deilmann EuropAmerica Cruises

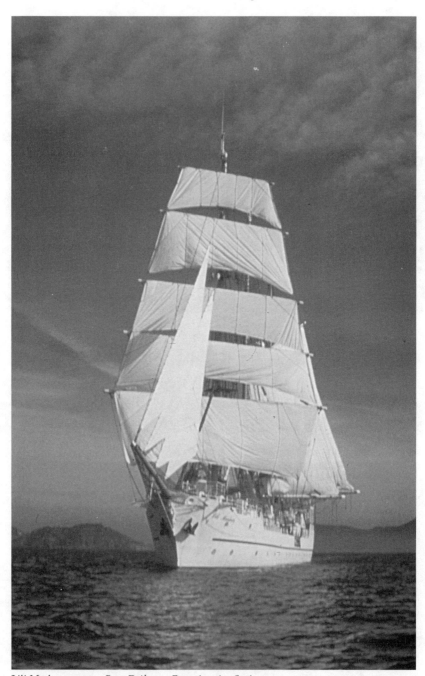

Lili Marleen, *courtesy Peter Deilmann EuropAmerica Cruises*

M/S MOZART

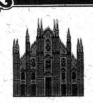

Welcome to Esztergom and Budapest

7:30-10:00 a.m. Full European breakfast buffet is served.

8:00 a.m. M.S. Mozart arrives in Esztergom.

8:45 a.m. Optional overland tour departs. (Visit Esztergom, the former residence of the Hungarian Kings. Explore all the wonders this beautiful city has to offer. Later in the day you arrive in Budapest where you re-embark on the Mozart.)

9:00 a.m. M.S. Mozart leaves Esztergom for Budapest.

9:00 a.m. If you do not wish to take the optional overland tour, stay on-board and settle into a cozy chair on deck while the Mozart glides along the Danube.

10:00 a.m. Hour long sessions with the masseur commence in the Fitness Center. (By appointment only)

11:00 a.m. Bouillon is served in the Cafe Amadeus.

11:00 a.m. Take a mid day dip in our indoor pool or enjoy the sauna.

12:30 p.m. Lunch is served in the Dining Room. (Buffet or 5-course meal)

12:30 p.m. Mozart docks in Budapest for overnight stay.

2:30 p.m. Optional tour departs. (This half day tour takes you by carriage through the fascinating landscape of the Puszta where you will see the famous Hungarian half-bred horses.)

2:30 p.m. Lecture on the sights and history of Budapest.

3:30 p.m. On deck activities.

4:00-4:45 p.m. Afternoon tea is served. (Piano background music)

5:00 p.m. Informational presentation on tomorrow's excursions.

7:00 p.m. Classical music presentation in the lounge. (Pre dinner cocktails available.)

7:30 p.m. **Dinner is served.**

9:30 p.m. Hungarian Folklore Show with a Gypsy band.

11:15 p.m. Late snack from the buffet.

11:45 p.m. Night cap at the Cafe Amadeus.

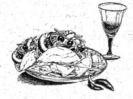

Courtesy Peter Deilmann EuropAmerica Cruises

CHEF'S SUGGESTION

Smoked Salmon with Cream Cheese
*
Bean Soup Serbian Style
*
Small Salad Plate with Carrots and Walnut Oil Dressing
*
Deep-Fried King Prawns with Sauce Gribiche and Chives Potatoes
*
Roast Saddle of Lamb "Provencale" with Rosemary Gravy,
French Beans, Half Tomato and Gratinated Potatoes "Dauphinoise"
*
Warm Apple Pie with Cinnamon Ice Cream

WINE SUGGESTION

1989 Nikolaihof im Weingebirge Federspiel
Grüner Veltliner
(Dry, Fruity, Spicy)
*
1989 Wehlener Sonnenuhr
Riesling Spätlese - Dry
(Spicy, Piquant Character, Elegant)
*
1988 Castello di Fagnano
Chianti Classico DOCG
(Fine Sourness, Intensive Colour)
*
1988 Château Picon
Bordeaux Supérieur AC
(Young Colour, Fruity)

Chef de Cuisine   Maître d'Hôtel
Manfred Schönleitner   Janos Gyulai

DINNER

Appetizers
Smoked Salmon with Cream Cheese
Pineapple Segments with Chicken Salad

Soups
Bean Soup Serbian Style
Cold Strawberry Soup with Maraschino

Salad
Small Salad Plate with Carrots and Walnut Oil Dressing

Fish
Deep-Fried King Prawns with Sauce Gribiche and Chives Potatoes

Granité
Granité of Melons

Main Dishes
Roast Saddle of Lamb "Provencale" with Rosemary Gravy,
French Beans, Half Tomato and Gratinated Potatoes "Dauphinoise"

Braised Small Cuttlet of Beef "Esterhazy"
Garden Vegetables and Buttered Noodles

Desserts
Warm Apple Pie with Cinnamon Ice Cream
Ice Pudding "Victoria" with Fruit Coulis

One of Today's Featured Ice Creams

Selection of International Cheese

Coffee / Tea

Bon Appetit!

Courtesy Peter Deilmann EuropAmerica Cruises

Gala Dinner

Sevruga Malossol Caviar and slices of Norwegian Salmon
in a Dill Mustard cream

* * *

Clear Oxtail soup with Sherry and Cheshire Cheese pastry

* * *

Sole with Cardinal sauce with Spinach and saffron
Potatoes

* * *

Pink Champagne Sorbet

* * *

Fillet Steak 'Chateau Excelsior' with white wine sauce,
vegetables and Pommes Duchesse

* * *

Cassisparfait in Vanilla Cream and Pistacchio sauce and
Fresh Fruits

* * *

Mocca

Courtesy Peter Deilmann EuropAmerica Cruises

THE DELTA QUEEN STEAMBOAT CO.
Robin Street Wharf

1380 Port of New Orleans Place

New Orleans, Louisiana 70130-1890

(800) 543-1949

(504) 585-0630 FAX

AMERICAN QUEEN: entered service 1995; 3,707 G.R.T.; 418' x 89'; 222 cabins; 436-passenger capacity; U.S. officers and crew; Mississippi and Ohio River cruises.

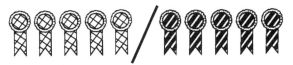

(Medical Facilities: C-9; P-0; N-0; WC; LJ; some crew trained in CPR.)

DELTA QUEEN: entered service 1927; refurbished 1947, 1989, 1993, and 1998; 3,360 G.R.T.; 285' x 605'; 174-passenger capacity; 87 cabins; U.S. officers and crew; Mississippi, Ohio, Tennessee, Cumberland, Atchafalaya, Illinois, Red, and Kanawha rivers, and the Intracoastal Waterway.

(Medical Facilities: C-O; P-O; N-O; WC; LJ; some crew trained in CPR.)

MISSISSIPPI QUEEN: entered service 1976; refurbished 1991 and 1996; 3,364 G.R.T.; 382' x 685'; 414-passenger capacity; 208 cabins; U.S. officers and crew; Mississippi, Ohio, Tennessee, and Cumberland River cruises.

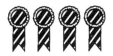

(Medical Facilities: C-1; P-0; N-0; WC; LJ; some crew trained in CPR.)

The *Delta Queen,* built in 1927, is one of America's only three authentic steam-powered overnight paddlewheelers. This venerable beauty with teak handrails, Tiffany-style stained glass windows, and brass fittings served as a Navy ferryboat during World War II and is so much a part of America's heritage that she is listed on the National Register of Historic Places and designated a National Historic Landmark. In 1947 she moved from California to the Mississippi River system, and her first sailing was from Cincinnati to Cairo, Illinois. The line is owned and operated by American Classic Voyages Company, which also owns American Hawaii Cruises but runs that line's ship as a separate operation.

Today the *Delta Queen* and her more modern sisters, the *Mississippi Queen* and *American Queen,* ply the waters of the Mississippi River and its tributaries and offer three- to fourteen-night cruises from New Orleans, Memphis, St. Louis, St. Paul, Nashville, Cincinnati, Louisville, Galveston, Pittsburgh, Chattanooga, and Ottawa (near Chicago), Illinois. Many of the cruises are based on themes such as "Big Band," "Dixie Fest," "Fall Foliage," "Kentucky Derby," and the like. The ports of call afford an opportunity to stretch your legs and discover American's heartland.

These are nostalgic, all-American cruises that the line promotes as "Steamboatin," wherein melodic riverboat tunes emanate from calliopes, a bright red paddlewheel churns up a frothy wake, Dixieland jazz bands entertain in the lounges, and Southern regional and Creole dishes are served in the dining rooms. A "riverlorian" offers historic lectures throughout the cruise. The Victorian decor, traditional and antique furnishings, appointments, and *objets d'art* in the public areas and guest rooms are tasteful and authentic and create the feelings of warmth and nostalgic "Mark Twain-era" Americana that the cruise line seeks to portray.

On the *Delta Queen,* all of the 87 cabins are outside, air-conditioned with private baths, and many include brass beds, stained-glass windows, and nineteenth- and early-twentieth-century furnishings. There are six suites, and twelve of the cabins have double or queen-size beds. The lower deck has a large dining room serving meals in two sittings, and the Texas Deck houses an entertainment lounge. There is no pool.

The *Mississippi Queen,* built in 1976, is designed to look like a classic riverboat with nineteenth-century decor, but it has less wood than her older sister. She features 207 cabins and 26 suites, more than half of which have outside verandas; a large dining room; a grand saloon; several lounges; a library; gift shop; theater; beauty salon; gym; a multitiered sun deck with a small bathing pool; and a good deal of entertainment ranging from dancing to the sound of big bands to Broadway show music and New Orleans-style jazz. Two of the rooms have king-size beds, and 14 have two single beds that can be converted to a king bed.

The waiters and cabin attendants are all from the United States and are relatively young and inexperienced as a crew on a cruising vessel; however they are very polite, friendly, and helpful.

The *American Queen,* the first steam-powered riverboat built in the past twenty years, commenced service in the summer of 1995. At a cost of $65 million, the steamboat is 418 feet long, with six decks accommodating 436 passengers in 222 cabins, 29 of which have verandas and three-quarters of which are outside. The decor and ambiance simulate the nineteenth century, but the vessel features many new amenities and comforts, including a small bathing pool, movie theater, and small gym. All of the cabins are elegantly furnished with Victorian period pieces, colorful floral fabrics, a great deal of wood, bathrooms circa 1920-1940, dressing tables and mirrors, ice buckets, telephones, piped-in music, and art. The guest accommodations have the appearance of hotel rooms in a grand Southern U.S. hotel rather than cabins on a steamboat. As you move up in categories from E to AAA, overall cabin size, sitting areas, and abundance of antiques increase. However, the single cabins are quite small and none of the accommodations have refrigerators, televisions, private room safes, lock drawers, hair dryers, or robes. The two-story "grand hotel style" dining room with stained glass-topped windows providing magnificent river views is located on the Main Deck of the steamboat and serves meals accompanied by piano music in two sittings. The food has improved over the past few years. Hearty, all-American breakfasts include a buffet of fresh fruits, melons, cereals, bakery items, egg dishes, and breakfast meats, as well as more intricate à la carte offerings. Multicourse dinners feature a choice of four entrees, and heart-healthy and vegetarian items are available. Hot dogs are served on deck all afternoon, freshly popped popcorn flows (with suds) at the Engine Room Bar (the location for sing-alongs and nightly entertainment), late-night theme buffets are offered about 11:00 P.M., and you can help yourself to fruit, coffee, tea, or cocoa in the Mark Twain Gallery around the clock. The unique, opulent Grand Saloon, flanked on the mezzanine level by private box seats, offers musical entertainment and dancing nightly. There is no gambling.

Prices vary with the length of the cruise. On the average, fares range from about $150 to $190 per person per night for a minimum cabin and up to $600 to $650 for the most expensive suite. A mid-priced outside cabin goes for about $375 per person, per night. Twenty-seven percent of the passengers are repeaters, and the median age is in the mid-sixties. Transportation to and from the boats is not included in the cruise fares. Although cruises generally commence in a major city near an airport, there are occasions where conditions on the rivers may require that the boat anchor some distance away. Be certain to verify the location of the vessel immediately before you depart for your cruise and, by and large, it is recommended that you have the cruise line make your air arrangements so that they will be responsible for any last-minute changes.

Strong Points:

An authentic, nostalgic, and wholesome "all-American" experience for mature adults who appreciate steamboating and U.S. history. The *American Queen* is an especially well-appointed and comfortable steamboat.

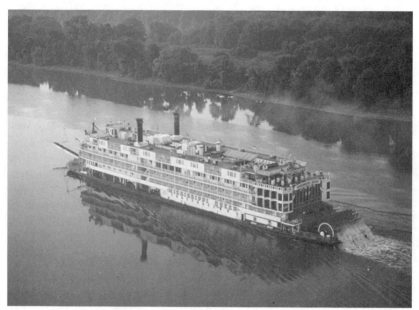

Courtesy The Delta Queen Steamboat Co.

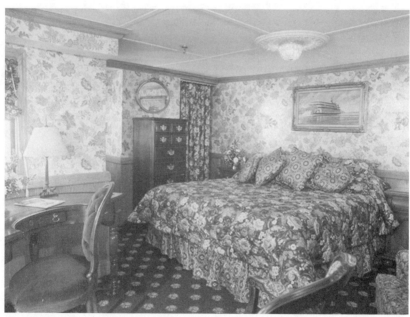

Courtesy The Delta Queen Steamboat Co.

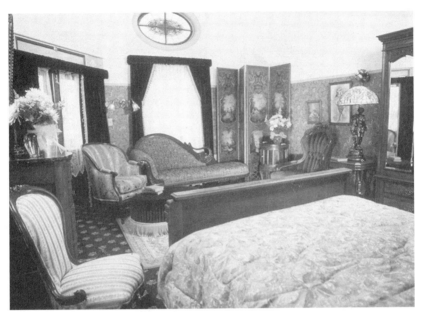

Courtesy The Delta Queen Steamboat Co.

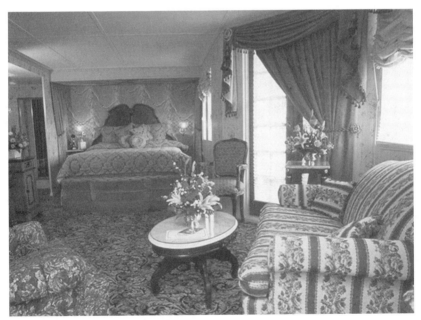

Courtesy The Delta Queen Steamboat Co.

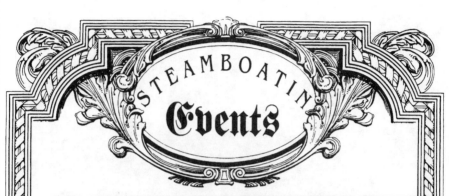

STEAMBOATIN

Events

ON THE BEAUTIFUL OHIO

| Sunday | On Board The American Queen | April 27, 1997 |

6 a.m. to 10 a.m. Enjoy Continental Breakfast in your bathrobe and slippers on the Front Porch of America. (Texas Deck, forward)

6:30 a.m. to 9 a.m. Breakfast is served in the J. M. White Dining Room, featuring an "a la carte" menu and a Buffet. Please enter through the Main Deck Lounge and the maitre d' will escort you to a table.

8 a.m. "Riverlorian River Chat" with *Lewis Hankins,* in the Grand Saloon. Coffee and Pastries will be served during the chat. (Also heard on Channel "D" in your cabin.) This morning's "River Chat" will be rebroadcast this afternoon at 4 p.m. on channel "C" in your cabin. Immediately following the "River Chat", Mariam will be telling you about our other cruises. Mariam will then be in the Main Deck Lounge to answer any questions.

8 a.m. to 3 p.m. & 5 p.m. to 9 p.m. The AQ Emporium is OPEN, on Cabin Deck, for your "Steamboatin' Shopping Enjoyment."

8:30 a.m. "Steamboatin' - Past, Present and Future" Join Mariam in the Grand Saloon for a special slide presentation and learn about our exciting plans for the future.

9 a.m. "The A.Q. A.M. Milers Club" Join *Chip* for a walk around the deck, at your own pace. Seven laps equals one mile. Meet on the Observation Deck, forward (weather permitting).

9:30 a.m. "Devotional Service" Join us for a non-denominational service in the Grand Saloon. Music by Dining Room Pianist *Tim Herbez.*

10:30 a.m. to 6 p.m. Hot Dogs with all the fixin's are available at the Calliope Bar. The Drink Of The Day is the "Oak Alley Julep" and the non-alcohol "Plantation Colada" for $2.00.

10:30 a.m. to 6 p.m. Soft serve ice cream is now available on the Front Porch of America.

10:30 a.m. "Musical Trivia Time" Quizmistress *Jennifer* asks the questions and you give the answers, in the Grand Saloon.

11:30 a.m. *Early Seating* Luncheon is served in the J. M. White Dining Room.

11:30 a.m. to 1:30 p.m. "Soup and Salad Bistro" on the Front Porch of America. Featuring Homemade Soups, a variety of Salads along with your favorite beverage, and something extra for the Sweet Tooth.

11:30 a.m. "Vessel Tour" (*Main Seating*) Would you like to learn your way around the American Queen *and* learn some interesting facts about our new grand lady of the river? Meet Mariam in the Mark Twain Gallery.

12:30 p.m. "Bingo! Bingo! Bingo!" Bring five dollars for each card you would like to play, as *Chip and Paula* call the lucky numbers in the Grand Saloon.

1:15 p.m. *Main Seating* Luncheon is served in the J. M. White Dining Room.

1:30 p.m. "Vessel Tour" (*Early Seating*) Would you like to learn your way around the American Queen *and* learn some interesting facts about our new grand lady of the river? Meet Mariam in the Mark Twain Gallery.

2:30 p.m. The Paddlewheel Steamboatin' Society of America Champagne and Punch Reception, for repeat passenger members only, please, will be held in the Grand Saloon. Join us for refreshments, meet the Captain, and swap stories with other members.

3 p.m. to 6 p.m. Mariam will be in her office off the Main Deck Lounge to discuss future Steamboatin' adventures.

3 p.m. "Photo Order Box" closes. Please have Photo orders in by this time.

3:30 p.m. "Liars Club" Join *Chip* with our panel of experts and try to catch them in a lie. Fun for all, and That's the Truth. In the Grand Saloon.

(continued on back)

THE EXPERIENCE OF A LIFETIME!

4 p.m. Rebroadcast of this morning's "Riverlorian River Chat" on channel "C" in your cabin.

4:30 p.m. "Cocktail Hour" Delicious Hors D'Oeuvres and your favorite beverage, In the Engine Room Bar.

4:45 p.m. "World's Greatest Sing-Along" Sound your 'Mi-Mi-Mi's' with *Steve Spracklen and Fred Dodd*, in the Engine Room Bar.

5:30 p.m. "Captain's Dinner" All *Early Seating* passengers. We ask that you arrive as the dinner bells chime, for Captain John Davitt has a very special toast from all of us to all of you. Dinner music by *Tim Herbez*.

7:15 p.m. SHOWTIME "Broadway Rhythm" For *Main Seating* guests, in the Grand Saloon.

8 p.m. "Captain's Dinner" All *Main Seating* passengers. We ask that you arrive as the dinner bells chime, for Captain John Davitt has a very special toast from all of us to all of you. Dinner music by *Tim Herbez*.

8:30 p.m. SHOWTIME "Broadway Rhythm" For *Early Seating* guests, in the Grand Saloon.

9 p.m. to 10 p.m. "Photographers" will be available in the Photo Gallery. (Cash Sales only, please.)

9:15 p.m. "Night Owls Club" with *Steve Spracklen and Fred Dodd* in the Engine Room Bar. Enjoy a "Cape Cod" for $2.00.

10 p.m. Dance to the sounds of *The Steamboat Syncopators*, in the Grand Saloon..

11 p.m. "Moonlight Buffet" is served in the Main Deck Lounge. Tonight's theme is *Seafood*.

Today's Movies-In The Theater

12:30 p.m. "Life on The Mississippi" (1 hr. 55 min.) hosted by *Fred.*

3:00 p.m. "Grumpier Old Men" (1 hr. 37 min.) hosted by *Bob.*

5:30 p.m. "Showboat" (1 hr. 48 min.) hosted by *Jennifer.*

9:30 p.m. "Showboat" (1 hr. 48 min.) hosted by *Paula.*

Tomorrow Morning's Schedule

Monday, April 27, 1997

6-8 a.m. Continental Breakfast is available in the Grand Saloon

6:30-8 a.m. Breakfast Buffet is served in the J.M. White Dining Room.

7-9 a.m. AQ Emporium will be open for any last minute purchases.

7-8 a.m. Photographers will be in the Photo Gallery. (Cash Sales only, please.)

Tonight In The Grand Saloon:

7:15 p.m.
for *Main Seating* Passengers
&
8:30 p.m.
for *Early Seating* Passengers

Broadway
Rhythm

Starring

**Paula Betlem, Fred Bishop,
Jennifer Davis, Chip Saporiti**

singing some of your
favorite songs from
Broadway Musicals,
Then and Now.

Accompanied By

**Chuck Easterling and
The Steamboat Syncopators**

9:30 & 10:30 p.m.
After the Shows we will feature dancing with
Chuck Easterling and the Steamboat Syncopators

The Engine Room Bar Presents:

"Night Owls Club"
9:15 p.m.

Steve Spracklen
The King of the Keyboard

&

Fred Dodd
The Sultan of Strings

All you "Night Owls" join
Steve and Fred for their special brand of
"Steamboatin' Entertainment."
THE LATE NIGHT PLACE TO BE!

Courtesy The Delta Queen Steamboat Co.

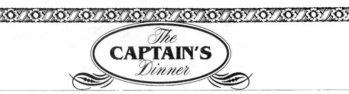

The CAPTAIN'S *Dinner*

❦ APPETIZER ❦
Shrimp Cocktail

❦ SOUPS ❦
Acadian Bisque
Petite Marmite

❦ SALADS ❦
Cæsar Salad • Steamboat Salad

❦ ENTRÉES ❦

Filet Mignon
Tenderloin Steak grilled and served with a rich red wine sauce.

Grilled Lamb Chops
Lean Lamb Chops on Couscous with a Vegetable Ratatouille.

Heart Healthy Dinner♥
Chicken Niçoise
Grilled Breast of Chicken with vegetable julienne and olives in a white wine broth.
Approximately: 250 Calories/ 95 mg Cholesterol/ 165 mg Sodium/ 6 gr Fat

---

Traditional River Fare
Braided Salmon and Flounder
Fillets of Salmon and Flounder braided together and
poached. Served with a Lemon Dill Beurre Blanc Sauce.

❦ BEVERAGES ❦
Freshly Brewed Coffee, Regular or Decaffeinated
Iced and Hot Tea
Milk • Soft Drinks

❦ DESSERTS ❦
The Chef's Sweets and Treats
Seasonal Fresh Fruit
Sherbets and Assorted Ice Creams

Courtesy The Delta Queen Steamboat Co.

DISNEY CRUISE LINE
210 Celebration Place

Celebration, Florida 34747

(800) 511-1333

(407) 566-7000

(407) 566-3751 FAX

DISNEY MAGIC: entered service 1998; 83,000 G.R.T.; 964' x 106'; 2,400-passenger capacity; 875 staterooms; European officers and international crew; three- and four-day cruises from Port Canaveral.

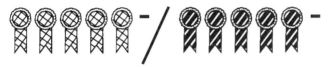

DISNEY WONDER: entered service 1999; 83,000 G.R.T.; 964' x 106'; 2,400-passenger capacity; 875 staterooms; European officers and international crew; three- and four-day cruises from Port Canaveral.

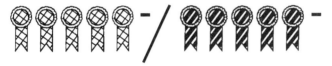

(Medical Facilities: C-12; P-2, CLS, MS; N-4; CM; PD; BC; EKG; TC; PO; EPC; OX; WC; OR; ICU; X; M; LJ.)

The state-of-the-art, unique, 83,000-ton *Disney Magic,* designed to be reminiscent of the classic ocean liners and capable of accommodating 2,400 passengers, entered service in July 1998, followed by *Disney Wonder* in August 1999.

The 875 larger-than-average staterooms range in size from 173 square feet up to the 899-square-foot Disney Suites. Seventy-three percent of the accommodations are outside and almost one-third have verandas. Most sleep at least three persons, while some accommodate four or five. All staterooms include tubs and showers, remote-control TVs, private safes, hair dryers, phones with voicemail message service, split bathrooms, and privacy dividers separating bedrooms from the sitting areas that convert to pull-down beds and sofas for the children. In addition there are two luxurious Disney suites and two 945-square-foot two-bedroom suites that can sleep five, as well as eighteen 614-square-foot one-bedroom suites, 14 of which sleep five and two that are wheel-chair accessible. The suites rival those on luxury-category ships. The line offers a dozen stateroom categories, air-sea packages, early booking discounts, and land packages that include visits to Walt

Disney World Resort. Although prices for the first two passengers in a stateroom for a three-night cruise range from $599 each for the least expensive inside cabin during value season, up to $2,789 per person for the Royal Suite in peak season, additional children sharing the accommodations pay minimum fare. The extra night on four-night cruises costs somewhat less than the first three. On the average, a 214-square-foot outside cabin on a three-night cruise goes for $1,034 per person, and a 268-square-foot cabin including a veranda for $1,284. Cabins, staterooms, and suites in all categories are a good deal larger and include more amenities than on most other cruise ships; however, they are designed to accommodate more passengers. The availability of a tub and shower and a mini-bar/refrigerator in the lower-cost categories is somewhat unique in the cruise industry.

All cruises include a visit to Castaway Cay, Disney's privately developed 1,000-acre island in the Bahamas, where guests will enjoy a protected lagoon for watersports, shops, dining pavilions, bicycles, and separate adults-only, family, and teen beaches. The ships are able to dock at the island and avoid time-consuming tender service.

The dining experience aboard these vessels is unique in that it permits guests to move to a different theme restaurant each night. Dinner companions and their wait staff move together to three different locations, including Lumiere's, a more traditional, Art Deco-motif dining room offering Continental/French cuisine; Parrot Cay, featuring Caribbean fare in a colorful, tropical decor; and Animator's Palate, a totally unique restaurant that transforms over the course of the evening from a room decorated solely in black and white to a kaleidoscope of lights and colors. Dining in these three venues is pleasant and has improved from the cruise line's inception, and will most likely get even better in the future.

Palo is a 138-seat alternative, adults-only, Italian specialty restaurant located atop ship, with windows out to the sea. This is definitely the choice for adults traveling without children. Reservations are required and it is advisable to book immediately upon coming on board. Here I found the dining experience top-notch, with gourmet Italian cuisine, an impressive wine list, and excellent presentation and service. In addition, families can opt for an indoor/outdoor café serving all three meals, snacks, and a buffet dinner for children; a hamburger, hot dog, and pizza grill near the pool; and an ice cream bar.

Public areas, which are traditional and nautical in decor, with numerous Disney-character and Art Deco accents, include an entire deck devoted to children and featuring age-specific supervised programs, children's pool, game arcade, teen club, play areas, and a full complement of children's counselors; three outdoor pools—one for families, a children's pool fashioned in the image of Mickey Mouse with an impressive water slide that is supervised, and a third with adjoining whirlpools exclusively for adults; a 1,022-seat theater for musical productions and a 268-seat cinema for Disney classics, first-run releases, and live entertainment; shopping opportunities with emphasis on Disney-signature items; several nightclubs and lounges including nightly improv presentations; a unique sports bar atop ship; an 8,500-square-foot, ocean-view, fully equipped gym and

Steiner health spa; and a promenade deck for jogging and walking. There is no casino, in keeping with the Disney family image. However, the separate adult pool, private beach on Castaway Cay, lounge areas, and the specialty adults-only Italian restaurant afford some sanctuary for cruisers traveling without children or wishing a few hours' respite. There are not many activities gauged to adult singles, couples, or older teens, and some may find this atypical for such a large cruise ship.

These ships offer a traditional Disney-style experience at sea that will appeal to families who enjoy a Disney vacation and wish to combine a short cruise with visits to the theme parks. Activities and entertainment are definitely directed to families and the younger set. Different activities are scheduled for the various children's age groups. Having cruised on the Magic's maiden voyage, and again five months later, it was evident that there was still need for some changes and fine-tuning. Disney has been garnering suggestions from passenger feedback and steadily making the modifications necessary to make it a top contender. These ships are presently receiving very positive passenger feedback from families experiencing their first cruise.

Strong Points:

This is an excellent family-oriented cruise for parents with young children, pre-teens and early teens, as well as Mickey Mouse junkies. Adults traveling without children may wish to adopt someone else's before coming aboard.

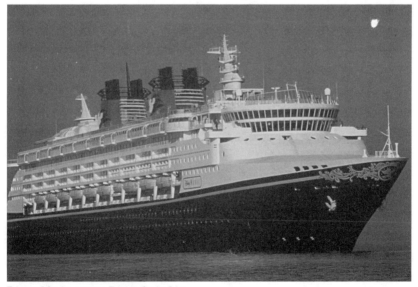

Disney Magic, *courtesy Disney Cruise Line*

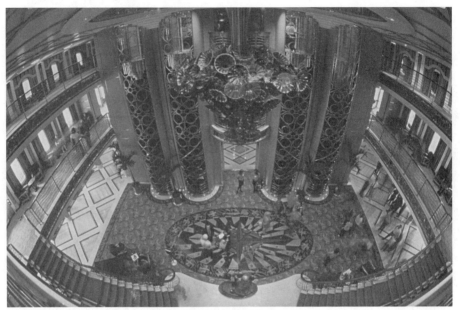

Grand Lobby on the Disney Magic, courtesy Disney Cruise Line

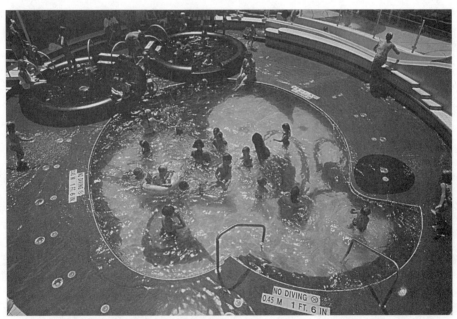

Kid's Pool on Disney Magic, courtesy Disney Cruise Line

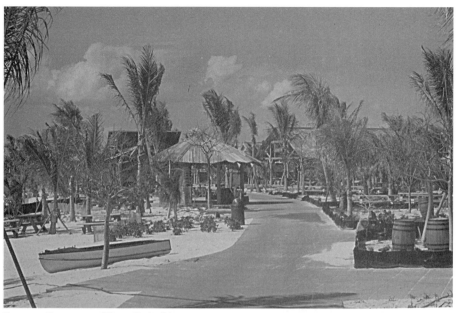

Castaway Cay, courtesy Disney Cruise Line

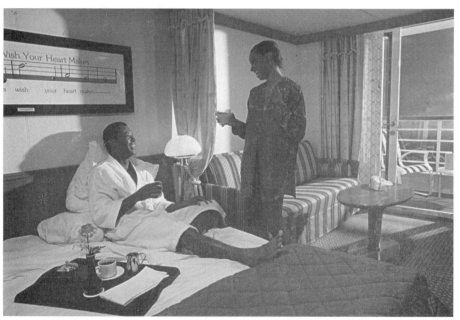

Guest Room, courtesy Disney Cruise Line

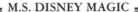

LUMIERE'S

"A dinner here is never second best."

*"Mesdames et Messieurs,
it is with the deepest pride and greatest pleasure
that we welcome you tonight. And now, we invite you to relax,
let us pull up a chair, as the Dining Room
proudly presents... your dinner."*

– LUMIERE

LES GRANDS PLATS

*"If you're stressed, it's fine dining we suggest...
We'll prepare and serve with flair a culinary cabaret!"*

POITRINE DE POULET FARCI A LA MOUSSE DE FOIE GRAS, SA SAUCE AU PORTO, POMME LYONNAISE
*Breast of Chicken Stuffed with Goose Liver, accompanied by a
Light Port Wine Sauce and Lyonnaise Potatoes*

JARRET D'AGNEAU BRAISÉ, SA RATATOUILLE PROVENCALE ET SES POMMES ECRASSES À L' HUILE D' OLIVE
Braised Shank of Lamb, Ratatouille and Crushed Potatoes with Olive Oil

FILET DE BOEUF AU POIVRE "GASTON"
*Beef Tenderloin with Green Peppercorn Sauce, served with Ratatouille
and Crushed Potatoes with Olive Oil*

LES PETITS FARCIS PROVENCAL
Stuffed Vegetables served with Spinach and a Coulis of Fresh Tomato

FILET DE BAR AUX TROIS SAVEURS ET SA SAUCE CHAMPAGNE
*Seabass Filet topped with Mushroom Duxelle, Tomato Concasse and Crusted with
Herbal Bread Crumbs on a Light Champagne Sauce*

LES DESSERTS

"Course by course, one by one 'til you shout enough! I'm done!"

BOURBON VANILLA CRÈME BRÛLÉE
Traditional French Vanilla Custard with a Caramelized Sugar Crust

SOUFFLÉ GLACÉ AU GRAND MARNIER
Frozen Souffle flavored with Grand Marnier Liquor served in a Chocolate Cup

GRATIN DE FRUITS ROUGE ET SON SABAYON AU KIRSCH
Seasonal Fruits Gratin with Cherry Liqueur Flavored Sabayon

MARQUISE AU CHOCOLAT ET SA CREME ANGLAISE MOKA
French Chocolate Cake served with Coffee Flavored Vanilla Sauce

ASSIETTE DE FROMAGES
A selection of Cheese and Crackers from our Pantry

LES DIGESTIFS

"Lift your glass, you've won your pass to be our guest."

As a digestif, we would like to recommend to you: Tia Maria, Vintage Port, Grand Marnier, Remy Martin Cognac or your favorite classic

LES CAFÉS ET LES THÉS

"While the candlelight's still glowing let us help you. We'll keep going."

Coffee or Decaffeinated Coffee, Tea or Herbal Tea

Please ask your server to recommend one of our specialty coffees.

© Disney

LES PETITS PLATS

"Try the grey stuff! It's delicious!"

ESCARGOTS BOURGUIGNONS
Burgundy Snails Baked with Mushrooms, Herbs and Garlic Butter

COCKTAIL DE FRUITS DE SAISON
Seasonal Fruits with Minted Yogurt

FEUILLETÉ D'ÉPINARDS ET D'ARTICHAUTS
Creamy Spinach and Artichoke served in Warm Puff Pastry

COCKTAIL DE CREVETTES "NEPTUNE"
Cocktail Shrimp along with Neptune Salad in a French Cocktail Dressing

TERRINE DU CHEF ET SA GARNITURE A L' ANCIENNE
Pate of Chicken with Red onion Jam, and Pear Chutney

LES SOUPES DU JOUR

"Don't be a beast! Use your spoon!"

SOUPE À L'OIGNON GRATINÉE
Oven-Baked Onion Soup

BISQUE DE HOMARD
Classical Lobster Bisque

LES SALADES

"A taste of provincial life!"

SALADE "LUMIÈRE"
Crisp Romaine and Iceberg Lettuces topped with Chopped Egg, Bacon Crumbles, Parmesan Cheese and Mustard Vinaigrette

SALADE NIÇOISE
Romaine Leaves with Green Beans, Tuna, Potatoes and Eggs in Nicoise Dressing

Courtesy Disney Cruise Line

PERSONAL NAVIGATOR®

M.S. DISNEY MAGIC
WELCOME TO NASSAU, BAHAMAS
Saturday, January 23, 1999

Arrival in Nassau: 8:00am
Approximate All Ashore: 9:00am

Onboard Time: 2:00am
Port Departure: 2:30am

Dining Experience

Breakfast

Lumiere's , Deck 3, Midship
Table Service 7:30am – 9:30am
Parrot Cay, Deck 3, Aft
"The Quick Breakfast" (Buffet & Table Service) 8:00am – 10:00am

Lunch

Lumiere's
Open-seating 12:00pm – 2:00pm
Parrot Cay
Open-seating 12:00pm – 2:00pm

Dinner

Lumiere's
Dinner 6:00pm (Main Seating) 8:30pm (Late Seating)
Suggested Dress: Jacket recommended, not required
Parrot Cay and Animator's Palate, Deck 4, Aft
Dinner 6:00pm (Main Seating) 8:30pm (Late Seating)
Suggested Dress: Casual (no shorts please)
Palo
Open from at 6:30pm
Reservations are required, cover charge applies
Suggested Dress: Jacket recommended, not required

Other Eateries

Early Bird Coffee	6:30am – 7:00am	Topsider Buffet, Starboard side, Aft
Buffet Breakfast	7:00am – 10:00am	Topsider Buffet, Deck 9, Aft
Lunch	12:00pm – 2:00pm	Topsider Buffet, Deck 9, Aft
Burgers and Hotdogs	12:00pm – 5:00pm	Pluto's, Deck 9, Midship
	6:00pm – 10:00pm	
Pizza, Pizza & Pizza	12:00pm – 6:00pm	Pinocchio's, Deck 9, Midship
	10:00pm – 1:00am	
Fresh ice cream	2:00pm – 6:00pm	Scoops, Deck 9, Midship
	7:00pm – 8:00pm	
Late-night Snacks	11:30pm – 1:00am	Promenade Lounge, Deck 3,
		Beat Street, Deck 3 & Studio Sea ,Deck 4

Bars & Lounges

Promenade Lounge	9:00am – 1:00am	Deck 3, Midship
Pinocchio's	11:00pm – 1:00am	Deck 9, Midship
Signal's	11:30am – 10:00pm	Deck 9, Forward
Outlook Bar	12:30pm – 6:00pm	Deck 10, Forward
Pluto's Bar	12:00pm – 5:00pm	Deck 9, Midship
	6:00pm – 10:00pm	
ESPN Skybox	12:00pm – 12:00am	Deck 11, Midship
Outlook Bar	2:00pm – 8:00pm	Deck 10, Forward
Sessions	5:00pm – 1:30am	Deck 3, Forward
Preludes	5:30pm – 11:30pm	Deck 4, Forward
Studio Sea	7:30pm – 1:30am	Deck 4, Midship
Rockin' Bar D	8:00pm – 2:00am	Deck 4, Midship
Offbeat	9:00pm – 1:00am	Deck 3, Forward

Shops & Services

Merchandise

Mickey's Mates	7:00pm – 12:00am	Deck 4, Midship
Treasure Ketch	7:00pm – 12:00am	Deck 4, Midship
Upbeat	7:00pm – 12:00am	Deck 3, Forward
ESPN Locker Room	7:00pm - 12:00am	Deck 10, Midship
Shore Excursion Deck	7:30am – 11:00am	Deck 3, Midship

Photography

Shutters *(photos only)*	4:00pm – 7:00am	Deck 4, Aft
(Photos & merchandise)	7:00pm – 12:00am	

Health and Beauty

Fitness Center	7:00am – 8:00pm	Deck 9, Forward
Vista Spa	8:00am – 8:00pm	Deck 9, Forward
Health Center	8:00am – 11:00am	Deck 1, Forward
	3:00pm – 7:00am	

SPECIAL PURCHASE	Disney Cruise Line	Today's Drink Special
Swiss Made	proudly presents	*Junkanoo Punch*
Designer Watches	*Hercules the Muse-ical*	*Colorful and fruitful*
$69.99	in the	*just like the Bahamas!*
	Walt Disney Theatre	
Tonight Only	Check your theatre ticket for your show time:	**$3.95**
Treasure Ketch Deck 4 Midship	6:15pm, 8:30pm or 10:30pm	$5.95 in a souvenir glass

---

Nassau: It's time to get off for a little sightseeing, a lot of shopping or a roll of the dice at one of Nassau's glimmering casinos. Enjoy a full day of soaking up the warm sun and rich, colonial heritage. U.S. currency is widely accepted in Nassau. Don't forget your Key to the World card as you disembark. Our gangways are located on Deck 1, Forward and Aft, Port side. Our Aft gangway is made to accommodate guests who are physically challenged. To check Nassau Shore Excursion availability, please see our Shore Excursion One Stop Desk or Guest Services no later than one hour prior to the scheduled departure time of the excursion. Visit Disney's Oceaneer Club or Lab for highlights of our children's offerings; program offerings available from 8:30am – 1:00am.

© DISNEY

Disney's Magical Events & Activities

6:00am – 10:00pm	**Mickey's Pool** is open for use	Deck 9, Aft
6:00am – 12:00am	The **Quiet Cove Pool** open for use (adults only)	Deck 9, Forward
6:00am – 12:00am	**Goofy's Pool** is open for use	Deck 9, Midship
8:30am – 9:15am	**Body Conditioning:** Firm and tone those muscles, Fitness Center	Deck 9, Forward
9:00am – 10:00am	**Bill W. Meeting.** Fantasia Conference Room (adults only)	Deck 2, Midship
9:00am – 10:00am	**Goofy Family Fitness:** Stretch with one of our wacky Disney friends at Wide World of Sports Deck	Deck 10, Forward
9:00am – 8:00pm	**Mickey's Slide** is open. (Height and age restrictions apply)	Deck 9, Midship
10:00am	**Skin Care & Make Up Seminar,** Vista Spa	Deck 9, Forward
11:00am	**Make Your "Bad Hair" Days a Thing of the Past,** Vista Spa	Deck 9, Forward
11:00am – 12:00pm	**Ping Pong Play:** Show off your ping pong talents at the Goofy Pool Port side	Deck 9, Midship

11:30am	**Disney Cruise Line** proudly presents *Island Magic* Stage Show featuring your favorite Disney friends **Buena Vista Theatre**	**Deck 5, Aft**

11:30am – 12:30pm	**Family Time:** Explore Oceaneer's Club as a family (children must be accompanied by and adult)	Deck 5, Midship
12:00pm – 3:00pm	**Bridge, Cards & More:** Relax and play in a cozy spot, Sessions	Deck 3, Forward
12:30pm – 1:30pm	**Animation Fun:** Learn to draw your favorite Disney characters in Animator's Palate	Deck 3, Aft
1:00pm – 3:00pm	**Guided Bridge Overlook Tour:** Check out the control center of the ship, Starboard side	Deck 9, Forward
2:00pm	**Movie:** *A Bug's Life* (G), Showing in the Buena Vista Theatre	Deck 5, Aft
2:00pm – 3:00pm	**DJs Clayton & Marty** create fun and games on the Deck Stage	Deck 9, Midship
3:30pm – 4:30pm	**Nautical Mystery Tour:** Discover clues that lead you all over the ship in search of clues, Topsider	Deck 9, Aft
3:30pm – 4:30pm	**Wine Tasting from Stem to Stern:** Sample wines in a relaxing atmosphere, Palo	Deck 10, Aft
	Cost: $12.00 Please reserve a place at Guest Services	
4:00pm	**CASTAWAY CAY SHORE TALK:** Discover the mysteries of Castaway Cay, Studio Sea	Deck 4, Midship
4:30pm – 5:30pm	**Volleyball Challenge:** Team up for a friendly game at Wide World of Sports Deck (adults only)	Deck 10, Forward
4:30pm – 5:15pm	**Low Impact Aerobics:** Increase your heart rate, Fitness Center	Deck 9, Forward
4:30pm – 6:00pm	**Character Appearances** at the *Disney Magic* gangway	Deck 1, Aft
5:00pm	**JACKPOT BINGO – Cash Prizes!** (Card sales 15 minutes prior) Rockin' Bar D (adults only)	Deck, 3, Forward
5:30pm – 6:30pm	**Portraits** taken in the Atrium Lobby – Don't forget to smile for our photographers!	Deck 3, Midship
6:00pm	**Movie:** *A Bug's Life* (G) at Buena Vista Theatre	Deck 5, Aft
6:30pm – 7:30pm	**Open Time:** Explore the Oceaneer's Club and Lab as a family (children must be accompanied by an adult)	Deck 5, Midship

Show Times: (Please check your show ticket) **6:15pm** **8:30pm** **10:30pm**	**Disney Cruise Line Entertainment** proudly presents *Hercules the Muse-ical* in the **Walt Disney Theatre**	**Deck 4, Forward**

7:30pm – 8:30pm	**Character Appearances:** Another opportunity to meet your favorite Disney friends in the Atrium	Deck 3, Midship

7:30pm	**Captain Hans Mateboer** cordially invites you to a **Welcome Aboard Cocktail Party** to be held in the Beat Street Area, Deck 3, Forward *(Please enter via the Atrium, Deck 3)*	**7:30pm**

7:45pm – 8:15pm	**So You Think You Know Your Music:** A great game with a lot of laughs at Studio Sea	Deck 4, Midship
7:45pm – 8:45pm	**Get your portraits** taken in the Atrium Lobby	Deck 3, Midship
8:00pm – 8:30pm	**Character Appearances** on Deck 4	Deck 4, Forward
8:15pm	**Movie:** *Water Boy* (PG-13) at Buena Vista Theatre	Deck 5, Aft
8:30pm – 10:00pm	**Character Appearances:** See some of your favorite Disney friends on Deck	Deck 4, Forward
8:30pm – 1:00am	**DJ Clayton** keeps the music alive at Studio Sea	Deck 4, Midship
8:30pm – 2:00am	**DJ Marty** spins the tunes at Rockin' Bar D (adults only)	Deck 3, Forward
9:30pm – 1:00am	**The Heart's Desire Band** serenade you on deck	Deck 9, Midship
9:45pm	**IMPROVISATIONAL COMEDY** at its best at Offbeat (adults only)	Deck 3, Forward
9:45pm – 10:45pm	**Get your portraits** taken in the Atrium Lobby	Deck 3, Midship
10:30pm	**Movie:** *Water Boy* (PG-13) at Buena Vista Theatre	Deck 5, Aft
10:30pm – 12:00am	**Charade of Stars:** It's a casting call for all karaoke talent at Studio Sea	Deck 4, Midship
10:45pm	**IMPROVISATIONAL COMEDY** sure to tickle your funny bone at Offbeat (adults only)	Deck 3, Forward
12:00am	**IMPROVISATIONAL COMEDY** at Offbeat (adults only)	Deck 3, Forward

Courtesy Disney Cruise Line

EUROPE CRUISE LINE/1ST CLASS HOLIDAYS

1010 University Avenue, C201

San Diego, California 92103

(619) 682-5114

(800) 923-3358

(619) 682-5117 FAX

BLUE DANUBE I and *II:* entered service 1995 and 1998; 1,500 G.R.T.; 360' x 38'; 144-passenger capacity; 72 cabins; Dutch officers and crew; cruises on Danube River.

RHINE PRINCESS: entered service 1983; refurbished 1992; 1,000 G.R.T.; 277' x 45'; 120-passenger capacity; 60 cabins; Dutch and British officers and crew; cruises in Holland and on Rhine River.

Europe Cruise Line/1st Class Holidays is a Dutch-owned company offering river cruises on the rivers and waterways of Northern Europe, with offices in the Netherlands, United Kingdom, Germany, Switzerland, and the United States. The company owns *Blue Danube I* and *II,* as well as *Rhine Princess* and *Diana,*, which is only used for charters. The line specializes in air, land, and cruise-tour packages.

The *Rhine Princess,* built in 1983 and refurbished in 1992, features 60 air-conditioned and heated outside cabins with twin or double beds, color televisions with in-house videos, direct-dial international telephones, radios, dressing table with mirrors, hair dryers and private toilets, some with showers and others with bath/shower combinations. Atop ship on Sun Deck are a whirlpool, outdoor swimming pool, and lounges. The next three decks house the sixty 124-square-foot cabins, the reception area, dining room, sauna, lounge, and bar.

Itineraries include tulip cruises in Holland in the spring and 7-night Rhine and Moselle River cruises between Amsterdam and Basel throughout the summer, ranging in price between $1,300 and $1,690 ($2,475 for a double-cabin suite).

Blue Danube I and *II* entered service in 1995 and 1998 respectively, offering cruises between Regensburg in German and Budapest, Hungary at prices between $1,625, and $2,195 ($3,290 for a double-cabin suite). Although there are differences in the design and locations, each vessel has seventy-two, 144-square-foot outside cabins. Each cabin includes twin or double beds, a closet and wardrobe, a large picture window, color television with cable and in-house movies, direct-dial telephones, small dressing tables with mirrors, a hair dryer, and bathrooms with either a shower or shower/tub combination. Cabins on the Promenade and Mozart decks offer the best views. Public areas encompass a large sundeck, with outdoor pool, a lounge, bar, attractive restaurant, a library, reception area, small fitness facility with sauna and whirlpool, and a golf simulator. Tours are offered at the various villages visited, and on several evenings a small combo performs for listening and dancing in the lounge.

Strong Points:

A relaxing, comfortable way to visit the charming cities and villages along the Rhine and Danube.

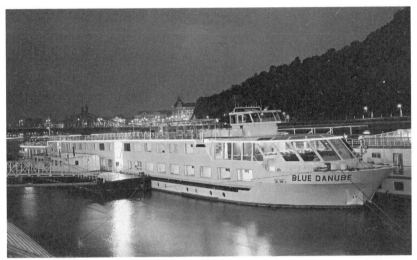

Blue Danube, *courtesy Europe Cruise Line/1st Class Holidays*

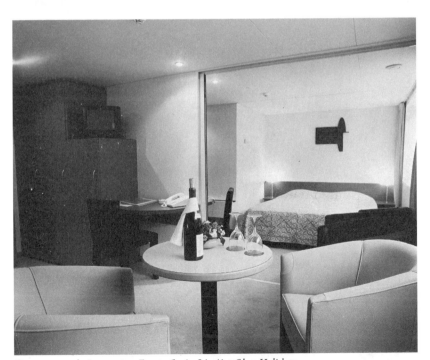

Guest accommodation, courtesy Europe Cruise Line/1st Class Holidays

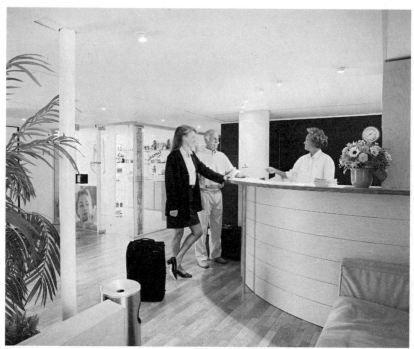

Reception area, courtesy Europe Cruise Line/1st Class Holidays

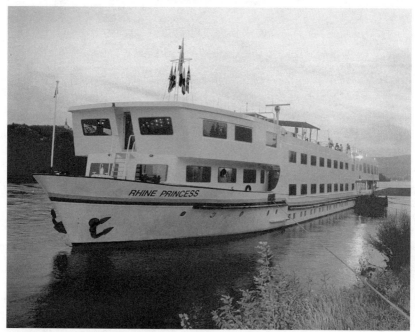

Courtesy Europe Cruise Line/1st Class Holidays

Dinner

Salad of smoked deerham and flageolet

***

Fillet of sole and gamba's with chinese vegetables

***

Spoom

***

Tournedos Rossini with almond potatoes and butter-beans

***

Raisins in brandy ice-cream with burned eggwhite

Courtesy Europe Cruise Line/1st Class Holidays

EUROPEAN WATERWAYS
140 E. 56th Street
New York, New York 10022
Tel. 800/217-4447

ACTIEF: entered service 1980; reconstructed 1989; 100' x 16.5'; 11-passenger capacity; 6 cabins; British officers and crew; cruises on River Thames, Great Britain.

ANJODI: refurbished 1997; 98'; 8-passenger capacity; 4 cabins; British and French officers and crew; cruises on canals in south of France.

BONA SPES: 75'; 10-passenger capacity; 5 cabins; British and Irish officers and crew; cruises upper Shannon in Ireland.

L'ART DE VIVRE: 100'; 8-passenger capacity; 4 cabins; French and English officers and crew; cruises in Burgundy and Chablis.

L'IMPRESSIONNISTE: entered service 1991; 128'; 12-passenger capacity; 6 cabins; British and French officers and crew; cruises in Burgundy and Provence.

LA JOIE DE VIVRE: entered service 1991; 128'; 10-passenger capacity; 5 cabins (a/c); British and French captain and crew; cruises in upper Loire.

LA REINE PEDAQUE: 128'; 12-passenger capacity; 6 cabins (a/c); British and French officers and crew; cruises in Burgundy.

LE BELLE EPOQUE: entered service 1995; 126'; 12-passenger capacity; 6 cabins (a/c); British and French officers and crew; cruises in Burgundy and Provence.

LE BON VIVANT: 126'; 8-passenger capacity; 4 cabins (a/c); British and French officers and crew; cruises in lower Burgundy.

NIAGRA: 100'; 6-passenger capacity; 3 cabins (a/c); British and French officers and crew; cruises in Burgundy.

NYMPHEA: refitted in 1996; 80'; 6-passenger capacity; 3 cabins; British and French officers and crew; cruises in Loire Valley.

ROSA: refitted in 1994; 100'; 8-passenger capacity; 4 cabins; British and French officers and crew; cruises in Armagnoc and southwest France.

European Waterways has owned and represented luxury hotel barges since 1974. All of the vessels they represent have been recently built or completely refurbished throughout with wood paneling, carpeting, and a blend of antique and traditional decor. All have central heating and some are fully air-conditioned.

With a capacity ranging from six to twelve passengers, each vessel has a combination salon, bar, and dining area with large windows for viewing the countryside and a partially-covered or umbrella-tabled sundeck lined with brightly colored flowers.

Accommodations range from small twin- and double-bedded staterooms to modest-size suites with sitting areas. All have small windows, closets, and drawers, with tiled bathrooms that include shower and sink, and some with tubs.

Each barge carries a fleet of bicycles for passengers to use along the waterway paths, as well as a library of books, games, and stereo tapes.

Dining is the highlight of each cruise, where highly trained chefs skilled in the tradition of French cuisine prepare epicurean meals for guests, with emphasis on the fabulous local cheeses, vintage wines, and fresh produce.

Included in the price that ranges from $1,390 to $3,990 are accommodations, all meals with wines, champagne welcome, open bar, sightseeing, and other facilities. Air fare and hot-air ballooning is not included.

During the day, passengers are offered tours to points of interest along the route, which could include medieval villages, museums, magnificent chateaux, abbeys, wine cellars, and open markets. Paths along the canals and waterways offer opportunities for long walks, jogging, and bicycle excursions.

Strong Points:

An intimate, tranquil cruise/barge experience with fine dining and excellent, friendly service.

FRENCH COUNTRY WATERWAYS, LTD.

P.O. Box 2195

Duxbury, Massachusetts 02331

(800) 222-1236

(781) 934-9048 FAX

ESPRIT: converted to hotel barge 1986; refurbished 1998; 280 G.R.T.; 128'; 18-passenger capacity; 9 staterooms; French and English crew; six-night cruises in Côte d'Or region of Burgundy between Dijon and St. Leger-Sur-Dheune.

HORIZON II: converted to barge hotel 1983/1984; refurbished 1999; 190 G.R.T.; 128'; 12-passenger capacity; 6 staterooms; French and English crew; six-night cruises in historic Burgundy between Venarey-les-Laumes and Tonnerre.

LIBERTE: converted to barge hotel 1992; refurbished 1999; 90 G.R.T.; 100'; 8-passenger capacity; 4 staterooms; French and English crew; six-night cruises in Nivernais region of Burgundy between Auxerre and Clamecy.

NENUPHAR: converted to barge hotel 1979; refurbished 1999; 280 G.R.T.; 128'; 12-passenger capacity; 6 suites; French and English crew; six-night cruises in upper Loire between Chatillon-Sur-Loire and Samois-Sur-Seine.

PRINCESS: built in 1973; refurbished 1998; 280 G.R.T.; 128'; eight-passenger capacity; 4 suites; French and English crew; six-night cruises in Champagne, Alsace-Lorraine, and Moselle Valley.
(Medical Facilities: Captains are certified in CPR and take a first-aid course. Motor vehicles travel with barge.)

Owned and managed by Jim and Pat Tyng, French Country Waterways, Ltd., offers barge cruises designed for sophisticated active travelers who wish to explore various charming regions of France in an intimate way. Itineraries vary, but include daily sightseeing excursions to medieval towns and cities, famous churches and chateaux, renowned vineyards with wine tastings, as well as options for hot-air balloon rides. French Country Waterways is unique in that it owns, operates and markets only its own vessels; whereas, the company's competitors do not own most of the barges, but only operate and/or market them.

The exceptionally friendly, well-educated captains and crews are fluent in English and French and admirably succeed in making passengers feel as though they are guests on a private floating home.

The barges, which are also available for individual and charter bookings, are refurbished annually and each has a sun deck, comfortable, homey, main salon that serves as a combination lounge, dining room, fully-stocked bar and library, as well as a fleet of bicycles for passenger-use ashore. The newest addition to the fleet is the eight-passenger *Princess*, which boasts large suites with king-size beds and spacious public areas.

All barges are tastefully furnished, air conditioned throughout, and suites and staterooms have private bathrooms with toilet and showers, vanities, hair dryers, and adequate closet/wardrobe space, as well as various amenities.

All-inclusive cruise prices, ranging from $2,895 to $4,395 per person, include all meals, as well as one meal ashore at a highly rated French restaurant that has received a two- or three-star rating in the Michelin Guide, open bar, estate bottled wines and delicious regional cheeses at lunch and dinner, all tours and excursions, and transfers to and from Paris or another main city. Restaurant visits in 2000 will include Lameloise in Chagny, L'Esperance in Vezelay, La Côte d'Or in Saulieu, Auberge des Templiers in Les Bezard, Le Cerf in Marlenheim, and Boyer's Les Crayers in Reims. (Auberge des Templier and Les Crayers are also two of the resorts included in *Stern's Guide to the Greatest Resorts of the World*.) Dining aboard the barges is exceptional, with excellent cuisine superbly prepared and presented by trained chefs who obtain fresh ingredients daily, and design menus based upon what appears most appealing at the local market.

A French County Waterways barge sojourn is a must for the seasoned cruiser who wishes to complete and enhance his or her cruise experiences and who can appreciate this very special type of cruise vacation.

Strong Points:

The epitome of an intimate, charming and tranquil barge/cruise experience with fine dining and exceptional, friendly service. This is also a good option for families or groups of friends wishing to charter the entire barge.

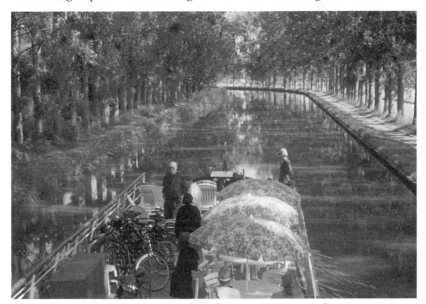

Horizon II *on Burgundy Canal, courtesy of French Country Waterways, Ltd.*

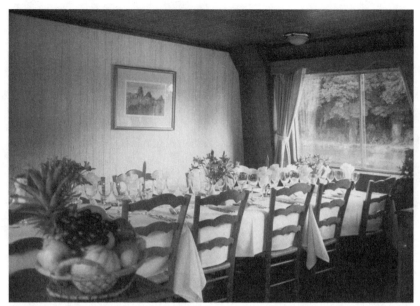

Dining room on Horizon II, *courtesy of French Country Waterways, Ltd.*

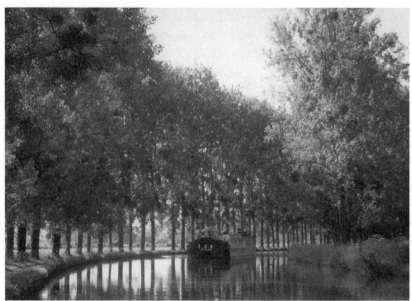

Horizon II *on Burgundy Canal, courtesy of French Country Waterways, Ltd.*

**FRENCH
COUNTRY
WATERWAYS,
LTD.**

Sample Menus from ESPRIT

Stephen Houchin, Chef

Petit Dejeuner (Breakfast)

Buffet service includes fresh fruit and juices, selection of cereals, yogurts, breads and pastries, coffee, tea, and chocolate.

Breads and croissants are brought aboard each morning from the village bakery near the barge's overnight mooring.

Dejeuner (Lunch)

Buffet service includes a variety of fresh salads, such as Salade Nicoise, Pasta with Seafood, Celeriac with Dijonnaise dressing, Tomatoes in Basil Vinaigrette. These are accompanied by a cold roast meat, such as filet of beef or roasted quail, and a hot tarte du jour, such as Tarte Provencal. A selection of three French cheeses and fresh fruit is presented to finish the meal.

Lunch is accompanied by a white and a red wine selected by the Captain.

Canal Cruises

Diner (Dinner)

Four course, candlelit meal consisting of an appetizer, main course, cheese course and dessert. The Captain selects appropriate white and red wines to accompany the meal. Sample menu:

Souffle de Fromage de Chevre,
Salade a l'huile de noix
(Rounds of baked goat cheese on a bed
of greens dressed with walnut oil)

Filet de Canard roti aux Olives
(Roasted duck breast with olives)

Choufleur et Marrons entier
(Cauliflower and chestnuts)
Pommes Gallete
(Oven browned, slivered potatoes)

Plateau des Fromages et Salade
(Selection of French cheeses and green salad)

Mousse Pralinee et l'Armagnac, Sauce Caramel
(Praline mousse flavored with Armagnac, caramel sauce)

Vin Blanc	Vin Rouge
Chablis Bougros,	Chassagne-Montrachet,
Grand Cru 1990	1er Cru 1989

P.O. Box 2195
Duxbury,
Massachusetts,
02331, U.S.A.

800-222-1236
(Nationwide)
617-934-2454
(In Massachusetts)

Fax 617-934-9048

Courtesy French Country Waterways, Ltd.

HAPAG-LLOYD

Europa: c/o Euro-Lloyd Tours
1640 Hempsted Turnpike
East Meadow, New York 11554
(800) 334-2724
(516) 794-1253
(516) 228-8258 FAX

Bremen and Hanseatic: c/o Radisson Seven Seas Cruises
600 Corporate Drive, Suite 410
Ft. Lauderdale, Florida 33334
(800) 333-3333
(305) 772-3763 FAX

ASTRA II: (formerly *Golden Odyssey*); entered service 1974; 10,563 G.R.T.; 426' x 63', 489-passenger capacity; 227 cabins; German officers and crew; various itineraries around Europe.

(Medical Facilities: No information furnished by cruise line.)

BREMEN: (formerly *Frontier Spirit*); entered service 1990; 6,752 G.R.T.; 336' x 56'; 164-passenger capacity; 82 cabins; European officers and crew; itineraries include ports around the world.

(Medical Facilities: No information furnished by the cruise line.)

M.S. *COLUMBUS:* entered service 1997; 14,903 G.R.T.; 472' x 70'; 418-passenger capacity; 205 cabins; German officers and crew; cruises in Great Lakes of U.S. and itineraries to be announced.

M.S. *EUROPA:* entered service 1999; 28,600 G.R.T.; 198 meters x 24 meters; 408-passenger capacity; 204 staterooms; German officers and crew; cruises to various locations around the world.

HANSEATIC: (See Radisson Seven Seas)

In 1970, Hapag-America and North German Lloyd lines merged. Both lines date back to the nineteenth century and have played a role in the development of cruising during the twentieth century. The M.S. *Europa* is the sixth ship of the original line to receive the same name. The fifth *Europa* was sold in 1998 and the present vessel entered service in 1999. In 1992, the U.S. marketing agent changed the company name to Euro-Lloyd Tours. The *Europa* is largely sold to the German market, with German being the official language on board and the Deutschmark the official currency.

Entering service in 1999, the new *Europa* includes many of the technological advances and creature comforts that appear in ships built in the late nineties. Atop ship on Deck 10 are 12 penthouse suites with 14 veranda suites below on Deck 9. The remaining staterooms and suites, are located on Decks 5, 6, and 7. All in all, 156 of the 204 accommodations have verandas, reflecting today's demand for this feature. All staterooms are quite large, measuring from 300 to 366 square feet (including verandas), with the two top suites reaching 666 square feet.

Deck 8 is the location of the pool, lido café and bar, several lounges, a cinema, and library. On Deck 7 are the two golf simulators, children's playroom, and vitality center, which includes a beauty salon, steam, sauna, massage solarium, and an exercise room. Deck 4 is the locale of all other public rooms, including the reception area, grand lounge, several other lounges and bars, boutiques and shops, the casino, the main dining room, and Italian and Oriental specialty restaurants.

The ship carries seven Zodiacs and offers itineraries around the world that are sold in segments.

Itineraries generally run from two to three weeks. At different times during the year, the ship offers cruises to the Caribbean, Mexican Riviera, Alaska, Mediterranean, North Sea, Baltic Sea, and South Pacific, as well as around the world.

The former *Frontier Spirit,* built for Explorer Cruising, is now marketed to the North American cruise market by Radisson Seven Seas Cruises and has been renamed the *Bremen.*

The ship has eighty-two, 149-square-foot, outside cabins featuring sitting and bedroom areas, closed-circuit TV, refrigerators, mini-bars, satellite telephone, hair dryers, and bathrobes. The two suites on Deck 7 and the six luxury staterooms on Deck 6 include private verandas.

Public areas and facilities include a library, several lounges, sauna, gym, swimming pool, observation lounge, a single-sitting dining room, bar, beauty parlor, infirmary, card/conference room, and exploration Zodiacs.

Built to cruise where other ships are unable to go, the *Bremen* visits such out-of-the-way destinations as the Antarctic and the deep Amazon and Orinoco rivers in South America, as well as the Red Sea, the Mediterranean, the Far East, and the South Pacific.

Prices vary, and frequently include 50 percent discounts for the second person, as well as early booking discounts.

The line also markets the 10,563-ton *Astra II,* formerly *Golden Odyssey,* and the 14,903-ton *Columbus.* The *Columbus* will be offering late summer and fall cruises in the Great Lakes of the U.S. Prices for these cruises range from $117 per person per night for an inside cabin for four, up to $376 per person per night for a two-berth suite with veranda.

Strong Points:

Europa: Accommodations, service, elegance, and itineraries.

Bremen: Small, luxury, yacht-like cruise ship with comfortable cabins, more public space than other small vessels, and outstanding itineraries.

HOLLAND AMERICA LINE
300 Elliott Avenue West
Seattle, Washington 98119
(800) 426-0327
(206) 281-1970

MAASDAM: entered service 1993; 55,451 G.R.T.; 720' x 101'; 1,266-passenger capacity; 633 cabins; Dutch officers, Indonesian and Filipino crew; cruises in the Caribbean, Panama Canal, European waters, Baltic Sea, Mediterranean, Black Sea, and transatlantic.

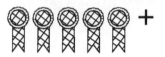

NIEUW AMSTERDAM: entered service 1983; 33,930 G.R.T.; 704' x 88'; 1,214-passenger capacity; 607 cabins; Dutch officers, Indonesian and Filipino crew; cruises to the Caribbean, Panama Canal, and Alaska.

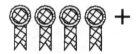

NOORDAM: entered service 1984; 33,930 G.R.T.; 704' x 88'; 1,214-passenger capacity; 607 cabins; Dutch officers, Indonesian and Filipino crew; cruises in the Panama Canal, Caribbean, South America, Europe, and trans-Atlantic.

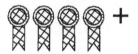

ROTTERDAM: entered service 1997; 59,652 G.R.T.; 722' x 103.5'; 1,316-passenger capacity (1,668 when every berth is filled); 659 cabins; Dutch officers, Indonesian and Filipino crew; cruises to Caribbean, Europe, Mediterranean, Baltic Sea, Panama Canal, Africa, South America, transatlantic, and around the world.

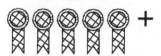

RYNDAM: entered service 1994; 55,451 G.R.T.; 720' x 101'; 1,266-passenger capacity; 633 cabins; Dutch officers, Indonesian and Filipino crew; cruises to Alaska and in Caribbean and Panama Canal.

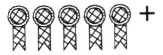

STATENDAM: entered service 1993; 55,451 G.R.T.; 720' x 101'; 1,266-passenger capacity; 633 cabins; Dutch officers, Indonesian and Filipino crew; cruises in Caribbean, Hawaii, Mexico, and Alaska.

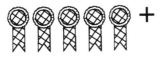

VEENDAM: entered service 1996; 55,451 G.R.T.; 722' x 103.5'; 1,266-passenger capacity; 633 cabins; British and Dutch officers, Indonesian and Filipino crew; cruises in Caribbean, Panama Canal, and Alaska.

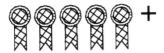

VOLENDAM: entered service 1999; 63,000 G.R.T.; 722' x 103.5'; 1,440-passenger capacity; 720 cabins; Dutch officers, Filipino and Indonesian crew; cruises to Caribbean, Panama Canal, and Alaska.

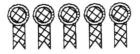

WESTERDAM: (formerly *Homeric*); entered service 1986; lengthened 1990; 53,872 G.R.T.; 798' x 95'; 1,494-passenger capacity; 747 cabins; Dutch officers, Indonesian and Filipino crew; cruises in the Caribbean, Panama Canal, and Alaska.

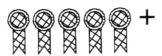

ZAANDAM: entered service 2000; 63,000 G.R.T.; 722' x 103.5'; 1,440-passenger capacity; 720 cabins; Dutch officers, Indonesian and Filipino crew; cruises in the Caribbean, Eastern Canada, and New England.

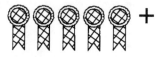 +

(Medical Facilities: P-1; EM, CLS, MS; N-3; CM; PD; BC (not full blood count); EKG; TC; PO; EPC; OX; WC; ICU; X; M; LJ; wheelchair accessible cabins *Rotterdam*-23, others 4 to 6.)

The Dutch owners started the Netherlands-America Steamship Company in 1872, and its first ocean liner, the original *Rotterdam,* made its maiden voyage to New York in 1873. In 1896, the company became known as Holland America Line. Westours, Incorporated, based in Seattle, Washington, had been selling Alaskan tours since 1947 and frequently leased Holland America ships. In 1974, Holland America Line/Westours became a subsidiary of the Dutch parent company. In 1989 the line was purchased by Carnival Corporation. Holland America owns Windstar Cruises but operates it as a separate division.

All of the ships today have Dutch or British officers holding the top jobs, with a mixed crew of Indonesians and Filipinos holding the positions of waiters, wine stewards, bartenders, and cabin attendants. Most cruisers find the crew attentive and anxious to please. Holland America Line has always featured a "tipping not required" policy; however, in practice many cruisers elect to tip their waiters and cabin stewards.

The *Rotterdam V,* built in the late fifties, was retired from service in 1997 and subsequently sold to Premier Cruise Line.

The sister ships, *Nieuw Amsterdam* and *Noordam,* were two of the more conveniently laid out, attractively designed, and tastefully furbished vessels built in the eighties. Historic art treasures, antique glassware, navigation instruments, and mosaics embellished the elegant fabrics and furnishings. However, these ships have not received major refurbishing since they entered service and though well-maintained, are no longer as elegant as the Holland America ships built in the nineties.

Each ship has 605 cabins, with 411 located outside and 194 inside. On the *Nieuw Amsterdam,* 121 of the cabins have king- or queen-size beds, as do 175 of the cabins on the *Noordam.* All staterooms have multichannel piped-in music, closed-circuit TVs, telephones, and well-appointed furniture and fabrics. Twenty suites are located in a private wing on Navigation Deck.

The least expensive cabins cost about $200 per person per day. Cabins average about $250, and suites go for more than $450. Third and fourth persons sharing a room pay only $100 per day. Although most fares on all Holland America ships do not include air travel, the line will arrange air at favorable rates.

The gigantic main dining room seats 700 at each of two sittings and offers ocean view windows. Full breakfasts, lunches, and midnight snacks are served buffet style at the large Lido restaurant for those wishing a more casual atmosphere. Hamburgers, hot dogs, and tacos are available at the Terrace Grill by the pool.

The *Westerdam* was built by Home Lines as the *Homeric* in 1986 and was one of the most attractively furnished ships in service at the time. She was purchased by Holland America in 1988 and given a $85-million expansion in 1989, increasing her tonnage to 53,872, her length from 671 feet to 798 feet, and her passenger capacity from 1,000 to 1,494. In addition to expanding the passenger facilities, a new 800-seat show lounge was added, as well as an expanded Lido buffet restaurant, a new sports deck and sunbathing area, and a new lounge, bar, and library. Accommodations in all of the deluxe and large outside cabin categories tend to be quite spacious, with generous sitting areas. There are nuances in size and decor as you move up from one price category to the next. During recent years, many of the cabins have been equipped with twin beds convertible to queen size; however cabins on the *Westerdam,* as on *Nieuw Amsterdam* and *Noordam,* do not have refrigerators, private safes, hair dryers, or balconies; and not much in the way of renovation or decoration to the standard cabins or public areas has taken place in recent years. All in all, the *Westerdam* is a "happening ship," offering more activities, musical entertainments, and spirit than on the newer vessels. Therefore, it is possibly the best choice for active cruisers under fifty.

On all vessels Holland America offers a full complement of activities and entertainment, including a good program for children known as Club HAL. You can expect movies, numerous live nightclub shows, several orchestras, deck sports, bridge and backgammon tournaments, dance lessons, gambling at the casinos, disco, romantic orchestras, golf lessons, trapshooting, wine tasting, formal teas, arts, crafts, bingo, horse racing, and audience-participation games. The median age on the three ships built in the eighties (especially on shorter cruises) tends to be lower than on the newer vessels, and activities and entertainment are geared to the more active cruiser. Further, the line has a larger budget on longer cruises and the quality of the entertainment and abundance of gourmet food offerings is directly proportional to the length of the cruise, the best being featured on the annual world cruise.

Although Holland America is constantly shifting the cruise grounds of these ships to accommodate the market, the ships generally sail to Alaska, Europe, Transcanal, the Caribbean, and Eastern Canada/New England.

Holland America added four new modern vessels in the mid-nineties. Each of the new ships is approximately 55,451 tons and carries 1,266 passengers in 633 staterooms, three-quarters of which are outside. The first of the new vessels, the *Statendam,* entered service in January 1993; the second, the *Maasdam,* in December 1993; the third, the *Ryndam,* in October 1994; and the fourth, the *Veendam,* in May 1996.

The 149 deluxe cabins and suites are located on Navigation and Verandah decks near the top of the ships and boast floor-to-ceiling windows, private verandas, whirlpool baths and showers, hair dryers, refrigerated mini-bars, VCRs, plush terry-cloth robes, personalized stationery, hors d'oeuvres in the suites, and maximum space and comfort. Most of the remaining accommodations are on the three lower decks and include two lower beds convertible to a queen-size bed, small sitting areas, decent closet space, multichannel music systems, telephones with voice mail, color TVs, private room safes, and hair dryers. Public facilities encompass eight passenger elevators; two outdoor pools; two outdoor, heated whirlpools; an elegant, dual-level dining room with tables adorned with fresh flowers, fine crystal, and Rosenthal china; a comfortable Lido Restaurant with exceptional buffets; a health spa with exercise and cardiovascular machines, sauna and steam rooms, a masseuse, a hair salon, and daily exercise and aerobics classes; a casino; a well-stocked library; card and game rooms; a comfortable movie theater; a large, two-level showroom; and numerous more intimate lounges.

Holland America's newest ship entered service in fall 1997, when the prior *Rotterdam* was retired. Appropriately, the ship was named *Rotterdam VI* (later known simply as *Rotterdam*) and is marketed as the company's new flagship. The vessel was built and designed especially for luxury, European and around-the-world voyages with the capability to sustain speeds up to 25 knots (20 percent faster than today's average cruise ships) to permit more hours in ports of call and shorter sailing time between ports.

At 59,652 tons and accommodating 1,316 passengers, she is the largest vessel in the fleet. She incorporates abundant use of woods and darker colors for a more classic feel; boasts an entire deck of suites with 180-square-foot verandas, including four 1,126-square-foot penthouse suites and thirty-six 565-square-foot suites with special concierge lounge and concierge services; offers an additional 120 deluxe 245-square-foot cabins with verandas, whirlpool bathtubs, refrigerators, VCRs, and other conveniences; includes a special alternative, 90-seat, intimate Italian restaurant that is opulent in decor, a spectacular, two-deck main dining room, and a two-deck show lounge; expensive art; and various other tasteful public areas and lounges as are found on all Holland America Line vessels. The layout of the ship is quite similar to the other vessels built in the nineties. For passengers opting to partake in the "suite life" (on Navigation Deck), the comfort and special amenities parallel those featured on luxury-market cruises.

The line purchased the 2,400-acre Bahamian island of Little San Salvador and developed a $16-million facility, completed in late 1997, naming it Half Moon Cay. In addition to a most enviable two-mile strand of white-sand beach, a snorkel area, and tender dock and sport area (offering kayaks, banana boats, Hobie catamarans, parasailing, Sunfish sailboats, and floating air mattresses), the development includes a shop, a Bahamian straw market, a food pavilion, several bars, numerous lounge chairs with umbrellas, and hiking trails. This is a major port of call for HAL ships with Caribbean itineraries.

In 1999 the *Volendam* and in 2000, the *Zaandam,* two modified sisters to the *Rotterdam* with some new innovations, came on line. The new ships, built by Fincantieri Shipyards in Italy at a price tag of approximately $300 million each, are 63,000 gross tons with passenger capacities of 1,440 each. The all-suite staterooms include 120 deluxe mini-suites with verandas, 385 large outside staterooms, and 133 large inside staterooms. The public areas are similar to those of the *Rotterdam.*

All Holland America Line's ships offer dining alternatives several evenings during each cruise in their Lido Restaurants between 7:00 and 8:30 P.M., with casual open seating, piano music, and tables set with linens, stemware, and flatware.

Strong Points:

Physical layout and decor of the vessels built in the nineties make them among the most attractively furbished ships afloat; activities, facilities, dining, and itineraries make for a solid cruise experience—one of the best in its market category. Higher-priced veranda and penthouse staterooms and suites on the four *"Statendam*-class" ships and on the *Rotterdam, Volendam,* and *Zaandam* are very large and comfortable, affording a superior experience similar to ships competing in the luxury cruise market.

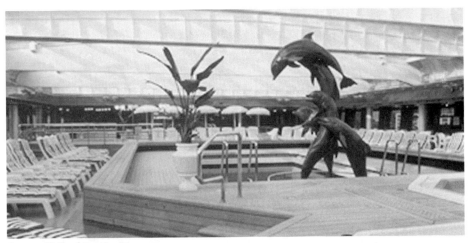

Courtesy Holland America Line

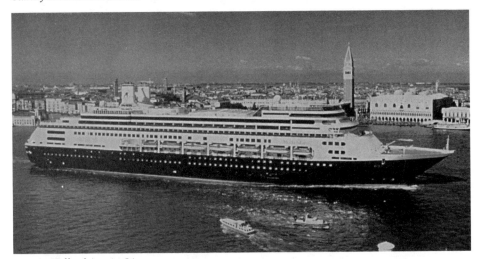

Courtesy Holland America Line

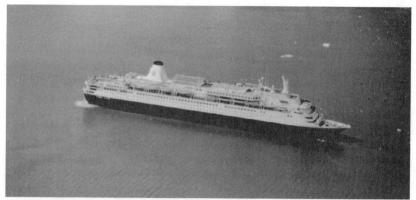

Courtesy Holland America Line

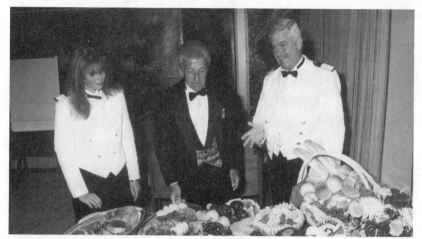

Courtesy Holland America Line

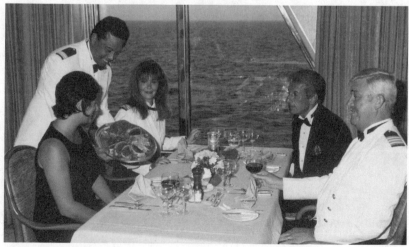

Courtesy Holland America Line

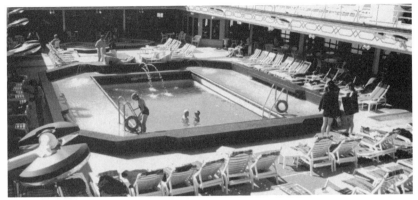

Courtesy Holland America Line

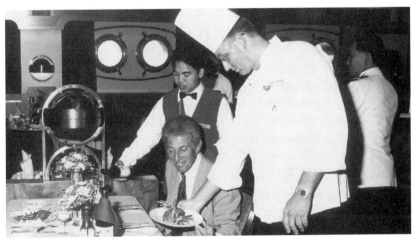

Courtesy Holland America Line

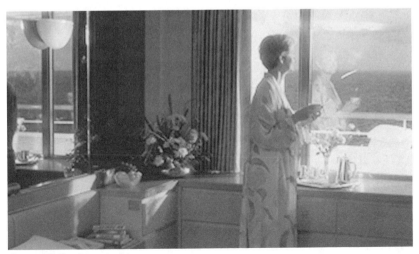

Courtesy Holland America Line

CHEF HOLGER FROHLICH RECOMMENDS

*a four course dinner for your enjoyment with wine
suggestions complementing the menu.*

DUCK RILLETTES WITH TRUFFLE
*this fine duck meat terrine is served with three berry
chutney, piquant red wine pear and kumquat*

THE KITCHEN SALAD
*Romaine lettuce served with garlic croutons, shredded red
cabbage, sliced cucumber and crumbled blue cheese*

FILET OF BEEF "WELLINGTON"
sauce Perigourdine, Marquise potato and pea pods

BAKED ALASKA WITH STRAWBERRY SAUCE

White:
Chardonnay Markham
$34.00/btl
Tonight: $30.60
Chardonnay, Lindeman
$21.00/btl
Tonight: $18.90
Red:
Cabernet Sauvignon,
R. Mondavi Coastal
$28.00/btl
Tonight: $25.20

APPETIZERS

CRUDITE FROM VEGETABLES
roasted bell pepper dip

MIXED MELON PEARLS
marinated with minted cassis syrup and on request with lemon sherbet

SMOKED TUNA
served with whole grain Wasabi vinaigrette

SHRIMP PLATTER
served with grapefruit sections and all American cocktail sauce

DUCK RILLETTES WITH TRUFFLE
*this fine duck meat terrine is served with three berry chutney, piquant
red wine pear and kumquat*

ITALIAN STYLE HAZELNUT CRUSTED CHICKEN FINGERS
honey mustard dressing

SOUPS

LOBSTER BISQUE WITH AGED BRANDY
topped with truffled cream

PETITE MARMITE
Consommé garnished with root vegetables, lean meat and chicken

CHILLED PAPAYA SOUP WITH TAPIOCA
served with watermelon sherbet

SALADS

STATENDAM SALAD
*escarole and iceberg served with jicamas,
cucumber and baby corn topped with balsamic olive oil vinaigrette*

THE KITCHEN SALAD
*Romaine lettuce served with garlic croutons,
shredded red cabbage, sliced cucumber and crumbled blue cheese*

Maitre d' Hotel: Ibnu Burhanuddin

ENTREES

BROILED LOBSTER TAIL WITH DRAWN BUTTER
honey glazed carrots, asparagus and tomato basil rice

FILET OF BEEF "WELLINGTON"
sauce Perigourdine, Marquise potato, peapods and grilled tomato

PANFRIED MAHI MAHI WITH MANGO RELISH
saffron risotto, baby carrots and chayote gratin

PASTA

GORGONZOLA AND WALNUT RAVIOLI
served with horseradish dill beurre blanc, crab meat, bay shrimps
and sprinkled with salmon, olives and broccoli
Also available as appetizer portion.

CORN KERNEL FRITTERS WITH SAUTÉED MUSHROOMS (VEGETARIAN)
served in a pool of tomato sauce
complemented with carrot julienne with mint and cauliflower florets

TODAYS SPA CUISINE

GRILLED CHICKEN BREAST
with fine herb sauce, cucumber, macaroni pasta, peapods,
yellow tear drop tomatoes, cucumber and tomato sauce

Baked potato with sour cream, chives and fresh bacon bits
will be served with any entrée upon your request.
Most dishes can be served without sauce.

Traditional favorite dressings available, plus todays special fat free
and low calorie dressings.

Executive Chef : Holger Frohlich

Courtesy Holland America Line

The day at a glance

8:00 am	The Ryndam docks at Bridgetown, Barbados.
8:00 am	♥ Walk-a-mile with our Fitness Advisor .... Lower Prom. Deck aft
8:00 am - 6:00 pm	Swimming Pools are open .... Lido & Navigation Deck aft
8:00 am - 9:30 am	Port Lecturer Elizabeth is available for questions .... Gangway
9:00 am	♥ Aerobic Exercises with our Fitness Advisor .... Ocean Spa
9:00 am	Man From Peking Quiz is available .... Reading Room
9:00 am - 5:00 pm	Books, Playing Cards and indoor games are available . Reading Room
10:00 am - 10:30 am	Morning Coffee is served .... Explorers Lounge
10:00 am - 6:00 pm	Jacuzzis are open .... Lido Deck
10:15 am	♥ Mixed Quoits Tournament with the Cruise Staff .... Sports Deck
10:30 am - 11:00 am	Lemonade is available .... Outside Decks
11:00 am	Scrabble Get-Together .... Explorers Lounge
11:30 am	♥ Ping Pong Get-Together .... Lower Promenade Deck forward
12:00 nn - 2:00 pm	The Wine Desk is open for dinner wine selection By the Ocean Bar
12:30 pm - 1:30 pm	Live Music with the Bridgetown Steel Band .... Lido Deck
2:15 pm	Informal Card Get-Together .... Card Room
2:45 pm	♥ Shuffleboard anyone? Meet the Cruise Staff .... Sports Deck
3:00 pm	♥ Learn the Art of Massage - bring a partner .... Ocean Spa
3:30 pm - 4:00 pm	Iced Tea is available .... Outside Decks
3:30 pm	Afternoon Tea is served .... Explorers Lounge
3:45 pm	♥ Great Wall of China Putting Challenge .... Ocean Bar
4:00 pm - 4:30 pm	♥ Walk-a-mile with our Fitness Advisor .... Lower Prom. Deck aft
4:30 pm	ALL ABOARD, the gangway is raised.
4:30 pm	Friends of Bill W. meet .... Lido Restaurant (portside)
4:30 pm	SNOWBALL CASH BINGO. The snowball stands at $1,386.00 ... . Vermeer Lounge
4:30 pm - 5:30 pm	Port Lecturer Elizabeth is available for questions .... Java Cafe
4:30 pm - 5:30 pm	Sailaway Music .... Navigation Deck
5:00 pm	The Ryndam sails for Guadeloupe (212 miles).
5:00 pm - 6:00 pm	Cocktail Hour .... Crow's Nest and Ocean Bar
7:00 pm & 11:30 pm	Silent Art Auction .... Java Cafe
7:15 pm - 8:15 pm	Cocktail Hour .... Crow's Nest and Ocean Bar
7:45 pm	Newlywed & Not So Newlywed Game Show .... Vermeer Lounge
8:30 pm	Showtime .... Vermeer Lounge
9:00 pm - 11:00 pm	Cigars Under The Stars .... Navigation Deck aft
9:45 pm	Name That Tune .... Piano Bar
10:15 pm	Showtime .... Vermeer Lounge
11:15 pm	Karaoke Time .... Crow's Nest
12:00 mn	D.J. Dance Music by request .... Crow's Nest

Port Capsule

Ship's Agent: Goddards Shipping & Tours Ltd.
Hincks Street
P.O. Box 1283
Bridgetown, Barbados
Tel: (809) 426-9918

Exchange Rate: U.S. $1.00 = 1.98 Barbadian Dollars
CAN $1.00 = 1.52 Barbadian Dollars
(U.S. Dollars are readily accepted in Barbados) Foreign currency obtained ashore cannot be re-exchanged on board.

Towels: We are pleased to provide you with towels for the beach. Please ask your cabin steward and he will provide you with towels.

Beaches: Carlisle Bay, Hilton Hotel & Crane Beach

Taxis: To Downtown $4.00   Hilton Hotel $8.00
Crane Beach $18.00   Harrison Cave $20.00
Fares to all locations are posted outside the terminal building, near the taxi pick-up.

Service Hours

FRONT OFFICE, (Information)
Promenade Deck: Open 24 hours.
FOR MEDICAL EMERGENCY dial 911.
SHORE EXCURSION OFFICE,
Promenade Deck: 4:00 pm-6:00 pm. Last chance to purchase or cancel tours for Guadeloupe.
Express order box available 24 hrs. a day.
CASINO, Upper Promenade Deck:
Slots: 5:30 pm - close.
Gaming Tables: 5:30 pm - close.
OCEAAN BOUTIQUES, Upper Prom. Deck:
6:00 pm - 10:30 pm.
PHOTO SHOP, Promenade Deck:
5:00 pm - 6:00 pm.
♥ **MASSAGE & BEAUTY SALON,**
Lido Deck: 8:00 am - 8:00 pm.
♥ **SAUNA & OCEAN SPA FITNESS**
CENTER, Lido Deck: 7:00 am - 8:00 pm.
ART GALLERY, Java Cafe:
Promenade Deck: 7:00 pm - 11:30 pm.
INFIRMARY (Dial 99),
A Deck port side forward.
Nurse on duty:
8:00 am - 12:00 nn & 2:00 pm - 6:00 pm.
Physician's consulting hours:
8:00 am - 9:00 am & 5:00 pm - 6:00 pm.
A fee is charged for a consultation.
GUEST RELATIONS MANAGER,
Promenade Deck:
8:30 am - 10:30 am & 3:00 pm - 5:00 pm.
INTERNATIONAL HOSPITALITY DESK,
Upper Promenade Deck Foyer:
4:30 pm - 5:00 pm.
JUICE BAR, Fitness Center, Lido Deck:
8:00 am - 11:00 am & 4:30 pm - 7:00 pm.
JAVA COFFEE CAFE, Promenade Deck:
9:00 am - 4:00 pm.

Dining Hours

BREAKFAST
Lido Restaurant
Early Coffee:	6:30 am
Continental Breakfast:	7:00 am - 11:00 am
Breakfast:	7:00 am - 10:00 am
Rotterdam Dining Room:	7:30 am - 9:00 am

LUNCH
Lido Restaurant
DUTCH LUNCH:	11:30 am - 2:00 pm

Lido Poolside:
Taco and Pasta Bar:	11:30 am - 2:30 pm
Hamburgers & Hot Dogs:	11:30 am - 5:00 pm
Rotterdam Dining Room:	Closed

DINNER
Rotterdam Dining Room
First Sitting	6:00 pm
Second Sitting	8:15 pm

ENGLISH LATE NIGHT SNACK
Lido Restaurant: 11:30 pm - 12:30 am

ICE CREAM PARLOR
Lido Restaurant
	11:30 am - 2:30 pm
	4:00 pm - 5:00 pm
	11:30 pm - 12:30 am

Coffee and Tea are available 24 hours in the Lido Restaurant.

Courtesy Holland America Line

K D RIVER CRUISES OF EUROPE
(formerly K D German Rhine Line)

USA—2500 Westchester Avenue   EUROPE—1 Frankenwerft

Purchase, New York 10577   50667 Cologne

(914) 696-3600   Germany (0221) 2088288

(800) 346-6525—Eastern U.S.

(800) 858-8587—Western U.S.

MS *AUSTRIA:* entered service 1971; 341' x 38'; 184-passenger capacity; 92 cabins; 4 decks; European officers and crew; Danube River cruises.

MS *BRITANNIA:* entered service 1969; refurbished 1991; 361' x 38'; 184-passenger capacity; 90 cabins, 2 suites; 4 decks; European officers and crew; Rhine River cruises.

MS *CLARA SCHUMANN:* entered service 1991; 312' x 36'; 124-passenger capacity; 62 cabins; 3 decks; German officers, European officers and crew; Elbe River cruises.

MS *DEUTSCHLAND:* entered service 1971; refurbished 1990; 1,180 G.R.T.; 361' x 38'; 184-passenger capacity; 90 cabins, 2 suites; 4 decks; European officers and crew; Rhine River cruises.

MS *HEINRICH HEINE:* entered service 1991; 104-passenger capacity; 51 cabins, 1 suite; 3 decks; European officers and crew; Danube River cruises.

MS *HELVETIA:* entered service 1962; refurbished 1994; 305' x 38'; 140-passenger capacity; 72 cabins; 4 decks; European officers and crew; Rhine and Moselle River cruises.

MS *ITALIA:* entered service 1971; 341' x 385'; 184-passenger capacity; 92 cabins; 4 decks; European officers and crew; Rhine and Moselle River cruises.

MS *THEODOR FONTANE:* entered service 1991; 312' x 36'; 120-passenger capacity; 63 cabins; 3 decks; European officers and crew; Saar, Moselle, Rhine, Main, or Neckar River cruises.

MS *WILHELM TELL:* entered service 1987; 311' x 34.5'; 100-passenger capacity; 52 cabins; European officers and crew; Danube River cruises.
(Medical Facilities: Information not provided.)

The predecessor of the present cruise line was formed back in 1826 and made up of a number of shareholders from Cologne (Köln). It operated passenger ships down the Rhine River between Basel and Rotterdam. By the middle of the nineteenth century, the emphasis was shifted to passenger excursion traffic from one city to another along the river. The original Köln Company subsequently merged with another corporation from Düsseldorf and became known as Köln Düsseldorfer, or K D German Rhine Line.

The first cruise boat with cabins was launched in 1960 and was soon followed by seven others. Four ships have been discontinued, and four new ships were built for cruising on the Elbe and Danube rivers, bringing the present fleet to nine. Today the line transports more than 1,400,000 passengers each year on day boats along the river, and tens of thousands more on cruises. K D also markets the cruises on the Seine and Rhône of French Cruise Lines (see separate section).

The line offers more than 500 cruises between April and October on their nine cruise vessels. Cruises on the *Deutschland* are represented and priced as "Exclusiv" cruises; the *Austria, Italia,* and *Britannia* and other ships offer somewhat lower priced and more informal cruises. Although the brochures recommend jackets and ties at dinner, the dress was casual during our most recent cruise on the Italia. On "Exclusiv" cruises, the dining-room service seemed better able to handle all the guests. Overall, passengers received more special treatment. On the other boats, lunch and dinner offerings are limited. Prices for liquors, wines, and soft drinks are quite high.

There are four passenger decks on each ship other than the *Clara Schumann, Heinrich Heine,* and *Theodor Fontane,* which only have three. The two lower decks contain all the double, outside cabins. The smallest of the boats, the *Wilhelm Tell,* has fifty cabins, and the two largest, the *Britannia* and *Deutschland,* each have ninety-two, including two large suites. Most of the cabins have two single beds, one of which converts to a sofa during the day (the other folding flat to the wall), an armchair, a table, a mirror, a shelf for knickknacks, a telephone, radio, hair dryer, an electrical outlet for hair dryers (you will need an adapter and converter to 220 volts), two small closets, a wash basin and medicine cabinet, a small toilet and shower compartment, a large picture window on the top passenger decks, and two smaller windows on the lower decks looking out at the passing scenery. There are a few cabins on each boat that contain bunk beds.

Overall, the space, beds, and bathrooms are much smaller than you will find in a standard cabin on most oceangoing cruise ships; however, they are ample and utilitarian. The friendly, European cabin stewardesses will take care of your laundry and other requests while keeping your cabin spotless. The purser's office is open all day and early evenings, and the officers and social host or hostess will coordinate your tours and provide all the information you will need.

The public areas are located on the Promenade Deck above the cabins, and they are very similar in shape and decor on all the boats. The main room is an observation lounge with comfortable chairs, couches, and tables. On the larger vessels, it is large enough to accommodate all the passengers for special programs, slide presentations, and evening dancing and entertainment. On smaller vessels, the space is very tight.

There is a cozy bar with several tables for cocktails, and a small reading room with newspapers and magazines.

The dining room is bright and cheery and, like every room on Promenade Deck, has floor-to-ceiling observation windows to assure passengers that they will not miss any scenery, irrespective of where they are sitting or what they may be doing. The purser/information office and a small souvenir shop are located on the Second Deck, and on seven of the boats there is a sauna on the Third Deck.

On top of the boat is outdoor deck space with areas to sun, sit, and view the sights. There are small, not very attractive, heated outdoor swimming pools on the *Deutschland* and the *Britannia,* and the *Heinrich Heine* has an indoor pool.

In the dining room, meals on Exclusiv cruises are efficiently served in one sitting by multilingual European waiters. German and Swiss chefs prepare diverse Continental dishes, and special requests usually can be arranged through the maître d'. The rather expensive wine list includes vintages from Germany, Switzerland, France, and Italy. As pointed out earlier, the dining experience varies considerably, and if gourmet-quality food and prompt service are an important factor, you will prefer the *Deutschland.* Like everywhere, you get what you pay for.

Most passengers take a K D cruise to relax, enjoy the scenic rivers, and visit the charming ports. Most Rhine River cruises hit four countries and are generally four nights and five days downstream from Basel to Amsterdam, and five nights and six days upstream from Amsterdam to Basel. Other river itineraries include two-night/three-day cruises from Cologne to Frankfurt, three-night/four-day cruises from Frankfurt to Trier, two-night/three-day cruises from Trier to Cologne, and various itineraries on the Elbe River between Hamburg and Prague and on the Danube between Nuremberg or Regensburg and Budapest. There are several special cruises offered, with both shorter and longer itineraries.

Embarkation is after 7:00 in the evening, with the ships departing early the following day. Although the itineraries vary, a sample Rhine itinerary would commence with embarkation in Basel on the first evening, followed by a gourmet buffet dinner, including patés, smoked salmon, seafood, cold meats, fresh cheeses, a few warm dishes, and pastries.

The following day the boat will arrive in Strasbourg, France, about 3:00 P.M., after passing through nine massive locks and offering a morning captain's welcome party, complete with champagne. Passengers can take the bus tour of the city, visiting historic monuments, the famous cathedral with its adjoining cafés and shops, or explore the city on their own.

On the second day, the boat disembarks in Speyer, and passengers may take a bus trip to the beautiful town of Heidelberg. Here, in addition to the old university, there are lovely old homes and buildings on hills along the Neckar River and the famous castle that houses the largest wine cask in the world. Passengers pick up the boat again in Gernsheim, from which point it continues on to Koblenz, arriving at 7:00 P.M. for an overnight stay.

The afternoon is spent cruising through the most picturesque portion of the river, where it narrows, passing a succession of medieval castles, the famous Lorelei Rock, and at Koblenz, the entrance to the Moselle. The next day the ship stops in the morning at Konigswinter and at 2:30 P.M., pulls into Cologne, where passengers can walk around the town and visit the magnificent Gothic cathedral. By 8:00 P.M., the boat docks for the night at the metropolitan city of Düsseldorf, permitting passengers to explore the colorful old town section of shops, beer gardens, and restaurants.

The final day, the boat sails to Amsterdam, where passengers disembark.

On the picturesque three-night/four-day cruise from Frankfurt to Trier, passengers embark after 7:00 P.M. and are offered a buffet dinner and an evening to stroll through Frankfurt. The next morning, the ship departs Frankfurt at 5:00 A.M. and arrives in Rudesheim at 9:45 A.M., docking until 11:45. After lunch, the ship cruises past the famous Lorelei Rock and visits Koblenz from 3:00 P.M. until 5:30 P.M. Departing Koblenz, she enters the Moselle and docks for the evening at Alken. On the following day, the ship visits the typical Moselle village of Cochem from 9:45 A.M. until 11:45 A.M. Cochem is the center of tourism on the Moselle, and has many shops, restaurants, guesthouses, and wine bars. The boat docks for the night by 7:30 P.M. at the most charming village on the Moselle, the fairy-tale land of Bernkastel-Kues, home of the world-famous Bernkastel Doktor vineyards and an excellent place to take leisurely strolls down cobblestone streets; enjoy a beer, a glass of wine, or meal at a charming old inn; or just breathe in the charm and beauty of this anachronism in the modern world.

The last day, the boat sails on to the ancient Roman city of Trier, the final destination, where you can take a bus tour to see the famous Porta Nigra (Black Gate), the imperial thermal baths, the amphitheater, and Roman basilica before disembarking.

The Elbe River cruises vary from four to seven nights and may visit such ports as Hamburg, Wittenberg, Magdeburg, Torgau, Meissen, Dresden, Bad Schandau, and Prague. Danube cruises of seven nights call at ports such as Regensburg, Passau, Linz, Melk, Durnstein, and Bratislava.

When the German mark was selling for 1.6 marks to one U.S. dollar, the fares on most cruises varied from $150 to $300 per person per night. Exclusiv cruises started at $380 per person for a cabin with twin beds on the lower deck and went as high as $1,140 for twin beds on the higher deck and $1,710 for a suite.

K D and its agents also market the *Arlene* and *Normandie,* operated by Aqua Viva Cruise Lines.

Strong Points:

This is a delightful, relaxing, and relatively inexpensive way to see this part of the world, as well as a good opportunity for Americans to meet and mingle with Europeans in intimate surroundings. On Exclusiv-class cruises, the food and service are excellent and on the other boats quite good; however, you will not find the same entertainment, activities, creature comforts, or dedication to please the passengers as exists on most oceangoing vessels.

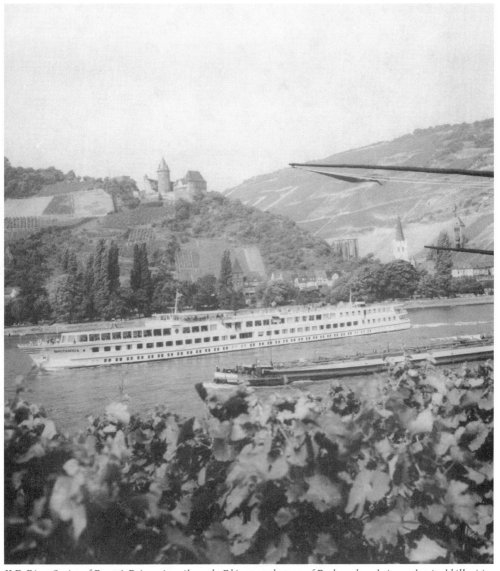

K D River Cruises of Europe's Britannia *sails on the Rhine past the town of Bacharach and vineyard-striped hills rising from the river. Above the town is Burg Stahleck, one of the most famous medieval castles on the Rhine; in the right foreground, the flagpoles of an ancient tollhouse. Courtesy K D River Cruises of Europe.*

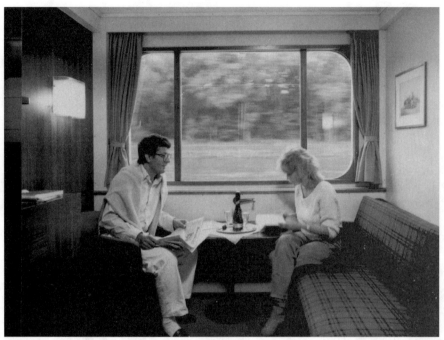

Courtesy K D River Cruises of Europe

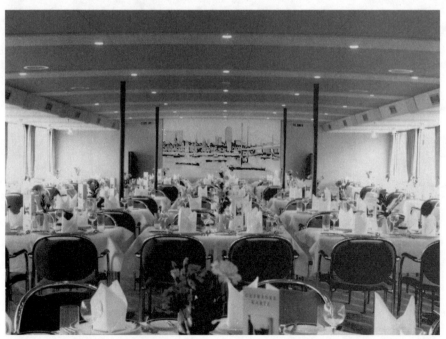

Courtesy K D River Cruises of Europe

Dinner

Melon cocktail
marinated with Port

***

Consommé
with vegetables

***

Salads in season
with a choice of dressings

***

Piccata of turkey "Milano style"
Tomato sauce
Home-made potato gnocchi
Paprika
or
Carved fillet of pork
Noodles
Fresh mushrooms
in cream sauce

***

Assorted cheese from the buffet

***

Cheesecake
with mandarins
or
Maracuja-orange cream

***

Coffee/Tea

If you have other wishes,
please ask the chief steward

BASLE – STRASBOURG

5.30 a.m.	**Departure from Basle,** Elsässer Rheinweg landing stage
7.30 a.m. to 9.30 a.m.	"à la carte" **breakfast** in the restaurant
9.00 a.m. to 11.00 a.m.	Which excursions would you like to go on today and tomorrow? Bookings can now be made at the **purser's office** for the following tours: ✱ a sight-seeing tour of Strasbourg today ✱ excursion to Heidelberg tomorrow
11.00 a.m.	You are invited by the captain to attend a **welcoming reception** in the observation lounge.
12.30 p.m.	**Lunch**
3.00 p.m. (approx.)	**Arrival in Strasbourg,** Gare Fluviale landing stage, Quai des Belges
3.00 p.m. to 6.30 p.m.	**Sight-seeing tour of Strasbourg** This extensive sight-seeing tour gives you a good insight into the fascinating historical monuments and other inter-esting aspects of this ancient Alsace city. The tour also includes a visit to Strasbourg's famous Gothic minster. Cost: DM 29.00.
4.00 p.m.	**Afternoon tea** in the observation lounge
7.00 p.m.	**Dinner**
9.00 p.m.	The day ends with a light-hearted **dance evening** on board ship. During the evening there will also be performances by local folk dancers.

STRASBOURG – BOPPARD

2.00 a.m.	**Departure from Strasbourg,** Gare Fluviale landing stage, Quai des Belges
7.30 a.m. to 9.30 a.m.	**Breakfast** in the restaurant
8.30 a.m.	The ship will dock briefly in **Speyer** to allow those passengers going on the excursion to Heidelberg to disembark.
8.30 a.m. to 12.15 p.m.	**Excursion to Heidelberg** The coach excursion to Heidelberg, a romantic university town which is rich in tradition, will last about three and a half hours. A sight-seeing tour of the city will be followed by a visit to the palace. In its cellar vault you will see the biggest wine cask in the world (221,726 litres). The palace terrace offers a magnificent panoramic view of Heidelberg. Cost: DM 38.00.
12.15 p.m.	The ship will dock briefly in **Gernsheim** to collect those passengers returning from the excursion to Heidelberg.
12.30 p.m.	**Lunch**
3.00 p.m. to 5.00 p.m.	Bookings can now be made at the **purser's office** for sight-seeing tours of Königswinter and Cologne tomorrow. You can also reserve a room at the Hotel Ramada Renaissance or Golden Tulip in Amsterdam.
4.00 p.m.	**Afternoon tea** in the observation lounge
5.00 p.m. (approx.)	The ship passes the **Loreley Rock**
5.30 p.m. (approx.)	**Arrival in Boppard** The "Pearl of the Middle Rhine" has many interesting sights not to mention a unique, 3 km long promenade.
7.00 p.m.	**Dinner**

MEDITERRANEAN SHIPPING CRUISES

420 Fifth Avenue

New York, New York 10018

(800) 666-9333

(212) 764-4800

(212) 764-1486 FAX

MELODY: (formerly *Star/Ship Atlantic* and *Atlantic*); entered service 1982; 36,500 G.R.T.; 672' x 90'; 1,500-passenger capacity; 586 cabins; international officers and crew; Caribbean and Mediterranean cruises.
(Medical Facilities: C-4; P-2; EM, CLS, MS; N-1; CM; PD; EKG; TC; OX; WC; OR; ICU; CCP; LJ.)

MONTEREY: (formerly *Free State Mariner* and *Monterey*); entered service 1952; refurbished 1991; 21,051 G.R.T.; 563' x 80'; 700-passenger capacity; 300 cabins; Italian officers and international crew; Mediterranean and South African cruises.
(Medical Facilities: C-300; P-1; EM, MS; N-1; CM; PD; EKG; TC; OX; WC; OR; M; CCP; LJ.)

RHAPSODY: (formerly *Cunard Princess*); entered service 1977; 17,495 G.R.T.; 536' x 75'; 962-passenger capacity; 425 cabins; Italian officers and international crew; Mediterranean and South American cruises.
(Medical Facilities: C-0; P-1; EM, MS; CM; PD; EKG; OX; WC; OR; M; CCP; LJ.)

SYMPHONY: (formerly *Enrico C* and *Enrico Costa*); entered service 1950; refurbished 1994; 16,500 G.R.T.; 579' x 73'; 664-passenger capacity; 332 cabins; Italian officers and international crew; Mediterranean and South African cruises.
(Medical Facilities: C-0; P-1; EM, MS; N-1; CM; PD; EKG; OX; WC; OR; X; M; CCP; LJ.)

Mediterranean Shipping Cruises is part of the giant Swiss shipping group MSC, which also operates a global fleet of container vessels. In 1990 MSC purchased an Italian cruise company, Starlauro, which owned one vessel, M.V. *Achille Lauro.* Between 1990 and 1995, Starlauro acquired M.V. *Monterey,* M.V. *Symphony,* and M.V. *Rhapsody.* In 1995 the name of the cruise line was changed to Mediterranean Shipping Cruises to take advantage of the reputation associated with the parent company. In 1997 it purchased the *Star/Ship Atlantic* from Premier Cruise Line and renamed her *Melody.*

Overall the line emphasizes Italian hospitality and ambiance and has largely serviced the Italian and European markets in the Mediterranean, South American, and South African cruise areas. During the winter, the line offers cruises in the Caribbean on the *Melody.*

Prices on the various vessels range from $100 per person per night for a minimum inside cabin with upper and lower berths to $325 for an outside suite. Air-sea packages are available.

The largest and most upscale ship in the cruise fleet is the newly acquired *Melody,* formerly *Star/Ship Atlantic* with Premier Cruise Line and *Atlantic* with Home Lines. When she was acquired by Premier, she received a $10-million refurbishment, which included remodeling by interior designer Michael Katzourakis; redesigning of the cabins that increased the ship's capacity from 1,100 to 1,500 by the addition of third, fourth, and fifth berths to the cabins to accommodate families; the addition of children's facilities, including a teen center, children's recreation centers, a video arcade, and an outdoor casual dining area; and enlargement of the main dining room, casino, and lounges.

There are 392 outside cabins, including 60 suites and 167 inside cabins. At the top of the ship on Sun Deck is the jogging track, which looks down to the terrace and pool on Pool Deck. Pool Deck is the location of two swimming pools, one outdoor and one indoor/outdoor, a health/fitness center, massage room, beauty salon, an outdoor café and buffet dining area, a piano lounge, and the ice-cream parlor. The main showroom, casino, photo gallery, video arcade, shops, and lounges, including Teen Center, are on Lounge deck; the theater is on Continental Deck and the Galaxy Dining Room is on Restaurant Deck. The children's Center is on Premier Deck. MSC will be carrying on its own remodeling. The *Melody* will offer Caribbean cruises during the winter and Mediterranean itineraries from Genoa during the warmer months.

The *Symphony,* originally *Provence* of the French Line, was acquired by Costa Cruises in 1964 (renamed *Enrico C* and later *Enrico Costa*), where it offered Mediterranean itineraries to a mostly Italian clientele for more than thirty-two years. Although she has been renovated and redecorated on numerous occasions throughout the years, the ship is an older vessel, does not have stabilizers, and all but the highest-category cabins are quite small. Atop on Sun Deck are a pool and buffet dining area. On Lounge Deck, immediately below, are most public rooms, including several lounges, bars, a cardroom, shops, a beauty center, tour office, and the main swimming pool/outside deck area. The higher-category cabins, disco, and hospital are on Promenade Deck, and the cinema, dining room, and balance of cabins are located on the bottom four decks. The *Symphony* offers cruises from Durban, South Africa, and Genoa, Italy.

The *Rhapsody,* formerly *Cunard Princess,* was acquired by MSC in 1995 and now offers summer itineraries in the Mediterranean and winter cruises in South America. On the top three decks are located the pools, health club, several lounges, theater, restaurant, casino, and upper-category cabins. The remainder of cabins are found on the bottom three decks, along with the purser's office, hairdresser, and shopping arcade. Cabins tend to be on the smaller side but about two-thirds are outside.

The venerable *Monterey* has had many lives, starting as a cargo liner in 1952, sailing for Matson Line from 1956 to 1971, for Pacific Far East from 1971 to 1978, and for Aloha Pacific Cruises from 1988 to 1989. Presently she sails in the Mediterranean during the warmer months and in South America during the winter. This ship is fully stabilized, air conditioned, and public facilities include a pool, restaurant, three lounges, three bars, a small casino, library, cinema, night-club, gym, sauna, hairdresser, boutiques, and a hospital. Those wishing more comfort will want to opt for one of the four suites on Promenade Deck or a deluxe outside twin on Boat Deck.

Strong Points:

Interesting and unusual itineraries, including areas of the world not regularly visited by most other cruise lines; Italian spirit and a chance to mingle with passengers from other countries.

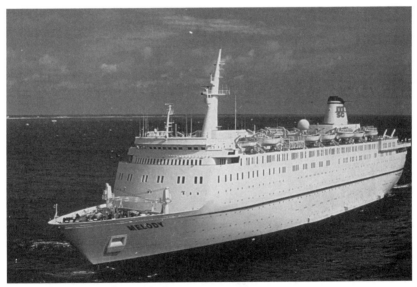

Courtesy Mediterranean Shipping Cruises

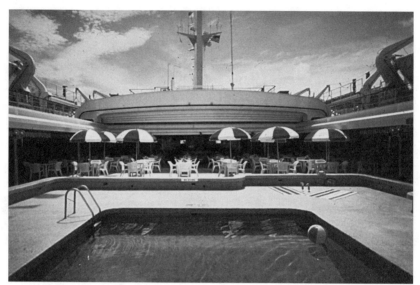

Courtesy Mediterranean Shipping Cruises

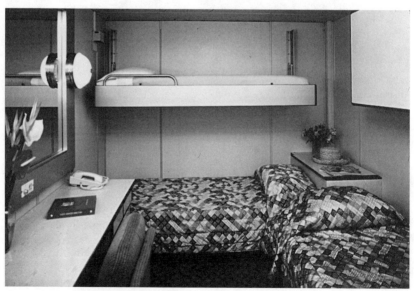

Courtesy Mediterranean Shipping Cruises

CHEF'S SUGGESTION

Cooked " Praga" ham with creamy horseradish sauce and dill pickles

"Linguine alle vongole veraci"

*Deep fried assorted fishes and squids with remoulade sauce
served with french fries*

"La pastiera" cake

GARDEN SIDE
Caribbean salad
*Raw carrots thinly sliced , zucchini sticks,diced tomatoes
cucumbers sticks marinated with olive oil and pimiento*

VEGETARIAN SANDWICH
*with lettuce, tomato, cucumbers and white beans
marinated in italian dressing*

LUNCH

Home made country toast is avaiable upon request

APPETIZERS
Cooked "Praga" ham with creamy horseradish sauce and dill pickles
Chicken salad with celery

SOUPS
Tomato cream soup " Pompadour "
Hungarian goulash soup

SALAD
Peppers and celery with diced apple on a bed of lettuce and carrots
Dressing : mayonnaise, french , blue cheese

THE ITALIAN TOUCH
"Linguine alle vongole veraci"
"Risotto Pastorella" with cooked ham and courgettes

MELODY BRUNCH
Omelette with vegetables ragout and mushrooms
served with rice

CATCH OF THE DAY
Deep fried assorted fishes and squids with remoulade sauce
served with french fries

MAIN COURSE
Chicken Genoa style
"Salmistrato di manzo bollito"
Brisket of beef served with boiled cabbage and vegetables,
steamed potatoes and horseradish cream

VEGETABLES - Selection of the day

DESSERTS
"La Pastiera" cake
Refreshing tropical sherbet
Vanilla , strawberry, chocolate ice cream

SELECTION OF INTERNATIONAL CHEESES
served with crackers

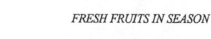

FRESH FRUITS IN SEASON

BEVERAGES
Freshly brewed regular or decafeinated coffee,
iced tea, assorted hot tea

Courtesy Mediterranean Shipping Cruises

M/S MELODY	WEDNESDAY, JANUARY 14th, 1998	AT SEA
The sun rises at 06.13		*... and sets at 18.07*

GOOD MORNING !

TONIGHT
(THE NIGHT BETWEEN TUESDAY 13th AND WEDNESDAY 14th JANUARY)
THE SHIP'S CLOCKS
WILL BE SET BACK BY ONE HOUR

NEWS FROM THE NAVIGATOR

At 06.00 a.m. we'll sail between the American Coast (on our right at approx. 40 milles) and the Cuba Coast (on our left at approx. 40 milles) and we'll enter the Mexican Gulf.

THE EXCURSION OFFICE

The Excursion Office is open so that you can book your excursions and collect your tickets:
09.00-12.00 for passengers from Bahamas, Restaurant and Oceanic Decks
16.00-19.00 for passengers from Continental, Premier and Lounge Decks

TODAY ON BOARD

Time	Activity	Location	Deck
09.00	GOOD MORNING FROM THE BRIDGE (Nautical News and Weather Forecast) with *Fabio*	in your cabin	radio channel no.3
09.00	MORNING WALK on the outer decks with Patrizio – meeting point:	Calypso Pool	Deck 7 (Pool)
09.15-09.45	GYMNASTICS and STRETCHING with Patrizio	Calypso Pool	Deck 6 (Lounge)
10.00	**COMPULSORY EMERGENCY LIFEBOAT BRIEFING** ENGLISH speaking guests .... (It is essential that you take your lifejacket to this briefing, which is mandatory under the International Convention for Safety of Life at Sea.) This talk is followed by a general outline of the cruise features and upcoming events.	Cinema, Deck 4 (Continental)	
10.30-12.00	PAINT-YOUR-OWN T-SHIRTS with Valentina and Daniela	Riviera Terrace	Deck 7 (Pool)
10.30-12.00	THE MINICLUB IS OPEN for all our youngest passengers	Pluto's Play House	Deck 5 (Premier)
11.00	Cooking Demonstration with Michele, the Maitre d'Hotel	Riviera Terrace	Deck 7 (Pool)
11.00	GAME IN THE SWIMMING-POOL with Rossina and Jurgen	Calypso Pool	Deck 7 (Pool)
11.00	CRAZY DANCE with the Entertainment Team	Junkanoo Lounge	Deck 6 (Lounge)
11.25	APERITIF GAME with the Entertainment Team	Riviera Terrace	Deck 7 (Pool)
11.30	AEROBICS with the Paris Paris Ballet	Junkanoo Lounge	Deck 6 (Lounge)
15.00	CARD TOURNAMENTS: "SCALA 40" with Vincenzo and Jurgen	Card Room	Deck 7 (Pool)
15.00-16.45	SIGN UP FOR THE **GRAND SLAM** A great new teem game with the Entertainment Team (teams made up of a minimum of 5 people and a maximum of 8)	Calypso Pool	**Deck 7 (Pool)**
15.00-17.00	PAINT-YOUR-OWN T-SHIRTS with Valentina and Daniela	Riviera Terrace	Deck 7 (Pool)
15.45	BELLY DANCING with Giorgia	Junkanoo Lounge	Deck 6 (Lounge)
16.00	GAME IN THE SWIMMING-POOL with Rossina and Jurgen	Calypso Pool	Deck 7 (Pool)
16.00-16.45	TEA AND CAKES (self-service) – music with the Elisir Duo	Riviera Terrace	Deck 7 (Pool)
16.00-16.45	TEA AND MUSIC - music with Piero	Sunrise Terrace	Deck 7 (Pool)
16.15	SOUTH AMERICAN DANCE with the Paris Paris Ballet	Junkanoo Lounge	Deck 6 (Lounge)
16.45	**GRAND SLAM BEGINS** A great new teem game with the Entertainment Team (teams made up of a minimum of 5 people and a maximum of 8)	Junkanoo Lounge	Deck 6(Lounge)

TONIGHT ON BOARD: GALA

Captain
Giovanni Massa
is delighted to invite all passengers to his "Welcome Cocktail Party"
which will take place this evening in the Club Universe

1st sitting: 17.30 2nd sitting: 19.30

Please use the entrance from the Casino.

1st Sitting: 18.30   **Galaxy Restaurant (Deck 2)** 2nd Sitting: 20.30
Welcome Gala Dinner

20.00-21.00	MUSIC with the *Night Passage* orchestra	Junkanoo Lounge Deck 6 (Lounge)
20.30-22.00	DANCING UNDER THE STARS with the *Duo Riviera*	Riviera Terrace Deck 7 (Pool)
20.30-22.30	**BABY DISCO**	Disco Teen Center Deck 6 (Lounge)

21.00   **Club Universe**   **23.00**

(Passengers from the 1st sitting)   **SHOW TIME**   (Passengers from the 2nd sitting)

"GALA VARIETY"

with Corlett's Puppets

David Dillon   Enrica Bacchia   Paris Paris Ballet

Passengers from the 1st sitting are kindly requested to vacate their seats before the beginning of the 2nd show, so that passengers from the 2nd sitting can enjoy the whole show from the start. The *Night Passage* orchestra will be waiting for you in the Junkanoo Lounge, *Duo Riviera* will be on the Riviera Terrace and *Duo Elisir* will be playing at the Blue Riband Club. Thank you very much for your collaboration.

21.30-23.30	ROMANTIC MUSIC with the *Duo Elisir*	Blue Riband Club Deck 7 (Pool)
21.30-22.15	DANCE MUSIC with the *Night Passage* orchestra	Junkanoo Lounge Deck 6 (Lounge)
21.45-23.00	DANCE MUSIC with the *Nello's Band*	Club Universe Deck 6 (Lounge)
22.00-23.00	MUSIC with *Piero*	Riviera Terrace Deck 7 (Pool)

22.15 – Junkanoo Lounge (Deck 6, Lounge)
CABARET CABARET
with the Entertainment Team

22.30-24.00	**TEEN MUSIC** - Music for teenagers	Disco Teen Center Deck 6 (Lounge)
22.45-00.30	DANCE MUSIC with the *Night Passage* orchestra	Junkanoo Lounge Deck 6 (Lounge)
23.00-01.30	DANCE MUSIC with the *Duo Riviera*	Riviera Terrace Deck 7 (Pool)
23.30-24.00	MUSIC with *Piero*	Blue Riband Club Deck 7 (Pool)
23.45-00.30	DANCING THE NIGHT AWAY with the *Nello's Band*	Club Universe Deck 6 (Lounge)
24.00-01.00	YOUR FAVORITE MUSIC with the *Duo Elisir*	Blue Riband Club Deck 7 (Pool)
24.00-.......	**DISCO MUSIC** with the D.J. *Ivan*	Disco Teen Center Deck 6 (Lounge)
00.45-01.30	**NIGHT MUSIC** – Piano Bar with Piero	Junkanoo Bar Deck 6 (Lounge)

TONIGHT'S DRESS CODE - FORMAL (GALA)

CINEMA (Deck 4 - Continental)

15.00	DIE BRÜCKEN AM FLUSS (129 Min.)	(German)
20.45 and 24.00	JUMANJI (100 min.)	(Italian)

TODAY'S MEAL TIMES

Coffee for early birds — 06.30-07.00
Satellite Café - Deck 7 (Pool)

BREAKFAST
Satellite Café (self-service buffet) — 07.00-10.00
Galaxy Restaurant (1st Sitting) — 07.30
Galaxy Restaurant (2nd Sitting) — 08.30
(The doors to the restaurant will be closed 15 minutes after the sitting commences.)

Breakfast in your cabin — 07.45-10.00
So as to improve our cabin service still further, we would like to inform all passengers that "Continental Breakfast" will be served in your cabin if you put out the special order card before 03.00 in the morning. Any orders placed after that time will take a little longer to prepare, and will arrive about half an hour later. We thank you for your kind collaboration in this matter.

Hot croissants at the Calyspo Bar — 10.00-11.30

LUNCH
Satellite Café (buffet self-service) — 12.15-14.00
Galaxy Restaurant (1st sitting) — 12.00
Galaxy Restaurant (2nd sitting) — 13.30

TEA AND CAKES
Riviera Terrace (Deck 7) Self-service — 16.00-16.45
Sunrise Terrace (Deck 7, Pool) — 16.00-16.45

Captain's Gala Dinner
Restaurant Galaxy (Deck 2) (1st sitting) — 18.30
Restaurant Galaxy (Deck 2) (2nd sitting) — 20.30
In order to guarantee the best service possible, we kindly ask all passengers to respect mealtimes. The doors to the restaurant will be closed 15 minutes after the sitting commences.

BUFFET: FLAMBE'
Riviera Terrace (Deck 7, Pool) — 23.45

ROOM SERVICE
Tel. 00 – Deck 5 (Premier) — 24 hours

PAYING AT THE BAR OR IN THE RESTAURANT WITH YOUR MAGNETIC CARD

ATTENTION !!!

Please show your card when you book excursions. The cost of excursions will NOT be debited to your card account, but it is necessary for issuing excursion tickets. You can then pay for your excursion tickets when you pick them up, either in cash or with any of the major credit cards (VISA, AMERICAN EXPRESS, DINERS, and MASTERCARD).

BAR OPENING HOURS

Junkanoo (Deck 6) — 12.00-01.30
Club Universe (Deck 6) — 09.00-12.00 / 18.00-01.00
Disco (Deck 6) — 22.30-03.00
Goombay (Deck 7, Riviera) — 09.00-02.00
Calypso Pool (Deck 7) — 07.00-19.00
Blue Riband Club (Deck 7) — 18.00-01.30

DIRECTORY OF SHIPBOARD SERVICES

INFORMATION OFFICE — 07.00-23.00
Tel. 04 - Deck 5 (Premier)
NIGHT CALLS - Tel. 00 — 23.00-07.00
SAFE BOXES — 08.00-12.00
Tel. 04 - Deck 5 (Premier) — 16.00-20.00
EXCURSION OFFICE — 09.00-12.00
Tel.1443/05 Deck 5, Premier — 16.00-19.00
BUREAU DE CHANGE — 10.00-12.00
Tel. 1446 - Deck 5, Premier — 17.00-19.00
RADIO STATION — 06.00-23.00
(closed in port) — at sea
Tel. 1249/1240 – Deck 8, Sun
MILKY WAY BOUTIQUE — 09.00-12.00
Tel. 1302 — 16.00-19.00
Deck 6, Lounge — 21.00-23.00
DUTY FREE SHOP — 09.00-12.00
Tel. 1305 — 16.00-19.00
Deck 6, Lounge — 21.00-23.00
SOUVENIR SHOP — 09.00-12.00
Tel. 1342 — 16.00-19.00
Deck 6, Lounge — 21.00-23.00
HAIR AND BEAUTY CENTER — 09.00-19.30
Deck 7, Pool - If you wish to fix an appointment, please feel free to go straight along to the Beauty Center. Thank you.
PHOTO GALLERY — 10.00-12.30
Tel. 1309 — 16.00-17.30
Deck 6, Lounge — 21.00-23.00
CASINO — 15.00-19.00
Deck 6, Lounge — 21.00-02.00
SLOT MACHINES — 10.00-02.00
Deck 6, Lounge
GYM - Tel.1400 — 08.00-12.00
Deck 7, Pool — 15.00-18.00
WITH INSTRUCTOR: — 10.30-11.30 / 15.00-17.00
HOSPITAL — 10.00-11.30
Tel.1333/03-Deck 2, Restaurant — 16.30-18.00
LIBRARY — 08.00-12.00
At the Information Office — 16.00-20.00
Deck 5, Premier
MINI CLUB – Pluto Lounge — 10.30-12.00
Tel. 1344 - Deck 5, Premier — 15.00-18.00

GENERAL EMERGENCY DRILL

A general emergency drill will take place today – English speaking passengers: at 10.00 in the cinema, Deck 4, Continental. In accordance with International Safety Regulations, all passengers must take part in this exercise. Please read the emergency instructions behind your cabin door carefully, take your lifejacket and proceed to your meeting point (specified above). Your participation is compulsory. During the exercise, all services on board will be closed.

PLAYING CARDS

You can buy playing cards at bars and boutiques on board. Playing cards for tournaments are provided by the animation team.

COCKTAIL DEL GIORNO

Banana Daiquiri — US$ 2.99
(Rum, lemon juice, banana)

COCKTAIL DELLA CROCIERA

Pink Lady — US$ 2.99

Courtesy Mediterranean Shipping Cruises

METROPOLITAN TOURING'S GALAPAGOS CRUISES

Adventure Associates

13150 Coit Rd., Suite 110

Dallas, Texas 75240

(800) 527-2500

(972) 907-0414

(972) 783-1286 FAX

ISABELA II: entered service 1989; 1,083 G.R.T.; 166' x 38'; 38-passenger capacity; 20 cabins; officers and crew mainly from Ecuador; three-, four-, and seven-night cruises around Galapagos Islands.

SANTA CRUZ: entered service 1979; refurbished 1998; 1,500 G.R.T.; 230' long; 90-passenger capacity; 45 cabins; officers and crew mainly from Ecuador; three-, four-, and seven-night cruises around the Galapagos Islands.

Metropolitan Touring operates the 1,500-ton, 90-passenger *Santa Cruz* and the 38-passenger *Isabela II,* as well as five smaller vessels offering three-, four-, and seven-night pleasure cruises exploring the flora and fauna of the Galapagos Islands, 600 miles offshore from Ecuador. Cruises on the *Santa Cruz* and *Isabela II* sail from Baltra Island.

On the Santa Cruz, 38 cabins are located outside and 6 inside. All cabins have twin lower beds, toilet and shower, a closet, and storage drawers. Seven cabins can accommodate three passengers and four cabins can accommodate four passengers.

The lounge, bar, dining room, purser's office, stores, and other cabins are located on Upper Deck, between Main and Boat decks. There is also a sun deck and observation area, but no pool.

The *Isabela II,* which began service in 1989, was built specifically for cruising in the Galapagos, with 20 outside air-conditioned cabins, each with private shower and toilet. This yacht-like vessel includes a large salon and bar area, a spacious dining room, separate reading and game rooms, and a sun deck with a Jacuzzi, deck chairs, and some exercise machines. She is considered more luxurious than the other ships.

The general atmosphere and dress code on all ships is casual, jackets not being required for men. There is little entertainment, and on most evenings, professional naturalists give lectures and slide presentations in order to brief passengers on the following day's activities.

The ships of Metropolitan Touring visit the islands of Barrington, Bartolome, Fernandina, Floreana, Hood, Isabela, James, North Seymour, Plaza, San Cristobal, Santa Cruz, Jervis, and Tower. Here passengers will take guided excursions and view sea lions, fur seals, penguins, flocks of flamingos, marine and land iguanas, giant tortoises, colonies of albatrosses, and such other rare birds as boobies, noddy terns, lava gulls, storm petrels, Darwin's finches, flightless cormorants, and frigates.

Strong Points:

This is heaven for naturalists and bird watchers who wish to pursue their hobby in comfort and in the companionship of other aficionados.

NORWEGIAN CRUISE LINE
95 Merrick Way
Coral Gables, Florida 33134
(800) 327-7030

S.S. *NORWAY:* (formerly S.S. *France*); entered service 1961; rebuilt for Caribbean service 1980; 76,049 G.R.T.; 1,035' x 110'; 2,032-passenger capacity; 932 cabins; Norwegian officers and international crew; cruise grounds to be determined. **(Category B/C—Not Rated)**

M.S. *NORWEGIAN CROWN:* (formerly *Crown Odyssey*); entered service 1988; 34,250 G.R.T.; 614' x 92'; 1,052-passenger capacity; 526 cabins; officers and international crew; cruise grounds to be determined. **(Category C—Not Rated)**

NORWEGIAN DREAM: (formerly *Dreamward*); entered service 1992; stretched in 1998; 50,760 G.R.T.; 754' x 94'; 1,748-passenger capacity; 874 cabins; Norwegian officers and international crew; cruise grounds to be determined. **(Category C—Not Rated)**

NORWEGIAN MAJESTY: (formerly *Royal Majesty*); 38,000 G.R.T.; 680' x 91' (stretched in 1999); 1,462 passenger capacity; 731 cabins; Norwegian officers and international crew; cruise grounds to be determined. **(Category C—Not Rated)**

NORWEGIAN SEA: (formerly M.S. *Seaward*); entered service 1988; 42,000 G.R.T.; 700' x 93'; 1,518-passenger capacity; 817 cabins; Norwegian officers and international crew; cruise grounds to be determined. **(Category C—Not Rated)**

NORWEGIAN SKY: entered service 1999; 76,000 G.R.T.; 2000-passenger capacity; 1001 cabins; Norwegian officers and international crew; cruise grounds to be determined. **(Category B/C—Not Rated)**

NORWEGIAN WIND: (formerly *Windward*); entered service 1993; stretched in 1998; 50,760 G.R.T.; 754' x 94'; 1,748-passenger capacity; 874 cabins; Norwegian officers and international crew; cruises from Miami to western Caribbean/cruise grounds to be determined. **(Category C—Not Rated)** (Medical Facilities: C-0; P-1; N-1; CM; PD; EKG; PO; OX; X.)

The Norwegian Cruise Line (NCL) is a subsidiary of the Oslo-based NCL Holding AS, formerly Klosters Rederi A/S, a shipping company owned by the

Kloster family since the turn of the century. In 1996 the name of the parent company was changed to Norwegian Cruise Line, Ltd. It was Knut Kloster and Ted Arison who initiated Caribbean cruises from Miami in 1966 with the introduction of the original M.S. *Sunward.* The relationship between Arison and Kloster ended in the early seventies, and Arison went on to form Carnival Cruise Line.

From 1968 to 1971, NCL introduced three similarly designed bread-and-butter cruise ships. First came the M.S. *Starward* in 1968, followed by the M.S. *Skyward* in 1969 and the M.S. *Southward* in 1971. All three ships were intended to bring the cruise experience to upper-middle-class and middle-class America. Historically, passengers received numerous meals, loads of food, continuous activities and entertainment, several popular ports of call, adequate service and accommodations, and the excitement of cruising at reasonable prices. All three ships ceased being operated by NCL during the nineties and were replaced with newer vessels.

The dinner menus on NCL ships are varied, featuring different theme nights with international offerings. Although there is quantity and variety, food preparation is simple and not gourmet. The cabin stewards and waiters are a mixture of Caribbean, Asian, or Central and South American. They are generally competent and efficient, but not on par with a European crew. Recently the NCL ships have introduced Le Bistro, an alternative open-seating, first-come, first-served Italian restaurant at no additional charge.

The itineraries have shifted over the years, but they normally cover three or four ports, including a beach party at one of NCL's privately owned island paradises in the Bahamas. In addition, all NCL ships feature a "Dive In" program, where passengers receive instruction and supervision in snorkeling, both aboard ship and while ashore.

NCL purchased the original S.S. *France* in 1979 and transformed her from a grand two-class transatlantic queen into the modern Caribbean megaship, the *Norway.* More than $100 million was spent on the original conversion, supervised by Danish naval architect Tage Wandborg, with the interior design by Angelo Donghia of New York.

The public areas include Fifth Avenue and the Champs Elysées, two separate promenades on opposite sides of International Deck lined with shops, lounges, an ice-cream parlor, an outdoor café, the information/purser's office, and the tour desk. There is sufficient outside deck space to offer two outdoor swimming pools (one of which is actually large enough to swim laps in); lido bars adjoining the pools; the Great Outdoor Restaurant, where optional breakfast and lunches are served; basketball courts; a jogging track; and golf-driving and trap-shooting facilities. On Dolphin Deck, the lowest passenger deck, is *Norway*'s Roman Spa, with marble floors and columns featuring eight massage rooms, an aquacise pool, a Jacuzzi, saunas, steam rooms, hairdressers, state-of-the-art exercise equipment, herbal therapy, body wraps, and skin exfoliates. There are two spectacular dining rooms, one with an upstairs balcony, along with public lounges and showrooms, ranging from the sophisticated International Lounge, the 840-seat Saga Theater, and state-of-the-art Dazzles Disco to the intimate, cozy Windjammer Lounge and a gigantic casino stocked with blackjack, craps, roulette tables, and hundreds of slot machines. There's even an art gallery.

The *Norway* offers more entertainment than is found on the other NCL ships. In addition to the usual deck parties, costume balls, dance instruction, variety shows, horse races, audience participation, bingo, and card tournaments, there are numerous specialty lectures, wine tastings, cosmetic classes, aerobics classes, fashion shows, and full-scale Broadway musical productions. There is a full-scale special program for children. Shore excursions for adults include organized beach parties, snorkeling expeditions, and party cruises.

In 1988 the 42,000-ton *Seaward* joined the fleet, accommodating 1,504 passengers, double occupancy. Originally it offered alternate three- and four-day itineraries from Miami. In 1995 it was repositioned to San Juan with three-, four-, and seven-day cruises to the southern Caribbean. In 1998 she was renamed *Norwegian Sea.*

There are two regular dining rooms, Le Bistro, an à la carte restaurant at the top of the ship, outdoor buffet restaurants, and an ice-cream parlor. Additionally, there are numerous lounges, a disco, a health club, two pools, shops, a piano bar, and a casino. The less-expensive cabins tend to be small and are located inside, on the bottom three decks of the ship.

Kloster, the parent company, purchased the Royal Viking Line during the eighties. In 1994, it sold off all of these ships, as well as the Royal Viking logo.

At 41,000 G.R.T., the *Dreamward* and *Windward* entered service in December 1992 and May 1993. In 1998 both ships were stretched and now each carries 1,748 passengers. The ships were then renamed *Norwegian Dream* and *Norwegian Wind.*

The 25,000-ton, 950-passenger *Leeward* was formerly a Baltic ferry that underwent a $60-million conversion to prepare it to take over the three- and four-day cruises from Miami. The ship left the fleet in 1999.

In the winter of 1990, the owners of NCL acquired Royal Cruise Line, which owned the *Queen Odyssey* (formerly *Royal Viking Queen*), *Crown Odyssey, Royal Odyssey* (formerly *Royal Viking Sea*), and *Star Odyssey* (formerly *Royal Viking Star*). However, in 1996, for financial reasons, Royal Cruise Line was closed and *Queen Odyssey* was sold to Seabourn and renamed the *Seabourn Legend;* the *Crown Odyssey* was transferred to NCL and renamed *Norwegian Crown.* The *Star Odyssey* was sold to Fred Olsen Lines and sails as the *Black Watch.* The *Royal Odyssey* sailed as the *Norwegian Star,* with seven-day cruises from Houston to the western Caribbean. The *Norwegian Star* has been deployed to serve the Australian cruise market commencing in 1999, in a joint venture with Norwegian Capricorn Line.

In 1997 the line purchased the *Royal Majesty* and *Crown Majesty* from Majesty Cruise Line. The ships were renamed *Norwegian Majesty* and *Norwegian Dynasty.* In 1997 NCL purchased the *Aida* from a German travel group and then leased her back until 2001.

A new 76,000-ton, 2,000-passenger ship to be named *Norwegian Sky* joined the fleet in August 1999.

As we go to print, schedules for the various ships have not been determined.

In the summer of 1998, Norwegian Cruise Line purchased Orient Lines but markets the line as a separate brand, with its existing management and staff.

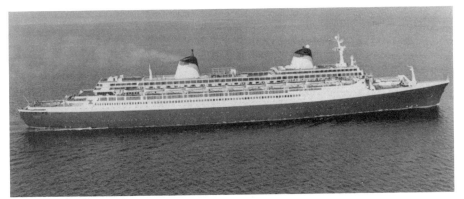

Courtesy Norwegian Cruise Line

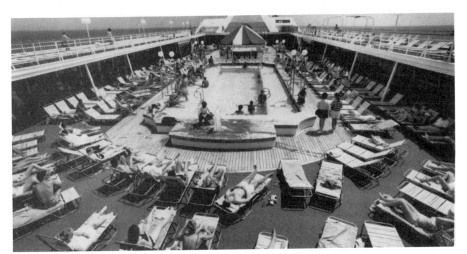

Courtesy Norwegian Cruise Line

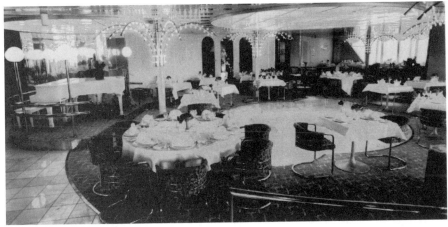

Courtesy Norwegian Cruise Line

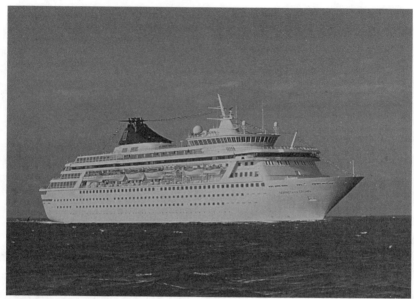

Courtesy Norwegian Cruise Line

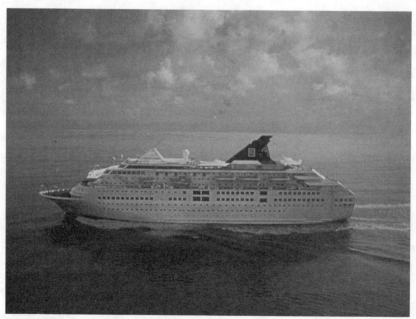

Courtesy Norwegian Cruise Line

Main Courses

Broiled Caribbean Lobster Tail
Complemented with Vegetables, Pommes Mousselin
and Lemon-Garlic Butter

Capellini alla Valdostana
Sautéed Shrimps and Mussels tossed with
Angelhair Pasta and Tarragon Sauce

Chicken "Oskar"
Broiled Chicken Breast crowned with Crab Meat, Asparagus
and Sauce Hollandaise, Cauliflower Cake with
Red Beet Mousse, Broccoli and Pommes Croquettes

Flamed Steak Diane
Grilled Striploin of Beef flamed with Cognac and completed
in the Classic Sauce. Cauliflower Cake with Red Beet Mousse,
Broccoli and Pommes Croquettes

Always Available

Grilled Chicken Breast
Steamed Vegetables   Baked Potato with Condiments

Vegetarian Entree

Grilled Vegetable "Strudel" with Basil-Pinenut Sauce

From Our Cheese Board

Variety of International Cheeses and Fruits

Desserts

Baked Alaska on Parade
A luminous Surprise performed by your brilliant Waiter

Petits Fours and Macaroons à la Chef de Patissier

From the Ice Cream Parlor

Vanilla, Chocolate, Strawberry, Pistachio, Pecan Ice Cream

Lemon, Pineapple, Orange Sherbet

Black Forest Ice Cream Coupe   Frozen Raspberry Yogurt

Beverages

Coffee, Decaffeinated Coffee, Espresso,
Cappuccino, Assorted Teas, Milk

* * *

Children's Menu and Kosher prepared items are available
These distinguished selections require time for preparation
Please consult your waiter for your advance order

ST/D7A/'98

Courtesy Norwegian Cruise Line

MORNING

Activities and Leisure

7:00am	Sun-Up Fitness Walk with your Sports Afloat Coordinator **Danielle**	Promenade Deck 6, Aft
7:40am	Stretch & Relax Class with your Sports Afloat Coordinator **Danielle**	Poolside Deck 9
8:00am	Water Aerobics with your Sports Afloat Coordinator **Danielle**	Poolside, Deck 9
9:00am	Lower Body Blast with your Sports Coordinator, **Danielle**	Poolside, Deck 9
9:00am-Noon	Morning Drink Special: Bloody Mary's, Screwdrivers and Mimosas for only $2.50!	All Open Bars
9:00am	**The Grandeur of Maya Civilization:** Numbers, Calendars, Pyramids and Ball Courts with your Enrichment Lecturer, **Joe Arbena**	Stardust Lounge, Deck 5
9:30am	**Port & Shopping Talk** with your Port & Cruise Consultant Information on Cancun & Cozumel, Mexico as well as Roatan	Cabaret Lounge, Deck 5
9:30am	**Craft Corner:** Flowered Combs with your Cruise Director's Staff	Oscar's Pub, Deck 5
10:00am	**Aromaspa Demonstration** Join us and learn all about the power of the sea and essential oils to sooth and firm the body.	Observatory Lounge, Deck 10
10:00am	Basketball Free Throw Contest with your Sports Afloat Coordinator **Danielle**	Deck 6, Aft
10:00am	Clay Pigeon & Trapshooting with a Norwegian Officer:	Deck 6, Aft
10:00am-Arrival	**MONTE CARLO CASINO - TABLES ARE OPEN**	Casino, Deck 5, Midship
10:30am	**Diamond Jackpot Bingo** Today we will be raffling off a diamond tennis bracelet to one Bingo player	Stardust Lounge, Deck 5
10:30am	**Partner Massage Demonstration** Come along with a friend or your partner and learn the techniques of relaxation.	Observatory Lounge, Deck 10
10:30am	*The Big Art Auction* – Preview is at 10:00am *Sponsored by Van Cleef & Arpels of Cozumel*	Oscar's Pub, Deck 5
Noon-1:00pm	Join *Joy* for some spicy Island sounds	Poolside, Deck 9

AFTERNOON

Activities and Leisure

1:00pm	**Welcome to Cancun** All guests on tour should refer to their tour ticket for meeting times and locations. If you are not on tour you will need a "Going Ashore" Tender Ticket. When you and your entire party are ready to go ashore, pick up your ticket from the Dive-In Desk on Deck 4. Please remain in the public areas until you hear your ticket number called (Please anticipate a possible waiting time and do not wait at the gangway). After the majority of guests are ashore, we will go on your own service. Please do not proceed to the gangway area until an announcement has been made. Tenders will run continuously throughout the day. You will not need a tender ticket to return to the ship. The gangway is located on Deck 1, Midship. Last tender from shoreside is at 9:30pm as the M/S Norwegian Sea sails for Cozumel, at 10:00pm.	Gangway, Deck 1 Aft
2:30pm	**Informal Bridge Play** with your fellow passengers	Butterfly Room, Deck 5
4:30pm	**Navigational Bridge Tour** with your Cruise Director's Staff	Stairwell, Deck 8, Forward
4:30-5:30pm	Join *Joy* for some spicy Island sounds	Poolside, Deck 9
5:00pm	Friends of Bill W. meet	Observatory Lounge, Deck 10
5:15pm	*Honeymooners Champagne Party*	Stardust Lounge, Deck 5
5:15pm	**Navigational Bridge Tour** with your Cruise Director's Staff	Stairwell, Deck 8, Forward
5:30pm	Join **Rabbi Seymour Rosen** for the second night of *Chanukah*	Gatsby's, Deck 10
5:30pm	Walk a Mile with a Smile with your Sports Afloat Coordinator, Danielle	Deck 6, Aft

EVENING

Dining and Entertainment

7:30-8:45pm	**ART GALLERY** is open. Meet **Chris**, your Art Director	Crystal Court, Deck 4
7:45-8:30pm	Listen to the smooth sounds of **Derek Lewis**	Oscar's Pub, Deck 5
8:00-8:45pm	Enjoy the musical talent of **Victor Reid**	Gatsby's, Deck 10
9:00 & 10:30pm	**COMEDY & MAGIC SHOWTIME** **Starring Doug Anderson**	Cabaret Lounge, Deck 5

9:30pm	**Last Tender from Shoreside to the M/S Norwegian Sea**
10:00pm	**The M/S Norwegian Sea sails for Cozumel**

10:00-10:45pm	**Country Music** - Enjoy acoustic country sounds with **Chip & Patrick** as they present **"Boots, Blues and Boogie"** **Drink Special:** Moonshine $2.75	Oscar's Pub, Deck 5
10:00pm-Close	Come & party with the musical talents of *Impromptu*	Stardust Lounge, Deck 5
10:00pm-Close	**Boomer's Party Zone** Our D.J. plays the hits and requests in our nightclub. (No one under 18 in the disco after 11:00pm) **Starting at Midnight Disco Special: buy one drink, and receive a raffle ticket at 12:30am we will start drawing for Free Drinks every 5 minutes!**	Boomer's, Deck 8
10:30pm-11:30pm	Get in the mood for our wonderful Texaribbean Carnival on deck with *Joy*	Poolside, Deck 9
10:30pm-Close	Late Night with **Victor Reid** at the keys. Enjoy our wine selection.	Gatsby's, Deck 10
10:45pm-Close	Relax in the pub with **Derek Lewis**	Oscar's Pub, Deck 5
11:00pm	**80's Night Party!** Join our **D.J.** and the late night crowd as they party 80's style!	Boomer's, Deck 8
11:30pm	**Texaribbean Night** Featuring: **Mariachi Band, Los Gallitos** from Cancun Mexico. Join your Cruise Director **Karen Campbell** & her staff for a fiesta under the stars **Drink Special** – Margarita Shaker for only $5.95	Poolside, Deck 9
Midnight-1:00am	**Texaribbean Buffet**	Poolside, Deck 9

REMINDERS:

LOTTO HOURS
**Win a cruise for 20 onboard the legendary S/S Norway and $25,000 in cash in our
Lottery or $1,000 instantly in our Pull Tabs!**
The Lottery Terminal is located in the Crystal Court on Deck 4
8:00pm - 8:30pm

Call Home

*Satellite Services: A call placed from your cabin will connect you in less than 30 seconds! Only $5.95 per minute for 1-800
numbers and calls to the U.S. & $6.95 per minute for International calls. Follow the dialing instructions posted in your cabin.*

Fine Dining - Le Bistro in the Palm Tree: Enjoy *unconventional dining and specially selected wines by the glass.
Continuous dinner service 6:00-11:00pm available every night. (No shorts please). Suggested Gratuity $5.00 per person. Sun
Deck 10, Aft.*

In Motion on the Ocean *Join our "In Motion on the Ocean" fitness program. Earn Sports Afloat tickets for
each fitness activity you attend throughout the cruise. Collect just ten (10) tickets and receive a free Sports Afloat T-shirt.*

Courtesy Norwegian Cruise Line

ORIENT LINES
1510 S.E. 17th Street, Suite 400

Ft. Lauderdale, Florida 33316

(800) 333-7300

(954) 527-6657 FAX

MARCO POLO: (formerly *Alexandr Pushkin*); entered service 1965; refurbished and reconstructed 1993; 22,080 G.R.T.; 578' x 77'; 800-passenger capacity; 426 cabins; European, Scandinavian, and Filipino officers and crew; itineraries in the Greek islands, New Zealand, Australia, the Mediterranean, Antarctica, Africa, India, Egypt, and Asia.

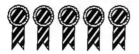

(Medical Facilities: C-2; P-1; EM, CLS, MS; CM; PD; BC; EKG; TC; PO; WC; OR; ICU; X; M; LJ.)

In 1991 Gerry Herrod, founder of Ocean Cruise Lines, purchased the Russian vessel *Alexandr Pushkin* and had her reconstructed in Perama, Greece, with the interiors being gutted and totally refurbished under the direction of well-known ship designers A & M Katzourakis. The end result is an attractive vessel with cabins and public areas reminiscent of the mid-size ships (15,000-30,000 G.R.T.) built in the late sixties to the early eighties. Like Herrod's former ships, the *Marco Polo* was designed to cruise to exotic destinations around the world, including cruises in the Indian Ocean from Africa to India and throughout the Mediterranean from Barcelona to the Black Sea. Constructed with a reinforced hull for adverse Arctic conditions and equipped with eight inflatable Zodiacs, the *Marco Polo* is one of the few exploration ships offering a full cruise experience with numerous facilities and a wide range of entertainments. In the summer of 1998, Norwegian Cruise Line acquired Orient Lines and indicated that it intends to market the line as a separate brand, maintaining the existing management and staff and adding one or more additional vessels to the fleet.

Seventy percent of the cabins are outside, average about 140 square feet in size, and include hair dryers, three-channel radios, private wall safes, and TVs with satellite news and in-house movies. The two deluxe suites have queen-size beds, tub and shower, and large separate sitting rooms, and cost about twice as much as a standard outside cabin. The four junior suites and eight "A" category deluxe cabins include larger bathrooms with a tub and shower, small sitting areas, refrigerators, and robes.

Raffles, the lido restaurant, serves a buffet breakfast and lunch daily both indoors and at umbrella-protected tables around the pool; depending on the cruising area, it often offers alternative dinners with various ethnic themes. The attractive Seven Seas Restaurant is located on one of the lower decks and features excellent Continental cuisine and American favorites.

A limited number of lounge chairs are available atop ship next to the three outdoor Jacuzzis; and additional lounges and steamer-style chairs are spread along Promenade and other decks. The small swimming pool is surrounded by the above-described tables and chairs for al fresco diners, and there are only a few lounges in this area. Outside deck areas are less generous than on many ships, reflecting the cruise line's emphasis on destinations and its expectation that most passengers will spend their days ashore.

The Steiner Spa and Fitness Center includes a beauty salon, an aerobics room, men's and women's locker rooms with saunas and showers, massage, beauty, and therapy treatment rooms, and a small exercise facility equipped with free weights and a limited number of cardiovascular machines. Unfortunately the one possible area for speed-walkers and joggers is very narrow and requires zigzagging around stairs and other obstacles.

Other tastefully decorated public indoor areas include a show lounge; the Polo Lounge and Bar, featuring nightly piano entertainment; the Charleston Club, an intimate lounge with late-night dancing; a library; a shopping arcade; a cardroom; a small, elegant casino; and a medical facility.

Itineraries encompass visits to the Greek islands, the Mediterranean, New Zealand, Australia, Africa, India, Antarctica, Egypt, and Asia.

Prices per person per day vary depending on the cruise. Per diems on the cruises in Europe are less expensive than on other itineraries: the suites located on the top decks run about $275-$460, average outside cabins run about $235, and the least expensive inside cabin costs about $165 (Europe). These prices include air, pre- or post-cruise hotel stays and transfers, resulting in an extremely attractive, all-inclusive cruise-tour package. Various air add-ons may apply, and those passengers not opting for air and/or the hotel stay receive a credit.

Overall, this is a traditional-style ship which, although reconstructed in 1993, does not offer the space, facilities, glamour, or glitz found on more modern vessels and cannot be compared to newly constructed ships or those competing in the premium and luxury cruise markets. However, it offers a friendly, full cruise experience with some of the most desired destinations, fine dining in its main restaurant, a variety of entertainments, and one of the industry's best values for a cruise-tour.

Strong Points:

Destination-oriented itineraries around the world on a more traditional-style, full-facility exploration-equipped ship with excellent cuisine at extremely competitive prices.

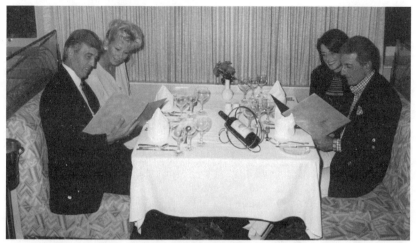

Courtesy Orient Lines

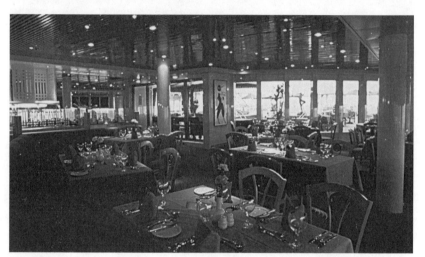

Courtesy Orient Lines

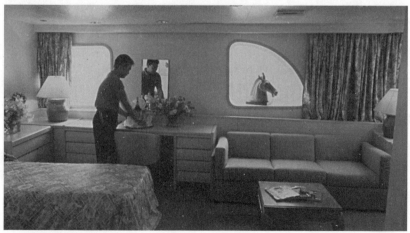

Courtesy Orient Lines

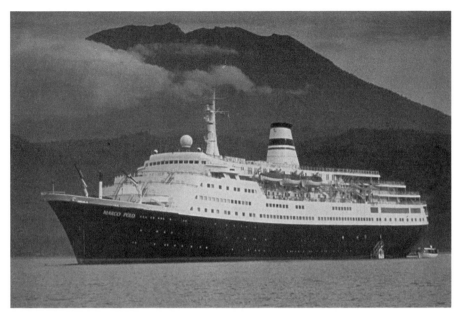

Courtesy Orient Lines

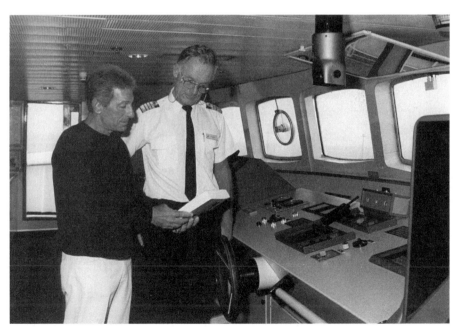

Courtesy Orient Lines

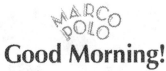

Good Morning!

———— YOUR DAY ON BOARD THE MARCO POLO ————

8.00am	Get in the Swim - The Pool is open	Belvedere Deck Aft
8.00am	TONE AND STRETCH - low impact class with **Janine**	Health Club
9.00am	**Fiona's**Crossword is at the Shore Excursion Desk (Answers in the Card Room before 5.00pm.).	Belvedere Deck
9.30am - 10.30am	The Library is open for the selection of books, or to have a chat with the Cruise Staff on duty.	Belvedere Deck
& 5.30pm - 6.30pm		
10.00am	The sports deck is open for shuffleboard	Promenade Deck
10.45am	SCRABBLE TOURNAMENT hosted by the **Cruise Staff**	Polo lounge
2.45pm	PARTY BRIDGE with your fellow passengers	Card Room
3.45pm	CHESS AND BACKGAMMON GET TOGETHER - challenge your fellow passengers.	Polo Lounge
4.00pm	ONE MILE WALK - take a breath of fresh air with **Janine**	Health Club
4.00pm	Afternoon tea is served	Raffles / Palm Court
4.00pm	TEAM TRIVIA hosted by the **Cruise Staff**.	Polo Lounge
4.45pm	GOLF CHIPPING CHALLENGE hosted by the **Cruise Staff**	Next to the Shore Excursion Desk
5.00pm	INTERDENOMINATIONAL SERVICE - conducted by **Rev. Payne**	Charleston Club
5.00pm	Friends of Bill W and Doctor Bob meeting.	Meeting Room

———— FROM THE SHORE EXCURSION OFFICE ————

PASSENGERS ON TOUR

Please relax in any of the public areas, open decks or your cabin and listen for disembarkation announcements according to your tour

(Please note, cabin radio should be set to channel 1 and the volume level raised to hear announcements in cabins.)

For your own comfort and safety DO NOT congregate at the gangway area.
This will cause unnecessary congestion and delays in departure.

Tours are expected to depart at the following times:

RHO 4	RHODES TOWN & ACROPOLIS OF LINDOS	8.00am
RHO 2	THE ACROPOLIS OF LINDOS	8.15am
RHO 1	MT. PHILERIMOS & RHODES TOWN	8.30am
RHO 3	OLD TOWN & GR. MASTER'S PALACE	1.30pm

Please remember your tour ticket which will be collected as you board the bus.

For security reasons all passengers should carry their own Cruise Card when going ashore.

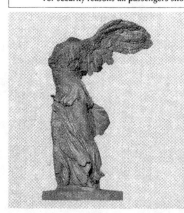

Rhodes became a centre of artistic activity from a very early date. A visit to the Archaeological Museum brings one into contact with the works of art produced on the island from the Mycenaen to the Roman period. The great artists, sculptors and painters whose names have survived - those of architects have not - are known to us because their reputation has found it's place in written tradition; the names of a of the sculptors are preserved on the bases of statues now lost, and just few of their works survive in copies dating from the Roman period. Not a single painting as survived. The names of over 100 artists from the last four centuries B.C. are known only from inscriptions. Many of them were Rhodians, but at the same time many foreigners from the coast of Asia Minor or from the rest of Greece worked in this important artistic centre.

Amongst originals from the 2nd century B.C., that have been attributed to Rhodian workshops are a bronze Sleeping Eros and the Victory of Samothrace, one of the finest surviving pieces of Greek art. It was dedicated by the Rhodians in the sanctuary of the Kabeiroi on Samothrace, after their victory over Antiochus III in 190 B.C., and was probably a work of Pythokritos, who also carved a boat in relief on the rock at Lindos. Victory is standing on her right foot on the prow of a boat that forms the base of the statue.

For Your Evening's Pleasure

5.30pm Main Sitting	Ambassador Lounge	7.30pm Late Sitting

ORIENT LINES' CAPTAIN'S RECEPTION
Captain Erik Bjurstedt requests the pleasure of your company.

The Captain will receive passengers at the Starboard side of the Ambassador Lounge.

 | 8.00pm – 9.00pm
9.45pm – Midnight | **John Daniel** with music and song to entertain you throughout the evening

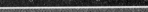

9.00pm	Ambassador Lounge	10.30pm

VARIETY SHOWTIME
starring

Multi-instrumentalist
Kenny Martyn
&
Comedy Star
Bernie Berns

Hosted by **Cruise Director, Steve Lewis**
Music **Gennadi Orchestra**

Please note the use of video cameras and audio recording equipment is prohibited during professional entertainment

CLUB	10.00pm – 11.30pm	**Romantic Swing Trio** play your favourite melodies for dancing
	11.45pm	*starring*
Charleston Cabaret		The "Classy Lassy" from Scotland **Maggi Ballantyne** music by the Gennadi Trio
	12.15am	The Club goes Disco with Music for the Young and Young-at-Heart

MPTV

Channel 1	CNN International, NBC or BBC World depending on satellite signal	8.00am- Midnight
Channel 2	'Air Force One' Harrison Ford, Gary Oldman	8.30am, 10.40am, 12.50pm, 3.00pm
	'City of Angels' Meg Ryan, Nicholas Cage	5.00pm, 7.00pm
	'The Truman Show' Jim Carrey, Ed Harris	9.00pm, 10.45pm
Channel 3	'Satellite Text News'	All Day
Channel 4	'Speed 2' Sandra Bullock, Jason Patrick	9.00am, 11.00am, 1.00pm, 3.00pm
	'Batman Forever' Val Kilmer	5.00pm, 7.00pm
	'Cat on a Hot Tin Roof' Liz Taylor, Paul Newman	9.00pm, 10.45pm
Channel 5	Tour Talk Fiona Beazley	All Day
	Video on Greece & Crete	
Channel 6	CNN International, NBC or BBC World depending on satellite signal	8.00am- Midnight

RADIO MP

Radio 1 - Ship's Announcements	**Radio 2** - Classical	**Radio 3** - Easy Listening

General Information

━━━━━━━ HOURS FOR TODAY ━━━━━━━

SERVICE

Public Telephone - Marco Polo Phone Cards are available from the Purser's Desk at a cost of $27 per card for 60 units (approx 3mins).

Purser's Office (☎ 300)	6.30am – 10.00pm
Information & Night Porter on duty (☎ 700)	**10.00pm – 6.30am**
Shore Excursion Desk (☎ 500)	7.15am - 7.45am
Deadline for Delos: 8.00pm	**6.30pm - 8.30pm**
Le Casino	Slots: 6.30pm - Close
	Tables: 8.30pm - Close
La Boutique / Shops	6.30pm - 11.00pm
Health Club	8.00am - 8.00pm
Beauty Centre & Gym Shop (☎ 732)	8.00am - 8.00pm
Photo Gallery	CLOSED
Radio Station(☎ 200)	6.30am – Midnight
For assistance with international telephone calls and faxes	
Medical Centre	9.00am – 10.00am
☎ 600 during clinic hours	6.00pm – 7.00pm
☎ 100 medical emergency	
Housekeeping ☎ 700	Wake-up Call ☎ 400

DINING

Seven Seas Restaurant

Breakfast	Open Sitting	6.30am - 9.00am
Luncheon		12.00 noon - 1.30pm
Captain's Dinner	Main Sitting	6.30pm
	Late Sitting	8.30pm

Raffles & Poolside

Continental Breakfast	6.00am – 10.00am
Breakfast Buffet	6.30am – 9.30am
Lunch Buffet & BBQ	12.00noon– 2.00pm
Afternoon Tea	4.00pm - 5.00pm
Poolside BBQ	7.00pm - 9.00pm

Palm Court

Afternoon Tea	4.00pm - 5.00pm

Charleston Deck

Late Night Snacks	11.30pm - 12.30pm

Polo Lounge

Goodnight Snacks	11.30pm – Midnight

BAR HOURS

Lido Bar	10.30am – 10.30pm
Polo Lounge	9.00am – 1.00am
Le Bar	5.30pm – Wee hours
Charleston Club	10.00pm – Wee hours
Ambassador Lounge	9.00pm - Midnight
Jacuzzi Bar	10.00am - Sunset

SHIP'S AGENT IN RHODES
Greek Star Co Ltd. Tourism Travel Agency
21 Kathopouli Str
851 00 Rhodes, Greece
Tel: (30-241) 23664 / 24986

HAPPY HOUR SPECIAL $2.75
Americano
5.30pm to 6.30pm — Sweet Vermouth, Campari, Club Soda
Rusty Nail
Scotch Whiskey, Drambuie — 7.30pm to 8.30pm
DRINK OF THE DAY $2.75
Baybreeze
Vodka, Cranberry Juice, Pineapple Juice

━━━━━━━ FOR YOUR INFORMATION ━━━━━━━

WINE
Wine orders for dinner may be given to the Wine Steward in the Purser's Lobby between 4.00pm and 5.00pm today.
BE A GOOD NEIGHBOUR - DO NOT DISTURB
We respectfully ask passengers who return to their cabins late at night, or rise early in the morning, to be considerate to others. Joggers - not before 8.00am or after 10.00pm please. You may be jogging over someone sleeping!
NEWSPAPERS IN THE LIBRARY
As we print only a limited number of copies of the Marco Polo Times, please return them to the Library after reading. Thank you.
HAVE YOU LOST ANYTHING?
We have a selection of hats, glasses and books at the Purser's Desk, why not stop by and see if we are holding your missing items?
WISH YOU WERE HERE....
When you have written your letters or postcards, take them to the Purser's Desk where they will be mailed at the next port of call. They will be charged to your shipboard account at $1 or 80c respectively.

SHIP'S CHART
Captain Erik Bjurstedt has donated a special chart of our cruise, which is on display at the Purser's Desk. This chart will be given in aid of a very special charity, supported by the members of our crew, the Marco Polo 'Children of the Philippines Foundation', an institution in Manila caring for homeless, abandoned and abused children. Raffle tickets, costing $3 each or two for $5 are available at the Purser's Desk, and can be charged to your shipboard account as a charity contribution. We hope that you will participate, to support a very worthwhile cause.
SMOKING
You are reminded that smoking is only permitted on the Port Side of the ship except, in the Charleston Club where we request that you smoke on the Starboard side. During showtime the Ambassador Lounge is a no smoking area. Elevators and hallways are no smoking areas.

Courtesy Orient Lines

Dinner

APPETIZERS

Jumbo Shrimp & Parsnip Crisps
on a Salad dressed with Nero Sauce

Avocado & Salmon Gâteau
*crowned with a soured Lemon Cream
and garnished with Sevruga Caviar*

Forest Terrine
served on a bed of Mixed Leaves

SOUPS

Cream of Celery

Consommé Mikado
garnished with Brunoise of Chicken and Tomato

ENTREES

Fillet Mignon
*served on a Brioche Crouton flavoured
with a smooth Parfait and laced with Madeira Sauce*

Delice of Salmon
with a Pinenut and Oatmeal Crust

Roast Norfolk Turkey
*offered with Sweet Potatoes and
Garden Vegetables, laced with natural pan jus*

Sauté of Duckling
finished with a sweet, dark Cherry Reduction

CHEESES

Selection of International Cheeses

DESSERTS

Baked Alaska on Parade

Pastry Chef's Iced Pralines

BEVERAGES

Coffee and Sablés à la Poche

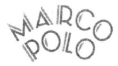

THE HEALTHY CHOICE

Our Chef has adapted a selection
of reduced fat & low salt dishes

Jumbo Shrimp & Parsnip Crisps
on a Salad dressed with Nero Sauce

•

Celery Soup

•

Roast Norfolk Turkey
with sweet Potatoes and steamed Vegetables

•

Pastry Chef's Iced Pralines

Our Wine Suggestions for Tonight's Dinner

6.	Laurent-Perrier Cuvée Rosé	$40.00
50.	Doluca Neusah 1996	$12.00
13.	Montagny 1er Cru, les Loges Vieilles Vignes 1994	$20.00
51.	Doluca Antik 1995	$14.00
27.	Haut-Médoc, Château Lamothe Bergeron 1990	$30.00

THE VEGETARIAN CHOICE

Vegetarian Avocado Gâteau
crowned with a soured Lemon Cream

•

Mixed Tossed Salad

•

Mushroom Risotto

•

Pastry Chef's Iced Pralines

At Sea, Tuesday 12th August 1997

Courtesy Orient Lines

P & O CRUISES

Shandwick	c/o Princess Cruises
3 Grosvenor Gardens	10100 Santa Monica Blvd.
London, SW1W 0BD	Los Angeles, California 90067
Tel: 0171-808-6600	
Fax: 0171-808-6700	

ARCADIA: (formerly *Fairmajesty* and *Star Princess*); entered service 1989; 63,524 G.R.T.; 811' x 105'; 1,500-passenger capacity; 748 cabins; international officers and crew. **(Category B—Not Rated)**

AURORA: will enter service 2000; 76,000 G.R.T.; 886' x 106'; 1,975-passenger capacity; 934 cabins; international officers and crew.

MINERVA: entered service 1996; 12,500 G.R.T.; 128 meters x 20 meters; 300-passenger capacity; 197 cabins. (Operated by Swan Hellenic.)

ORIANA: entered service 1995; 69,153 G.R.T.; 853' x 106'; 1,800-passenger capacity; 914 cabins; British officers and mixed crew; cruises around the world and around Europe. **(Category B—Not Rated)**

VICTORIA: (formerly *Kungsholm* and *Sea Princess*); entered service 1966; refurbished 1978 and 1986; 27,620 G.R.T.; 660' x 87'; 726-passenger capacity; 370 cabins; British officers and mixed crew; cruises around the world. **(Category C—Not Rated)**

(Medical Facilities: [For all ships] C-0; P-2 [except *Victoria* has one]; EM, CLS, MS; N-4 [except *Victoria* has 2-3]; CM; PD; BC; EKG; TC; PO; EPC; OX; WC; OR; ICU; X; M; CCP.)

P & O (The Peninsular and Oriental Navigation Company) dates back to 1837 and is one of the oldest, most prestigious lines in the history of cruising. P & O purchased Princess Cruises in 1974 and ran most of its ships under the Princess flag during the 1980s. P & O markets the *Victoria* (formerly named *Sea Princess*) and *Oriana* under the P & O banner (*Canberra* left the line in 1997), with the major promotion to the British and European cruisers. P & O's Swan Hellenic division operates the *Minerva,* which replaces the *Orpheus* and offers eleven- to fifteen-day cultural cruises to the Mediterranean, Aegean, Red, and Black seas, as well as cruises around Britain, Scandinavia, and the Baltic.

Star Princess of Princess Cruises was refurbished and renamed *Arcadia;* she entered service for P & O Cruises in 1997.

The *Victoria* was inaugurated into service in 1966 as the *Kungsholm,* the pride of the now-defunct Swedish America Line. After a short stint for Flagship Cruises, she was acquired by P & O in 1978, refurbished, and renamed *Sea Princess.* However, she was not transferred to the Princess operation until 1986, where she remained until 1991, after which she returned to P & O. Recently she was renamed *Victoria.*

This is a ship of the sixties, with many spacious cabins, high ceilings, and real wood in the public areas. There are 370 accommodations, including 6 suites with double beds. Eighty-four cabins are on the inside, and 36 will accommodate a third person. Atop the ship on Lido Deck are two outdoor pools, the sun area, the Lido buffet, and the Carib Lounge. Directly below are the main show lounge, theater, boutiques, bars, and numerous cabins. Below, on A Deck, are the purser's office, the 6 suites, and the more expensive accommodations. The remaining cabins are on B, C, and D decks; the dining room is also on C Deck; and the indoor pool, sauna, Jacuzzi, and spa are at the bottom of the ship, on E Deck.

Prices on the *Victoria* range from approximately $190 per person per night for an inside cabin up to $655 for a luxury suite, with $260 being about average for an outside cabin.

The *Oriana* was the first P & O (non-Princess division) ship built in decades, and was designed to be marketed primarily to the British as an upscale, more modern vessel than *Victoria.* At 69,000 tons, 850 feet long, and with accommodations for up to 1,800 passengers, it is the largest ship in the P & O fleet, and has received a most enthusiastic reception by British cruisers wishing to sail on this more updated high-tech vessel capable of speeds up to 25 knots. The ten passenger decks are serviced by ten elevators and include eleven categories of cabins and suites including eight 500-square-foot suites with private balconies, 16 deluxe 300-square-foot cabins with private balconies, 590 cabins with twin beds that are convertible to double beds (94 have balconies and 254 are inside), 112 doubles also sold as singles, and 132 three- and four-berth cabins. Half the cabins have bathtubs and all have color TVs, radios, refrigerators, direct-dial telephones, and personal safes—all in keeping with the ships built in the nineties.

Atop ship is the observation lounge. Immediately beneath is the health spa with sauna, steam, whirlpools, massage and beauty-treatment rooms, and exercise and aerobics facilities. Adjacent is a large swimming pool, a vast sun deck area, and an indoor-outdoor lido buffet breakfast-and-lunch restaurant with an adjoining bar. The majority of cabins and suites are located on the next three decks.

Then comes D Deck, where you will find the Curzon Room, an alternate lounge for concerts, dining, and afternoon tea; the library; the cardroom; writing room; 189-seat, tiered cinema; video arcade; teen disco; the Peter Pan children's playroom; and children's pool area. On Promenade Deck, next below, is the 650-seat production theater, photo gallery, several bars and lounges, a casino, slot machine area, and disco. E Deck, below that, is the site of 81 cabins, the two dining rooms, and the bottom of the atrium area where the shops are located. The remaining cabins and reception desk are located on F Deck, and the medical center and night nursery are on G Deck.

Do not expect the overall experience to be the same as that found on P & O's Princess Cruises subsidiary. Dining is geared to British tastes, and the clientele tend not to have experienced the more deluxe cruise lines and therefore are more accepting. The waiters are largely from Goa and other areas in India.

From January through April, the vessels offer world cruises departing from Southampton, with the option to purchase segments of various lengths.

Arcadia, formerly the *Star Princess,* at 63,524 tons and measuring 811' x 105', entered service in 1989. She can accommodate 1,500 passengers in 748 cabins located on fourteen decks. There are 583 cabins outside and 165 inside, with 14 luxury suites and 36 junior suites, all of which feature terrace-verandas. All cabins have twin beds that convert to doubles and four-channel radio and color TV. One hundred fifty cabins have pull-out upper berths. There are three swimming pools, one with a swim-up bar, and four poolside Jacuzzis, an 800-seat two-level horse-shoe-shaped main showroom with a retractable stage, running track, a multitiered main dining room, a state-of-the-art gym/aerobics/sauna-massage center, a 270-degree glass-domed observation lounge, children's facilities, and a pizzeria. This ship was transferred to the P & O fleet in September 1997.

Because most of the passengers are British and there is a cross-section of cruisers from other European countries and around the world, the ships offer a chance for North Americans to mix with people of other nationalities.

In the spring of 1997 P & O ordered a new 76,000-ton, 1,975-passenger ship named *Aurora* and to be delivered in 2000. The 934 cabins will include two-deck penthouse suites, 10 suites with balconies, 18 mini-suites with balconies, 368 additional staterooms and cabins with balconies, and 22 cabins that accommodate disabled passengers. All cabins will include coffee and tea-making facilities, refrigerators, private safes, color televisions, direct-dial telephones, and twin beds convertible to queens. Among several dining options, a bistro-style restaurant will be open 24 hours a day. The ship will also feature expanded facilities for children and teens.

Strong Points:

Exceptional around-the-world itineraries at considerably lower prices than the more luxurious cruise lines. The ships especially appeal to a British clientele.

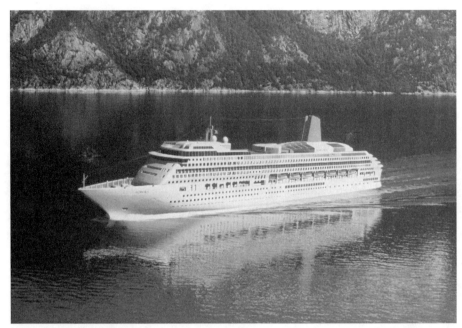

Aurora, *courtesy P & O Cruises*

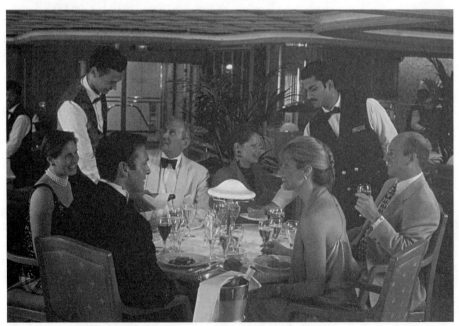

Restaurant on Oriana, *courtesy P & O Cruises*

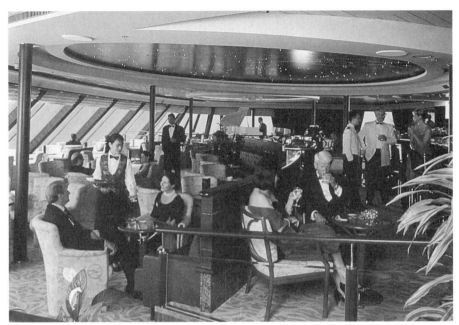

Crows Nest Bar on Oriana, *courtesy P & O Cruises*

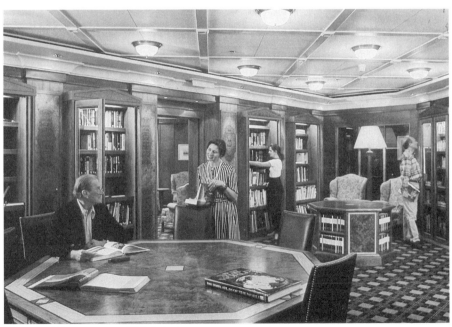

Library on Oriana, *courtesy of P & O Cruises*

ORIANA

D5

Your Executive Chef is Ralph Winzinger

From the Wine Cellar

White:
Crown of Crowns Liebfraumilch Langenbach - £8.50

Red:
Merlot Errazuriz - Chile - £7.50

Coffee and Liqueurs are also available in the Crows Nest,
The Curzon Room and Tiffany's

So much on, crunch on, take your muncheon
Breakfast, supper, dinner, luncheon!
Robert Browning

ᴎ Denotes vegetarian choice
✿ indicates dishes which may be served with or without a sauce

A matter of choice
Fish can be served either as a fish course or main course
Large portions are available on request, please notify your Steward

❀ Gravadlax of Salmon with a Light Dill and Mustard Sauce

ઢ Corn on the Cob with Melted Butter

Caesar Salad

❖

ઢ Cream of Asparagus

Essence of Beef with Oxtail and toasted Pine Kernels

❖

Medallions of Monkfish with Noodles
enriched with butter, lemon zest and parsley

❀ Roast Rib of Beef with Yorkshire Pudding, Gravy and Roast Potatoes

❀ Sauté of Lamb's Kidneys with Creamed Spinach and Dijon Mustard Sauce

Panfried Breast of Chicken
with ginger, spring onions and braised bok choy topped with sesame seeds

ઢ Vegetable Roulade with a Tomato Coulis

Fine Beans   Panache of Vegetables   Savoyarde and Boiled Potatoes

❖

❀ Warm Apple and Cherry Strudel with Crème Anglaise
Banana and Pecan Nut Sundae
❀ Peppered Pineapple with a Sauce of Crème de Cacao with Vanilla Ice Cream
Vanilla, Mint Choc Chip and Strawberry Ice Creams
Sweet Sauces: Butterscotch Chocolate Melba
Fresh Fruit Salad
Mango Sorbet

❖

A selection of British and Continental Cheeses with Biscuits

Fresh Fruit

❖

Freshly Brewed Coffee   De-Caffeinated   Espresso   Cappuccino   Speciality Teas
After Dinner Mints

Fresh from the Bakery
White, Wholemeal, Malted Wheat and Sun Dried Tomato Rolls

Courtesy P & O Cruises

Sunday, 18th October 1998

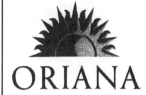

ORIANA TODAY

8.30pm & 10.30pm
Theatre Royal

The Stadium Theatre Company
proudly presents

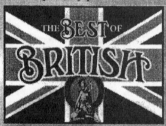

A cavalcade of favourite music, laughter and stars
from the very best of British radio and television
entertainment over the years - including
'Workers Playtime',
'Sunday Night at the London Palladium',
'Last Night of the Proms' and 'Celtdance'.

9.00pm - 12.45am
Pacific Lounge

with

Kenny Johnson & Northwind

and

Neon Moon

We begin the evening at 9.00pm with **Neon Moon** and 10.45pm
with a chance to practice any new line dances you have learnt.
Then at 9.45pm and 11.45pm **Kenny Johnson & Northwind** continue the country
theme as they play the hits for you to dance or relax to.
A must for all country fans!

9.30pm Tunes in Tiffany's
Stave off your thirst as you hear *Alan Christie* tinkle those ivories tonight in *Tiffany's*.

9.45pm With a View to Dancing
By Design will be pleased to have your company in the *Crow's Nest* whether you are dancing or enjoying their great sound.

9.45pm Boulevard Entertain
In the mood for dancing? *Boulevard* make some of the best sounds around that'll get you up on your feet dancing to the beat. *Harlequins*

10.30pm Syndicate Quiz
Get the fizz if you win the quiz. Come and join in the fun at tonight's teaser. *Crichton's*

10.45pm Checkmate
Continue dancing the night away to more great music in *Harlequins*.

10.45pm Alan Christie's Request Time
More music from our superb pianist as he plays familiar favourites in the *Crow's Nest*.

11.15pm Prepare to Party with Boulevard
Our guest band pull out all the stops to keep you up on your feet dancing to their fabulous beat in *Harlequins*. Remember the night is still young!

11.30pm Dance to the Duo
Sweet sounds from *By Design* as they take you through to a brand new day. *Crow's Nest*

12.15am Disco Dance Date
Our Debonair DJ will be spinning the discs as all you disco dollies boogie into tomorrow. *Harlequins*

12.30am Late Night Date
Scale the heights to the Room with a View where *By Design* make the midnight melodies. *Crow's Nest*

SUPERLATIVE TRAVEL

Clive Peterson, Tour Director will be available in the Crow's Nest between 10.00am and 11.00am to answer any queries you may have.

GOLF GET TOGETHER

Although we do not officially organise golf tours, any passengers who wish to play in port or borrow any clubs should meet *Pete* at noon in *Crichton's*.

WITHOUT RESERVATIONS

'Without reservations' means you may sit at any table on either sitting in either restaurant, subject to availability. When meals are served without reservations' the port side window tables are designated smoking areas.

TOURS OFFICE

Open 8.30am to noon, and 3.30pm to 5.30pm. *Jackie* and *Nikki* will be available to assist you with bookings.

BOOKINGS FOR TOURS IN TENERIFE MUST CLOSE A T 5.30PM THIS EVENING

TENERIFE
Tour E - Taganana Village and Mercedes Forest, due to a landslide this tour has had to be cancelled.

PORT ENHANCEMENT TALKS - TENERIFE AND GRAN CANARIA
Chaplin's Cinema 11.15am and 4.45pm.
Today *Greville* will describe in his illustrated talk our visits to the Canary Islands of Tenerife and Gran Canaria. There are two large cities to explore and also some spectacular tours to consider.
These talks can also be viewed on *channel 3* of the cabin TV circuit.

FOOD COMMENT FORMS

For your convenience we have installed outside the Peninsular and Oriental Restaurants passenger comment boxes and forms so that should you wish to express a concern or some satisfaction you are more than welcome.
There is also a box in the Conservatory on the port side by the doors to the lifts.

WINE TALK

At 11.00am in the *Curzon Room*, Head Wine Steward *Bisht Satinder* will be giving an informative illustrated talk on some of the wines served on Oriana.

SPECIAL OFFER

Later in the cruise we will be offering the following special take ashore bottle offers.

Whyte & MacKay Special Scotch Whisky
£6.50 per litre

Beefeater London Gin
£6.50 per litre

Please hand a completed and signed bar chit to your Cabin Steward who will deliver the bottle to your cabin towards the end of the cruise.

CHAPLIN'S CINEMA

11.15am & 4.45pm
Port Enhancement Talk - Tenerife and Gran Canaria

2.30pm
Songwriter
Drama starring Willie Nelson and Kris Kristofferson
Running time 91 minutes, certificate 15

6.00pm
Children's Magic Show

8.30pm & 10.30pm
A Perfect Murder
Drama with Michael Douglas and Gwyneth Paltrow
Running time 105 minutes, certificate 15

DINING HOURS

CONSERVATORY

Early Bird	6.30am to 7.00am
Hot Breakfast	7.00am to 10.00am
Continental Breakfast	10.00am to 11.00am
Buffet Luncheon	noon to 2.00pm
Afternoon Tea	3.30pm to 4.30pm
Children's Tea	5.15pm to 5.45pm
	(starboard side only)

PENINSULAR & ORIENTAL RESTAURANTS
Breakfast - *without reservations*
First sitting - *Doors close at 8.15am* 8.00am
Second sitting - *Doors close at 9.15am* ... 9.00am

Luncheon - *without reservations*
First sitting - *Doors close at 12.30pm* ... 12.15pm
Second sitting - *Doors close at 1.45pm* ... 1.30pm

Afternoon Tea
Peninsular Restaurant only . 4.00pm to 4.45pm

Dinner - *with reservations*
First sitting 6.30pm
Second sitting 8.30pm

Oriana Sandwich Bar
Peninsular Restaurant only
.... 11.30pm to midnight

PIZZERIA AL FRESCO

Continuous service .... from Noon to 7.00pm

LIBRARY

9.00am - 12.30pm
2.30pm - 5.30pm
9.30pm - 10.30pm

IN THE BARS

Andersons	11.00am until 2.00pm & 5.00pm until late
Crow's Nest	11.00am until 2.00pm & 5.00pm until late
Harlequins	10.30am to noon & 8.30pm until late
Lord's Tavern	11.00am until late
Pacific Lounge	4.00pm to 5.00pm & 8.30pm until late
Riviera Bar	9.00am until 7.00pm
Splash Bar	11.00am until 6.00pm
Terrace Bar	9.00am until 7.00pm
Tiffany's	9.00am until noon & 5.00pm until midnight

Passengers under 18 years of age will not be served alcoholic beverages. Please understand that you may be requested to show identification indicating date of birth.

Cocktail of the Day
Brandy Alexander   £1.50
Smooth and creamy, with brandy, Creme de Cacao and cream.

Virgin Cocktail
Orchard Dream Fizz   90p
A blend of apple juice, grapefruit juice, a dash of Grenadine and soda.

Speciality Coffee
French Café   £1.20
Cointreau.

TODAY'S EVENTS

7.55am **Navigator's Early Morning Call**
Tune into TV *channel 8* for the *Navigator's* early morning broadcast with up to date weather, geographical details and other points of interest. This will also be broadcast over the open decks.

9.00am **Social Short Tennis**
A chance to make a racket and have a ball. Any players wishing for a friendly game should meet in the *Sun Deck Nets* at this time.

9.45am **Choir Practice**
Let's hear those harmonies. *Cathy* takes you through the hymns for this morning's service. *Theatre Royal*

9.45am **Keep Fit**
No time to waste, so just make haste and lose those inches from your waist. Join *Alison* in *Harlequins.*

10.00am **Walk & Talk**
Ramble as you amble around the Promenade. Meet outside the *Pacific Lounge.*

10.00am **Games Handout**
A chance for you to monopolise the games cupboard as you search for your favourites. *Library*

10.00am **Hand and Nail Care Demonstration**
Dry, brittle or cracked nails, or your nails simply won't grow? Join Steiner the nail care experts today and find a way to beautiful hands. *Medina Room*

10.15am
Theatre Royal
Ship's Church Service
This morning's service will be conducted by **Captain Colin Campbell**. There will a collection made for marine charities

10.30am **Coffee Chat**
Thirsty for conversation. Time to relax for a while with a cuppa and a chat with some of the team in the *Curzon Room.*

10.30am **Travelling Alone Get Together**
Don't sit there feeling all alone, we're here to make you feel at home. *Tiffany's*

10.30am **American Line Dancing for First Sitting Passengers**
Calling all Beginner Bootscooters. Hold on to your holster and make for *Harlequins* as today *Chris* will be revising what you learnt yesterday before starting on a fun new dance. Yeehah!

10.45am **Ship in a Bottle with Ted Machin and Norman Rogers**
Assembly of the ship continues with the mainsail and rigging lines being finalised and secured. *Crow's Nest*

11.00am **Wine Talk**
Head Wine Steward **Bisht Santinder** will be giving an informative illustrated talk on the wine served on Oriana with particular reference to some of the interesting bin ends available. *Curzon Room*

11.00am **Deck Quoits**
Make it your target to compete in this morning's game. *Deck 13 Aft*

11.00am **Shuffleboard**
Shuffle along and try your luck, will yours be the winning puck. *Deck 13 Aft*

11.00am
Pacific Lounge
'Madeira Wine'
An informal lecture by *Ana Isabel Dantas* of The Old Blandy Wine Lodge Madeira Wine Company. Win a fabulous prize of some Madeira wine. Complete the quiz sheet in your cabin and return it to the *Reception Desk* by 6.00pm on the 18th October. Prizes will be announced at 10.30am on the 19th in the *Pacific Lounge.*

11.00am **Short Tennis Competition**
See if you can net yourself a prize in this morning's game. Suitable footwear must be worn. *Sun Deck Nets*

11.00am **Couples Massage Demonstration**
Let our experts teach you how to ease away those aches and pains. *Oasis Spa*

11.00am **Masonic Meeting**
All Brethren are invited to meet at this time in the *Iberia Room.*

11.15am **American Line Dancing for Second Sitting Passengers**
Calling all Beginner Bootscooters. *Chris* repeats his earlier class in *Harlequins.* Yeehah!

11.15am **Daily Tote**
Come and guess how far Oriana has steamed from noon yesterday until noon today. 50p a go. Cash only please - bet you win! *Lord's Tavern*

11.15am **Port Enhancement Talk - Tenerife and Gran Canaria**
Greville Rimbault gives an informative, illustrated talk on Tenerife and Gran Canaria. This will be repeated at 4.45pm and can also be seen on *channel 3* of your cabin circuits. *Chaplin's Cinema*

11.30am
Lord's Tavern
Singalong with Checkmate
The trio choose those cheery songs that'll get you humming along.

Noon **Announcement from the Bridge**
Details of ship's position, present and predicted weather, and mileage report. Have you won the Daily Tote? If so collect your winnings from *Lord's Tavern.*

Noon **Golf Get Together**
Crichton's

Noon
Crow's Nest
Sounds of Jazz
The Rick Laughlin Trio jazz up your lunchtime as they play for your listening pleasure.

2.00pm **Eye and Neck Care Seminar**
The eyes and neck area are very delicate and unfortunately show visibly early signs of the ageing process. Join your on board therapist for the correct advice today. *Medina Room*

2.30pm **Bridge Get Together**
Anyone wishing to play rubber bridge should meet in *Crichton's* at this time.

2.45pm **Adult Cricket**
Don't be caught out. Join us for an afternoon game in the *Sun Deck Nets.*

2.45pm **Whist Drive**
It's on the cards you'll be able to get a game in *Crichton's Aft.*

2.45pm **Make-up Made Easy with Viv Foley**
Viv shows you how to do make-up easily with no fuss. *Viv* will also look at eye shapes. Please bring a lipstick with you. *Crow's Nest.*

2.45pm **Advanced Line Dancing with Dawn Jordan**
Dawn revises what you learnt yesterday before tackling another new dance. *Harlequins*

2.45pm **Shuffleboard**
Paddle up and make your way to *Deck 13 Aft* where you can try your luck with the puck.

2.45pm **Beginner's Dance Class**
If you missed yesterday's class, it's not too late. Join *Ian* and *Ruth* as they continue their light hearted instruction. Today they will revise your basic steps in the Social Foxtrot and Cha Cha Cha. Also at today's class, have fun with the Merengue. *Pacific Lounge*

3.00pm **Perfume Talk**
Join *Hayley* as she describes the various perfumes available from the Knightsbridge Shop on board. *Iberia Room*

3.00pm **Deck Quoits**
Make it your aim to join one of the team for this competition and you could be on target for a prize. *Deck 13 Aft*

3.15pm **Aromaspa Demonstration**
The ultimate in body wraps, using the richness of seaweed combined with aromatherapy oils. This is followed by a facial and half body massage. Learn more about it with our specialist. *Oasis Spa*

3.30pm **Games Handout**
All of your favourites will be available from the *Library.*

4.00pm **Social Short Tennis**
See if you can meet your match and maybe net yourself a P&O prize. *Sun Deck Nets*

4.00pm **Ship in a Bottle with Ted Machin and Norman Rogers**
This afternoon's class is devoted to those who require a little help. *Crow's Nest*

4.15pm **Jackpot Bingo**
Hughie and the team will be calling out the lucky numbers and today it could be you. *Pacific Lounge*

4.15pm **Captain's Coketail Party**
Captain Colin Campbell meets our younger cruisers in *Harlequins.* All adults are welcome to attend.

4.45pm **Port Enhancement Talk - Tenerife and Gran Canaria**
Greville Rimbault repeats his informative talk on Tenerife and Gran Canaria. *Chaplin's Cinema*

5.15pm **Colours for Men and Women with Viv Foley**
Viv repeats her talk on colours and how the right colours make you look healthy and successful. *Medina Room*

5.30pm **Individual Quiz**
Twenty teasers to test the grey matter and if you have the highest score a prize could be yours. *Crichton's*

5.30pm **Football**
Can we corner you into joining in a fun kick around in the *Sun Deck Nets?*

5.45pm **Cocktail Set**
Alan Christie's music takes you to new heights in the *Crow's Nest* as you enjoy an aperitif and *Rick Laughlin* plays in *Tiffany's.*

6.00pm **Radio Oriana**
The *Pete Le Gros* radio show will be playing your requests and keeping you up to date with the activities on board so tune into *channel 6* on your cabin circuits and 7317 is the number to call.

7.45pm **Cocktail Melodies**
Alan Christie makes the music in the 'room at the top' as you enjoy the sounds and the views around and **Gary Jones** plays in *Tiffany's.*

8.30pm & 10.30pm
Theatre Royal
The Stadium Theatre Company presents BEST OF BRITISH

9.00pm - 12.45am
Pacific Lounge
COUNTRY MUSIC SPECIAL with Kenny Johnson & Northwind and Neon Moon

9.00pm **A Step in Time**
Checkmate ask you to put on your dancing shoes and dance the night away in *Harlequins.*

PREMIER CRUISES

901 South America Way

Miami, Florida 33132

(800) 992-4299

(305) 358-5122

(305) 358-4807 FAX

OCEANIC (THE BIG RED BOAT): (formerly *Oceanic* and *Star/Ship Oceanic*); entered service 1965; refurbished 1985 and 1993; 38,772 G.R.T.; 782' x 96'; 1,800-passenger capacity; 574 cabins; international officers and crew; three- and four-night cruises from Port Canaveral to the Bahamas.

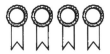

(Medical Facilities: C-0; P-1; CLS, MS; N-2; CM; PD; EKG; TC; PO; EPC; OX; WC; OR; ICU; LJ.)

SS *ISLANDBREEZE:* (formerly *S. A. Vaal, Transvaal Castle,* and *Festivale*); entered service 1961; refurbished 1978, 1986, 1995, and 1997; 38,175 G.R.T.; 760' x 90'; 1,146-passenger capacity; 583 cabins; international officers and crew; seven-night southeast and southwest Caribbean itineraries from Santo Domingo.

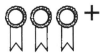

OCEANBREEZE: (formerly *Azure Seas*); entered service 1955; refurbished 1980, 1992, and 1997; 21,486 G.R.T.; 604' x 78'; 776-passenger capacity; 388 cabins; international officers and crew; seven-night cruises from Jamaica to Panama Canal, and Central and South America (under charter 1999 and 2000).

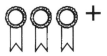

REMBRANDT: (formerly *Rotterdam*); entered service 1959; refurbished 1969, 1972, 1987, 1990, and 1997; 38,650 G.R.T.; 748' x 94'; 1,075-passenger capacity; 565 cabins; international officers and crew.

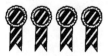

(Medical Facilities: P-1; CLS, MS; N-2; CM; PD; BC; EKG; TC; PO; EPC; OX; WC; OR; ICU; X; M; CCP; LJ.)

SEABREEZE 1: (formerly *Starship Royale* and *Federico C*); entered service 1958; refurbished 1982, 1989, 1990, and 1991; 21,000 G.R.T.; 605' x 79'; 840-passenger capacity; 421 cabins; international officers and crew; alternate seven-day cruises from Miami to eastern and western Caribbean and summer cruises from New York.

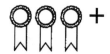

SEAWIND CROWN: (formerly *Infante Dom Henrique* and *Vasco Da Gama*); entered service 1961; renovated 1989, 1994, and 1997; 23,306 G.R.T.; 642' x 81'; 724-passenger capacity; 362 cabins; international officers and crew; seven-night cruises from Aruba.

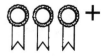

(Medical Facilities: C-2; P-1; EM, CLS, MS; N-1; CM; PD; EKG; TC; PO; EPC; OX; WC; OR; ICU; CCP.)

The predecessor Premier Cruise Line was founded in 1983 with the intent of running three- and four-night cruises to the Bahamas from Port Canaveral in conjunction with land packages to Walt Disney World and the Kennedy Space Center.

Premier first purchased the *Federico C* from Costa Cruise Lines, refurbished her, and put her in service as the *Star/Ship Royale* in 1984. Next came the purchase of the *Oceanic* from Home Lines for $20 million. After investing another $10 million into refurbishing and interior designs by Michael Katzourakis, the *Oceanic,* with a new red exterior, joined the *Royale* in April 1986.

Early in 1989, the *Royale* was transferred to Dolphin Cruise Line and the *Atlantic,* formerly of Home Lines, and the *Majestic,* formerly the *Sun Princess* of Princess Cruises, were added to the Premier fleet. In January 1995 the *Majestic* was leased to another cruise line, and in 1997 the *Atlantic* was sold to Mediterranean Shipping Cruises.

Dolphin Cruise Line commenced cruise operations in 1984 with the *Dolphin VI,* which it leased from Paquet Cruises. In 1989 Dolphin Cruise Line purchased the S/S *Royale* from Premier, the former *Federico C* of Costa Line, refurbished her, and renamed the ship *Seabreeze.* In 1992 the 740-passenger *Azure Seas* was acquired from Admiral Cruises and renamed *Oceanbreeze.* In 1996 the *Islandbreeze* was acquired from Carnival Cruise Lines, where it had sailed as the *Festivale.*

The *Seawind Crown* was converted from the cruise ship *Vasco Da Gama* in 1989 and acquired by Cruise Holdings, Inc., in 1991. In 1997 Cruise Holdings, Inc. entered into agreements with Premier Cruise Line, Seawind Cruise Line, and Dolphin Cruise Line to combine their ships under one banner, to be known as Premier Cruises. After a multimillion-dollar refurbishment of the vessels and a consolidation of finance, administration, sales, marketing, and on-board passenger services, the new line commenced operations in September 1997 as "Premier Cruises."

At the same time, it acquired the *Rotterdam* from Holland America Lines and renamed her *Rembrandt.*

The Big Red Boat caters to the family trade, offering attractive family holidays consisting of three- or four-night sailings to the Bahamas, a tour of the Kennedy Space Center or the U.S. Astronauts' Hall of Fame, and the balance of the week at Disney World or Universal Studios and Sea World. Of course, the cruise can be booked separately. A number of the cabins can accommodate five family members.

A minimum cabin on the three-night weekend cruise goes for $99-$199 per person per night (including port charges), an outside cabin from $136-$263, and a deluxe ocean-view suite for $336. Third, fourth, and fifth passengers sharing the cabin pay $99 per night and children 2-9 only $66. The air-sea-land packages are very attractive.

Formerly the *Oceanic,* the pride and joy of the Home Lines, was one of the largest and most popular ships sailing the Caribbean in the 1960s and 1970s. The ship received a second major refurbishment in 1992 and 1993; however, cabins and public indoor and outdoor areas do not have the modern look of the ships built in the eighties and nineties. Typical of ships of its vintage, a majority of the cabins (338 of the 574) are inside. There are 65 suites. The 8 largest, located atop the ship on Sun Deck, are quite large, with two bathrooms, balconies, and a separate parlor that converts into a second bedroom.

Also on Sun Deck are a jogging track and a small fitness room. On Pool Deck there are two small swimming pools surrounded by outdoor dining tables and chairs, a whirlpool, and a few lounges. The pool and outdoor dining area can be enclosed by a retractable glass megadome in bad weather. There is no steam or sauna, and outdoor lounges are limited. Sunrise Terrace and Satellite Cafe, the locations for buffet breakfasts and lunches, as well as the ice-cream parlor, are also located on Pool Deck.

The children's recreation center is on Premier Deck, and on Lounge Deck are the 600-seat Broadway Showroom; the Starlight Cabaret, site of late-night dancing and entertainment; the Heroes and Legends Pub; the cruise tour office; the Lucky Star Casino; the Space Station Teen Center, which has video games; and an enclosed veranda. Most of the cabins are located on Premier and Continental, Restaurants, Atlantic, and Bahamas decks. The 7 Continents Restaurant seats 750 passengers and offers meals in two seatings.

On a recent cruise on the *Oceanic,* I was impressed with the quality of the food and service in the dining room but not at the Satellite Cafe, as well as the cruise's overall appeal to the entire family. Originally, the ship featured Walt Disney characters at special events throughout the cruise; however, with Disney entering the cruise market, Looney Tunes characters have been substituted under an agreement with Warner Brothers. Youth counselors provide supervised activities and special programs for the youngsters.

The Big Red Boat presently offers Monday and Friday departures to Nassau and Port Lucaya in the Bahamas. At a fraction of the cost of the more upscale Disney ships, the *Big Red Boat* offers a less expensive, no-frills option for families seeking a short cruise from Port Canaveral.

The *Seawind Crown* commenced seven-night cruises from Aruba to Curaçao, Margarita Island, Barbados, and St. Lucia in October of 1991.

Originally built as a Portuguese ocean liner, *Infante Dom Henrique* was converted to the cruise ship *Vasco Da Gama* at a cost of $40 million in 1989. In 1994 fifty new staterooms were added, and various public areas were remodeled. All cabins were renovated and include refrigerators, TVs, and hair dryers. The 2 deluxe suites, measuring 500 square feet each, and the 6 additional suites atop the ship are the most desirable accommodations, and include additional amenities and up to $240 worth of free shore excursions.

The outside deck area includes two swimming pools, a bar, and an area to walk or jog. Entertainment and dancing take place in the large show lounge, the more intimate Panorama Lounge, and the disco. Activities and entertainment parallel those of most other cruise ships.

Because her home base is in Aruba, passengers from the U.S. will require a full day of travel in each direction. However, once aboard, ship passengers have ample time to visit four of the Caribbean's more desirable ports (Curacao, Caracas, Barbados, and St. Lucia), which are not accessible on seven-day cruises from Miami.

On-board facilities include two swimming pools, a sauna, beauty salon, volleyball court, a fitness room, a casino, cinema, boutiques, and several bars, nightclubs, and lounges.

Dolphin Cruise Line commenced cruise operations in 1984 with the *Dolphin IV,* which it leased from Paquet Cruises. In 1989 Dolphin Cruise Line purchased the S/S *Royale,* the former *Federico C* of Costa Line, from Premier. The ship was refurbished, renamed *Seabreeze 1,* and presently offers seven-day cruises from Miami to the eastern and western Caribbean.

In 1992 the 740-passenger *Azure Seas* was acquired from Admiral Cruises and renamed *Oceanbreeze.* Commencing in 1998, she offers seven-night cruises from

Jamaica to the Panama Canal and Central and South America. In 1999 and 2000 she is under charter to another company.

The *Islandbreeze* was acquired from Carnival Cruise Lines in 1996, where it had formerly sailed as the *Festivale*. During the summer she is under charter; however, during the rest of the year she offers southeast and southwest Caribbean itineraries from Santo Domingo.

Cruise-only prices for seven-night cruises on all Premier ships start at $1,198 per person, with top suites going for $2,398. The ships also offer attractive pre- and post-cruise land packages (which are free for passengers in the higher state-room categories), as well as air add-ons from major U.S. gateways.

Dining on these ships was historically a notch above its competitors. Considering the full range of activities and entertainment, these ships offer an excellent bargain in the economy-cruise marketplace. However, these are older ships, and cabins in all categories are quite small, plumbing is not always state of the art, the overall service staff is not as well honed as on premium and luxury category vessels, and the ships physically pale when compared with those built in the eighties and nineties.

Strong Points:

The *Big Red Boat* offers an excellent no-frills family vacation with above-average food, service, and entertainment for an economy category ship. All of the Premier ships offer full-fledged cruise experiences at bargain prices on older vessels. The *Rembrandt* was a very respected grande dame when it sailed as the *Rotterdam* for Holland America, and still retains much of its traditional ocean-liner charm.

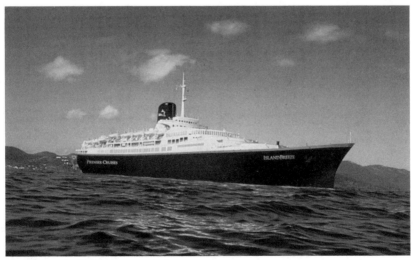

Courtesy Premier Cruises

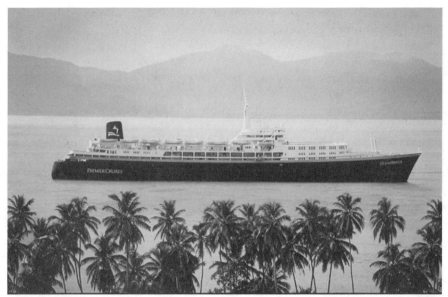

Courtesy Premier Cruises

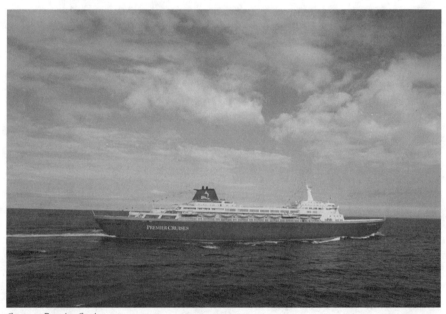

Courtesy Premier Cruises

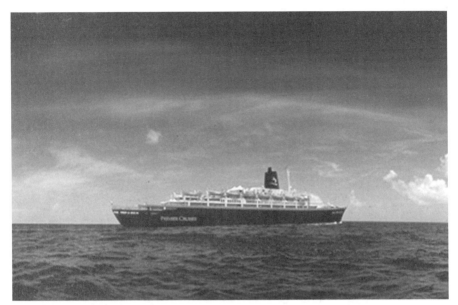

Courtesy Premier Cruises

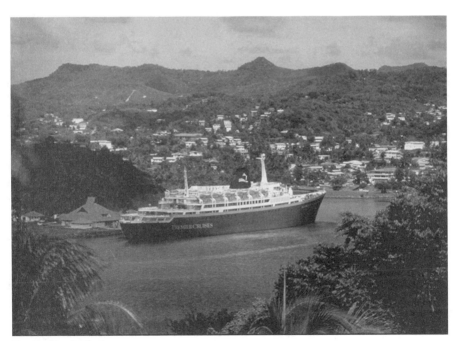

Courtesy Premier Cruises

MENU

Appetizers

Pineapple Gondola
Fresh Pineapple wedge with shredded Coconut

Duck Terrine with Truffle served with a Red
Wine Onion Confit

Escargot a la Bourguignonne

Soup

Chicken Bouillon Fragrant with Tarragon

Lobster Bisque with Cognac

Spiced Chilled Fruit Soup

Salads

Garden Mixed Greens with Sliced Tomatoes and Cucumbers

Mimosa Salad with Lettuce, Chopped boiled Egg, Alfalfa Sprouts
and Cherry Tomatoes

Choice of Dressings
Goombay, Ranch, Red Wine, Vinaigrette

O–D2

Entrees

Catch of the Day
Your waiter will explain today's catch and its preparation
Suggested Wine: Kendall Jackson Chardonnay, Vinters Reserve $28.00

Linguine
Tossed with Light Cream Sauce, Prosciutto and Basil Leaves
Suggested Wine: Trapiche Chardonnay $18.00

Broiled Lobster Tail
Served with Tarragon Butter Sauce
Suggested Wine: Pouilly-Fuissé

Veal Cutlet Natural
Pan Fried with a Ragout of Forest Mushrooms
Suggested Wine: Deloach Merlot $25.00

Beef Tournedos
Tenderloin of Beef grilled to your preference, with Eggplant and Anchovy Fillet offered with Green Peppercorn Sauce
Suggested Wine: Raymond Cabernet Sauvignon $28.00

Vegetarian
Stir Fried Vegetables with Potato Pie

Fresh Vegetables and Potatoes to accompany the Entrees

Today's Deserts Presented by your Waiter

Coffee   Tea   Iced Tea   Milk

O-D2

Courtesy Premier Cruises

Welcome to Port Lucaya!

Welcome to beautiful Port Lucaya, Grand Bahama Island. We will begin our tendering operation to this beautiful new port, upon arrival at 8:30 AM. Port Lucaya offers a wide array of activities for the exploring tourist. From sight-seeing or casino action, we hope you enjoy the Bahamas newest destination, Port Lucaya. **Looney Tunes tuck-in or personal visit for your children. Just call the Bugs Hot Line "BUGS" (2847). (Limited availability)**

Time		Activities	Location
6:00	- 7:30	Early Riser's Coffee and Danish.	Satellite Cafe
6:00 am	-11:00 pm	Exercise Room Open.	Sun Deck
7:30		Main Seating Breakfast is served.	Seven Continents
7:30	- 10:30 am	Pool Side Buffet Breakfast.	Satellite Cafe
7:30		Walk a Mile with your Fitness Director.	Gym
8:00	- 8:45 am	Yoga, stretch and relaxation.	Tiki Bar
8:00	- 8:30 pm	**Steiners Hair & Beauty Salon open.** Mini facials for only $20.00! Combos available for $59.00! French braids–$10.00	Continental Deck
8:00	- 10:30 am	**SPLASHDOWN/TOUR DESK OPEN FOR PORT LUCAYA SNORKELING AND TOURS.** Stroller rentals also available.	Lounge Deck
8:30		**TENDERING OPERATION BEGINS TO PORT LUCAYA.** All tender procedures and issuing of tender tickets will take place in the Broadway Showroom. All tender tickets will be issued on a first come, first serve basis. Once you have your ticket, remain in the Broadway Showroom until your time of departure. (There is no charge for the ticket.) Don't forget to purchase your bottle of water in the Broadway Showroom before you go ashore. Please pay careful attention to the departure announcements.	Broadway Showroom
8:30		Splashdown Snorkeling trip meets.	Starlight Cabaret
8:45		Late Seating Breakfast is served.	Seven Continents
9:00	- 10:15	Step Areobics and cardiobox. Join your Fitness Director!	Tiki Bar
9:00	- 11:30 am	Shooting Star Photo Gallery Open for photos and videos.	Lounge Deck Aft
9:00		Galley Tour Tickets available at the Tour Desk. Come look "behind the scenes!"	Lounge Deck
9:30	- 10:30	**Meet & Greet with our Looney Tunes Characters!**	Broadway Showroom Lby
11:00		Personal Training available.	Gym
12:00	- 1:30 pm	Open Seating Lunch is served.	Seven Continents
1:30	- 3:00 pm	Buffet Lunch is served pool side on board the Star/Ship Oceanic.	Satellite Cafe
2:00	- 5:00 pm	Big Dipper Ice Cream Parlor Open. Make your own Sundae.	Pool Deck
3:00		Calling all Bridge Players!	Library
3:30	- 6:00 pm	Foot and Ankle Massage...only $20.00!	Pool Deck
4:00	- 12:00 am	Shooting Star Photo Gallery Open for photos and videos!	Lounge Deck Aft
4:00		**Juggling Workshop!** Join our Master Juggler as he teaches you how to juggle!	Lucky Star Lounge
4:15	- 5:15 pm	Afternoon Tea and Cakes.	Sunrise Terrace
4:30		**Grandfather's Beer Bash!** Calling all Grandpa's!	Heroes & Legends
4:30		**Grandmothers Brag Party!** Meet for tea with your Social Hostess, Jeannie!	Sunrise Terrace
4:30	- 5:00 pm	**Autograph Session with the Looney Tunes Characters.**	Broadway Showroom Lby
4:45		**FAMILY CASH SNOWBALL BINGO!** Jackpot could be well over $1000.	Broadway Showroom
5:00	- 7:00 pm	Music with "Steamer!" (Well drinks–$3.00 & Margaritas!)	Lucky Star Lounge
5:15	- 6:15 pm	Sail away party with "Natural Vibes!"	Tiki Bar
5:30		**DISEMBARKATION TALK.** Join your Cruise Director, Bob, for this brief, fun and informative meeting. At least one family member should attend.	Broadway Showroom
5:30	- 6:30 pm	Final adjustments at Tour Desk. Pick up your dolphin T-shirts.	Lounge Deck
5:30	- 6:30 pm	**SPLASHDOWN SNORKELERS!** Join your Splashdown Divers. Pick up your Splashdown Certificate. Splashdown T-shirts available.	Tour Desk
6:00		THE S/S OCEANIC SAILS FOR PORT CANAVERAL. LAST TENDER LEAVES PORT LUCAYA AT 5:30 PM!	
6:00		**Lucky Star Casino Open!** (Slots & Gaming Tables) Win card special–$10!	Lounge Deck

| 8:30 | (Main) | Premier Presents, direct from Las Vegas: | Broadway Showroom MC: Bob Brizendine |
| 10:30 | (Late) | *Starring: The Blues Brothers, Bobby Darin & Elvis Presley* | *Also a special Farewell from the Crew!* |

9:30	- 10:30 pm	Final adjustments at Tour Desk. Pick up your dolphin T-shirts.	Lounge Deck
9:30	- 10:30 pm	Port Lecturer, Nikki, is available for questions.	Tour Desk
9:30	- 12:30 am	Music with "Ray & Carla!" Come party the night away!	Lucky Star Lounge
9:30	- 10:30 pm	Late night snacks...pizza, ice cream and cookies.	Ice Cream Parlor
9:30	- ????	Poker Game starts! 7 card stud poker game. ($2–$5 limit)	Lucky Star Lounge
9:30		Party under the stars with "Natural Vibes!" (Drink Specials)	Tiki Bar
9:30		**BIG BAHAMA DERBY & FAMILY CASH SNOWBALL BINGO!** Bet on your favorite horse! Followed by Big Money Bingo! The Jackpot must go!	Broadway Showroom
10:00	- 12:00 am	Join "Marilyn Wood" for some great tunes.	Tropicana Lounge
10:00	- ????	Farewell Karaoke Show Time! Come and be a Star! (Adults Only!)	Heroes & Legends Pub
10:00	- ????	Let's jam to the music, back when it was still Rock 'n Roll!	Starlight Cabaret
11:30	- 12:30 am	Pizza Time! (16 oz. Draft Beer–$2.25!)	Heroes & Legends Pub
11:30		**BAHAMA BEACH PARTY!** Dance under the stars with the Cruise Staff and "Natural Vibes!" Bahamas Mamas and Yellow Bird drink specials only $3.00!	Lounge Deck Aft (Starlight Cabaret If bad weather)
11:45		**KENO DRAWING! Win up to $50,000.00!**	Lucky Star Lounge
12:00	- 1:00 am	**INTERNATIONAL MIDNIGHT BUFFET.**	Seven Continents

FRIDAY, ARRIVAL PORT CANAVERAL

The Star/Ship Oceanic arrives in Port Canaveral at 7:00 AM. DISEMBARKATION BEGINS AT APPROXIMATELY 9:00 AM. GUESTS WILL DISEMBARK FROM THE BROADWAY SHOWROOM.

6:00	- 8:00 am	Purser's Credit Desk Open.	Atlantic Deck
6:00	- 9:30 am	Coffee, Danish and Juices Only.	Satellite Cafe
7:00	- 7:45 am	Splashdown Desk Open for last minute business.	Lounge Deck
7:00		Main Seating Breakfast is Served.	Seven Continents
7:00	- 9:00 am	**TOUR DESK OPEN.** Last chance for Jungle Safari Tour Tickets!	Lounge Deck
7:30	- 10:00 am	Shooting Star Photo Gallery open for last minute photos and videos.	Lounge Deck Aft
7:55		**COMMENT CARD DRAWING! WIN A FREE CRUISE!**	Broadway Showroom
8:00		**DON'T MISS CRUISE BINGO! WIN A FREE CRUISE FOR TWO!**	Broadway Showroom
8:00		Lucky Star Lounge Open.	Lounge Deck Fwd.
8:15		Late Seating Breakfast is Served.	Seven Continents

NOTE: Farewell...Premier Cruise Lines trust that you have enjoyed this cruise and will have many a pleasant hour reliving your time on board the Star/Ship Oceanic. It has been our pleasure serving you and we sincerely hope that the future will bring us the opportunity of sailing with you again. We won't say good bye but "A Happy Landing!"

– Sincerely, Captain A. Passas

TODAY'S FEATURED MOVIE ON CHANNEL 6 & 13

"Ransom" & "James And The Giant Peach" ....

...... 8:00 AM, 12:00 Noon, 3:00 PM, 6:00 PM, 9:00 PM & 12:00 AM

Disembarkation Information will be shown continuously on channel 34 on your in-cabin TV

HELPFUL HINTS ON TIPPING

Dining Room Waiter	$12.00 Per Person
Busboy	$6.00 Per Person
Cabin Steward	$12.00 Per Person
Head Waiter	$3.00 Per Person

These gratuities for services rendered should be extended on the last night of the cruise. Some personnel are tipped as service is rendered; for example: Bar Waiter, Bartender, Wine Steward and Bell Boy.

PORT LUCAYA TENDER SCHEDULE

Tenders from the Star/Ship Oceanic to the Marketplace and from the Marketplace to the Star/Ship Oceanic

8:30 am*	11:00 am*	1:30 pm	4:00 pm
9:00 am*	11:30 am*	2:00 pm	4:30 pm
9:30 am*	12:00 pm*	2:30 pm	5:00 pm
10:00 am*	12:30 pm	3:00 pm	5:30 pm
10:30 am*	1:00 pm	3:30 pm	

*Tender Tickets will be required for these tenders. Please pick them up in the Broadway Showroom and remain there until you are called. All other tenders will depart from the Atlantic Deck, Midship; no tender tickets required. No tickets required from Marketplace to the Star/Ship Oceanic.

All tenders based on space availability and subject to change. The Lucaya Marketplace features island entertainment, shopping, a straw market and restaurants. The ship will sail at 6:00 pm. Last tender is at 5:30 pm. Tender ride takes approximately 20 minutes between Star/Ship Oceanic and the Marketplace.

Ask our Tour Staff about our Friday morning Jungle Safari and Airboat Family Adventure.

Courtesy Premier Cruises

PRINCESS CRUISES

10100 Santa Monica Boulevard

Los Angeles, California 90067

(800) 421-0522

(310) 284-2844 FAX

CROWN PRINCESS and *REGAL PRINCESS: Crown Princess* entered service in 1990 and *Regal Princess* entered service in 1991; 70,000 G.R.T.; 805' x 115'; 1,590-passenger capacity; 795 cabins; Italian officers, British and Italian staff, and international crew; cruises in the Caribbean, Alaska, Panama Canal, Hawaii-Tahiti, Mexico, and Costa Rica.

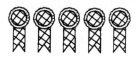

(Medical Facilities: C-10; P-2; EM, CLS, MS; N-5 [*Regal*], N-3 [*Crown*]; CM; PD; BC; EKG; TC; PO; EPC; OX; WC; OR [*Crown* only]; ICU; X; M; CCP.)

GRAND PRINCESS: entered service 1998; 109,000 G.R.T.; 935' x 118'; 2,600-passenger capacity; 1,300 cabins; British and Italian officers, international crew; Caribbean and European itineraries.

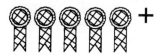

(Medical Facilities: C-28; P-2; EM, CLS, MS; N-3; CM; PD; BC; EKG; TC; PO; EPC; OX; WC; OR; ICU; X; M; CCP; TM.)

PACIFIC PRINCESS: (formerly *Sea Venture*); entered service 1970; renovated 1992; 20,000 G.R.T.; 550' x 80'; 640-passenger capacity; 320 cabins; British officers, international crew; cruises to Europe, Africa, and the Middle East.

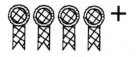

(Medical Facilities: C-2; P-1; EM, CLS, MS; N-2 to 3; CM; PD; BC; EKG; TC; PO; EPC; OX; WC; OR; ICU; X; M; CCP.)

ROYAL PRINCESS: entered service 1984; 44,348 G.R.T.; 761' x 95'; 1,200-passenger capacity; 600 cabins; British officers, international crew; cruises to Europe, Canada/New England, and South America.

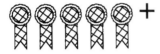

(Medical Facilities: C-4; P-2; EM, CLS, MS; N-3; CM; PD; BC; EKG; TC; PO; EPC; OX; WC; OR; ICU; X; M; CCP.)

SKY PRINCESS: (formerly *Fairsky*); entered service 1984; 46,314 G.R.T.; 789' x 91'; 1,200-passenger capacity; 600 cabins; British and Italian officers, international crew; cruises in Alaska, Asia, South Pacific, and Hawaii-Tahiti.

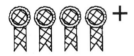

(Medical Facilities: C-6; P-2; EM, CLS, MS; N-3; CM; PD; BC; EKG; TC; PO; EPC; OX; WC; OR; ICU; X; M; CCP.)

SUN PRINCESS, DAWN PRINCESS, SEA PRINCESS, and *OCEAN PRINCESS:* entered service late 1995, May 1997, December 1998, and 2000 respectively; 77,000 G.R.T.; 856' x 106'; 1,950-passenger capacity; 975 cabins; British and Italian officers and staff, international crew; cruises to Caribbean, Panama Canal, and Alaska.

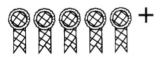

(Medical Facilities: C-19; P-2; EM, CLS, MS; N-3; CM; PD; BC; EKG; TC; PO; EPC; OX; WC; OR; ICU; X; M; CCP.)

*All ships can accommodate passengers performing peritonial dialysis, as well as holmodialysis groups accompanied by nephrologist, dialysis nurses, and technicians.

The London-based Peninsular and Oriental Steam Navigation Company (P & O) dates back to the early 1800s and is one of the oldest, largest, and most prestigious lines in the history of cruising. During the first three-quarters of the twentieth century, numerous vessels sailed under the P & O flag. However, most of them were sold after P & O purchased Princess Cruises in 1974.

Princess was originally formed by Stanley McDonald. In 1965, he chartered the 6,000-ton *Princess Patricia* and initiated cruises from California to ports on the west coast of Mexico. Thereafter, in 1967, with the charter of the *Princess Italia,* the itineraries were expanded to include spring and summer sailings to Canada and Alaska.

The *Princess Carla* was chartered in 1968 for a short period. In 1971 came a major upgrade when McDonald chartered Flagship Line's *Island Venture,* renaming her the *Island Princess.* When P & O acquired Princess in 1974, they purchased the *Island Princess,* and soon afterward also purchased her sister ship, the *Sea Venture,* which subsequently became famous as the *Pacific Princess*—television's "Love Boat." During the same period, P & O changed the name of its *Spirit of London* to the *Sun Princess* and designated her for seven-day cruises in the Caribbean and Alaskan markets.

"The Love Boat" television series brought cruising into the living rooms of millions of Americans whose prior nautical experience had not gone beyond a rowboat. The show not only gave a gigantic shot in the arm to the cruise industry as a whole, but also made Princess Cruises a household word. Although on most sailings, passengers will not rub elbows with Captain Stubing, Julie, Gopher, Doc, or Isaac, the television series did film several segments each year on board. Ironically, I have found the real-life captains, officers, and crew on Princess ships to be among the most friendly and efficient staff sailing today. (In 1998, an update of the original series returned to television screens around the world, initially filming aboard *Sun Princess.*)

The success of the line gave rise to the addition of the popular 44,000-ton *Royal Princess* in 1984, as well as the transfer of P & O's *Sea Princess* to the Princess group and Caribbean market in 1986. (The *Sea Princess* was returned to P & O for European cruises in 1991.)

In 1988, Princess acquired Sitmar Cruises, changed the name of its vessels, and instantaneously added four new ships to its rapidly expanding empire. At the same time, the *Sun Princess* was transferred to Premier Cruise Line (not to be confused with the new *Sun Princess* that entered service in 1995).

Sitmar had entered the North American cruise industry in 1971 with two refurbished Cunard ships, the *Fairsea (Fair Princess)* and *Fairwind (Dawn Princess).* Their spacious cabins, friendly and efficient Italian service, excellent cuisine, and special children's facilities and programs combined to make these two of the most popular ships of the seventies. The 46,000-ton *Fairsky (Sky Princess)* was added in 1984, and in 1989 the 62,500-ton *Star Princess* became the largest vessel in the then-combined Princess-Sitmar fleets. Two new 70,000-ton vessels, the *Crown Princess* and the *Regal Princess,* were added in 1990 and 1991, respectively.

In 1993 the *Fair Princess* was sold and the original *Dawn Princess* was withdrawn from service and temporarily replaced when the line leased the former *Royal Viking Sky,* renaming her *Golden Princess.* This lease expired in September 1996, and the ship was returned to the Birka Line. In the mid-nineties Princess committed more than $1 billion to the construction of five gigantic superliners. The 77,000-ton *Sun Princess, Dawn Princess,* and *Sea Princess* entered service in 1995, 1997, and 1998 respectively. The 109,000-ton *Grand Princess* commenced cruising in 1998, and the 77,000-ton *Ocean Princess* is scheduled to enter service in 2000. These five ships will add 10,400 berths to the Princess fleet and will increase the passengers sailing with the line annually to more than one million. Two additional "Grand Princess"-class ships have been ordered for delivery in 2001.

Itineraries for the ships vary from year to year and in 1998 included more than 200 different ports around the globe. The line offers not only Caribbean, Mexican Riviera, Panama Canal, Alaska, South America/Amazon, Canada/New England, and Colonial America cruises, but Mediterranean, North Sea-Baltic, Hawaii/Tahiti, South Pacific, India, Africa, Holy Land, and Far East cruises as well. Since Princess makes a practice of following the pulse of the marketplace, it is best to recheck itineraries each season.

As of 2000, Princess is one of the three largest cruise lines, with ten vessels servicing more than 10 percent of the cruise market.

The *Island Princess* and *Pacific Princess* were built as identical sister ships, only differing a bit in decor. When they entered service in the early seventies, they were considered the gems of the industry, which was then leaning toward constructing new vessels in the 15,000- to 25,000-ton range. Cruisers were delighted with the tasteful decor in the public rooms on Riviera Deck, the romantic lounges with Austrian shades, the dramatic staircase that rises to the information and purser's offices, the ultracomfortable theater, and the retractable sun dome over the mid-ship pool area. The biggest weakness is the size of the standard cabins. Although comfortable, smartly decorated, and adequate, they are not as large as standard cabins on other luxury ships. The deluxe rooms and suites are larger and more desirable if you are willing to pay the price. Both vessels received multimillion-dollar face-lifts in 1992. The ships were built without full casinos; however, there are gambling areas aboard. In 1999 the *Island Princess* was sold.

The *Royal Princess* was one of the most innovative ships built in the 1980s. All staterooms are outside cabins with large picture windows, closed-circuit, color TVs, refrigerators, private wall safes, tubs and showers, and twin beds that can be converted to doubles. One hundred and fifty of the rooms have outside verandas. The 12 deluxe and 2 super-deluxe suites are magnificent, with larger verandas perfect for enjoying breakfast, before-dinner cocktails while the sun sets at sea, or just stargazing before bed. All of the cabins and suites are located on the top decks, with most public rooms below. This is the reverse of most other ships and represents an emphasis on passenger accommodations. The decorations are truly elegant, with considerable brass, glass, wood, art, and soft-toned fabric. There is one immense dining room that seats all the passengers in two sittings. In addition, there is a larger-than-average swimming pool for laps, smaller wading pools and Jacuzzis, a 1/4-mile jogging track, a large casino, and a 360-degree panorama lounge on the top deck that presently converts to a disco at night. Here again, the greatest weakness is the size of the standard staterooms, which come off narrow and not terribly spacious. Designing the ships so that all passengers have exterior cabins was not without its trade-offs.

The *Sky Princess,* one of the original Sitmar ships, can accommodate 1,200 passengers in 600 cabins and suites, three-fifths being located outside. Two hundred eighty-two of the rooms can be booked as triples or quads. There are 10 deluxe and 28 mini-suites with twin beds that can be converted to doubles, and all suites have refrigerators. The deluxe suites also have terrace-verandas. Every cabin has a four-channeled radio, color TV, and telephone.

The *Sky Princess* has a showroom that seats 800 passengers and intimate lounges for romantic dancing, piano lounges for before- and after-dinner cocktails, a disco, casino, special pizza parlor, pools, gyms, saunas, and shops. For the small fry, there are special counselors, craft programs, a children's pool, soda fountain, and playroom with babysitting available. For the teens, there are video game rooms, a pizza parlor, a special teen disco, and varying programs. A multimillion-dollar refurbishment program took place in 1989 for the *Sky* and included new showrooms and face-lifts for many of the public areas. Personal safes were installed in her cabins.

The *Star Princess,* which entered service in 1989, was transferred to the P & O fleet in September 1997 and renamed *Arcadia.*

The 70,000-ton *Crown Princess,* with a unique exterior design by the award-winning Italian architect Renzo Piano, entered service in 1990, and her sister, the *Regal Princess,* in 1991. One hundred eighty-four of the 795 staterooms have outside balconies, 50 are suites, and all staterooms have two twin beds that can be converted to one queen bed, five-channel remote-controlled color TV, four music channels, large closets with separate dressing areas, guest safes, refrigerators, and card keys for cabin access. The average cabin on these ships is somewhat larger than the average cabins found on the other Princess ships.

At the top of the *Crown Princess* and *Regal Princess* on Sun Deck are the Observation Lounge, nightclub, and casino under one roof. A jogging track is also located on this deck. On Lido Deck are two swimming pools, whirlpools, a bar, a buffet restaurant serving breakfast and lunch, and a pizzeria. The next four decks—Aloha, Baya, Caribe, and Dolphin—are the location for the more expensive accommodations. There are also several lounges on Dolphin Deck. Next comes Promenade Deck, with its 740-seat multitiered Show Lounge, the dining room, the shopping arcade, and several bars and smaller lounges. On Emerald Deck are a shopping arcade, cinema, and more staterooms. The balance of the cabins are on Plaza and Fiesta decks, with the disco, fitness center, and beauty shop on Holiday Deck, the bottom passenger level. The fitness center includes an aerobics room, weights, and exercise machines; men's and women's steam, sauna, and massage areas; and a hairdressing salon.

When the sleek, 856-foot, 14-story, 77,000-ton *Sun Princess* made its debut in December 1995, it was the largest cruise ship in service. Passenger capacity was limited to 1,950 (somewhat less than its behemoth competitors), which is in keeping with Princess Cruises' intention to provide a more intimate, less crowded cruise experience aboard a giant ship while still offering more dining, entertainment, and lounging options. The abundance of soft woods, brass, fine fabrics, and art-work—together with the dramatic central atrium area and design in the public rooms—makes this and its sister ship the most attractive in the Princess fleet.

In terms of cabins, 603 of the 975 passenger accommodations are outside, 410 have balconies, and 19 are wheelchair accessible. Standard staterooms are not large; however, they are cleverly designed and tastefully appointed and include two twin beds that convert to a queen; electronic wall safes; refrigerators; remote-control color TV with CNN, in-house movies, and three music channels; terry-cloth robes; hair dryers; and ample drawer and closet space. The 32 deluxe mini-suites and 6 ultra-deluxe full suites are considerably more spacious, have larger balconies, and include bathrooms with Jacuzzi tubs. There are self-serve laundry facilities on every stateroom deck.

The *Sun Princess* offers numerous dining and entertainment options, which include two elegant, formal dining rooms; a 24-hour lido café featuring breakfast, lunch, and tea-time buffets and an alternative à la carte dinner menu; a pizzeria; a patisserie; a hamburger-hot dog grill; an ice-cream bar; 24-hour room service; and a champagne, wine, and caviar bar that is one of the seven more intimate lounges aboard. Two 500-seat show lounges provide a diversity of evening entertainment while avoiding crowding passengers into a single multilevel facility. Other public rooms and areas adorned with 2.5 million dollars of art include an attractive casino; a library; a cardroom; seven duty-free shops; five swimming pools and five whirlpools; an expansive walking-jogging track (3 1/2 times around to a mile); and a marvelous spa-fitness area with a fully equipped gym, aerobics room, his and hers sauna and steam rooms, a variety of massage and spa treatment rooms, whirlpools, a beauty salon, and computerized golf simulator. In its tradition of appealing to the family trade, *Princess* has built a unique cyberspace center for teens ages thirteen to sixteen, a fully equipped and supervised fun zone for toddlers, and a state-of-the-art disco.

The *Dawn Princess* and *Sea Princess,* the *Sun's* sister ships, commenced service in 1997 and 1998 respectively and are identical except for the art, decorations, and nomenclature of the various public rooms. A fourth sister ship, to be named *Ocean Princess,* is scheduled to enter service in early 2000.

The 109,000-ton *Grand Princess* entered service in the spring of 1998, offering Mediterranean cruises through the end of the summer and then repositioning to the Caribbean during the fall and winter seasons.

Seven hundred and ten of the 1,300 staterooms boast private balconies, and include 28 full- and 180 mini-suites with butler service. 28 accommodations are wheelchair accessible. The 372 inside cabins at 160 square feet seemed a bit small, especially when they are occupied by a third or fourth passenger. Standard outside cabins vary from 165 to 210 square feet and increase by an additional 45 square feet if they have balconies. Although the cabins and bathrooms are not very large, all have twin beds that convert to queens, refrigerators, color televisions with CNN and in-house movies, hair dryers, terry robes, and electronic safes. The mini-suites, measuring 325 square feet (balcony included), have a second television, larger sitting area with sofa bed, and a walk-in dressing area adjacent to a bathroom with tub and shower. The full suites have separate parlors, wet bars, larger split bathrooms, and walk-in closets and as expected are the most desirable accommodations aboard ship.

The *Grand Princess* offers a wide range of dining venues which include three Italian-Renaissance-style main dining rooms with sitting areas divided for greater intimacy, Sabatini's, a more casual Italian Trattoria, Painted Desert, featuring southwestern-style menus (both open for lunch and dinner), and the 24-hour Horizon Court, an alternate dining facility offering buffet breakfasts and lunches and bistro-style full-service dinners. On Lido Deck, passengers can enjoy the hamburger/hot dog grill and the pizza counter, as well as ice cream creations. Room service is available around the clock.

Indoor and outdoor public facilities are mind-boggling and include: the 748-seat Princess Theater with lavish nightly productions, a 13,500-square-foot casino, numerous additional lounges offering entertainment, dancing, and piano music, dozens of bars, a library, a writing room, a cardroom, a business center, a wedding chapel for marriages and vow renewals, a sport bar, a coffee-champagne-caviar bar, several boutiques, three regular swimming pools (one of which has a retractable dome for inclement weather), a children's pool and playground area, a pool with infused current for exercise swimming, several whirlpools, a golf center with a 9-hole putting green and golf simulator machine, a fitness center with cardiovascular equipment, aerobics rooms, massage and beauty treatment rooms, a beauty salon, sauna and steam rooms and locker facilities, a sport court for tennis, basketball, and volleyball, a small jogging track, youth and teen centers, a virtual reality center with motion-based simulator rides, a hospital with tele-medical machines, and atop ship a glass-enclosed moving sidewalk ascending to Skywalkers Disco and Observation Lounge that provides the feeling of entering a spaceship.

Most public areas are broken up into multiple sections in order to downplay the immensity of the vessel. In spite of multiple exits for disembarkation of the ship and tenders and numerous elevators, traffic can be heavily backed up at peak times.

Many of the areas, such as the sauna-steam-shower complex, the fitness center, the outside deck lounges, the jogging track, and the outside lido dining tables appeared inadequate to accommodate all passengers on a day at sea. However, overall this is truly a "resort at sea," with vast facilities and options offering something that will appeal to all age groups and a diverse segment of the cruising population.

Prices vary somewhat from ship to ship, being higher on European and Far East sailings. Minimum cabins on all the ships cost about $175 to $225 per person per day, average cabins cost about $250 to $350, and the suites and mini-suites range from $300 to $750. There is only a supplement for single occupancy of double cabins, and there are reductions for third and fourth passengers sharing a room. Numerous air-sea packages are available, and Princess features significant discounts on early bookings, referred to as "love boat savers."

In 1994, Princess introduced many new amenities in the staterooms on all vessels, including hair dryers, electronic safes, and white terry-cloth robes. As the line adds more larger vessels (ships that enter service over 77,000 tons), which Princess refers to as "Grand Class" ships, the smaller vessels built in the seventies will most likely be sold. It is anticipated that by the year 2000, 85 percent of the line's berths will have been delivered in the nineties, making Princess one of the most modern lines in the market. In keeping with innovations throughout the industry, "Grand Class" vessels offer butler service in all suites and mini-suites. In recent years Princess has placed more emphasis on shore excursions, offering a vast array of options including air, sea, and land tours that afford opportunities to get close to the natural environs and sample the best sightseeing each area has to offer.

Princess competes in the premium cruise market and offers a well-rounded cruise experience. There is an overall ambiance, desire to please, and lack of stuffiness not present on many other luxury liners. All Princess ships have exceptional special facilities and programs for youngsters and a full range of activities and entertainment, making them ideal choices for families. Most passengers are very pleased with the blend of luxury, fun, food, and service.

Strong Points:

Attractive vessels, activities, entertainment, ambiance, itineraries, and a well-rounded, upscale cruise experience. The "Grand Class" ships are extremely well-appointed and among the most glamorous in the industry.

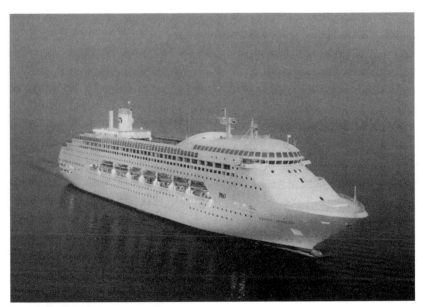

Courtesy Princess Cruises

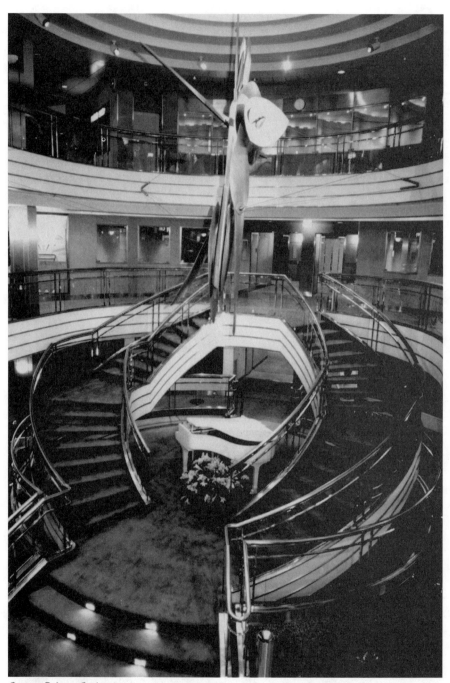

Courtesy Princess Cruises

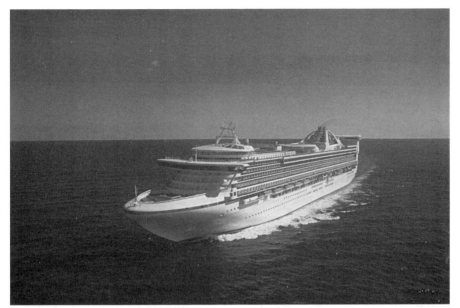

Grand Princess, *courtesy Princess Cruises*

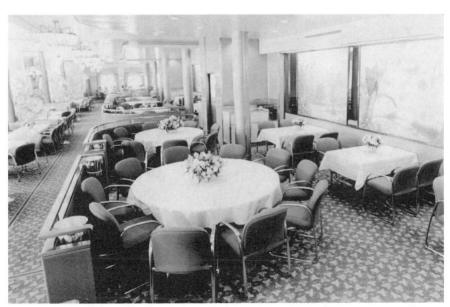

Courtesy Princess Cruises

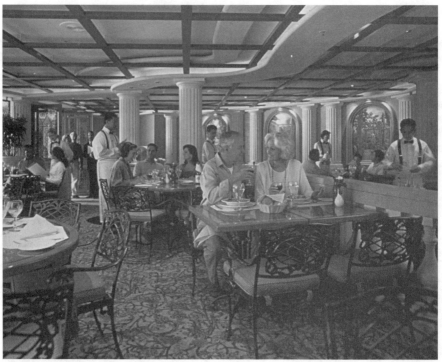

Sabatini Restaurant, courtesy Princess Cruises

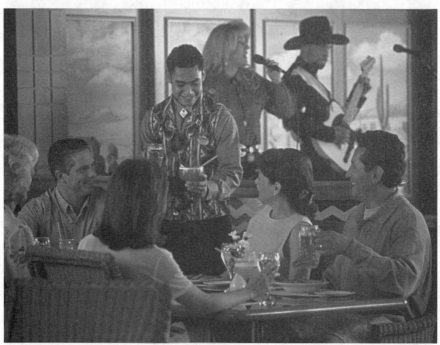

Painted Desert Restaurant, courtesy Princess Cruises

GRAND PRINCESS PRINCESS CRUISES

It's more than a cruise, it's the Love Boat

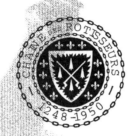

Captain's Gala Dinner

HEALTHY CHOICE MENU

Our Healthy Choice Menu reflects today's awareness of
lighter, more balanced diets. In response to these
nutritional needs, Princess Cruises offers dishes that are
low in cholesterol, fat and sodium, but high in flavor.

DOUBLE CHICKEN BROTH WITH VERMICELLI AND SCALLIONS

RADICCHIO, BOSTON LETTUCE AND TOMATO SALAD

SAUTEED BABY TURBOT WITH SNOW PEAS AND CRUSTY NEW POTATOES

VEGETARIAN MENU

GOLDEN FRESH FRUIT COLLECTION WITH KIRSCH

ROASTED GARLIC BISQUE WITH ROSEMARY

RADICCHIO, BOSTON LETTUCE AND TOMATO SALAD

RAVIOLI DI RICOTTA WITH FRESH TOMATO SAUCE

ASSORTED INTERNATIONAL CHEESE AND CRACKERS

SEASONAL FRESH FRUIT PLATE

APPETIZERS
Caviar Tartlet with Alaskan Salmon Roe
Jumbo Shrimp Cocktail with Calypso Sauce
Golden Fresh Fruit Collection with Kirsch

SOUPS
Double Chicken Broth with Vermicelli and Scallions
Roasted Garlic Bisque with Rosemary
Jellied Beef Consommé Madrilène with Celery Julienne

SALAD
Radicchio, Boston Lettuce and Tomato
Thousand Island Dressing, Balsamic Vinaigrette or Low-Fat House Italian

PRINCESS FAVORITE
Ravioli con Salsa di Funghi Porcini
Pasta Squares Filled with Meat in a Creamy Mushroom Sauce

ENTRÉES
Sautéed Baby Turbot with Saffron Dip
With Snow Peas, Glazed Carrots and Crusty New Potatoes

Broiled Lobster Tail
On the Shell with Melted Lemon Butter and Rice Pilaf

Royal Pheasant in Pan Juices
An Oven Roast with Brussels Sprouts, Champignons and Parisienne Potatoes

Beef Wellington
*Puff Pastry-Wrapped Tenderloin in a Black Truffle Madeira Sauce
with Baby Vegetables and Duchess Potatoes*

YOUR SOMMELIER SUGGESTS

	Glass	Bottle
Chilled Kremlyovskaya Vodka	$4.25	
Chardonnay Kendall Jackson, Lake County	$6.00	$24.00
Pinot Noir Coastal Robert Mondavi, North Coast	$5.00	$19.00
Chardonnay Kenwood, Sonoma		$32.00
Brunello di Montalcino (DOCG), Toscana		$39.00

7/D5 C

Courtesy Princess Cruises

GRAND PRINCESS

GRAND PRINCESS	ST. THOMAS	TONIGHT'S DRESS:
WEDNESDAY, OCTOBER 7, 1998	SUNRISE: 6:12AM SUNSET: 6:04PM	CASUAL

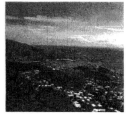

WELCOME TO
ST. THOMAS, U.S.V.I.

I t is both foreign and familiar. Exotic flowers with such delightful names a Clashie Melashi and Jump Up and Kiss Me grow next to fast-food restaurants and supermarkets. The scent of jasmine and frangipani fill the air, and Hollywood movies fill the television screens.

Welcome to the U.S. Virgin Islands, the "American Paradise," a unique blend of island magic and American practicality. Capital of the island group, the green, mountainous St. Thomas offers every sport imaginable—snorkeling, flightseeing, golfing, hiking, sailing. From the beautiful scenery to the unsurpassed sunsets, St. Thomas is as inviting as a cool, Caribbean breeze.

Spotlight On... The Purser's Office

With Grand Class Cruising we are committed to further enhance our services to you by introducing the following for your traveling needs.

Purser's Desk, deck 5 - Open 8:00am-8:00pm
Purser's Desk, deck 6 - Open 24 hours

At both locations our team of Officers will always be more than happy to assist you in any possible way including the following services:

- General Enquiries
- Lost and Found
- Shipboard Account queries
- Purchase of Postage Stamps
- Cashing of Traveler's checks and Personal checks.

CURRENCY EXCHANGE MACHINES

Grand Princess is the first ship to have state-of-the-art Currency Machines, designed in Italy specially for Princess Cruises. These two machines, situated on either side of deck 6 Purser's Desk, are available 24 hours a day for you to change money. They accept most currencies, and will always dispense U.S. Dollars.

Spotlight On... Skywalkers

This futuristic nightclub, suspended 150 feet above the sea on Deck 17 is as unique as the moving Skywalk travelator that brings you to its doorstep. Inside, the lighting and sound effects are stunning. Overhead, fiber-optic and metallic stars twinkle in a gold celestial expanse, shot with neon flashes. The room's high-tech upholstery combines copper-colored leather and silver-shot fabric for a look that's equally inviting during the daylight hours.

GOOD MORNING!

7:00am   **GRAND PRINCESS IS EXPECTED TO ARRIVE IN ST. THOMAS, U.S.V.I.**

SHIP'S SECURITY NOTICE

In order to prevent unauthorized persons boarding the ship, you are asked to carry your "Cruise/Key Card" ashore with you. You will be asked to produce this at the gangway when you leave the ship and again when you return onboard. We kindly ask that you do not bring onboard any parcels from unknown people. You may also be asked to open parcels or handbags which you are carrying. We are sure you will appreciate that this security is in the best interest of all concerned.

ADVENTURES ASHORE TOUR OFFICE
Located on Plaza Deck, Deck 5
7:00am to 10:00am & 4:00pm to 6:00pm
Bookings for St. Maarten close at 10:00am today
Car Rental Reservations for Fort Lauderdale close at 6:00pm tonight

Please refer to your tour tickets for exact meeting times and locations today.
For further information about our Shore Excursions, stop by the Tour Office during our opening hours. Our 24-hour drop box is available for out-of-hours bookings, tickets are delivered directly to your stateroom. You may also tune into Channel 21 of your stateroom television.
Port & Shopping Lecturer, Laura, is available at the Tour Office between 5:30pm and 6:00pm for questions.

NEW WAVES SNORKEL RENTAL HOURS
7:30am to 8:00am and 5:00pm to 6:00pm
Located on Sun Deck, Deck 15 Forward, Starboardside (next to Sea Breeze Bar)
Snorkeling Equipment Rental and sales available including
cameras, fish food, mask de-fog & much more.
The New Waves Instructors can be contacted at the Tour Office between 4:00pm & 6:00pm

---

CAPTAIN'S CIRCLE HOSPITALITY DESK HOURS
8:00am to 10:00am - Atrium Lobby, Deck 5 Portside

Captain's Circle members, your packets with your pin, sticker and logbook will be delivered to your cabin this evening at turndown.

Please stop by if you have never received a Captain's Circle membership card or is you have an address change. Have a great day in St. Thomas!

FUNZONE	9:00am to 5:00pm & 7:00pm-10:00pm	*for Babysitting*
	7:00pm to10:00pm	*for activities*
OFF LIMITS	10:00am-12 Noon, 2:00pm to 5:00pm and	
	7:00pm to 1:00am for activities	

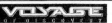

VOYAGE OF DISCOVERY - Deck 15 Aft
Open today: 7:00pm - Late
ALPINE RACERS
Hot outside? Bring a friend and cool off by racing each other on the Alpine Racers
50% OFF between 7:00pm and 10:00pm
Your stateroom Keycard may be used to buy a $20 game card.
Game prices range from 50¢ to $3.00

DAYTIME ACTIVITIES

CRUISERCISE FITNESS PROGRAM
Your Cruisercise Manager **Jenée** has a fun exercise program aimed at getting you on the road to good health and fitness. For each activity you attend you will receive Cruisercise Cash which you trade for Cruisercise Logo articles in the ship's boutique. So start collecting today!

7:30am	Walk-A-Mile	Deck 7 Aft, Starboardside
7:45am	Stair Climb	Aft Staircase, Deck 7
4:30pm	Hi/Lo Aerobics	Spa Studio, Deck 15 Forward
5:30pm	Walk-A-Mile	Deck 7 Aft, Starboardside
6:00pm	Abs, Abs, Abs!!!	Spa Studio, Deck 15 Forward
6:15pm	Stretch & Relax	Spa Studio, Deck 15 Forward

7:30am-8:00am	**New Waves Dive Locker Is Open** for snorkel rental equipment and sales, including cameras, fish food, mask de-fog and much more.	
	Sun Deck 15 Starboard Side, next to Sea Breeze Bar	
8:15am	**Port & Shopping Lecturer, Laura,** will be available for questions at the gangway Don't forget your **Port Guides!**	
8:00am-8:00pm	**Library and C.D. Rom** - Open throughout the day. The Cruise Staff will be on duty between 11:00am and Noon and again between 5:00pm and 6:00pm. A Quiet Corner, Deck 5	
9:00am-11:00am & 3:30pm-6:30pm	**Princess Links** - Open for putting or golf simulator! For reservations (golf simulator only) please refer to page 18 of your stateroom portfolio. Deck 16 Midships	

9:45am
CREW EMERGENCY STATIONS

At 9:45am this morning, alarm bells will be sounded and broadcasts made as the crew are exercised in their Emergency Duties. During the exercise, all passenger services will cease. On hearing the General Emergency Stations signal, which consists of at least seven short blasts followed by one long blast on the ship's whistle and alarms, any passengers remaining onboard are strongly encouraged, on this occasion only, to go to the Explorers Lounge on Deck 7. Here you will be shown a safety related video. It will not be necessary for you to take your lifejacket to the Drill. Please keep clear of the outside area of Promenade Deck during this exercise.

11:15am	**Brunchtime Trivia** - The Cruise Staff prepares you a mental minefield. The Explorers Lounge, Deck 7
11:30am-1:30pm	**Lunchtime Melodies** - in the Atrium with the Grand Princess musicians. Atrium Lobby, Decks, 5, 6 & 7
Noon-3:00pm	**Basketball Play** Sports Court, Deck 16 Forward

---

1:00pm until 3:00pm
TOUR OF THE NAVIGATIONAL BRIDGE
The Cruise Staff escort you to the nerve center of Grand Princess.
For security reasons, the use of video cameras will not be allowed.
Please meet in the Lido Deck 14, Forward Lobby, by elevators.

2:15pm	**Shuffleboard Play** - Test your skills at this traditional ship's pastime. Sun Deck 15 Aft
2:30pm	**Informal Cards & Games Get-together** Players Card Room, Deck 5
3:00pm	**Paddle Tennis** - Sports action on center court. Sports Court, Deck16 Forward
3:30pm	**Afternoon Tea** - Light snacks served in a traditional musical atmosphere. Da Vinci Dining Room, Deck 6
4:30pm	**Outburst Challenge** - A fun game of verbal explosions. Explorers Lounge, Deck 7
5:00pm-6:00pm	**New Waves Dive Locker Is Open** for snorkel rental/returns & sales, including cameras, fish food, mask de-fog and much more. Sun Deck 15 Starboard Side, next to Sea Breeze Bar
5:30pm	**Friends of Dr. Bob and Bill W. Meeting** Wedding Chapel, Deck 7

5:30pm	**ALL PASSENGERS ON BOARD PLEASE!**
6:00pm	**GRAND PRINCESS SAILS FOR ST. MAARTEN**

5:30pm to 6:45pm - Decks 12, 14, 15 & 16 Aft

Sunset Sailaway on Deck
After the heat of the day relax with a cooling cocktail, beautiful sunset
and the soothing sounds of **Pantastic Steel Band.**

Princess Theater, Deck 7 Forward
EVENING MOVIE
7:45pm & 10:45pm

THE HORSE WHISPERER
STARRING: Robert Redford
Rated PG-13 168 min.

PRE-DINNER MUSIC
FOR YOUR LISTENING AND DANCING PLEASURE

5:45PM ONWARDS - WHEELHOUSE BAR, DECK 7
PATRICIA DEAN TRIO & JOHN DE HAAS

5:45PM TO 8:30PM - ATRIUM LOBBY, DECK 5
GAZSI BAND

7:00PM-7:45PM & 9:30PM-10:45PM
PAINTED DESERT, DECK 7
DAVID & DANIELLE

TONIGHT'S ENTERTAINMENT
This Evening's Suggested Dress is Casual/Island Attire

FOR YOUR LISTENING AND DANCING PLEASURE

VISTA LOUNGE

PROMENADE DECK 7 AFT
PRE-SHOW DANCING 6:45PM & 8:30PM
SHOW TIMES:
7:00PM (2ND SITTING)
8:45PM (1ST SITTING)
TONIGHT ONLY!
PRINCESS CRUISES PRESENTS

"NEW YORK NEW YORK"

STARRING
LAURIE WELLS & JAMES CAMPBELL
PLUS
THE GRAND PRINCESS DANCERS
M.C. RUSSELL GRIFFIN
MUSICAL BACKING:
GORDON HOUGH AND THE VISTA SHOWBAND
AUDIO OR VIDEO TAPING IS NOT ALLOWED DUE TO
COPYRIGHT. NO RESERVATION OF SEATS PLEASE.

EXPLORERS LOUNGE

PROMENADE DECK 7 AMIDSHIPS
CONTINUOUS LIVE ENTERTAINMENT
FROM 8:00PM TILL LATE
8:45PM & 10:45PM

"CABARET SHOWTIME"

TONIGHT ONLY!
STARRING
COMEDIAN/JUGGLER

DAN BENNETT

M.C. MAURY KELLEY

—— **ALSO** ——

8:00PM AND 9:15PM TILL LATE
DANCING WITH

TON TON PHOENIX

THE PROMENADE LOUNGE
DECK 7 MIDSHIPS
9:30PM TILL LATE

JONATHAN HUNT
entertains in his own
unique style.

WHEELHOUSE BAR
DECK 7
5:45PM ONWARDS

PATRICIA DEAN TRIO
and
JOHN DE HAAS
Invite you for an intimate evening
of music and dancing

SKYWALKERS NIGHTCLUB
DECK 17 AFT
11:00PM TILL LATE

"ISLAND FIESTA"
D.J. Viviano continues the Island Night theme
with more Island, Latin and Caribbean disco music.

Courtesy Princess Cruises

RADISSON SEVEN SEAS CRUISES
600 Corporate Drive, Suite 410
Ft. Lauderdale, Florida 33334
(800) 333-3333
(305) 772-3763 FAX

M/S *HANSEATIC:* entered service 1993; 9,000 G.R.T.; 403' x 59'; 184-passenger capacity; 90 cabins; European officers and crew; Antarctica and other exotic destinations around the world. (Category B—Not Rated)

M/S *PAUL GAUGUIN:* entered service 1997; 18,800 G.R.T.; 513' x 71'; 320-passenger capacity; 160 cabins; French officers, international crew; cruises in French Polynesia.

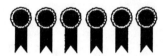

SSC *RADISSON DIAMOND:* entered service 1992; 20,295 G.R.T.; 420' x 103'; 350-passenger capacity; 177 cabins; international officers and crew; cruises in the Caribbean, Transcanal, Mediterranean, and Northern Europe.

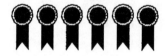

M/S *SEVEN SEAS NAVIGATOR:* entered service 1999; 30,000 G.R.T.; 560' x 81'; 490-passenger capacity; 245 suites; international officers and crew; cruises in Mediterrean, Caribbean, Panama Canal, and South America. (Category A— Not Rated)

SONG OF FLOWER: (formerly *Explorer Starship*); entered service 1986; refurbished 1990; 8,282 G.R.T.; 180-passenger capacity; 107 cabins; Norwegian officers, European crew; cruises southern Asia, Arabia, Australia, and New Zealand in winter; Mediterranean, Western Europe, Scandinavia, and the Baltic Republics in the summer.

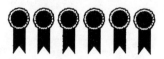

(Medical Facilities for *Paul Gauguin, Radisson Diamond,* and *Song of Flower* include: C-0 [except 2 on *Radisson Diamond*]; P-1; EM, CLS, MS; N-1; CM; PD; EKG; TC; PO; EPC (On *Radisson Diamond* only); OX; WC; OR; ICU; M (Not on *Song Of Flower*); CCP, LJ.)

In January 1995 Diamond Cruises and Seven Seas Cruise Line merged and became Radisson Seven Seas Cruises. The emphasis of the company is destination cruising. In January 1997 the cruise line was acquired by Carlson Hospitality Worldwide. In 1998 it embarked upon a joint venture with Monte Carlo-based V. Ships (part of Vlasof Group, which formerly owned Sitmar Cruises) to build five new ships.

Radisson Hotels Worldwide made its debut into the cruise industry in May 1992 with the revolutionary, $125-million, twin-hull, ultradeluxe *Radisson Diamond*. The vessel competes in the luxury cruise market, specializing in cruises for leisure travelers as well as offering special facilities for corporate conferences and incentive groups. Although group and full-ship charter rates run somewhat less, the average cruise fare is $550 to $700 per person per night (based on double occupancy).

During the spring, summer, and early fall, the ship offers seven- to eleven-day cruises to various European ports on the Atlantic and Mediterranean. During the remainder of the year, the *Diamond* offers a series of Caribbean, Panama Canal, and Costa Rica cruises.

Technologically, the ship is the trendsetter for the cruise industry into the twenty-first century. The unique stabilization of the twin hulls results in unparalleled comfort and stability, furnishing less motion and a quieter, more comfortable cruise for its discriminating clientele. The ship's modern air-conditioned tenders are designed to provide passengers organized sightseeing excursions, and its hydraulically operated, free-floating retractable marina features a stage area for watersports, including water-skiing, jet boats, and small sailboats. The marina pool opens directly into the sea, permitting passengers the experience of swimming in the open waters or in the more protected area around the marina platform.

Interior design of the vessel is by award-winning designer Vincent Kwok and features a blend of subtle contemporary and Art Deco styles with fabrics imported from around the world, black ebony and brass handrails on the elegant staircases leading to the observation deck, and two five-story glass-enclosed elevators rising above the magnificent atrium-style lobby.

Each of the 175 posh staterooms is approximately 243 square feet; 123 feature private balconies, and the remainder have floor-to-ceiling bay windows with larger lounging areas. The 2 master suites measure 511 square feet. Every accommodation includes a queen-size bed convertible to two twins, a spacious sitting area with sofa and chairs, a full-length mirror and wardrobe, considerable storage space, remote-controlled color TV with five channels (including CNN) and VCR and stereo attachments, refrigerator and bar stocked with complimentary liquors and soft drinks, a private wall safe, direct-dial ship-to-shore telephones, and large bathrooms with marble vanities, hair dryers, bathtubs with showers, terry-cloth robes, and personal amenities. These are among the most well-designed and comfortable guest accommodations afloat.

The elegant Grand Dining Room, with its floor-to-ceiling glass windows looking out to sea, features open seating, complimentary house wines, and the opportunity to choose from numerous dinner entrees that change daily and always include a selection of prime meats, fresh fish, and seafood. The variety of offerings is amazing and the entire dining experience is more akin to a sophisticated European restaurant rather than a cruise ship. The indoor/outdoor Lido Deck restaurant with a brasserie format serves four meals each day, with a wide range of both buffet and à la carte selections. In the evening, it converts to a romantic Italian specialty restaurant, Don Vito's, with strolling musicians, a multicourse tasting menu that changes each evening, and complimentary Italian wines. One evening on each cruise, there is an outdoor barbecue by the pool. There is 24-hour room service, and private banquets and business meals can be arranged.

The conference facilities located on the bottom two passenger decks include a 2,050-square-foot auditorium/ballroom that can be divided into six breakout rooms. For your business meeting or conference, there are state-of-the-art audio-visual equipment and communication facilities, secretarial services, fax machines, computer rooms, and a publishing center.

Atop the ship is an impressive health and beauty spa-fitness center surrounded by an oval, soft-composition jogging/walking track. The spa offers steam, sauna, massage, herbal wraps, skin-care treatments, and a gym with exercise and cardio-vascular equipment and free weights. The extremely attractive outside deck area below on Deck 10 features a swimming pool, an outdoor whirlpool, a spacious sunbathing area, a bar, and the Lido Deck Restaurant. Other sport facilities in addition to the marina and fitness center include a golf driving range with nets, a putting green, shuffleboard, and table tennis.

Public facilities consist of an intimate lounge; a small casino offering Caribbean stud poker, blackjack, roulette, and slots; a library stocked with books and videos; a boutique and gift shop; and the 230-seat bi-level Windows Lounge at the bow of the ship, which affords passengers an elegant, comfortable place to enjoy the panoramic view of the sea. An orchestra plays dance music each evening in the Windows Lounge, a piano player performs in the dining room and at the piano bar in the Club, and there are several individual performances and production numbers during the cruise. Windows converts to disco entertainment later in the evening. Overall, activities and entertainment are somewhat limited, emulating the environment on the small luxury cruise ships. Passengers are encouraged to do their own thing rather than participate in around-the-clock activities. The ship is also a trendsetter with its advanced security system and outstanding tender service.

Originally owned by Exploration Cruise Line, *Song of Flower* was purchased by "K" Line and underwent a seven-million-dollar refurbishment. Although initially marketed to the Japanese from Singapore, in 1991 the company changed its focus to the North American market and established its U.S. headquarters in San Francisco. Passenger complement is predominately North Americans, with a few Europeans, Asians, and Australians. Officers are European, the stewardesses are Scandinavian, and the exceptional dining room staff is European. Service throughout the ship is flawless.

Fine wines, premium liquor, and soft drinks served in public rooms or provided in the staterooms are included in the cruise fare. Dining features a single open sitting. Gratuities are neither expected nor accepted.

Breakfast and lunch are offered in your cabin, in the beautifully appointed main dining room, and buffet style on deck by the pool. The buffet selections are far more upscale than on most ships. Throughout the day, the friendly service staff roams the decks and public rooms to offer the guests their choice of beverages. Room service is available around the clock.

Dinners are multicourse extravaganzas with expensive hors d'oeuvres such as caviar, Norwegian salmon, escargot, and prawns; imaginative soups and salads; choice of four gourmet entrees; and several desserts. The white and red wines offered *gratis* change nightly and are always a vintage selection that would cost upwards of $35 a bottle in a restaurant. In 1997 a new alternative-dining restaurant, named Angelo's, was added to complement the single open-seating dining aboard ship.

The staterooms vary in size and design, ranging from 183 square feet to 398 square feet for a two-room suite. All staterooms include refrigerated bars, color TVs with VCRs, lock drawers, and hair dryers. There are 20 suites, 10 of which feature verandas. The veranda suites are the most desirable, with the largest and brightest bedroom areas. Standard staterooms—although not large for a luxury ship—are well-equipped and provide decent storage. There is a large main lounge for lectures and entertainment, a more intimate nightclub/disco for nightly dancing, the Observation Lounge, a small casino, a boutique, a video library, and a health club consisting of a small exercise room with cardiovascular equipment and a sauna. Per diem prices range from $350 up to $690 per person per day.

Asia, Australia, and New Zealand program prices include shore excursion programs and airfare from seventy-eight North American cities. For European programs, optional shore excursions are available, and airfare add-ons range from $195 to $295.

Considering the attractive free air-sea packages and free shore excursion programs in Asia, the complimentary wines, liquors, and champagne, and the exceptional cuisine and service, those opting for the less-expensive cabins cannot duplicate the experience for the price on any other cruise ship.

The line also markets the 188-passenger *Hanseatic,* one of the newest and most sophisticated "soft adventure" passenger ships, designed to ply the waters of the Antarctic and other polar destinations, as well as Russia, Alaska, the Northwest Passage, Galapagos, South America, South Africa, and the Seychelles. Built in 1993 at 9,000 tons, she can accommodate 188 passengers in 90 cabins.

In late 1997, the 18,800 ton, 320-passenger *Paul Gauguin* joined the fleet, offering seven-night Polynesian cruises. The ship is owned by French investors, but Radisson Seven Seas Cruises operates the ship and handles sales and marketing.

The 160 staterooms, including 7 suites, measure from 200 square feet up to 456 square feet, half with private balconies. All accommodations include full-size bathtub and shower, cotton robes, hair dryers, television with in-house movies and programs, VCR attachments, private safes, direct-dial telephones, refrigerators stocked with soft drinks and an initial supply of the guests' choice of complimentary liquors, wardrobes, and a vanity-desk. Vanities both in the staterooms and bathrooms include numerous mirrors affording multisided views.

Unlike most of the other upscale vessels under 20,000 tons, the staterooms on *Paul Gauguin* are not similar in size. There are eight categories, and the space and comfort levels are directly proportionate to what you pay. Thus, passengers booking in "Category F" for about $450 per person per night share a 200-square-foot stateroom with two portholes, a small sitting area, and reduced storage space; whereas "Category C" guests paying approximately $615 per night receive a veranda, tub/shower combination, and additional storage; while guests opting for a 300-square-foot "Category A" stateroom at $715 per night or one of the 332-square-foot Grand Suites at $915 per night receive more closet and storage, more spacious sitting areas, and larger outside verandas. All categories of accommodations are cleverly designed and decorated with attractive dark wood and chrome cabinetry, floor-to-ceiling mirrored walls, and tasteful fabrics.

Single open-seating dining is offered in three restaurants. The opulent L' Etoile is reminiscent of a grand Parisian restaurant and features multicourse, Continental dinner menus. The specialty restaurant, La Veranda, with menus and cuisine designed by Michelin two-star chef Jean-Pierre Vigato, owner of Apicius in Paris, alternates gourmet French dinners with Italian specialties each evening, to accompanying piano music. La Veranda is also open for breakfast and lunch, as is the indoor-outdoor Le Grill by the pool. In the evenings Le Grill features grilled fish, seafood, and steaks under the stars.

A late-risers' Continental breakfast and afternoon high tea are served at La Palette, an observation lounge that converts to a disco late in the evening. Complimentary wines from around the world are offered at mealtimes in all restaurants, and classified vintages are available at an additional charge. The quality of the cuisine throughout the vessel is exceptional. The Connoisseur Club, which has a spiral staircase descending to La Veranda, offers special before-dinner cocktail parties for La Veranda dinner guests, and after dinner it is a popular haven for those wishing to indulge in imported cigars, fine wines, liqueurs, and brandies. Hors d'oeuvres are featured in all lounges before dinner, and numerous complimentary cocktail parties take place during each cruise.

Facilities aboard include the Grand Salon, the setting for lectures, movies, dancing and nightly entertainment, a casino, a cardroom, a photo shop, a boutique, the restaurants and lounges described above, an outdoor pool, numerous bars, a sea-level marina, a small exercise room, Carita Spa (which offers massage and beauty treatments), a steam room, and a hairdressing facility.

In August of 1999, the line's newest vessel, the M/S *Seven Seas Navigator,* debuted. This 30,000-ton, 560-foot-long vessel accommodates 490 guests in

245 suites. Standard suites measure 301 square feet, 10 deluxe suites measure 538 square feet, and 4 grand suites provide 1,238 square feet of luxury. Ninety percent of the suites have balconies, and the vessel offers an alternative restaurant featuring Italian cuisine at the Porto Fino Grill. After spending her inaugural summer season in the Mediterranean she will reposition to the U.S. in October for a 50-night "Circle South America" voyage. We are eager to review what promises to be an exceptional vessel.

Radisson Seven Seas cruises and V. ships have announced their intentions to add three new ships in 2000, 2001, and 2002, commencing with a 46,000 G.R.T., 713 feet by 95 feet, 720-passenger ship to be named *Seven Seas Mariner*. The ship is scheduled to have a French captain, French and European senior officers, and four different dining venues operating worldwide itineraries.

Strong Points:

Song of Flower offers an intimate, small-luxury-ship experience with exotic itineraries, superior food, impeccable service, and comfortable accommodations at very competitive prices. This is the best buy in the luxury-cruise class.

Radisson Diamond and *Paul Gauguin* also offer luxury, more intimate cruise experiences on exceptionally comfortable, well-appointed, mid-size vessels with more facilities; very utilitarian, tasteful staterooms; a vast variety of exceptional meal offerings; and exciting itineraries with more hours in port. The *Paul Gauguin* cruise in French Polynesia is an excellent choice for honeymooners.

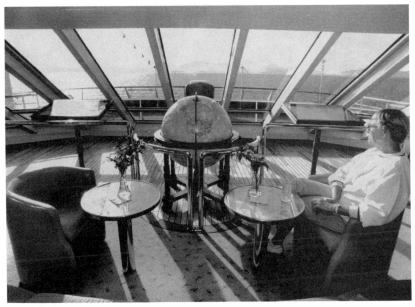

Song of Flower, *courtesy Radisson Seven Seas Cruises*

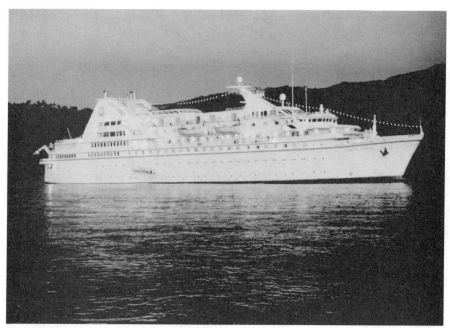

Song of Flower, *courtesy Radisson Seven Seas Cruises*

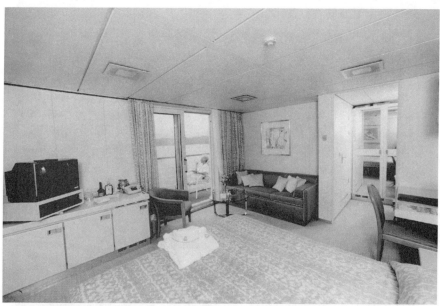

Song of Flower, *courtesy Radisson Seven Seas Cruises*

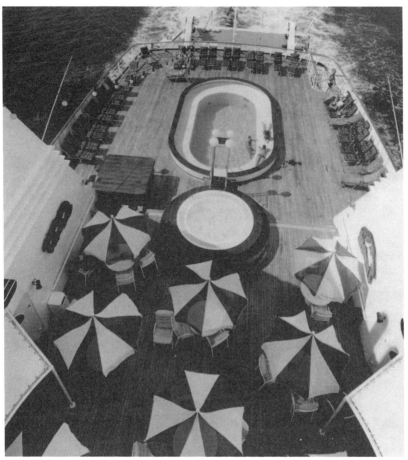

Song of Flower, *courtesy Radisson Seven Seas Cruises*

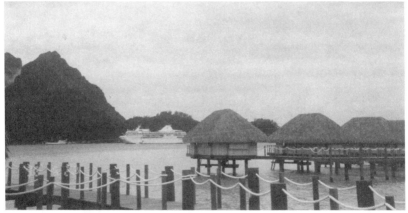

Paul Gauguin, *courtesy Radisson Seven Seas Cruises*

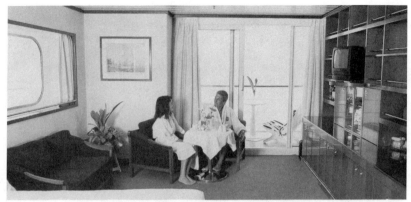

Paul Gauguin, *courtesy Radisson Seven Seas Cruises*

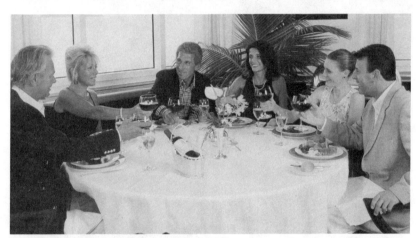

Paul Gauguin, *courtesy Radisson Seven Seas Cruises*

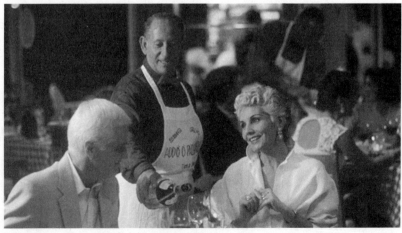

Paul Gauguin, *courtesy Radisson Seven Seas Cruises*

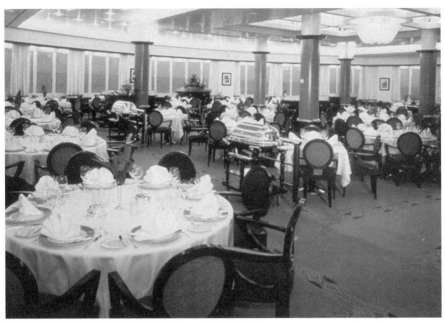

Paul Gauguin, *courtesy Radisson Seven Seas Cruises*

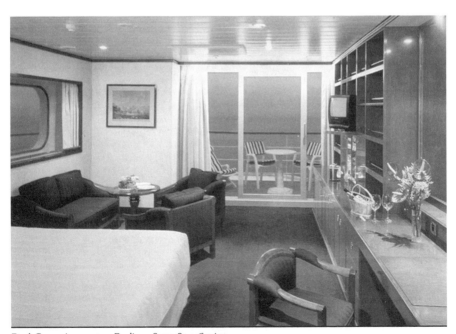

Paul Gauguin, *courtesy Radisson Seven Seas Cruises*

DINNER MENU

SPECIAL FROM THE BAKERY
Engadiner Walnut Bread

COLD APPETIZERS
Fresh Sea Bass in Lime and Cilantro
Baby Chicken and Shrimp Salad, Balsamic Vinaigrette
Thai Marinated Vegetables with Crab
Glaced Grapefruit with Dark Rum

HOT APPETIZER
Texas Cornfritters with Fruit Salsa

SOUPS
Consomme Double Carmen
French Onion Soup, Cheese Croutons
Chilled Pear Soup with Cognac Cream and Prosciutto

SALADS
Lettuce, Sliced Bell Peppers and Baby Corn, Cheese Dressing
Salad Irma Four Season

ENTREES

FISH
Atlantic Halibut Swedish Style

SHELL FISH
Broiled Lobster Tail with Melon, Beurre Rouge

MEAT
Roast Rib Eye with Yorkshirepudding
Supreme of Duckling, Cassis Sauce

FROM THE GRILL
Veal Steak with Light Creamy Tarragon Sauce

TODAY'S WOK
"Suki Yaki" Beef, Fresh Vegetables Julienne, Shrimp and Noodles

PASTA
Penne Rigate with Scallop and Spinach Sauce

DESSERTS

Mixed Berry Tarte
Chocolate Charlotte with Amaretto Sauce
Black Bing Cherry Jubilee Flambee
Freshly Made Fruit Sherbets and Frozen Yoghurt

ICE COFFEE

"Elizabeth"
Coffee Ice Cream with Drambuie, Sauce Caramel
and Whipped Cream

ICE CREAMS

Vanilla - Choc Choc Mint - Chocolate
Hot Chocolate Sauce - Hot Blackberry Sauce

PETIT FOURS

CHEESE AND CRACKERS

From the Cart

CHEF'S RECOMMENDATION

Texas Cornfritters with Fruit Salsa

* * *

Supreme of Duckling with Cassis Sauce

* * *

Viennese Bing Cherry Jubilee Flambee

SIMPLICITY

Fresh Marinated Sea Bass in Lime and Cilantro
Plain Broiled Lobster
Glazed Grapefruit

Courtesy Radisson Seven Seas Cruises

BORA BORA ~ APRIL 1ST, 1998

EXECUTIVE CHEF MARIO VALERA'S SUGGESTIONS

Salmon & Scallop "Carpaccio"
Parmesan flakes and Balsamic dressing

Potage "Malakoff"
cream of tomato, potato and spinach

Roast Rack Of Spring Lamb "Dijonnaise"
panaché of fresh vegetables and potato gratin, mint gravy

Brazo De Mercedez
Spanish roulade filled with meringue

POLYNESIAN WOK SPECIALITY
Lobster "Siam"
stir-fried with spicy lemon sauce with Jasmine rice

VEGETARIAN

Sautéed Tofu
stir-fried vegetables, steamed rice

CUISINE LÉGÈRE

Roast Quail "Paesana"
*with boiled vegetables and
parsley potatoes*

SELECTION OF INTERNATIONAL CHEESES
Available from the trolley
served with Port Wine

*To enjoy a fine Cognac or Liqueur, you may retire to our
Connoisseur Club on Deck 7 "après dîner"*

COMPLIMENTARY WINE
FOR THIS EVENING

Red: *Château le Sartre 1995*
"Cabernet Sauvignon & Merlot"
Bordeaux, France
White: *Château La Tour Leognan 1995*
"Sauvignon Blanc & Semillon"
Bordeaux, France

HEAD SOMMELIER'S WINE
SUGGESTION

Red : *Penfold Bin 389, 1993*
Cabernet Sauvignon & Shiraz
Barossa Valley, South Australia
$35.00
White :*Rosemount Semillon Chardonnay 1996*
Semillon Chardonnay
Rosemount Estate, South Eastern Australia
$16.00

RADISSON SEVEN SEAS
CRUISES

COLD APPETIZERS

Chilled Jumbo Shrimps
with American cocktail sauce

Red Bell Pepper Mousse
on broccoli coulis

Iced Cantaloupe Fruit Cup
with Midori liqueur

HOT APPETIZERS

Deep-fried Brie Cheese
with strawberry compote

SOUPS

Double Beef Consommé "Monté Carlo"
with foie gras "jeton"

Chilled Cream Of Doria
chilled cream of cucumber

SALADS

"Niçoise"
*marinated tuna, potato, string beans, anchovy and hard boiled egg
on lettuce leaves*

Panaché Of Garden Salads
your choice of low fat and homemade dressings

ENTRÉES

**Grilled Fillet Of Fresh Grouper
"Marinière"**
*with selected garden vegetables and steamed
potatoes*

Tortiglioni Alla "Bolognese"

pasta tossed with meat sauce

Broiled Entrecôte "Bercy"
with marrow and herb butter

DESSERTS AND OTHER TREATS

Gâteau Opéra
sponge cake layers with mocca and chocolate cream

Cherry Streusel
with vanilla ice cream

TONIGHT'S ICED COFFEE

"Mount Mc Kinley"
vanilla ice cream, vodka, mixed berries, whipped cream

PREMIUM ICE CREAMS

Pistachio Almonds - Peaches & Cream - Banana

FROZEN YOGURT

Vanilla - Chocolate

Petits Fours

Maître D'Hôtel Enzo Mazzali	RADISSON SEVEN SEAS CRUISES	**Executive Chef** Mario Valera

Showtime 10:00pm Grand Salon
Featuring your Cruise Director
Billy Phillips
Music by **Siglo**

MOVIES

Channel 28 -	Bridge Camera
Channel 30 -	Ship's Information & Anouncements **(If you wish to hear anouncements in your Stateroom,Switch to this Channel).**
Channel 31 -	The Great Gatsby
Channel 32 -	L A Confidential
Channel 34 -	Time Cop

Showtimes at 10:00am * 2:00pm * 5:00pm * 8:00pm *11:00pm

MOVIES

Le Cercle du Paul Gauguin
is open tonight at 5:30pm, featuring Blackjack lessons upon opening. Come in and learn the ***winning way*** *for the most popular game in the world.*

Bridge Visits

Navigational Bridge visits will be offered:

Tuesday — 2:00pm
Wednesday — 2:00pm
Thursday — 10:00am
Friday — 2:00pm

Please sign up at the Reception Desk, Deck 4 (15 per trip)

La Boutique
Today, for this Cruise only. We have a special discount on Cartier & Tag Watches, Tee Shirts & Swimwear.

Room Service
(Dial 999)
24 Hours

Hospital Hours
Open Daily
8:30-10:00am
5:00-7:00pm

In case of Emergency
Dial 0

Wakeup Call
Dial 66

CARITA SPA

Experience the deep relaxation with our
Harmonipunture Treatment
Feel refreshed and energized in body and a calm serenity in your mind

For appointments dial 933

What's happening aboard...

Roberto, our host of La Veranda, is there taking resevations for our alternativedinning experience.

Our Maitre'D Enzo Mazzali, will take your bookings for Le Grill Dinner "Al Fresco", daily during breakfast & lunch.

Good Morning

	m/s Paul Gauguin has remained at anchor through the night.	
8:00am	Morning stretch class with the ship's staff.	Pool Deck 8
8:30am	Walkathon. 13 Laps = One mile	Pool Deck 8
9:00am	Board Games available till 9:00pm.	The tables deck 5 midships
10:00am	Big Screen Movie: **"Peacemaker'**. Starring George Clooney	Grand Salon 5
11:00am	**Last Tender from shore. m/s Paul Gauguin sails for Raiatea.**	
11:00am	**Sailaway music.** Join *Les Gauguines* on deck as we depart Rangiroa.	Pool Deck 8

Good Afternoon

2:00pm	Deck Quiz. Join the ships staff for a fun Quiz.	Poolbar area Deck 8
2:30pm	Golf Putting Tournament. With Les Gauguines.	Sun Deck 9
3:00pm	Flower Lei making class with Les Gauguines.	Pool Deck 8
3:15pm	**Lecture by Bernhard Rickenbach.** An Ex Patriot in Polynesia.	Grand Salon 5
3:30pm	Fitness Center Orientation with our Sports Staff.	Fitness Center 6
4:00pm	Low Impact Aerobics, with the ships staff.	Pool Deck 8
4:00-5:00pm	Afternoon tea is served with music by Gail.	La Palette 8
4:30pm	**Black Pearl presentation.** An introduction of Sibani byRani.	Grand Salon Deck 5
5:30pm	**Blackjack Lessons.** Le Cercle Casino.	Casino Deck 5
5:30pm	**Honeymooners,** meet Sarah.	La Palette Deck 8

Good Evening

DRESS THIS EVENING: **COUNTRY CLUB CASUAL**

6:00PM-8:00PM	COCTAILS WITH MUSIC BY SIGLO.	GRAND SALON DECK 5
6:30-7:30pm	Cocktails are served with music by Gail.	La Palette Deck 8
7:00-9:30pm	L'Etoile is Open for Dinner. Maitre D' Enzo Mazzali and Executive Chef Mario Valera in attendance.	Deck 5
7:30pm	Le Grill opens for Dinner " Al Fresco ". Reservations only.	Deck 8
8:00pm	La Veranda opens for "A Taste of Italy". Reservations only.	Deck 6
9:00pm-close	Connoisseur Club opens for Cognacs and Cigars.	Deck 7
10:00pm	**Showtime. Featuring your Cruise Director Billy Phillips** Music by **Siglo.**	Grand Salon Deck 5
10:00pm	**Gail Penny** Entertains at the Piano.	La Palette Deck 8
11:30pm	Disco Time. Boogie on down with our **DJ AnDee.**	La Palette Deck 8

Courtesy Radisson Seven Seas Cruises

RENAISSANCE CRUISES, INC.
1800 Eller Drive
Suite 300
P.O. Box 350307
Ft. Lauderdale, Florida 33335
(800) 525-2450

R-1, R-2, R-3, and *R-4:* entered service July 1998, November 1998, September 1999, and December 1999, respectively; 30,200 G.R.T.; 594' x 84'; 684-passenger capacity; 342 staterooms and suites; British and European officers, international crew; smoke-free vessels; *R-1* and *R-2* offer cruises in eastern and western Mediterranean, Greek islands, and Israel; *R-3* and *R-4* sail in Tahiti and the South Pacific.

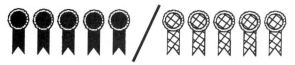

(Medical Facilities for all R Class ships: C-0; P-1; CLS, MS; N-1; CM; PD; BC; EKG; TC; PO; EPC; OX; WC; OR; ICU; X; M; CCP; TM.)

RENAISSANCE VII and *VIII:* entered service 1992; 4,500 G.R.T.; 297' x 50'; 114-passenger capacity; 57 suites; Italian officers, mixed international crew; cruises in Greek islands, western Mediterranean, Scandinavia, and Asia.

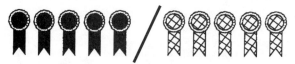

(Medical Facilities: C-0; P-1; CLS, MS; N-0; PD; EKG, OX; WC; CCP.)

Through 1997 Renaissance Cruises, Inc., operated a fleet of eight yacht-like vessels (built in Italy) that commenced service between 1989 and 1992. In 1996 and 1997, R Cruises, an affiliated company, ordered four new 684-passenger ships (the *R-1, R-2, R-3,* and *R-4*), and sold six of the original eight vessels. *R-1* offers year-round cruise tours between Athens and Istanbul to the Greek islands, Israel, and other Mediterranean ports, and *R-2's* initial itinerary is between Barcelona and Lisbon. Cruise fares include air transfers and pre- and post-cruise overnight stays at first-class or deluxe hotels in Athens, Istanbul, Barcelona, and Lisbon.

Renaissance VII and *VIII* are identical yacht-like vessels, with a capacity to accommodate 114 passengers in 57 outside suites ranging in size from 210 to 287 square feet.

The four most expensive suites are located on Explorer Deck atop each ship and feature private verandas. Eight additional suites on Erikson Deck also feature private verandas. All suites are beautifully appointed and include twin beds that convert to queens, modern bathrooms with marble vanities, hair dryers, robes, teak floors, remote-control color TVs and VCRs, refrigerated mini-bars, separate lounging and entertainment areas, either private safes or security lock drawers, and generous closet/storage space. All suites on each ship are located at the forward part of the ship and all public rooms at the stern. This layout guarantees quiet and privacy.

The ships' public areas are elaborately furnished and have wide corridors and staircases. These areas include a small outdoor pool, an outdoor dining facility for alfresco breakfast and lunch buffets, a beauty salon, a book and video library, a small casino, a club and piano bar, a domed lounge, a hospital, and the most attractively furnished dining rooms to be found on any ship afloat, featuring open seating with international cuisine and impressive service. The menu generally includes popular choices such as lobster, smoked salmon, and imported cheeses, with such items as Caesar salad, steak, chicken, and seafood entrees available at every meal.

In the evenings there is a three-piece band in the Lounge, a piano player in the more intimate Club, a blackjack table, several slot machines, and a large selection of videos that can be taken back to your suite for private viewing. Do not expect the usual range of cruise-ship entertainment.

The two smaller Renaissance ships offer cruises throughout the eastern and western Mediterranean, cruises from the Mediterranean up to Scandinavia, cruises in Scandinavia, and cruises calling at ports in the Far East and Asia. Most cruises are from five to eight days, with options to combine back-to-back itineraries in modular segments, permitting exploration of more ports.

In August 1996 R Cruises announced plans to construct two 684-passenger cruise ships. *R-1,* the first in the series of "R Class" vessels, began sailing in July 1998, followed by *R-2* in November 1998. Both offer ten- to sixteen-day cruise tours in the Mediterranean and Greek Isles. In March 1997, Renaissance Cruises also commissioned the building of two additional "R Class" ships, *R-3* and *R-4,* to be home-ported in Tahiti. *R-3* and *R-4* will explore the exotic splendor of the South Pacific year-round on ten-day itineraries. These new ships, in this observer's opinion, are the most elegantly and tastefully decorated ships currently in service, and could be described as a Ritz-Carlton or Four Seasons Hotel at sea. Corridors are laden with floral-runner-style carpets similar to those found in grand hotels; stairways are adorned with antiques and works of art; and lounges and all three dining rooms are furnished with rich, dark woods, as well as very expensive classical period French and English furnishings, and wall and window treatments. The decor throughout the vessels was ingeniously orchestrated to create a feeling of understated elegance and grand refinement without a hint of glitz or ostentation. Ten "Owner's" suites on each ship range in size from 533 to 598 square feet, with 253 to 364-square-foot private wrap-around balconies, two televisions, separate living rooms with dining areas, bedrooms, guest baths, and all marble master bathrooms with whirlpool tub. Fifty-two suites, averaging 260 square feet, include 72-square-foot private balconies, comfortably furnished sitting areas, bathtubs, and refrigerated mini-bars. An additional 170 outside staterooms averaging 173 square feet also offer 43-square-foot private balconies. All 342 tastefully appointed suites and staterooms on each ship feature a choice of twin- or queen-size bed configuration, remote-controlled satellite TV, individual stateroom temperature controls, ample wardrobe and storage space, hair dryers, and mini-safes. Presently robes and refrigerators are only found in the higher category staterooms and suites.

The ships' public areas are designed to offer the elegance, refinement, and amenities of the great ocean liners of the past. The public rooms, while spacious, maintain the intimacy and high service standards for which Renaissance Cruises' fleet is known.

Open-seating dining is offered between 6:30 and 9:00 P.M. at a choice of four uniquely different restaurants. The informal Panorama Buffet offers breakfast, lunch, and dinner buffets, as well as grilled items from the poolside barbecue and piping-hot pizza from the pizzeria. This is one of the best buffet operations at sea, with attentive service. Traditional formal breakfasts, lunches, and dinners with piano music in the evenings are the specialty of The Club, the largest of the dinner venues, offering a variety of Continental cuisine. World-class chefs prepare Italian regional dishes in the romantic Italian Restaurant, while The Grill, with warm décor and dark woods reminiscent of a grill room in London, specializes in prime steaks, seafood, and fine wines. All restaurants offer multiple, gourmet courses, imaginatively presented with impeccable service and spectacular ocean views through floor-to-ceiling windows. For a light snack, Sweets serves specialty coffees and desserts. High tea is offered each afternoon, and late-night snacks each evening. 24-hour room service is also available.

In contrast to its smaller vessels, a full array of cruise-ship entertainment and activities is available on board the "R Class ships." Cabaret-style shows, music, dancing, and popular entertainers are highlighted in the Cabaret Lounge; the Sports Club, which also serves as an observation lounge, boasts continuous big-screen live news and sports coverage along a 12-TV video wall, together with music and gaming machines and dancing. There is also an elegant Las Vegas-style casino, complete with blackjack, roulette, and slot machines, as well as an extraordinarily furbished library, and card and game room.

A fully equipped health and fitness facility and a world-class spa which provides holistic body treatments, massage, thalassotherapy whirlpool treatments, an attractive outdoor saltwater pool with two adjoining freshwater heated whirlpools, an oval jogging track above the lido area, and expansive decks with comfortable lounges also enhance the on-board experience. There is no sauna; however, for $20 per day guests can use the steam room, small thalassotherapy pool, and private deck area.

Renaissance Cruises appeals to well-heeled but value-conscious active cruisers wanting luxury while being destination-oriented. Service is attentive and friendly, comparable to its competition in the luxury cruise-ship market. With prices ranging from $270 to $699 per person per day depending on the ship, season, and cabin category, including round-trip airfare and deluxe hotel stays, Renaissance Cruises is considerably less expensive than its upscale competitors and an excellent buy in the premium segment of the cruise industry.

The emphasis is on offering its customers sensational itineraries all over the world. The ships sail mostly at night, which affords more time during the day to explore the ports of call. All itineraries include complimentary round-trip air, pre- and post-cruise stays at five-star hotels, and all ground transportation. Passengers not requiring the air or hotel accommodations are given a credit from their cruise fare. Taking everything into consideration, Renaissance Cruises is an exceptional value.

Strong Points:

The vessels of Renaissance Cruises offer exceptional itineraries; desirable pre-and post-cruise hotel stays; beautifully appointed spacious accommodations; fine dining; and outstanding service at extremely competitive prices—adding up to the best cruise-tour vacation value in the premium cruise market. The new "R Class" ships are among the most warmly and elegantly furbished vessels presently in service.

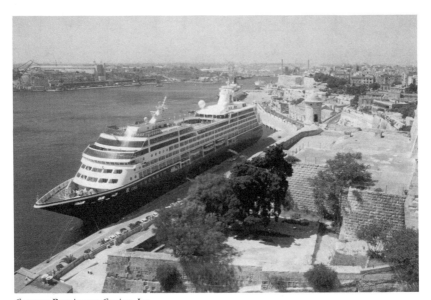

Courtesy Renaissance Cruises, Inc.

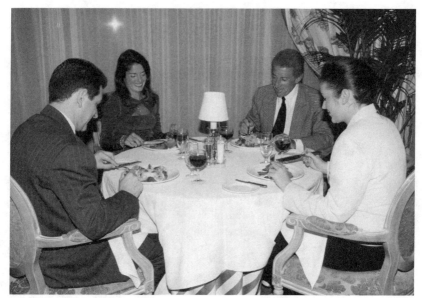

Courtesy Renaissance Cruises, Inc.

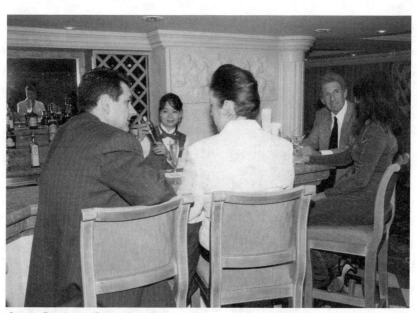

Courtesy Renaissance Cruises, Inc.

APPETIZERS

Fresh Starburst Fruit Medley

Norwegian Smoked Salmon, Onion Rings, Capers and Lemon

Sauteed Mushrooms on Pastry Pillow, Herbed Sauce

SOUPS

Cream of Pencil Asparagus

French Onion with Three-Cheese Croutons

SALADS

Curly Endive with Walnuts, Pears and Goat Cheese

Vine Ripened Tomato, Fennel with Seasonal Mesclun

VEGETARIAN

Brown Rice with Ginger and Green Banana

Served with Peas, Eggplants, Red Bell Pepper,
chopped Tomato and Green Beans, enhanced with a Curry Sauce

ENTREES

Chef's Fresh Pasta
Your Waiter will describe tonight's Selection

Baked Supreme of Halibut
With a White Butter Sauce and fragrant Black Beans

Crisply Roasted Raspberry Duck
Presented with slivered Potatoes, and aged Balsamic Vinegar

(❦) Veal Scallopine Marsala
With roasted Shallots and Celery

Grilled Tournedos of Beef
*With sliced Artichoke, Cocotte Potato,
laced in rich Chardonnay Demi-glace*

Selection of Fresh Market Vegetables

(❦) *indicates Health Conscious selection*

ENTREES

Chef's Fresh Pasta
Your Waiter will describe tonight's Selection

Baked Supreme of Halibut
With a White Butter Sauce and fragrant Black Beans

Crisply Roasted Raspberry Duck
Presented with slivered Potatoes, and aged Balsamic Vinegar

(❧) Veal Scallopine Marsala
With roasted Shallots and Celery

Grilled Tournedos of Beef
*With sliced Artichoke, Cocotte Potato,
laced in rich Chardonnay Demi-glace*

Selection of Fresh Market Vegetables

(❧) *indicates Health Conscious selection*

RENAISSANCE CRUISES, INC.

DAILY PROGRAM
Monday, November 2, 1998
Ashdod, Israel

GOOD MORNING

7:00	**R1 is scheduled to dock in Ashdod, Israel.**	
8:00	**R1's Daily Challenge.** Pick up today's quiz or crossword.	Reception (4)
10:00 & 4:00	**Meet your fellow Bridge Players** for an informal game.	Card Room (9)
10:15	**Checkers Challenge.** Meet your fellow guests for a game.	Library (10)

GOOD AFTERNOON

1:00	**Board Games Available.** Meet your fellow guests.	Library (10)
1:15	**Golf Chipping.** Meet the Cruise Staff on the Green.	Sun Deck (11)
2:00	**Ping Pong Challenge** with the Cruise Staff.	Poolside (9)
5:30	**Today's Daily Challenge Solutions.**	Reception (4)

GOOD EVENING

7:15-8:00	Dance to the Beautiful Sounds & Make Your Requests With the ♪**Renaissance Orchestra** Under the Direction of Michael Lalonde.	Sports Bar (10)
7:00-9:00	**Dine & Dance** to the Piano Music of Ron Van Dyke.	Club Restaurant (5)

Renaissance Cruises Proudly Spotlights Ashdod's Local Entertainers

8:15 & 10:00	Cabaret Lounge (5)

Featuring

The Traditions of Israel

Come and Enjoy this Folkloric Show!

Celebrate the music and movement of the Israeli Culture and all it has to offer!

9:15	**Name That "TV Tune" Trivia** Join your Assistant Cruise Director Bryan for a nostalgic walk down memory lane. Test your knowledge of all the classic TV Tunes & Shows.	Cabaret Lounge (5)
9:30-10:30	**The Piano Romance of Broadway** with Ron Van Dyke.	Upper Hall (5)
10:30-11:45	**Late Night** The Renaissance Orchestra Presents **"Dance the Night Away"** Relive some of the greatest dance music of all time.	Sports Bar (10)

Courtesy Renaissance Cruises, Inc.

RIVERS OF EUROPE/DANUBE CRUISES AUSTRIA
11802 Washington Boulevard
Unit 121
Los Angeles, California 90066
(800) 999-0226
(310) 397-3899
(310) 397-5139 FAX

M/S *AMADEUS I* and *II:* entered service 1997 and 1998 respectively; 110 meters x 11.4 meters; 154-passenger capacity; 77 cabins; international crew; cruises on Danube to the Black Sea.

M/S *CEZANNE I:* entered service 1993; 356' x 33'; 102-passenger capacity; 52 cabins; European crew; Rhône and Saône River cruises.

M/S *CEZANNE II:* entered service 1999; 2,500 G.R.T.; 118.5 meters x 11.2 meters; 146-passenger capacity; 72 cabins; cruises from Rome to Rhône River at Avignon.

M/S *DELTASTAR:* entered service 1992, renovated 1996; 1,550 G.R.T.; 107.5 meters x 12.8 meters; Romanian crew; 80 cabins.

M/S *NIAGRA:* 100'; 6-passenger capacity; 3 cabins; a/c; French and English crew; 6-night cruises in Burgundy area of France.

M/S *REINE PEDAQUE:* 128', 12-passenger capacity; 6 cabins; a/c; French and English crew; 6-night cruises in Burgundy, France.

M/S *RIVER CLOUD:* entered service 1996; 360' x 37'; 98-passenger capacity; 49 cabins; German/Austrian crew; cruises on Main-Danube Canal and the Danube.

M/S *ROUSSE:* entered service 1984, renovated 1993; 1,295 G.R.T.; 106 meters x 16 meters; 98 cabins; Bulgarian crew.

Dr. W. Lueftner Reisen is the owner of the new M/S *Amadeus I* and *II* and operator for the two Eastern European vessels M/S *Rousse* and M/S *Deltastar;* Sea Cloud Cruises is the owner of the M/S *River Cloud;* and Provence Line is the owner of the M/S *Cezanne I* and *II;* all of which are represented in the United States by Rivers of Europe/Danube Cruises Austria in Los Angeles. The ships sail between April and October, with special cruises over Christmas and New Year's.

The M/S *Amadeus I* and *II* are the most modern vessels on the European waterways. Atop ship is the sun deck, the location of a heated swimming pool with deck chairs, a small bar, and a life-size chess game. Exercise classes are offered here every morning. Next comes Mozart Deck with its Panorama Bar, with large windows permitting unobstructed views, the dining room, the hairdresser, gift shop, luxury conference area, and reception. The 77 cabins, which include 2 apartments, are spread along Mozart Deck and the next two descending decks.

In the evenings, the ship's orchestra entertains with dance music, and occasionally there are other musicians brought aboard. The 75 cabins and 2 apartments, located on three decks, are air conditioned and heated and include color TVs with video channels, radios, international direct-dial telephones, hair dryers, and two twin beds that can be arranged together. The restaurant features international cuisine in one sitting.

Itineraries include ten days on the Danube between Passau and the Black Sea and eight-day cruises between Nuremberg and Budapest, cruising on the famous Main-Danube Canal and the Danube. Prices range from $135 to $300 per person per day, depending on the season and cabin location.

M/S *Rousse* and M/S *Deltastar* travel on the Danube in the German, Austrian, Slovakian, and Hungarian sectors, with some cruises going all the way to the Black Sea. Prices range from $97 to $270 per person per day, again depending on the season and cabin location.

M/S *River Cloud* is one of the newer deluxe vessels on the European waterways. Atop ship is the sun deck, the location of a putting green, deck chairs, a small bar, and a life-size chess game. Exercise classes are offered here every morning. Next comes Promenade Deck with its gym—equipped with two stationary bicycles, one stair climber, different sizes of free weights, and a sauna; the dining room; junior suites; the hairdresser; gift shop; library; reception; and lounge. The standard cabins are spread along Cabin Deck.

In the evenings, the ship's pianist entertains with dance music, and, as on the two *Amadeus* ships, occasionally there are other musicians brought aboard. The 33 cabins and 6 junior suites, located on two decks, are air conditioned and heated and include color TVs with video channels, radios, international direct-dial telephones, electronic safe, hair dryers, and two twin beds (can be arranged together in some cabins) or one queen-size bed (two mattresses/one box spring) in all standard cabins or one queen-size bed (two mattresses/one box spring) in all junior suites. The restaurant features international cuisine in one sitting.

The itinerary is eight days on the Main-Danube Canal and the Danube between Nuremberg and Budapest. Prices range from $140 to $289 per person per day, depending on the season and cabin location.

Coming on line in 1993 from the Benetti shipyard in Viareggio, Italy, the M/S *Cezanne I* is one of the most modern and attractive boats plying the rivers of Europe. The open deck atop the vessel has lounge chairs and generous space for sunning as well as two heated Jacuzzis, and a life-size chess game. Exercise classes are offered here every morning. Next comes Prelude Deck with its circular reception hall, Four Seasons Restaurant, attractive 2,376-square-foot Dolce Vita Lounge with conference facilities and adjoining bar, gift shop, and 12 cabins. The four 178-square-foot cabins with queen beds and the nine 162-square-foot twin-bedded cabins have large picture windows; whereas the remaining 41 accommodations spread along Nocturne Deck only have portholes and range in size between 125 and 142 square feet.

All accommodations are air conditioned and heated and include large wardrobes, desks, bedside tables, color TVs with video channels, radios, international direct-dial telephones, private safes, and lovely marble bathrooms with showers, fully mirrored vanities, toilets, and storage space. Also on Nocturne Deck are a sauna, fitness center, and lounge.

Itineraries include eight, five, and four days on the Rhone between Lyon and Arles, as well as theme cruises. Prices range from $200 to $344 per person per day, depending on the season and cabin location.

The menus are impressive, with numerous selections and emphasis on French cuisine and wines with international alternatives.

Entering service in 1999, the M/S *Cezanne II* is a truly unique cruise vessel combining the power and capacity of an ocean-going sea liner with the intimacy and characteristics of a riverboat. She accommodates up to 146 passengers in 68 cabins and 4 spacious suites. The official languages aboard ship are English, French, and Italian, and the cuisine is French and Italian. Atop ship is the Sun Deck, featuring a jogging track, putting green, chess board, bar, and wading pool. The deck below is the location of the restaurant, bar, lounge, and casino. The two lower decks house the staterooms, suites, fitness/sauna, swimming pool, and hairdresser/beauty center. Passengers embark either in Rome or Avignon, and the vessel divides the itinerary between calls at such Mediterranean ports as Viareggio (for Florence, Pisa, and Siena) and Monte Carlo, as well as inland Rhône river cities such as Arle. Seven-night cruises range in price from $1,190 to $3,800 in low season and from $2,920 to $4,920 in high season.

Strong Points:

The M/S *Amadeus I* and *II,* like the *Mozart,* offer an upscale riverboat experience covering the most scenic and desired areas along the Danube River.

M/S *Cezanne I* and M/S *River Cloud* are newly constructed deluxe riverboats with expanded facilities offering upscale cruising for their respective itineraries.

M/S *Cezanne II* offers a unique combination of an ocean cruise coupled with a riverboat experience.

The M/S *Rousse* and *Deltastar* offer a more inexpensive opportunity to explore this area.

Rivers of Europe also represents all of Peter Deilmann's ships: *Mozart, Danube Princess, Prussian Princess, Dresden, Konigstein, Princess de Provence,* and *Lili Marleen,* (all covered earlier), as well as two barges, M/S *Niagra* and M/S *Reine Pedaque.*

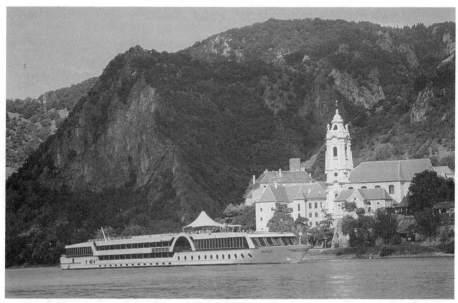

Amadeus *on Danube, courtesy Rivers of Europe/Danube Cruises Austria*

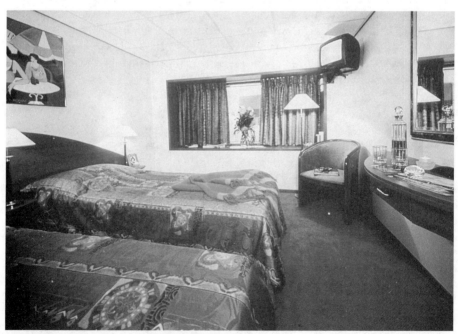

Amadeus *cabin, courtesy Rivers of Europe/Danube Cruises Austria*

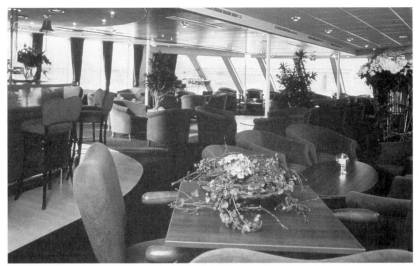

Amadeus *lounge, courtesy Rivers of Europe/Danube Cruises Austria*

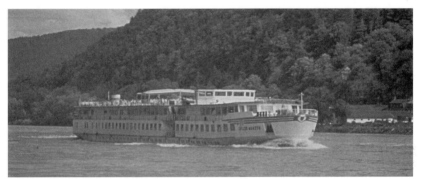

Delta Star, *courtesy Rivers of Europe/Danube Cruises Austria*

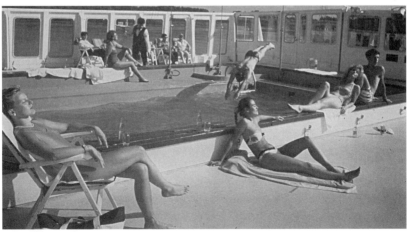

Upper deck of Rousse, *courtesy Rivers of Europe/Danube Cruises Austria*

—— CEZANNE ——

Les Entrées - *Appetisers*

Bouquet d'asperges printanier Mousseline froide à la ciboulette
Selection of fresh asparagus served with a cream and chive sauce

Feuille de jambon de Parme à l'Italienne
Thinly sliced Parma ham served with chilled melon

Papeton d'Aubergines et son coulis de tomate relevé au pistou
Traditional braised eggplant served with a fresh tomato and basil dressing

Rosace maraîchère au Magret de canard séché et ses billes de melon macérées
Delicate salad served with wafer-thin slices of cured breast of duck and pearls of melon

Terrine de Veau et Mozzarella en persillade vinaigrette Balsamic
Veal and mozzarella terrine spiced with parsley and garlic,
served with a balsamic vinegar dressing

Marinade de Saumon au jus d'olive des Baux
Thin slices of fresh salmon marinated with fresh herbs and delicate olive oil

Potage Cultivateur
Thick seasonal vegetable soup

Chaudron du Pêcheur
A richly garnished Mediterranean fish soup

Tagliatelles al Pesto alla Genovese
Broad pasta served with the traditional fragrant pesto sauce
and freshly grated parmesan cheese

Nid de pâtes et Morillettes
A nest of fine pasta served with delicate morel-mushrooms

Les Poissons - *Fish Courses*

Ragoût de Lotte à la Provençale

Monkfish steamed in a rich red wine sauce

Suprême de Turbotin en bourride

Turbot poached in stock enriched with egg and garlic
to form a velvet sauce

Escalope de Saumon mi-cuit au fumet de Morilles

Slice of prime salmon delicately braised in stock
flavoured with morel-mushrooms

Ensoleiade de Rougets juste poêlés,
à l'infusion de thym

Lightly sauteed fillets of red mullet,
accompanied by a thyme infused butter sauce

Les Viandes - *Meat Courses*

Crépinelle de Bœuf en robe Languedocienne

Fillet of beef topped with a crispy olive paste

Tranche de gigot d'Agneau à l'os,
jus à la menthe fraîche

Roast leg of lamb with fresh mint gravy

Rouelle de volaille farcie, crème à l'ail

Stuffed breast of chicken accompanied by a garlic-cream sauce

Magret de canard, jus épicé

Sliced breast of duck with a lightly spiced gravy

Les Grillades - *From the Grill*

Faux-filet grillé, Beurre Avignonnais
Prime sirloin steak with a herbal butter prepared with olives and shallots

Filet de Bœuf grillé
Grilled fillet of beef

Médaillon de Veau grillé
Grilled medaillons of veal

Ronde de gigot d'Agneau grillé
Grilled leg of lamb

Poisson - *Fish*

Dos de Saumon Verdurette
Fillet of salmon, served with a fresh garden herb sauce
prepared with olive oil and tomatoes

Sélection de Fromages de France
Make your choice from our cheeseplatter

Chariot de Desserts
A choice from our extensive dessert trolley

I.C.B. S.A. CHRÉTIEN - 04 42 07 39 09

Courtesy Rivers of Europe/Danube Cruises Austria

ROYAL CARIBBEAN INTERNATIONAL
1050 Caribbean Way
Miami, Florida 33132
(800) 526-RCCL

ENCHANTMENT OF THE SEAS: entered service 1997; 74,140 G.R.T.; 916' x 106'; 2,446-passenger capacity (1,950 double occupancy); 975 cabins; Norwegian and international officers and crew; seven-night cruises in eastern and western Caribbean from Miami. The home port changes to Port Everglades in April 2000.

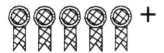

GRANDEUR OF THE SEAS: entered service 1996; 74,140 G.R.T.; 916' x 106'; 2,446-passenger capacity (1,950 double occupancy); 975 cabins; Norwegian and international officers and crew; seven-night cruises in eastern Caribbean from Miami.

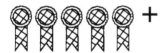

LEGEND OF THE SEAS: entered service 1995; 69,130 G.R.T.; 867' x 105'; 2,076-passenger capacity (1,800 double occupancy); 900 cabins; Norwegian and international officers and crew; Hawaii, Panama Canal, Mexican Riviera, Mediterranean, Europe, Middle East, Far East, Australia, and New Zealand.

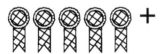

MAJESTY OF THE SEAS: entered service 1992; 73,941 G.R.T.; 880' x 106'; 2,744-passenger capacity (2,350 double occupancy); 1,175 cabins; Norwegian and international officers and crew; three-and four-night cruises to the Bahamas (after May 2000).

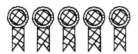

MONARCH OF THE SEAS: entered service 1991; 73,941 G.R.T.; 880' x 106'; 2,744-passenger capacity (2,350 double occupancy); 1,175 cabins; Norwegian and international officers and crew; seven-night southern Caribbean cruises from San Juan.

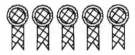

NORDIC EMPRESS: entered service 1990; 48,563 G.R.T.; 692' x 100'; 2,020-passenger capacity (1,600 double occupancy); 800 cabins; international officers and crew; three- and four-night cruises from San Juan to the southern Caribbean, and seven-night cruises to Bermuda from New York in the summer.

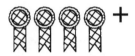

RHAPSODY OF THE SEAS: entered service 1997; 78,491 G.R.T.; 915' x 106'; 2,435-passenger capacity (2,000 double occupancy); 1,000 cabins; Norwegian and international officers and crew; southern Caribbean, Hawaii, Mexican Riviera, and Alaska cruises.

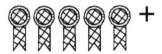

SOVEREIGN OF THE SEAS: entered service 1988; 73,192 G.R.T.; 880' x 106'; 2,850-passenger capacity (2,250 double occupancy); 1,125 cabins; Norwegian and international officers and crew; three- and four-night cruises from Miami to the Bahamas and from Port Canaveral to the Bahamas.

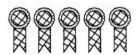

SPLENDOUR OF THE SEAS: entered service 1996; 69,130 G.R.T.; 867' x 105'; 2,076-passenger capacity (1,800 double occupancy); 900 cabins; Norwegian and international officers and crew; Caribbean and European cruises.

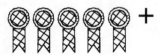

VIKING SERENADE: (formerly *Stardancer*); entered service 1982; refurbished 1986 and 1989; rebuilt 1991; 40,132 G.R.T.; 623' x 89'; 1,863-passenger capacity (1,500 double occupancy); 750 cabins; international officers and crew; three- and four-night cruises from Los Angeles to Baja, Mexico.

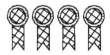

VISION OF THE SEAS: entered service 1998; 78,491 G.R.T.; 915' x 106'; 2,435-passenger capacity (2,000 double occupancy); 1,000 cabins; Norwegian and international officers and crew; cruises to Caribbean and Transcanal between San Juan and Acapulco, Hawaii, and Alaska.

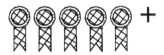

VOYAGER OF THE SEAS: entered service fall 1999; 142,000 G.R.T.; 1,021' x 158'; 3,838-passenger capacity (3,114 double occupancy); 1,557 cabins; Norwegian and international officers, international crew; seven-night cruises in Western Caribbean from Miami. **(Category B—Not Rated)**

(Medical Facilities: RCI advises that all ships have full medical facilities and equipment and are staffed with highly qualified physicians and nurses trained in trauma, emergency medicine, and general practice; however the cruise line has a policy of not providing specifics and suggests passengers concerned contact the medical department of the cruise line prior to sailing.)

Note: Actual passenger capacity on all ships will vary and on most cruises is less when there are only two passengers in a cabin. Thus, doubling the number of cabins is reflective of usual passenger capacity.

   Royal Caribbean International (formerly Royal Caribbean Cruise Line and referred to hereinafter for convenience as RCI) was founded in 1969 by three Norwegian shipping companies. Today it is a publicly held company traded on the New York and Oslo Stock Exchanges under "RCL." Its first vessel, *Song of Norway,* entered service in 1970 (sold in 1996), followed by *Nordic Prince* in 1971 (sold in early 1995), *Sun Viking* in 1972 (sold in 1978), and *Song of America* in 1982 (sold in 1998). All four ships were built in Finland and designed for cruising the Caribbean. The first of RCI's new breed of ships, *Sovereign of the Seas,* entered service in 1988, followed by *Nordic Empress* in 1990 and *Monarch of the Seas* and *Majesty of the Seas* in 1992. Commencing with *Legend of the Seas* in 1995, RCI introduced its

"Vision Class" fleet with many improvements and innovations from prior vessels. *Splendour of the Seas* and *Grandeur of the Seas* followed in 1996, along with *Enchantment of the Seas* and *Rhapsody of the Seas* in 1997 and *Vision of the Seas* in 1998, bringing the line's passenger berth count up to approximately 24,000.

In June 1997 RCI's parent company acquired the highly acclaimed Celebrity Cruise Lines, Inc.; however, each line continues to operate as a separate brand.

Cruise fares vary slightly from ship to ship and on different itineraries. The least expensive, inside cabin on all the ships goes for about $190 per person per day, graduating to $250 to $320 per day for an average cabin without a veranda, and $450 to $550 per day per person for a deluxe stateroom or mini-suite with a veranda. The top-of-the-line Royal Suite on each ship will set you back from $650-$1,000 per day per person. Add about $36 per day per person ($250 per week) for the air-sea packages. Additional parties sharing cabins pay about $100 per day. Prices on the new "Eagle Class" ships will run slightly higher, and discounts ranging from 20 percent to 33 percent are available for early bookings (9-12 months in advance).

Unlike most cruise lines, there are numerous suites, staterooms, and cabins in each price category, and the gradual increase in price from one category to the next buys you more space and not just a more desirable location.

At its inception, RCI was well known for providing fine cuisine, fine dining room service, and a large variety of activities and entertainment. In recent years, RCI has expanded its marketing program throughout the world, visits over 125 ports of call worldwide, and provides daily programs, shore excursions lists, and other on-board material in Spanish, German, Italian, French, and Portuguese. As a result, the line has attracted a more international mix of passengers. The number of non-U.S.-Canadian cruisers will vary between 10 percent and 33 percent, depending upon the itinerary and port of embarkation.

In 1988 the 73,192-ton *Sovereign of the Seas* joined the fleet as the largest cruise ship then in service. She is capable of carrying 2,276 passengers in 1,138 cabins, 722 of which are located on the outside of the ship. All passenger cabins are forward and entertainment areas are aft of a dynamic central atrium area (the Centrum), creating an exceptionally quiet cabin zone. The 8 regular suites and the 4 deluxe larger suites are all located high above the sea on Bridge Deck, together with 50 deluxe outside staterooms. The remaining cabins are spread among eight other lower decks. All beds in all staterooms can be converted to double beds.

At the very top of the ship, 11 stories above sea level, is the panoramic 360-degree Viking Crown Lounge, accessible by special lift. The upper level of the Windjammer Cafe and the Mast Bar are on Compass Deck. The main entrance to the café is below on the Sun Deck, and this indoor-outdoor restaurant is the site for breakfast and lunch buffets. Also on the Sun Deck are two swimming pools, a bar, and the children's center with video games. The gymnasium and men's and women's saunas are on the Bridge Deck, and immediately below is the Anything Goes (state-of-the-art) Disco. The Music Man Show Lounge on the Mariner Deck seats 675 and the twin-level Follies Lounge seats 1,050. Besides the upper level of the main lounge, the Promenade Deck includes Finian's Rainbow Lounge for dancing, The Touch of Class Champagne Bar, a library, and cardroom. On the Show-time Deck are the first level of the Main Lounge, the casino, and the Boutiques of Centrum. The Purser's desk and Kismet Dining Room are on the Main Deck, the Gigi Dining Room is on A Deck, and two cinemas are on B Deck. The ship is currently offering three- and four-night cruises from Miami to the Bahamas, but will relocate to Port Canaveral for the spring 2000 season.

Viking Serenade was transferred to RCI in 1989 after its purchase of Admiral Cruises, Inc. Formerly known as the *Stardancer,* the ship will continue to be positioned in the Pacific, offering three- and four-day cruises from Los Angeles to Baja, Mexico. The ship was built in France by Scandinavia World Cruises in 1982 and was originally intended as a cruise ship with the capacity to transport automobiles. Stanley McDonald purchased the ship in 1985 for Sundance Cruises and instituted an expensive redecoration. In 1986 Admiral Cruises was formed as a result of a merger between Eastern, Western, and Sundance cruise lines. In 1991 RCI spent $75 million on completely rebuilding the ship, adding another dining room, a 360-degree panoramic lounge atop the ship, and numerous cabins.

Though older and less modern than on RCI's newer vessels, the staterooms and public areas are very attractively furnished in warm, soft tones. The public lounges are beautifully decorated, and the main pool area, with its sliding glass roof, is also outstanding. The cabins, although small, are unusually well appointed, and include twin beds that convert to doubles, color TVs, three-station radios, dressing tables and mirrors, modern lighting systems, good dresser and closet space, and modern bathrooms with ample shelving (seldom found on cruise ships).

At the top of the ship on the Sun Deck are the large pool area with a jogging path around the sliding glass roof; two outdoor Jacuzzis; the Windjammer Cafe, where a buffet breakfast or lunch can be enjoyed alfresco; and a health club with exercise equipment, sauna, massage, tanning bed, and children's room. Next comes the Club Deck, the location of several shops, a lounge, and more cabins. Below on the Cabaret Deck are the main show lounge, the casino, a bar, and cabins. On the bottom three decks are the remaining cabins, the two dining rooms, and conference facilities.

Nordic Empress, at 48,563 tons and accommodating 1,600 passengers double occupancy or 2,020 when all berths are filled, entered service during the summer of 1990. For many years it competed in the Miami to Bahamas three- and four-night cruise market. Presently it resides in San Juan, offering three- and four-night cruises to the southern Caribbean and in the summer she moves to New York, offering seven-night cruises to Bermuda. Like *Sovereign of the Seas,* it has a dramatic atrium lobby (nine decks high) called the Centrum, which connects with many of the ship's public rooms, including the unique two-level dining room. For alfresco dining, a wide-open, indoor/outdoor café offers a variety of food services, including midnight buffets under the stars.

There are seven lounges with public areas, including a two-level show lounge complete with balcony opera boxes; a two-level inverted amphitheater surrounded by glass, which converts from a daytime observatory to a state-of-the-art disco at night; a two-level casino; a jogging track; four whirlpools; a health club; a computerized golf room; and a shopping mall.

In 1991, the 73,941-ton *Monarch of the Seas* joined the fleet, followed by *Majesty of the Seas* in 1992. The ships' designs are similar to *Sovereign of the Seas*, with several innovations and improvements, including the addition of balconies in 62 of the suites and superior staterooms. The 2,354-passenger *Monarch* offers seven-night cruise vacations from San Juan to the southern Caribbean, and the identical *Majesty* features seven-night cruises from San Juan, changing to three- and four-night cruises from Miami to the Bahamas in the spring of 2000.

In May 1995 the 70,000-ton, 2,076-passenger *Legend of the Seas*, the first of the "Vision Class" ships, entered service, with emphasis on windows overlooking the sea, a seven-deck atrium topped off by a two-deck skylight attached to a 250-seat observation lounge/nightclub, facilities that include an 18-hole miniature golf course, a state-of-the-art spa and fully equipped fitness center, an 118-foot swimming pool, an indoor-outdoor pool with sliding glass roof, special youth and teen facilities, and public areas, with numerous innovations and improvements from the lines' prior megaships. Twenty-five percent of the staterooms and suites have private verandas, and all cabins convert to double-bed configurations. In 1996 the sister ship, *Splendour of the Seas*, joined the fleet. *Grandeur of the Seas*, which entered service in late 1996, *Enchantment of the Seas* and *Rhapsody of the Seas*, which entered service in 1997, and *Vision of the Seas*, in 1998, are all somewhat similar to *Legend of the Seas* and boast extremely exquisite designs, fabrics, and artwork.

These are among the most attractively furbished larger ships in service. Passengers can appreciate the elegant main lobbies, stairwells, and wide corridors with their abundance of wood, brass, marble, glass, and exquisite sculptures and artwork; the spacious elevators and public washrooms; the unique casinos; the lavish spa area with its numerous facilities; the opulent shopping plaza; the selection of theme lounges and bars; the lovely, comfortable two-story dining rooms and show lounges; giant panoramic observation lounges; special facilities for children and teens; and gigantic lido-pool complexes. A standard cabin is quite adequate and includes a small sitting area, two double or one queen bed, a private safe, a remote-control television, a mirrored make-up area, and small bathroom. All staterooms and suites on decks 7 and 8 are spacious and include nice-sized patios. The 19 full suites and 1 Royal suite on Deck 8 have larger sitting areas and balconies, refrigerator/mini-bars, and beautiful marble bathrooms with double vanities, tubs, showers, and robes. All accommodations on *Rhapsody of the Seas* and *Vision of the Seas* are a bit larger. On all of the Vision Class ships the smallest inside cabin is at least 135 square feet, average outside cabins without balconies range from 153 to 193 square feet, staterooms and regular suites with balconies from 236 to 630 square feet, and the Royal Suites over 1,100 square feet.

All of RCI's 70,000+-ton ships offer the same caliber of cruise experience; i.e., they are megaships lavishly furnished with a multitude of activities, facilities, and entertainment options. The dining rooms feature a variety of items nightly with multicourse, rotating menus and concerned service. The Windjammer Cafés offer a casual dining alternative for all three meals, with a good selection of choices.

The line is in the process of constructing three 142,000-gross-ton, 1,019-foot-long, 1,550-cabin, 3,114-passenger "Eagle Class" megaships, scheduled for completion in the fall of 1999, 2000, and 2002, respectively. The first will be named *Voyager of the Seas* and will offer seven-night Western Caribbean itineraries from Miami. These will be the largest ships ever built and will feature innovations such as an ice rink, a television studio, a 400-seat conference facility, an in-line skating track, a golf driving range, a rock-climbing wall, a 25,000-square-foot, world-class spa, a 1,350-seat theater spanning five decks, a three-level dining room with separate themed dining areas, plus numerous alternative dining options and greatly expanded youth facilities. Staterooms in all categories have been expanded in size, 50 percent have balconies, and each is equipped with generous storage, a mini-bar, hair dryer and 19-inch T.V. The second "Eagle Class" ship will be named *Explorer of the Seas* and will offer seven-night Eastern Caribbean itineraries from Miami.

Strong Points:

Beautifully appointed megaships offering spacious, attractive accommodations, a large variety of facilities, activities, and entertainments, as well as enjoyable dining experiences. All in all, RCI is a strong competitor in the premium cruise market.

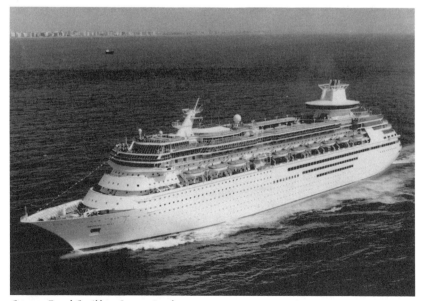

Courtesy Royal Caribbean International

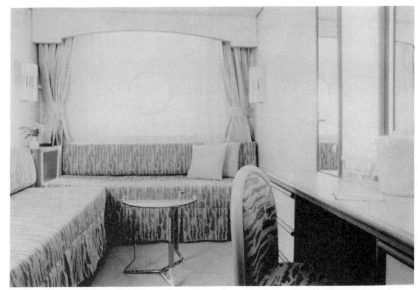

Courtesy Royal Caribbean International

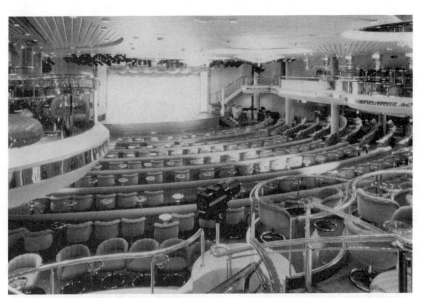

Courtesy Royal Caribbean International

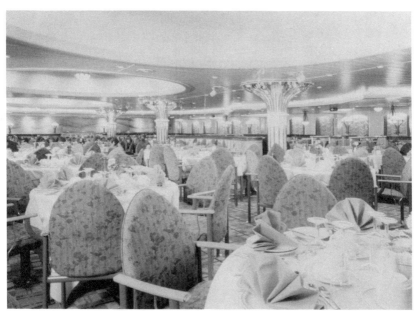

Courtesy Royal Caribbean International

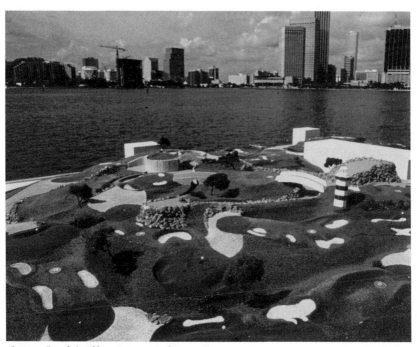

Courtesy Royal Caribbean International

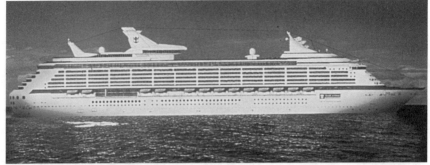

Voyager of the Seas, *courtesy Royal Caribbean International*

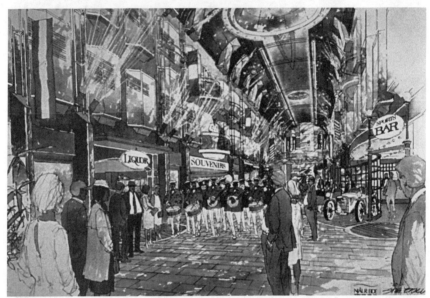

Voyager of the Seas, *courtesy Royal Caribbean International*

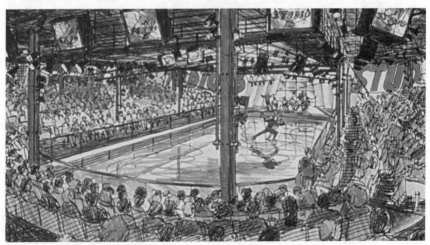

Voyager of the Seas, *courtesy Royal Caribbean International*

CAPTAIN'S FAREWELL DINNER

M/S *Vision of the Seas*

APPETIZERS

Complement of Fresh Fruit, water chestnuts and bean shoots
Chilled Poached Fillet of Sole with marinated salmon on a couscous salad
Mole Pablano, chicken slivers with a chilled Mexican chocolate flavored chili sauce
Baked Escargots Bourguignone

SOUPS

Waterzooi Soup with chicken, carrots, celery and onions
Barley Broth and Vegetables
Vichyssoise, chilled potato and leek with chives

SALAD

Assorted Baby Lettuce with celery, radish, alfalfa sprouts and tomatoes served with your choice of French dressing, parsley vinaigrette or fat free raspberry vinaigrette

"Iceberg Lettuce seasonally available upon request"

PASTA

Sautéed Ravioli with roasted shallots and fresh stewed tomato concasse with dill and romano cheese

MAIN COURSE

Grilled Fillet of Snapper with sauteed cassava and patti pan squash with a savory rice pilaf

Breaded Veal Chop with spinach and a marsala saffron rissoto

Roasted Duck with a rhubarb sauce, served with a wild rice and roasted pepper pilaf, chayotte squash and peas

Pan Seared Filet Mignon with a wild mushroom ragout and carrots

Artichoke Bottoms, tomatoes, garlic, zucchini with fettucini with toasted pine nuts

"Shallow Poached or Grilled Chicken Breast, Sirloin Steak or Salmon, as well as Baked Potato or Pilaf of Rice available"

CHEESE

Selective Cheese from the board

Signature dishes created by our Master Chefs

ROSEMARY & SHALLOTS

*R*osemary has the reputation for strengthening the memory. It has become the emblem of fidelity for lovers. In times past, it was worn around the neck as a powerful charm against witches' spells.

*S*hallots originated in Asia Minor and became an onion substitute because of its softer taste and aroma. Mild flavored shallot balls are highly prized for use in soups and stews, in salads and salad dressings and are an important ingredient in French recipes.

SHIP SHAPE

Our Ship Shape Menu has been carefully developed to meet Healthy Dietary Guidelines, limiting total calories from fat.

Mole Pablano, chicken slivers with a chilled Mexican chocolate flavored chili sauce
Calories: 86 ; Fat: .50 g;

Barley Broth and Vegetables
Calories: 71 ; Fat: .87 g:

Assorted Baby Lettuce with Celery, Radish, Alfalfa Sprouts and Tomatoes served with fat free raspberry vinaigrette
Calories: 80 ; Fat: 0 g:

Grilled Fillet of Snapper with sauteed cassava and patti pan squash with a savory rice pilaf
Calories: 352 ; Fat: 5 g:

Crisp Napoleon
Calories: 140 ; Fat: 2.1 g:

DESSERTS

Your Waiter will present you with our menu of specially selected desserts.

BEVERAGES

Coffee freshly brewed, regular or decaffeinated
Tea   Herb Tea   Hot Chocolate
Milk   Soft Drinks

"In an effort to support worldwide conservation measures, ice water is served upon request only."

WINE

Our recommendations for tonight are listed under the following categories on the wine list

Light, Dry White Wines

Full Bodied, Moderately Tannic Red Wines

D-9/10DAYS
D-10/11DAYS
9.98

Courtesy Royal Caribbean International

Today At A Glance

Thursday

MORNING

8:00 a.m.		THE M/S VISION OF THE SEAS IS DUE TO ARRIVE AT CHARLOTTE AMALIE, ST. THOMAS, U.S.V.I. - When the ship has been cleared by the local authorities, guests may disembark the vessel. Location of Gangway will be announced upon arrival. All guests on tour are reminded to meet at your respective departure locations.
REMINDER:		PLEASE REMEMBER YOUR BOARDING CARD AND TOUR TICKETS.
8:00 a.m.	- 8:20 a.m.	SUNRISE STRETCH CLASS - The perfect way to start your day. Some Enchanted Evening Lounge, Deck 6. $
8:00 a.m.	- 9:30 a.m.	YOUR PORT AND SHOPPING LECTURER, TOM is available at the gangway to answer any questions on St. Thomas and for Island Maps.
8:00 a.m.	- 5:00 p.m.	SIGN-UP FOR SABBATH SERVICES - Any members of the Jewish faith wishing to attend "Oneg Shabbat" services tomorrow evening, please sign-up today at the Shore Excursion Desk, Deck 5
8:30 a.m.	- 8:50 a.m.	GUTBUSTERS - Tone that Tummy! Some Enchanted Evening Lounge, Deck 6. $
9:00 a.m.	- 9:45 a.m.	BEGINNERS STEP AEROBIC - ShipShape Center, Deck 10 Aft. $
9:00 a.m.	- 4:00 p.m.	ROYAL CARIBBEAN'S EXCLUSIVE "CROWN & ANCHOR CLUB" IS OPEN - Be sure to visit this air-conditioned restored Danish Warehouse, Hibiscus Alley, Downtown Charlotte Amalie.
9:00 a.m.	- 8:00 p.m.	SPORTS DECK OPEN - Ping Pong and Shuffleboard equipment will be available for informal play. Deck 9 & 10 Aft.
9:00 a.m.	- 10:30 a.m.	EARLY BIRD EYE - OPENERS - Bloody Marys & Screwdrivers $2.95 - Schooner Bar Deck 6.
9:00 a.m.	- 5:00 p.m.	CARD AND BOARD GAMES ARE AVAILABLE - Explorer's Court, Deck 8.
9:00 a.m.	- 5:00 p.m.	LIBRARY IS OPEN AND TRIVIA SHEETS ARE AVAILABLE - Deck 7, Centrum.
9:15 a.m.	- 9:45 a.m.	WALK-A-THON - Meet by the Glass Elevators, Centrum, Deck 10. $
10:15 a.m.	Sharp!	STAYING ON BOARD TODAY? - Looking for something to do? Meet other guests and a Cruise Staff in the Card Room, Deck 7 Centrum.

AFTERNOON

2:30 p.m.		INFORMAL BACKGAMMON, CHECKERS AND BRIDGE PLAY - Join your Cruise Staff and team up with other guests staying on board. Card Room, Centrum, Deck 7.
3:30 p.m.	- 4:15 p.m.	CARIBBEAN MUSIC with our Calypso Band - Poolside, Deck 9.
4:30 p.m.	- 4:50 p.m.	SIT TO BE FIT - Exercise in your chair. Some Enchanted Evening Lounge, Deck 6. $
4:30 p.m.	- 5:15 p.m.	TUMS, BUNS & THIGHS - ShipShape Center, Deck 10. $
4:30 p.m.	- 5:15 p.m.	CARIBBEAN MUSIC with our Calypso Band - Poolside, Deck 9.
5:00 p.m.	- 5:30 p.m.	AFTERNOON WALKATHON - Meet inside by the Glass Elevators, Centrum, Deck 10. $
5:00 p.m.	- 6:00 p.m.	FRIENDS OF BILL W. MEETING - Library, Deck 7, Centrum.
5:00 p.m.	- 11:00 p.m.	PHOTO GALLERY IS OPEN - Centrum, Deck 6.
5:15 p.m.	- 6:00 p.m.	PIANO MELODIES with David McFarland - Schooner Bar, Deck 6.
5:15 p.m.	- 6:15 p.m.	DANCING MUSIC with the "Tami Novak Trio" - Champagne Terrace, Centrum, Deck 4.

EVENING

5:30 p.m.		ALL GUESTS ARE REQUESTED TO BE BACK ON BOARD.
5:30 p.m.	- 6:15 p.m.	SAIL-AWAY CARIBBEAN MUSIC with our Calypso Band - Poolside, Deck 9.
5:30 p.m.	- 6:30 p.m.	2 FOR 1 HOUSEBRANDS in the Some Enchanted Evening Lounge, Deck 6.
5:30 p.m.	- 6:30 p.m.	ROMANTIC SERENADES with the "Rosario Strings" - Viking Crown Lounge, Deck 11.
5:30 p.m.	- 8:30 p.m.	FLOWER SALE - Deck 6, Next to the Photo Gallery in the Centrum.

5:30 p.m. - 6:00 p.m.	*SINGLES GET-ACQUAINTED GATHERING*
Deck 9 Forward	an informal get-together of all guests traveling alone
Outside the Windjammer Café	Meet your Cruise Staff for coffee and tea.

$ = Indicates 1 ShipShape Dollar is earned for participation.

Thursday

6:00 p.m.		THE M/S VISION OF THE SEAS IS EXPECTED TO SAIL FOR WILLEMSTAD, CURACAO. *(455 Nautical Miles).*
6:30 p.m.	- 7:15 p.m.	CARIBBEAN MUSIC with our **Calypso Band** - Poolside, Deck 9.
6:30 p.m.	- 11:00 p.m.	TAX & DUTY FREE SHOPS ARE OPEN - Centrum, Deck 6.
6:30 p.m.	- 11:00 p.m.	PHOTO SHOP IS OPEN - Centrum, Deck 6.

6:30 p.m. - Till Late
Deck 5

CASINO ROYALE
The Casino opens for your gaming pleasure.
Featuring Slots, Blackjack, Craps and Caribbean Stud Poker.

7:00 p.m.	- 7:45 p.m.	DANCE MUSIC with **"Masquerade"** - Some Enchanted Evening Lounge, Deck 6.
7:30 p.m.	- 8:30 p.m.	PORT & SHOPPING LECTURER, TOM, is available for all your shopping questions. Shore Excursion Desk, Deck 5.
7:45 p.m.	- 8:30 p.m.	ROMANTIC SERENADES with the **"Rosario Strings"** - Viking Crown Lounge, Deck 11.
7:45 p.m.	- 8:45 p.m.	DANCING MUSIC with the **"Tami Novak Trio"** - Champagne Terrace, Centrum, Deck 4.
8:00 p.m.	- 8:45 p.m.	PIANO BAR ENTERTAINMENT with **David McFarland** - Schooner Bar, Deck 6.

8:30 p.m. Main Seating
10:30 p.m. Second Seating
Decks 5 & 6

Masquerade Theater
proudly presents
CELEBRITY SHOWTIME
Starring
HERB REED AND THE PLATTERS

10:00 p.m. - 11:00 p.m.
Some Enchanted Evening
Lounge, Deck 6

KARAOKE SING ALONG
Pick a song and sing-a-long. Over 500 to choose from.
Wanted: Singers & Spectators

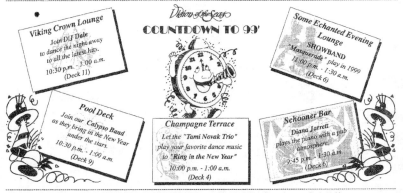

Vision of the Seas
COUNTDOWN TO 99'

Viking Crown Lounge
Join DJ Dale to dance the night away to all the latest hits.
10:30 p.m. - 3:00 a.m.
(Deck 11)

Some Enchanted Evening Lounge
SHOWBAND
"Masquerade" play in 1999
11:00 p.m. - 1:30 a.m.
(Deck 6)

Pool Deck
Join our Calypso Band as they bring in the New Year under the stars.
10:30 p.m. - 1:00 a.m.
(Deck 9)

Champagne Terrace
Let the "Tami Novak Trio" play your favorite dance music to "Ring in the New Year"
10:00 p.m. - 1:00 a.m.
(Deck 4)

Schooner Bar
Diana Jarrett plays the piano with a pub atmosphere.
9:45 p.m. - 1:30 a.m.
(Deck 6)

10:30 p.m. - 3:00 a.m. **DANCING TO THE TOP DISCS (Minimum age 18)** - Viking Crown Lounge, Deck 11 Aft.

Film Developing
Don't just tell your friends about your cruise, *SHOW THEM!* We offer same day professional film developing. Simply drop your film into the Film Drop Boxes in the Photo Gallery by Noon and your prints will be ready after 6:00 p.m.

HERB REED & THE PLATTERS
Herb Reed, the original bass singer, is who organized and named the group "The Platters". The Platters were inducted into the Rock & Roll Hall of Fame in 1990 with such hits as "Only You", "Smoke Gets In Your Eyes", "Twilight Time" and "The Great Pretender". We invite you to enjoy their timeless music tonight, in the Masquerade Theater, Decks 5 & 6.

CASINO *Royale*
WELCOMES YOU after sailing from St. Thomas, U.S.V.I. Come and Try your luck!
SLOTS & TABLES OPEN
6:30 p.m. - Till Late
GOOD LUCK!!

GUEST SERVICES

Purser's Office, Deck 5 (Dial 0)	Open 24 Hours
Room Service/Bell Station (Dial 53)	Open 24 Hours
Beauty Salon, Deck 9 (Dial 6850)	8:00 a.m. - 8:00 p.m.

24 hour notice of cancellation must be given to avoid a 50% cancellation charge at the Salon & ShipShape Center.

Sauna / Massage, Deck 9 (Dial 6850)	8:00 a.m. - 8:00 p.m.
ShipShape Center Deck 9 (Dial 6850)	7:00 a.m. - 8:00 p.m.
Casino Royale, Deck 5	6:30 p.m. - Till Late
Tax & Duty-Free Shops of the Centrum, Deck 6	6:30 p.m. - 11:00 p.m.
Photo Gallery, Deck 6 (Dial 6794)	5:00 p.m. - 11:00 p.m.
Photo Shop, Deck 6 (Dial 6789)	6:30 p.m. - 11:00 p.m.
Shore Excursion, Deck 5 (Dial 59)	8:00 a.m. - 10:00 a.m.
	7:30 p.m. - 8:30 p.m.
Library	9:00 a.m. - 5:00 p.m.
Reading Area	Open 24 Hours
Swimming Pools	7:00 a.m. - 8:00 p.m.
Medical Facility, Deck 1 (Dial 51)	8:00 a.m. - 12 Noon
	2:00 p.m. - 6:00 p.m.
Doctor's Office Hours	9:00 a.m. - 10:00 a.m.
	4:00 p.m. - 5:00 p.m.
After Hours Nurse on Call	Dial 51
In Extreme Emergency Only	**DIAL 911**

Telecommunications *(Ship to Shore Calls)*
Consult the Directory next to the phone in your cabin. $15.50 per minute

Ships Telephone	874-363-676-111
	874-363-676-211
Ships Fax	874-663-676-020
	874-363-676-220

WAKE UP CALL

To program a wake up call on your telephone, just dial:
56 (wait for voice prompt) then dial four digits of time you wish to wake up.
Number 1 for A.M.   Number 2 for P.M.

FOR EXAMPLE

6:00 a.m.	=	56	(voice prompt)	+	0600	+	1
10:45 a.m.	=	56	(voice prompt)	+	1045	+	1
7:00 p.m.	=	56	(voice prompt)	+	0700	+	2
3:30 p.m.	=	56	(voice prompt)	+	0330	+	2

To Cancel = 56 (voice prompt) + 2

SAME DAY FILM PROCESSING

Drop film in before noon and pick up at 6:00 p.m.
Drop boxes located on Decks 5, 6.

SHIP'S AGENT:

The West Indian Company, Ltd.
Longbay Havensite
Charlotte Amalie, St. Thomas, U.S.V.I. 00801
Phone: 809.776.4170

TODAY'S TOUR DEPARTURES

ST. THOMAS, U.S.V.I.

7:45 a.m.	Golf Ahoy! Mahogany Run G.C.	Outside on the Pier
8:45 a.m.	Atlantis Submarine-A	Schooner Bar, Dock 6
	Coral World & Mountain Top-A	Masquerade Theater, Deck 5
9:00 a.m.	St. Thomas Sightseeing Tour-A	Masquerade Theater, Deck 5
	Buck Island Sail & Snorkel- A	Schooner Bar, Deck 6
	Champagne Catamaran Sailaway	Schooner Bar, Deck 6
9:30 a.m.	Scuba Adventure	Outside on the Pier
	Virgin Islands Seaplane	Schooner Bar, Deck 6
11:00 a.m.	St. Thomas Helicopter	Schooner Bar, Deck 6
12:15 p.m.	Scenic St. John Sea & Snorkel	Masquerade Theater, Deck 5
	Scenic St. John Snuba Adventure	Masquerade Theater, Deck 5
12:45 p.m.	Island Bike Adventure	Outside on the Pier
	Coral World & Mountain Top-B	Masquerade Theater, Deck 5
1:00 p.m.	St. Thomas Sightseeing Tour-B	Masquerade Theater, Deck 5
	Kon-Tiki Party Tour	Outside on the Pier
	Buck Island Sail & Snorkel-B	Schooner Bar, Deck 6
	Catamaran Sailing & Snorkeling	Schooner Bar, Deck 6
	Coral World & Snorkeling Tour	Masquerade Theater, Deck 5
1:15 p.m.	St. John Island Tour	Masquerade Theater, Deck 5
	St. John Beach Tour	Masquerade Theater, Deck 5
1:30 p.m.	Kayak Marine Sanctuary Tour	Outside on the Pier
2:45 p.m.	Atlantis Submarine-B	Schooner Bar, Deck 6
Anytime	Paradise Point Tramway	10 Minute Walk to Tramway

*Exact gangway location to be announced upon arrival.

Please remember your tour tickets. All tours depart punctually.
Please meet at least 10 minutes prior to the listed departure times.
Members of the Staff will be in the lounges and on the pier to assist you.

INTERNATIONAL HOST

Guests requiring language assistance are invited to meet with our International Host, **Barbara Weisen** between 5:00 p.m. - 6:30 p.m. at the Purser's Square, Deck 5, Centrum. **(Spanish, German & Greek)**

ST. THOMAS CROWN & ANCHOR SOCIETY CLUB HIBISCUS ALLEY

Visit Royal Caribbean International's exclusive Crown & Anchor Club located in the heart of downtown Charlotte Amalie in Hibiscus Alley. Relax in the air-conditioned beauty of a restored Danish warehouse, purchase beverages and snacks, or call home from the AT&T calling station. Open until 4:00 p.m. Please see shopping map for exact location.

ANNOUNCEMENT IN CABINS

Please be advised that you are able to control non-emergency announcements coming into your cabin by using the "Info-Channel" control knob, located near the vanity. For more information, please contact your cabin attendant.

MAIL YOUR POSTCARDS TODAY!

Purser's Desk, Deck 5. Ship Postcards available for purchase.

JOGGING ON DECK

We kindly ask all guests to refrain from jogging on Deck 5 in consideration of fellow guests in the cabins below. Please utilize the Jogging Track on Deck 10.

SAVE THE WAVES

Royal Caribbean International requests that all guests kindly refrain from throwing **ANYTHING** overboard both in port and at sea. Please deposit trash in the proper receptacles/ashtrays located throughout the vessel. We're doing everything we can to protect the fragile ecological balance of the oceans that support cruising . . . and we're grateful for your cooperation in this effort.

GW-032/12.30.96

Courtesy Royal Caribbean International

ROYAL OLYMPIC CRUISES
(c/o Sun Line Cruises, Inc.)

One Rockefeller Plaza, Suite 315

New York, New York 10020

(800) 872-6400

(212) 397-6400

(212) 765-9685 FAX

ODYSSEUS: (formerly *Aqua Marine*); entered service 1962; refurbished 1996; 12,000 G.R.T.; 483' x 61'; 400-passenger capacity; 224 cabins; Greek officers and crew; Mediterranean, European, and Baltic cruises.

OLYMPIC COUNTESS: (formerly *Cunard Countess*); entered service 1976; 17,593 G.R.T.; 536' x 75'; 796-passenger capacity; 398 cabins; Greek officers and crew; Mediterranean and Greek island cruises, and also cruises the Orinoco River and in the West Indies.

ORPHEUS: (formerly *Munster* and *Thesus*); entered service 1952; refurbished 1983 and 1987; 5,092 G.R.T.; 364' x 50'; 280-passenger capacity; 152 cabins; Greek officers and crew; seven-day Aegean and Ionian Sea cruises in summer.

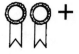

STELLA OCEANIS: (formerly *Aphrodite*); entered service in 1966; rebuilt and refurbished in 1967; 5,500 G.R.T.; 350' x 53'; 300-passenger capacity; 159 cabins; Greek officers and crew; Mediterranean-Greek island cruises in summer; Red Sea cruises in winter.

STELLA SOLARIS: (formerly *Camboge* and *Bunte Kuh*); entered service in 1953; rebuilt and refurbished in 1963, 1973, 1994, 1995, and 1996; 18,000 G.R.T.; 544' x 72'; 620-passenger capacity; 329 cabins; Greek officers and crew; Mediterranean-Greek island and Black Sea cruises in the summer; Caribbean-South America-Amazon River cruises in fall and winter.

TRITON: (formerly *Sunward II* and *Cunard Adventurer*); entered service 1971; refurbished 1991; 14,100 G.R.T.; 484' x 71'; 694-passenger capacity; 348 cabins; Greek officers and crew; Greek island cruises.

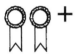

WORLD RENAISSANCE: entered service 1966; refurbished 1978, 1987, and 1998; 12,000 G.R.T.; 492' x 69'; 457-passenger capacity; 242 cabins; Greek officers and crew; Mediterranean and Greek island cruises.

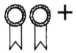

(Medical Facilities: Information not provided by cruise line.)

Royal Olympic Cruises is a conglomerate formed by the owners of Sun Line and Epirotiki. The ships are operated as two distinct products or brand names.

The late Charalambos Keusseoglou founded Sun Line in the late fifties, having received his prior experience in the cruise industry as vice-president of Home Lines. His intention was to create luxury cruising in the Mediterranean. Originally, the line had two small ships named the *Stella Maris* and *Stella Solaris I.* These were replaced with the *Stella Maris II* in 1966, the *Stella Oceanis* in 1967, and the second *Stella Solaris* in 1973. Marriott Corporation acquired an interest in 1971, which it retained for two decades.

Epirotiki, a family-owned Greek shipping company, dates back to the mid-nineteenth century, when it operated sailing vessels and transported goods and passengers to Mediterranean ports. In the 1930s Epirotiki began marketing Greek island cruises and operated a ferry service to Italy. Today, brothers George and Andreas Potamianos of the former Epirotiki line and the Keusseoglou family of the former Sun Line reign over the largest Greek-flag fleet of cruise ships in the world.

The line excels at "bread-and-butter" cruises on older, partially renovated ships that offer an abundance of popular ports, busy itineraries, and good food and service in the budget cruise market. These are not luxury cruise ships, and accommodations and public areas may not be comparable to some of the more expensive cruise liners.

Although the ships will be marketed under the Royal Olympic Cruise umbrella, there will be two brands, i.e., "the blue ships of Sun Line," which will encompass *Stella Solaris, Stella Oceanis,* and *Odysseus;* and "the white ships of Epirotiki," which include *Triton, Orpheus,* and *Olympic.*

Royal Olympic Cruises also manages the *Stella Maris, Jason, Neptune,* and *Argonaut;* however, these ships are used primarily for charters in different geographic areas.

The fleet will operate three-, four-, seven-, and fourteen-day cruises to the Greek islands, Turkey, Egypt, Israel, and Black Sea and various European destinations during the summer months; and various itineraries in the Caribbean, South America, Amazon, and Orinoco River in winter.

The Greek crew adds a definite Greek flavor to the cruises, with numerous Greek dishes being served in the dining rooms and Greek theme nights that include Greek dancing and entertainment. Activities aboard these ships range from aerobics, dance classes, bridge, Greek lessons, enhancement lectures, backgammon, trap shooting, bingo, and cooking lessons, to the usual shipboard entertainment.

On my most recent cruise on the *Stella Solaris* and my inspection of the *Stella Oceanis,* it was apparent that the ships were in need of some major refurbishing, redecorating, and modernizing. However, the passengers all seemed delighted by the ambiance of the Greek crew, the casual, fun atmosphere, and interesting itineraries. The *Stella Solaris* is the flagship of the line. Although built in 1953 in France as the *Camboge,* a passenger/cargo liner, she was rebuilt and converted for luxury cruising and entered service for Sun Line in 1973. In 1994, 1995, and 1996, some major refurbishing took place on this ship.

At the top of the *Stella Solaris* is the Lido Deck, with its unique "figure eight" pool and sunning area. On Boat Deck are located the deluxe suites and reading and cardrooms. All of the suites have a separate sitting area, TV, and bathtubs; and some have double beds. On Solaris Deck is the main show lounge, an intimate and attractive piano bar lounge, bar and casino room, dining room, and gallery. Next comes Golden Deck, with a new 2,600-square-foot health spa and massage rooms, as well as cabins. The remaining staterooms are found on Ruby, Emerald, and Sapphire decks, where the cinema is located. The disco is at the bottom of the ship. Deluxe suites cost $390 per person per night, with superior outside cabins costing $290 and minimum inside cabins starting at $190.

Children under twelve sharing a cabin with their parents, and third and fourth persons sharing a cabin, receive reduced rates.

In the winter she offers cruises from Florida and Galveston, Texas, to the Panama Canal, Amazon River, and South America. She spends her summers sailing the Greek islands and eastern Mediterranean, offering seven- and fourteen-day itineraries to the Greek islands, Turkey, Israel, Black Sea, and Egypt.

The *Stella Oceanis,* at 5,500 tons, is considerably smaller and more intimate. The somewhat limited public areas include the Aphrodite Restaurant, a show lounge, observation bar/lounge, a cinema, casino, shops, beauty salon, barber shop, an outdoor pool, sun deck area, hospital, and laundry. There are 10 suites that are located near the top of the ship on Lido Deck with the Plaka Taverna. The pool is above, and beneath is Oceanis Deck, the location of most public rooms, including the show lounge, restaurant, and casino. The remaining cabins are on the bottom three decks. During the spring, summer, and fall, the *Stella Oceanis* offers seven-day cruises from Piraeus, Greece, to the Greek islands and Turkey.

The *Triton* was built by Cunard in 1971 and called the *Adventurer*. Norwegian Cruise Line purchased the ship in 1977, refurbished her, and placed her into the three- and four-day Miami to Bahamas market. Epirotiki acquired and refurbished the ship in 1991. Currently, the *Triton* is scheduled to do seven-day cruises from Piraeus to the Greek islands and Turkey. The passenger cabins are located on the three lower decks, with 20 suites on Apollo Deck next to the dining room. The pool and lido area is also on this deck. Above on Ouranos Deck are the lounge and a few inside rooms, and atop ship on Hera and Zeus decks are the theater, small casino, and nightclub.

The 5,000-ton, 280-passenger *Orpheus* was built in 1952 as the *Munster,* and was refurbished in 1983 and 1987. She includes a small swimming pool and a lounge, and 117 of her 144 cabins are outside.

The *Odysseus* entered service in 1962 as the *Aqua Marine* and was refurbished in 1996. Three-quarters of the 224 cabins are outside and 2 suites feature double beds. Public facilities, other than the dining room, are located on the top three decks and include a small gym, beauty salon, a tiny pool, a small casino, a library, cardroom, main lounge, and nightclub.

The line frequently changes the itineraries of its vessels. When sailing in the eastern Mediterranean, Greek islands, and South America, it offers some excellent opportunities to visit numerous ports at relatively low fares while enjoying good food and service.

In the spring of 1998, Royal Olympic purchased the former *Cunard Countess* (built in 1976) and renamed the 840-passenger vessel the *Olympic Countess.* At the same time, the line purchased the former *World Renaissance,* a 900-passenger ship that began service for Paquet Line in 1966. The former *Olympic* (originally named the *Carnivale*) was sold earlier that year.

The line has contracted to build two 25,000-ton, 800-passenger ships for delivery in 2000 and 2001. These ships will be able to achieve a speed of 27 knots, with interior designs by M. Katzourakis, 400 staterooms with 48 suites, a multi-level showroom, a coffee bar, wine-tasting café, nightclub, casino, spa, conference room, library, cardroom, terrace grill, and the amenities offered by many of the mass-market cruise lines.

Strong Points:

For the price, passengers get better food, service, and more ports than on many competitors, especially other Greek ships cruising the Greek islands.

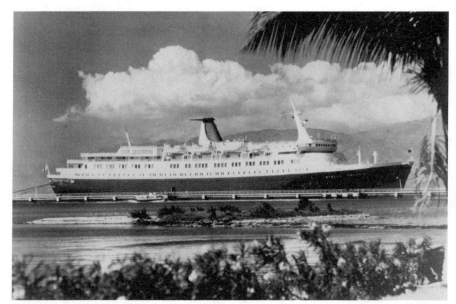

Courtesy Royal Olympic Cruises

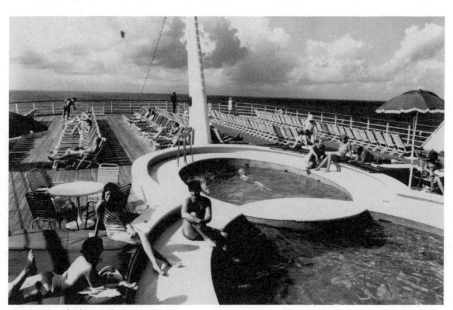

Courtesy Royal Olympic Cruises

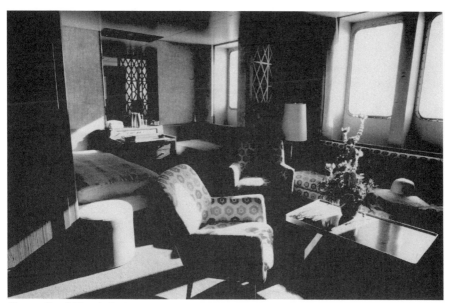

Courtesy Royal Olympic Cruises

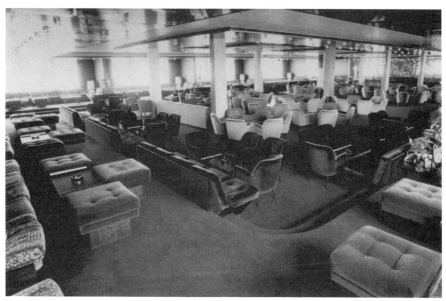

Courtesy Royal Olympic Cruises

DINNER

JUICES
Orange, Apple, V-8 Cocktail

APPETIZERS
Salad of Seafood "Port au Prince"
Breast of Smoked Turkey on Melon

SOUPS
Cream of Vegetables
Clear Soup "Mimosa"

FARINACEOUS
Spaghetti alla "Bolognese" with a Rich Meat Sauce

FISH
Broiled Salmon Steak "Medici" with Bearnaise Sauce

ENTREES
Chicken Curry with Italian Rice
Braised Leg of Lamb with Thyme
Grilled Kansas Sirloin Steak "Café de Paris"

COLD DISH
Paste Salad with Parma Ham

VEGETABLES AND STARCH
Hearts of Celery with Gravy
Broccoli with Noisette Butter
Sauteed Potatoes with Onion
Buttered Potatoes

SALADS
Salad Panachee
Salad of Beetroots

DRESSINGS
French, Italian, Roquefort, Thousand Island

CHEESES
A Selection of Cheeses from the Board

DESSERTS
Fruits with Mousse of Yogurt and Meringue
Profiteroles with Choco Sauce
Bavarian Apple Struedel
A Selection of Ice Cream

STEWED FRUIT
Apricots, Pears, Prunes

FRESH FRUIT
A Choice of Seasonal Fruits

BEVERAGES
Coffee, Sanka, Nescafé, Iced Coffee,
Tea, Ceylon Tea, Iced Tea

The Wine Steward will be happy to assist in choosing your wine

Courtesy Royal Olympic Cruises

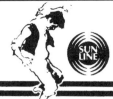

STELLA SOLARIS ™ **WEDNESDAY**
Istanbul, Turkey
Arr: 7.00am - Dep: 7.00pm

SAY IT IN GREEK
"F. Harry Stow"...which means..."Thank you"
"Pah-rah-kah-lo"...which means..."Please" or "You are welcome"

6.30am	The PURSER'S OFFICE opens. Solaris Deck.
7.00am	**TSS STELLA SOLARIS IS DUE TO ARRIVE IN ISTANBUL, Turkey.**
7.00am - 10.00am	The HOSPITALITY DESK opens for passengers remaining on board who would like to play backgammon, etc. Solaris Deck.
7.30am	HOLY MASS with Father Frugoli, S.J. in the Theater. Sapphire Deck.
8.00am	DEPARTURE OF THE EXCURSION TO ISTANBUL with Lunch on board. Please wait for the announcements before coming to the gangway and remember to take your Excursion Ticket, your Safety Identification Card and TURKISH LANDING CARD with you.
8.15am	DEPARTURE OF THE EXCURSION TO ISTANBUL with Lunch Ashore. Please wait for the announcements before coming to the gangway and remember to take your Excursion Ticket, your Safety Identification Card and TURKISH LANDING CARD with you.
8.30am	DEPARTURE OF THE EXCURSION TO ISTANBUL/BOSPHORUS with Lunch Ashore. Please wait for the announcements before coming to the gangway and remember to take your Excursion Ticket, your Safety Identification Card and TURKISH LANDING CARD with you.
12.00Nn - 1.00pm	COCKTAIL MUSIC. Lido Cafe. Lido Deck.
1.30pm - 2.30pm	The HOSPITALITY DESK opens for information. Foyer. Solaris Deck.
4.00pm	MOVIE... The synopsis will be posted on the Bulletin Board. Theater. Sapphire Deck.
6.00pm - 7.00pm	MUSICAL COCKTAILS. Piano Bar. Solaris Deck.

| 6.30pm | **ALL ABOARD PLEASE!!!** At 7.00pm, TSS STELLA SOLARIS SAILS FOR KUSADASI, Turkey ... **320 nautical miles** |

7.45pm - 8.45pm	MUSICAL COCKTAILS. Grill Bar. Solaris Deck.
8.15pm	BINGO !!! Come and try your luck for cash prizes. Solaris Lounge. Solaris Deck.

8.30pm -	12.30am	Continuous music for your dancing and listening pleasure. Solaris Lounge. Solaris Deck.

9.00pm
&
10.45pm

*** SHOW TIME ***
Early Sitting Passengers. Solaris Lounge.
Late Sitting Passengers. Solaris Lounge.

10.15pm   MOVIE... The synopsis will be posted on the Bulletin Board. Theater. Sapphire Deck.

10.30pm   The TAVERNA opens its doors until the wee hours. Pizza will be offered after Midnight. Main Deck Aft.

11.30pm   "SPOT SHOW" Grill Bar. Solaris Deck.

11.30pm   *** A SALUTE TO THE FABULOUS 50's ***
Twist Contest. Taverna. Main Deck Aft.

*** The suggested attire for this evening is ... CASUAL ***
(Shirt and slacks for gentlemen and similar attire for ladies)

!!! KA-LI NIKTA - GOOD NIGHT !!!

TODAY'S MEAL HOURS:

6.00am -	7.00am	EARLY RISERS' COFFEE. Lido Cafe.
6.30am -	8.30am	BREAKFAST BUFFET and A LA CARTE. Open sitting. Dining Room. Continental Breakfast is served in cabins until 10.00am.
12.00Nn -	2.00pm	OPEN SITTING LUNCHEON. Dining Room.
	4.00pm	TEA TIME. Solaris Piano Bar.
	7.00pm	DINNER is served. Early sitting. Dining Room.
	8.45pm	DINNER is served. Late sitting. Dining Room.
11.30pm -	12.30am	LIGHT NIGHT SNACKS. Lido Cafe.

SHIP'S SERVICES:

PURSER'S OFFICE	6.30am - 8.00pm
HOSPITAL	7.00am - 9.00am / 6.00pm - 8.00pm
BOUTIQUE	7.00pm - 11.00pm
BEAUTY SALON	9.00am - 11.00am / 5.00pm - 8.00pm
SAUNA/MASSAGE	8.00am - 10.00am / 4.00pm - 7.00pm
BLACKJACK TABLES	8.00pm - 2.00am
MONTECARLO SLOT MACH.	7.30pm - 12.30am
RADIO ROOM	Open at sea / Closed in port
PHOTO SHOP	9.00pm - 11.00pm
EXCURSION OFFICE	7.00pm - 9.00pm

*** TURKISH LANDING CARDS ***

These will be distributed immediately AFTER formalities have been completed by the local authorities on arrival at Istanbul. All passengers must collect their TURKISH LANDING CARD from the Purser's Office from 7.00am onwards. These cards will be collected at the gangway upon your return to the vessel prior to sailing.

*** LOOKING AHEAD... Our MASQUERADE will take place tomorrow evening. Start planning your costume now!!! Your aim is to be the winner of one of the three prize categories.....
.....MOST ARTISTIC.....MOST HUMOROUS.....MOST ORIGINAL.....

Courtesy Royal Olympic Cruises

SEA AIR HOLIDAYS, LTD.

733 Summer Street

Stamford, Connecticut 06901

(800) 732-6247

M.V. *QUEEN OF HOLLAND:* entered service 1995; 146-passenger capacity; 73 cabins; Dutch officers and crew; cruises on the Rhine, Danube, and waterways of Holland.

M.V. *ROYAL STAR:* 200-passenger capacity; cruises in Indian Ocean from Mombasa, Kenya.
(Medical Facilities: These vessels do not carry physicians or nurses, according to the cruise line.)

Sea Air Holidays, Ltd., formed in 1979, is the U.S. marketing agent for various riverboats and barges that are owned by foreign companies and traverse the rivers of Europe. Because the different vessels have different ownership and management, it would be incorrect to assume that the experience on each is the same. The physical condition and facilities of each boat determine your comfort; however, the attitude and training of the staff affect your enjoyment.

The newest boat is the *Queen of Holland.* On the deck where you enter is located the information desk; a large, nicely appointed lounge and bar; a small salon; and the higher-priced accommodations. On the deck below are the remaining cabins, a comfortable restaurant, a sauna-whirlpool area, and a small kiosk. Atop each boat is an observation deck with lounge chairs and deck games.

There is some entertainment on board, and the meals include numerous courses but limited selections. The cabins, although modern, are typical of riverboats, with limited storage space and small bathrooms. The twin beds fold up during the day, with one converting to a couch. Each accommodation is air conditioned and includes a hair dryer, a mini-bar, telephone, a private safe, a radio, a color TV, and large picture windows that open.

Because Sea Air Holidays has full charter of the *Queen of Holland,* the on-board crew, entertainment, and food are maintained with the utmost quality by the company.

Waterways of Holland cruises depart from Amsterdam and include stops at Ubrecht, Schoonhoven, Zierikzee, Verre, Zijpe, Hoorn, Wik, and Volendam.

The company also markets cruises through France on the 22-passenger *Lafayette,* the 12-passenger *La Reine Pedanque,* the 6-passenger *Niagara,* the 20-passenger *Litote,* the 22-passenger *Lorraine,* the 50-passenger *Chardonnay* (newly built for the 1999 season), the 24-passenger *L'Escargot,* the 24-passenger *Chanterelle,* and the 51-passenger *Anacoluthe,* as well as Galapagos Island cruises on the M.V. *Santa Cruz, Corinthian,* and *Isabela II* (see Metropolitan Touring).

Sea Air Holidays has expanded its product line for 1998-99 to include additional global destinations.

The M.V. *Royal Star* is a 200-passenger-capacity vessel with teak decks, polished wood, and gleaming brass. She is equipped with deck chairs for sunbathing, a sauna, small gymnasium, cardroom, and a lounge. Morning coffee and tea are served in your cabin, and a buffet breakfast is offered on deck or in the Belvedere Restaurant. Lunch is served on deck or in the restaurant, and dinner is served in two seatings. Cabins have private shower and toilets, telephones, adequate storage, and either a porthole or window. Suites are equipped with mini-bars and hair dryers.

The *Royal Star* sails from Mombasa, Kenya in the Indian Ocean. Ports of call include Mahe and Praslin in the Seychelles, as well as Nose Be, Madagascar, and Zanzibar, Tanzania.

Strong Points:

Queen of Holland offers a comfortable, relaxed way to explore the charming villages along the various rivers and waterways in Europe.

SHERATON NILE CRUISES
48 B Giza Street

P.O. Box 125

Orman Tower Boulevard

Giza, Egypt

ATON, TUT, ANNI, and *HOTP:* identical sister ships built in 1979; renovated 1989; 178-passenger capacity; 83 cabins; Egyptian officers and crew; three- to seven-night cruises between Aswan and Luxor, Egypt.

(Medical Facilities: No information was provided by the cruise line.)

These four identical cruisers were built in Norway in 1979 and are the largest riverboats along the Nile. They are operated by Sheraton Hotels in Egypt. All of the cabins and suites are quite spacious by riverboat standards and are located on the outside of the boat, thus offering panoramic views of the passing scenery. They are air conditioned, with private toilet and shower. The public areas include four decks. At the top is the sun deck and swimming pool. The lounge is on A Deck, the dining room and souvenir shop on B Deck, the reception on C Deck, and the cabins and suites are spread among A, B, C, and D decks.

A typical seven-night itinerary includes visits to Kitchener's Island and the Agha Khan Mausoleum, the High Dam, Old Dam and Granite Quarries, the Phitae Temple, Kom Ombo Temple, Edfu Temple, Esna Temple, Karnak and Luxor Temples, Abydos Temple, Dendera Temple, and Luxor.

The food is a mixture of Oriental and Western, and sightseeing is included in the price of about $200 per night per person in the summer and $300 per night in the winter.

Strong Points:
Itineraries and accommodations.

SILJA LINE

Europe: Mannerheimintie 2   USA: General Sales Agent

00100 Helsinki   Bergen Line, Inc.

Finland   405 Park Ave.

Tel: 358-0-180-41   New York, New York 10022

Fax: 358-0-1804-402   Tel: 1-800-323-7436

Fax: 212-319-1390

SILJA EUROPA: entered service 1993; 59,914 G.R.T.; 662' x 105'; 3,000-passenger capacity; 1,194 cabins; Finnish officers and crew; day and night cruises between Turku and Stockholm.

SILJA FESTIVAL: entered service 1986; 34,419 G.R.T.; 551' x 90.5'; 2,000-passenger capacity; 588 cabins; Finnish officers and crew; day and night cruises between Turku and Stockholm.

SILJA FINNJET: entered service 1977; 25,900 G.R.T.; 698' x 83'; 1,584-passenger capacity; 565 cabins; Finnish officers and crew; cruises between Travemunde and Helsinki. **(Category D—Not Rated)**

SILJA SERENADE: entered service 1990; 58,376 G.R.T.; 660' x 130'; 2,500-passenger capacity; 984 cabins; Finnish officers and crew; day and night cruises between Helsinki and Stockholm.

SILJA SYMPHONY: entered service 1991; 58,376 G.R.T.; 660' x 130'; 2,500-passenger capacity; 984 cabins; Finnish officers and crew; overnight cruises between Helsinki and Stockholm.

WASA QUEEN: entered service 1975; 16,500 G.R.T.; 156 meters x 22 meters; 1,600-passenger capacity; 314 cabins; Finnish officers and crew; cruises between Tallin, Estonia, and Helsinki, Finland. **(Category D—Not Rated)**

(Medical Facilities: No information was provided by the cruise line.)

Silja Line is part of the Silja Group.

The *Silja Europa* and *Silja Festival* offer either day or night sailings between Turku, Finland, and Stockholm, Sweden (taking nine to twelve hours), and range in price for someone sharing a double cabin from $35 to $115 for a night sailing and $40 to $125 for a day sailing. Cars are additional.

The *Silja Europa* is the world's largest cruise ferry. All cabins are air conditioned and include telephone, radio alarm clocks, TV (except in the lowest category), and toilets with showers. Cabins are small and storage space is limited. I wouldn't recommend anything less than a Silja-class cabin for cruisers requiring a modicum of comfort.

Dining options aboard the *Europa* range from a self-serve café, a McDonald's at Sea, an all-you-can-eat Food Market up to a 670-seat smorgasbord-style buffet, and à la carte steak, seafood, and gourmet restaurants. The Bon Vivant, the most upscale and expensive dining room, offers Continental cuisine and fine wines.

After dinner, cruisers can enjoy a movie, so-so live entertainment, disco and pop dancing, a music pub, gambling at a casino, or duty-free shopping. The facilities aboard include a small, indoor swimming pool; sauna; three whirlpools; a children's pool; conference rooms and VIP meeting facilities; and a children's playground.

The voyage between Helsinki and Stockholm offered on the *Symphony* and *Serenade* departs at 6 P.M. and arrives at 8:30 A.M. the next morning.

On all the ships Scandinavians make up the majority of the passengers, with a smattering of travelers from other European countries, Asians, and North Americans. Announcements are in numerous languages. There is an abundance of families including small children.

The *Silja Finnjet* sails from Helsinki to Travemunde, Germany, in 22 hours, with fares running from $103 to $659 per person for passengers sharing a double cabin plus $110 to $150 for a car. Restaurants range from a cafeteria and Scandinavian buffet to an à la carte Continental dining room. As on the other ships, the facilities include duty-free shops, a pool, solarium, sauna and massage area, a movie theater, children's playroom, conference rooms, a casino, and a lounge with live entertainment.

The above sailings offer an economical alternative means of transportation between the countries they service and are especially ideal for travelers with automobiles. The seasoned cruiser must be prepared to make many allowances. Overall comfort, food, and service are not comparable to that found on typical cruise ships.

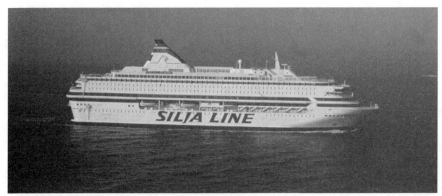

Courtesy Silja Line

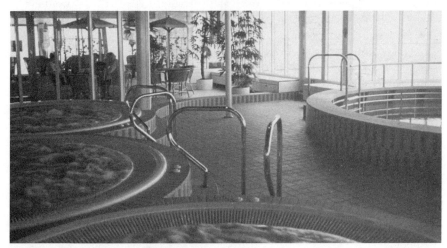

Sun Flower Oasis Spa, *courtesy Silja Line*

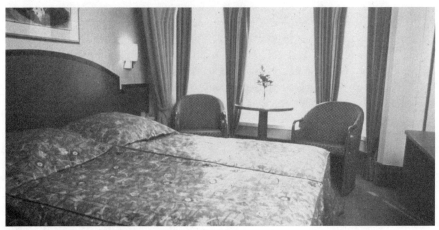

Silja-class cabin on the Silja Europa, *courtesy Silja Line*

SILVERSEA CRUISES, LTD.
110 E. Broward Boulevard
Fort Lauderdale, Florida 33301
(800) 722-6655

SILVER CLOUD: entered service 1994; 16,700 G.R.T.; 514' x 71'; 296-passenger capacity; 148 suites; Italian officers, European staff; cruises in Europe, the Baltic Sea, Scandinavia, Canada, North America, South America, and the Caribbean.

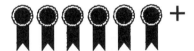

SILVER WIND: entered service 1995; 16,700 G.R.T.; 514' x 71'; 296-passenger capacity; 148 suites; Italian officers, European staff; cruises in the Mediterranean, Europe, the Far East, and the South Pacific.

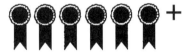

(Medical Facilities for both ships: C-148; P-1; EM, CLS, MS; CM; PD; BC; EKG; TC; PO; EPC; WC; OR; ICU; X; M; CCP; LJ.)

Note: Six+ black ribbons is the highest rating given in this edition to ships in the deluxe market category.

In 1994 the Lefebvre family of Rome and the Vlasov group of Monaco, previously co-owners of Sitmar Cruises, entered the deluxe cruise market with two new 16,000+-ton vessels that compete with Seabourn, Cunard, Renaissance, Crystal, and Radisson Seven Seas. The cruise line boasts all-suite ships, three-quarters of which feature spacious teak verandas. Although the majority of the line's staterooms are "Veranda Suites" (295 square feet in size including the veranda), other suites range in size from 240 to 1,315 square feet. Air-sea fares are among the industry's "most inclusive" and somewhat less than many of the line's competitors.

The intent of Silversea Cruises was to create the optimum ship—small enough to sail intriguing waterways unavailable to most of the larger vessels while also providing a smooth, comfortable ride in deep-water cruising. In addition, these ships offer the intimacy, service, and nuances found on many of the smaller deluxe cruise ships while also affording all of the facilities, amenities, and activities available on the larger cruise ships.

These ships have the most advanced nautical architecture and maritime equipment, which renders them very steady at high speeds and highly maneuverable. Design and decor were conceived by Norwegian architects whose credits include most of the other small luxury cruise ships as well as RCCL's megaliners. In addition to glass doors leading out to verandas in 75 percent of the suites and floor-to-ceiling glass windows in the remaining 25 percent, each suite features spacious storage; a walk-in closet; mirrored dressing table; writing desk; twin beds (convertible to queen); a separate sitting area; stocked refrigerator; electronic wall safe; remote-controlled TV with videocassette player; a large umbrella; all-marble bathrooms with tub, shower, hair dryer, and 110- and 220-volt outlets; and plush terry-cloth robes with slippers. Guests desiring more space than the standard Vista or Veranda Suites can opt for one of 3 "Silver Suites" (528 square feet), the "two-bedroom Owner's Suite" (887 square feet), a "two-bedroom Royal Suite" (985 square feet), or a "two-bedroom Grand Suite" (1,315 square feet). These larger suites sell for considerably more than the Vista or Veranda Suite and feature additional amenities such as a whirlpool tub, greater private veranda space, a CD player, and a comfortable dining area, as well as deluxe bathroom amenities.

The line offers one of the most inclusive cruise packages currently available in the ultraluxury cruise market. Air-sea fares include port charges, all gratuities, alcoholic and nonalcoholic beverages (both in your suite and throughout the ship), fine wines with lunch and dinner, round-trip air transportation, a deluxe pre-cruise hotel stay, as well as transfers, porterage, and complimentary shuttle-bus service to the city center in most ports of call. Although there is a charge for shore excursions, select sailings feature a special complimentary "Silversea Experience"—a customized shore event available only to Silversea guests—which can range from a traditional street party in Mykonos with wine, dancing, and singing, to a formal soirée in one of St. Petersburg's lavish nineteenth-century palaces. Also included in the fare are special "in-suite" touches, such as fresh fruit and flowers, personalized stationery, lunch and dinner menus and satellite newsletters delivered daily, and a bottle of chilled Moet & Chandon champagne to greet you upon arrival. In addition, your cruise tickets, baggage tags, and itineraries arrive before the cruise in a handsome, zippered leather portfolio.

Dining options range from casual to elegant, with open seating in both the more casual indoor/outdoor Terrace Cafe as well as in the more formal restaurant. Twenty-four-hour in-suite dining is also offered, with course-by-course dinner service available. (Gratuities are not expected.) Both the more formal restaurant and the Terrace Cafe are elegantly furnished and afford a good deal of space between tables, a well-controlled sound level, and exceptional food and service. The Terrace Cafe offers an alternative option for dinner with Italian theme dinners, and occasionally dinners representative of the cruising region. The formal restaurant features selected menu items created in conjunction with the famed Le Cordon Bleu Culinary Academy. Special theme parties and dinner dancing are featured on each sailing, and mature gentleman hosts are available as dance and bridge partners on selected sailings. Public areas also offer guests a great variety of choices and include a multilevel show lounge with full-scale entertainment throughout the cruise; a panorama lounge; a library stocked with books, periodicals, and reference materials as well as videos and a CD-ROM computer system; a bar/nightclub; full casino with roulette, blackjack, and slots; a health spa with masseuse, beauty salon, sauna, and well-equipped exercise facility; cardroom; outdoor pool and two heated whirlpools; and a sun deck observation area.

Worldwide itineraries offer cruises that can be booked from 5 to 50 days.

Officers and staff on board Silversea ships are highly experienced, and many have extensive tenure with other upscale and premium cruise lines. Italian officers create a warm and friendly on-board ambiance, Scandinavian stewardesses provide efficient and hospitable suite service, and a northern European hotel staff, together with an international support staff, provides gracious on-board dining.

A new partnership with *National Geographic Traveler* offers guests the opportunity to travel aboard select sailings with noted *National Geographic* journalists and photographers who will host lectures and shore excursions to give guests a more complete view of the history, culture, and geography of the lands they visit. The line will also continue its Culinary Extravaganza cruises, created in conjunction with the renowned Le Cordon Bleu Culinary Academy, during which master chefs from the famed school will give cooking presentations, wine tastings, floral demonstrations, and seminars on the art of French table setting.

Silversea has plans for two additional new ships to enter service in 2000 and 2001, respectively. As currently designed, they will be approximately 25,000 G.R.T. and accommodate 390 passengers.

Strong Points:

Silversea offers the ultimate in a luxury, yacht-like cruise experience with imaginative gourmet cuisine, sumptuous accommodations, and impeccable service on vessels somewhat larger than its competitors, with more public area space and expanded facilities, activities and entertainment, and exotic itineraries. Many critics rate Silversea as "the best."

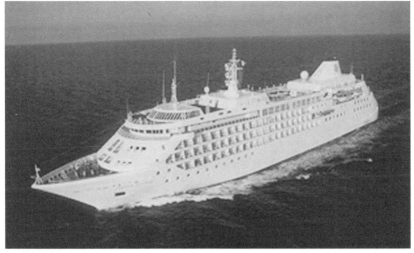

Courtesy Silversea Cruises, Ltd.

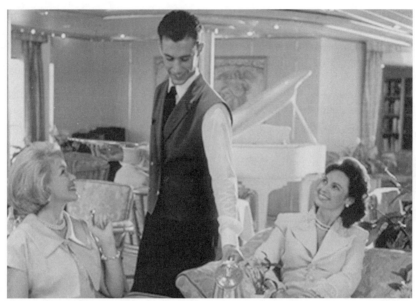

Courtesy Silversea Cruises, Ltd.

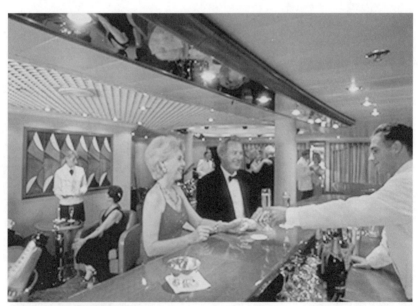

Courtesy Silversea Cruises, Ltd.

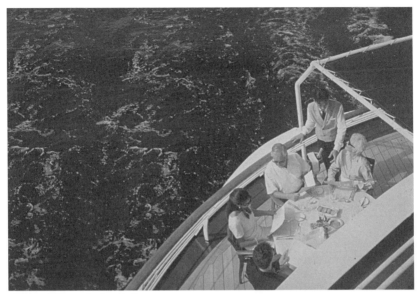

Courtesy Silversea Cruises, Ltd.

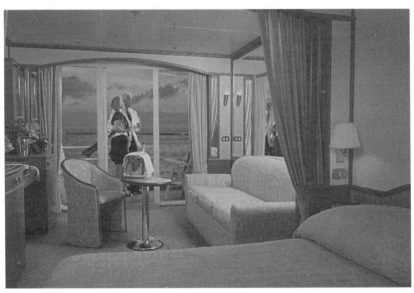

Courtesy Silversea Cruises, Ltd.

En Route to Alexandria, Egypt

Monday, June 9, 1997

LUNCHEON IN THE RESTAURANT

APPETIZERS

Half an Avocado with Poached Salmon

Served with Yogurt Chive Sauce

Vegetable Antipasto

Marinated Bell Peppers, Eggplant, Artichokes, Mushrooms and Zucchini with Grissini Sticks

PASTA DISH

Spaghetti alla Checca

Spaghetti Pasta with Fresh Tomatoes, Herbs and Mozzarella Cheese

FROM THE TUREEN

Italian Minestrone

Chilled Cream of Banana Soup

FRESH FROM THE GARDEN

Watercress Salad, Chopped Bacon and Eggs with French Dressing

Creamy Potato Salad with Bell Peppers and Spring Onions

FROM THE COLD KITCHEN

Silversea's Chef Salad

Mixed Lettuce with Avocado, Tomato Wedges, Sliced Warm Chicken and Crisp Bacon
Served with Thousand Island Dressing

SANDWICH OF THE DAY

Grilled Turkey Sandwich with Sauce Marie Louise

Served on Whole-wheat Bread with Iceberg Lettuce and Tomatoes
Served with French Fried Potatoes and Marinated Lettuce

MAIN COURSES

Broiled Fresh Local Fish Fillet in a Vegetable Dill Sauce

Served with Fresh Vegetables and Chive Potatoes

Beef Stufato al Lemon

Braised Beef in Lemon Flavored Red Wine Sauce
Served with Garden Fresh Vegetables and Polenta Gnocchi

SPECIALITY FROM ASIA

Marinated Stir-Fried Chicken Chow Mein

Marinated with Ginger, Garlic, Sambal, Soy Sauce and Oyster Sauce

Served with Fried Mie Noodles and Stir-Fried Chinese Vegetables

In Port: Alexandria, Egypt
Monday, June 9, 1997

French Dinner Dance in the Restaurant

Appetizers
Gratinated Escargots in a Garlic Herb Butter

Salade Landaise
Mixed Salad with Duck Liver, Smoked Duck, Asparagus and Baby Corn

Chilled Fruit Cup with Calvados

Pasta Dish
Lumache or Macaroni aux artichauds, lardons et thym frais
Lumache Pasta or Macaroni with Artichokes, Bacon and Fresh Thyme

From The Tureen
French Onion Soup with Cheese Croutons

Chilled Vichyssoise

Fresh From The Garden
Mixed Garden Greens with French Dressing, Garnished with Alfalfa Sprouts and Red Radishes

Marinated Green Beans with Artichokes and Walnut Vinaigrette

Sorbet
Refreshing Cassis-Fig Sorbet

Vegetarian Dish
Mille Feuille à la Niçoise
Layers of Puff Pastry with Oyster Mushrooms and Ratatouille

Main Courses
Dover Sole and Salmon Paupiette with Sauce Duglère
Served on a Bed of Fresh Spinach
Accompanied by Parisienne Potatoes and Vegetables

Roast Rack of Lamb with a Herb Crust
Served with Ratatouille Niçoise and Green Beans
Accompanied by Gratinated Potatoes and Natural Gravy

Silversea Signature Dish
Stuffed Chicken Breast Wrapped in Zucchini Slices
Served with Natural Gravy, Sautéed Potatoes and Carrots

From the Grill
Grilled Calf's Liver à la Lyonnaise
Served with Onions Confit with Xeres Vinegar and Veal Jus
Accompanied by Potatoes Mousseline, Carrots and Green Beans

DAILY PROGRAM

TUESDAY, JUNE 10, 1997   SUNRISE: 5:57 A.M. / SUNSET: 8.05 P.M.

GOOD MORNING

7:00	**ALX-3 "Cairo & The Great Pyramids" tour departs**	**Pierside**
8:00	Walk-a-Mile with Fitness Instructor Shae	Walking Track (9)
8:30	The Silver Quiz is available - Prize points will be awarded to the first, most correct form returned before 3 p.m.	Tour Desk (6)
8:30	Morning Stretch workout with Shae	Fitness Center (7)
9:00	Sit and Be Fit, armchair aerobics with the Fitness Instructor	Parisian Lounge (6)
9:30	Bridge Lecture: "Takeout Doubles and Overcalls" with Edward and Helen Halluska	Card Room (6)
9:30	Language Class: Learn some basic words and phrases in Italian with Michèle	The Bar (5)
10:00	"Can We Talk?!" Enjoy a friendly chat with the Social Staff	Panorama Lounge (8)
10:15	Golf Putting: Compete for prize points with Michèle	The Bar (5)
11:00	Shuffleboard Competition: A traditional shipboard game with the Social Staff	Poolside (8)
11:00	**Wine Tasting: Our Head Sommelier, Brian O'Brien shares with you some secrets of the trade and lets you sample a specially chosen selection**	**Panorama Lounge (8)**
12:00	Midday Melodies with the music of Jerry Blaine	Panorama Lounge (8)
12:05	Information from the Bridge by the Captain	Public Address System
2:00	Duplicate and Rubber Bridge with your Bridge Directors Ed and Helen	Card Room (6)
3:00	Scrabble Tournament for Prize Points, judged by the Social Staff	Panorama Lounge (8)
3:00	*DOCUMENTARY HOUR:* "Karnak - The Hidden History" **Egyptologists continue to unravel the mysteries of the Ancient Egyptians and their hieroglyphs, and have come up with some surprising revelations (45 mins)**	**Parisian Lounge (6)**
3:15	Dance Class: Today it's the "Waltz!" with Gentleman Host George	The Bar (5)
3:30	Water Vollayball: Splashing good fun for the whole family with the social staff	The Pool (8)
3:30	Craft Class: The art of making silk roses with Michèle	The Bar (5)
4:00	Step to the Beat with Fitness Instructor Shae	Fitness Center (7)
4:00	Afternoon Tea is served with Jerry playing for you at the piano	Panorama Lounge (8)
4:00	A teatime crossword puzzle is available. Please see the social staff	Panorama Lounge (8)
4:30	TeaTime Team Trivia with Michèle, for more Prize Points	Panorama Lounge (8)
5:00	Phenomenal Abdominals with Fitness Instructor Shae	Fitness Center (7)

GOOD EVENING - DRESS CODE: CASUAL

7:00	**Dock in Port Said, Egypt, to pick-up guests from the Cairo tour**	
7:00	Enjoy cocktails and piano music of Jerry Blaine	Panorama Lounge (8)
7:00	Music for dancing to the *The Silver Wind Quartet*	The Bar (5)
7:30	**All aboard, as the *Silver Wind* sets sail for Limassol, Cyprus**	
10:15	**EVENING SHOWTIME:** *JERRY BLAINE presents:* A unique tribute to the "Music of the Movies" with a cast of thousands appearing on the big screen, from Charlie Chaplin to Tom Cruise	**Parisian Lounge (6)**
11:00	Dance to the fabulous music of *The Silver Wind Quartet*	The Bar (5)
11:15	**Liar's Club !!** Who's lying? Who's telling the truth? See if you can beat our panel of 'untruth tellers', **Julie, Nigel and Margaret** in this word game with a difference. **Darius** tries to keep order!!	Panorama Lounge (8)

Courtesy Silversea Cruises, Ltd.

SONESTA HOTELS AND NILE CRUISES

c/o Sonesta International

200 Clarendon Street

Boston, Massachusetts 02116

U.S. and Canada (800) 766-3782

U.K. 0800898410

NILE GODDESS: entered service 1989; renovated 1995; 130-passenger capacity; 65 cabins; Egyptian crew; four- and six-night cruises up and down the Nile.

SUN GODDESS: entered service 1993; 124-passenger capacity; 62 cabins; Egyptian crew; four- and six-night cruises up and down the Nile.

(Medical Facilities: No information was provided by the cruise line.)

Sonesta Hotels is presently marketing its new upscale riverboat, the *Nile Goddess,* which was built in 1989 and totally renovated in 1995. Its five decks include a pool with an adjoining lounge, recreation area, barbecue area, a show lounge, bar, game room, shop, disco, and restaurant. The one-sitting restaurant provides buffet meals.

There are 63 cabins and 2 presidential suites with their own private lounge. All cabins are air-conditioned and include private phones, two-channel music systems, a TV with video player, mini-bars, safety deposit boxes, and bathrooms with bathtubs and showers.

The *Sun Goddess* was built and added to the fleet in 1993. The public areas are similar to the *Nile Goddess* and include a Turkish bath. The ship has 58 cabins and 4 suites with the same facilities and amenities as its sister ship.

Both ships sail between Luxor and Aswan, Egypt, on alternate four- and six-night cruises. Shore excursions visit the Temples of Karnak and Luxor, the Valley of Kings and Queens, the Temple of Queen Hatshepsut, the Colossi of Memnon, the Temple of Dandara in Kena, the Temple of Horus in Edfu, the Temple of Sobek and Haroeris in Kom Ombo, the Agha Khan Mausoleum, the High Dam granite quarries, and the Temple of Philae in Aswan.

Strong Points:

New, modern riverboats offering in-depth Nile cruises.

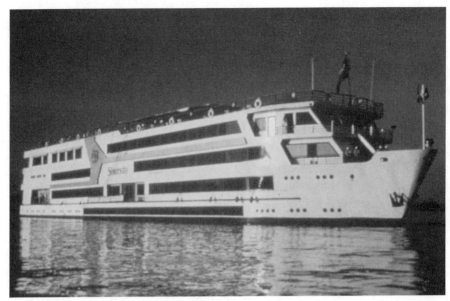

The Nile Goddess, *courtesy Sonesta Hotels and Nile Cruises*

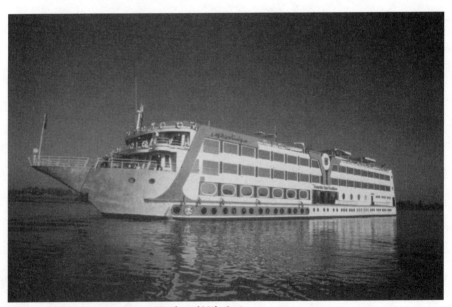

The Sun Goddess, *courtesy Sonesta Hotels and Nile Cruises*

STAR CLIPPERS, INC.

4104 S. Salzedo Avenue

Coral Gables, Florida 33146

(800) 442-0551

ROYAL CLIPPER: entered service 2000; 5,000 G.R.T.; 439' x 54'; 246-passenger capacity; 112 cabins; Belgian and European officers, international crew; seven- and fourteen-day Caribbean cruises in the winter from Barbados and Mediterranean cruises in the summer from Cannes. **(Category B—Not Rated)**

STAR CLIPPER: entered service 1992; 3,025 G.R.T.; 360' x 50'; 170-passenger capacity; 85 cabins; Belgian and European officers, international crew; seven- and fourteen-day Caribbean cruises from Barbados, with alternating itineraries to the Grenadines, the Windward Islands, and the Virgin Islands.

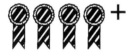

STAR FLYER: entered service 1991; 3,025 G.R.T.; 360' x 50'; 170-passenger capacity; 85 cabins; Belgian and European officers, international crew; cruises in Caribbean, Mediterranean, and Southeast Asia.

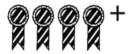

(Medical Facilities: C-0; P (on trans-ocean cruises only); N-1.)

In 1991 Mikael Krafft, a Swedish shipping and real-estate entrepreneur and the founder and managing owner of Star Clippers, embarked on the concept of bringing to the cruise market yacht-like sailboats that actually sail more than operate their engines. The cruise line emphasizes enjoying a sailing vessel, being close to the sea, participating in water sports, and visiting great beaches in a casual yet comfortable shipboard environment. Do not expect to be pampered, and many conveniences and amenities standard on traditional cruise ships are not present.

These are the tallest sailing ships afloat, with 36,000 square feet of Dacron sail flying from four towering masts, the highest rising 226 feet. The ships feature a unique, anti-rolling system designed to keep them upright and stable for sailing and while at anchor.

Eighty-five air-conditioned staterooms accommodate 170 passengers. Two are small, inside cabins with upper and lower berths. The remainder measure about

120 square feet and are outside, with two twin beds that convert to a double bed, TV that plays in-house videos, radios, lighted dressing table with mirror and stool, small closets with shelving and built-in personal safes, cellular satellite telephone with direct dialing, and small bathrooms with showers, toilets, hair dryers, and mirrors. The eight more expensive cabins located on Main and Sun decks are a wee bit larger and include refrigerators, full windows, and larger bathrooms with Jacuzzi tubs and shower attachments.

Public areas, entertainment, and on-board activities are very limited, as is information about the ports of call. However, every day the officers permit passengers to participate in hoisting and lowering the sails and steering the vessel. Atop ship on Sun Deck, surrounded by the sails, are two small swimming pools and the lounge chairs. Main Deck, below, is the location of six of the larger cabins, the piano bar lounge, the library, and the sheltered outdoor tropical bar—the hub of activity on the ship. The dining room and half of the remaining cabins are on Clipper Deck; the other remaining cabins are located on Commodore Deck.

The attractive dining room seats all passengers at an open sitting. Breakfast and lunch are served buffet style, and a five-course dinner features a limited number of offerings. The atmosphere is casual, and jackets are never required. At midnight the chef prepares a special snack that is served in the piano bar.

At least once each cruise, there is a barbecue lunch and beach party at a private, secluded beach with watersports and games. An extensive watersport program is available daily as well. The watersport staff supervises scuba, snorkeling, banana-boat rides, and small-craft sailing.

Although the exact future itineraries for the two ships are not written in stone, the cruise line anticipates positioning one ship in the Caribbean during the fall, winter, and spring; and two ships in the Mediterranean during the warmer summer months. Home ports will most likely be Barbados in the Caribbean and Cannes, Athens, and Kusadasi in the Mediterranean. The Caribbean itinerary includes some of the best beach stops in the British Leeward Islands and in the Grenadines and the Windward Islands. In the Mediterranean, the ships call at several of the northern Mediterranean islands as well as the more picturesque ports along the coast, including Greek and Turkish ports. When cruising in Southeast Asian waters, alternating home ports for one-way, seven-day cruises are Phuket, Thailand, and Singapore. Ports of call include some of the most picturesque and pristine Thai and Malaysian beaches, which are among the most beautiful in the world. The ships are often under charter to private groups, and you must check in advance to be certain the cruise date you select is open to the general public.

Rates run from approximately $200 per person per day for a standard outside cabin with double or twin beds up to $350 per person per day for one of the larger cabins on Main or Sun decks. The cruise line will arrange air from most U.S. cities for an average cost of $700 in the Caribbean, $1,100 in the Mediterranean, and $1,500 in Asia. Star Clippers, Inc., is also marketed throughout Europe, so you can expect a large percentage of the travelers to be European, even in the Caribbean.

The new 5,000-gross-ton, 42-sail *Royal Clipper* will enter service in spring 2000. Somewhat larger than the other vessels, it will offer 2 owner's suites and 14 regular suites with verandas. The 7-day and 14-day itineraries will be offered in the

Caribbean from Barbados during the late fall and winter and in the Mediterranean from Cannes throughout the remainder of the year. Renderings of the public areas indicate that the accommodations and public areas will be a great deal more upscale than on the other vessels.

Strong Points:

A more intimate, hands-on sail/cruise experience to great beach destinations and offbeat small ports in a casual environment at middle-market prices, but with less entertainment, service, creature comforts, pampering, and amenities than found on the other, more traditional smaller cruise ships—a must for real sailors! We anxiously await our review of the new vessel.

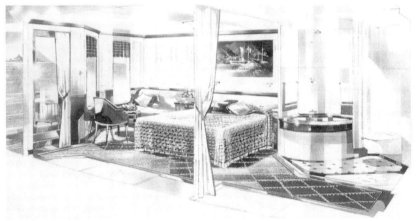

Veranda Suite, Royal Clipper, *courtesy Star Clippers, Inc.*

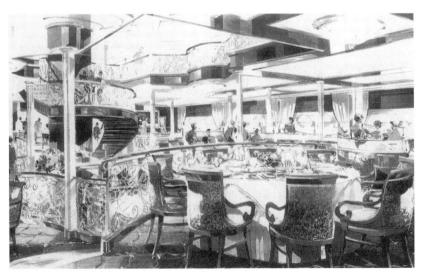

Dining Room, Royal Clipper, *courtesy Star Clippers, Inc.*

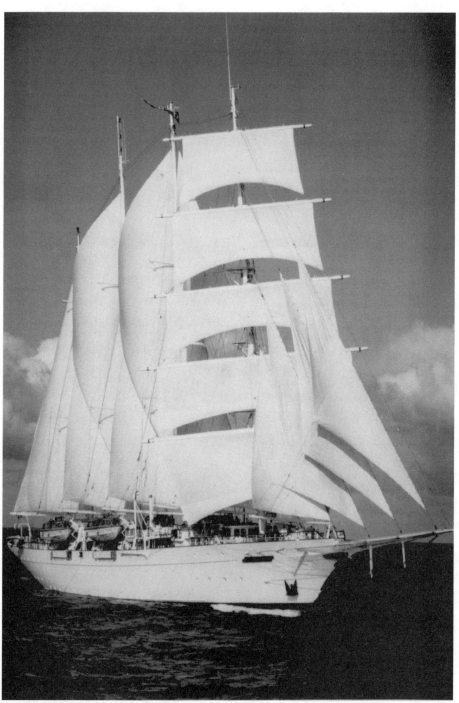

Farewell Dinner

Appetizers

Escargots en Burre Garlic

Asparagus Wrapped in Smoked Salmon

Soup

Cream of Mushroom

Salad

Dill Cucumber Salad

Entrees

Caribbean Lobster Tail, Drawn Butter

Grilled Sirloin
Choice Angus Sirloin Topped with Sauteed Mushrooms

To complement your entree

Baked Stuffed Potatoes   Mandarin Style Vegetable Medley

Buttered Baby Lima Beans

Desserts

Kiwi Crepe

Cheesecake, Raspberry Sauce

Courtesy Star Clippers, Inc.

*W*ednesday, 26th *F*ebruary 1997
*L*angkawi / *M*alaysia
08.00 - 17.30

Captain: Gerhard Lichfett   *Cruise Director/Hotel Manager: Peter Kissner*

*L*angkawi

*Langkawi is the biggest island in Malaysia with tax free
shopping, water sports and an active night life. The
temperature varies between 23 - 33 degree Celsius.
Beaches range from white to amber to black. And the
water is generally pure blue. If you are tired from the
beach visitors can pass the time gambling in the casino.*

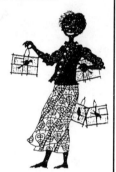

*M*ealtimes

06.30-10.30	Early Bird Breakfast	Piano Bar
07.30-09.30	Breakfast Buffet	Clipper Dining Room
13.00-14.30	Luncheon Buffet	Clipper Dining Room
17.00	Happy Hour with hors d'oeuvre	Tropical Bar
19.30-21.45	Dinner is served	Clipper Dining Room
23.00	Late Night Snack Special	Sundeck

*V*ideoprogram *C*hannel 3 & 10

	Channel 10 (English)	Channel 3 (German/French)
10.30	„Surviving the game" (96 min.)	„Pret a Porter" (128 min.) (D)
14.00	„Death and a Maiden" (103 min.)	„Forever Young" (98 min.) (D)
17.00	„Mad Max" (107 min.)	„Jenseits von Eden" (108 min.) (D)
22.00	„Indiana Jones & the Temple of Doom"	„Bodyguard" (124 min.) (D)

Activities

08.00	**SPV Star Flyer anchors off Langkawi / Malaysia**	
08.30	Start of the excursion: „ Culture Tour"	
	Return approx. 13.30	
09.00	Captain's story time behind the bridge	Sundeck
09.30-16.30	Water sport activities (details on the black board)	Tropical Bar
17.00	Last tender back to the vessel - All guests aboard!	
	Please check-in your key-tag!	
17.30	**SPV Star Flyer sets sail towards Malacca / Malaysia**	
17.00-18.00	Musical carrousel with Geza	Tropical Bar
19.00	Cocktail melodies on the piano	Piano Bar
21.30	Dance under the stars of Malaysia	Sundeck
22.00	Come in a traditional Toga - join our **Toga-Party**	
22.00	We have a **Pool-Party!!** One free drink for everybody	
	who joins us in the pool.	Sundeck

Notes

* Currency: Malaysia Ringitt / 1 US = approx. 2,4 Baht / Dollars are mainly accepted
* Agency: MSA Shipping Comp. / Langkawi / Tel. 9591007
* Name of our anchorage: Tanjung Rhu - There is no jetty at Tanjung Rhu, please be prepared
  for a wet landing.
* Tenderschedule: Each half hour one tender from the ship to the Langkawi and back.
  Last tender to the ship: **17.00 h**
* Visit our Sloop Shop, we are looking forward to be to your assistance.
* On Thursday evening we have a talent show. Do you like to participate? Do you have talents
  as singer, magician, comedian or any other talents you like to perform for us. Please contact
  Peter or Geza for a rehearsal? Don't be shy, just take part!

We wish you an exciting day in Langkawi

Courtesy Star Clippers, Inc.

STAR CRUISES

391B Orchard Road

#13-01 Ngee Ann City Tower B

Singapore 238874

(011) 65-733-6988

(011) 65-733-3622 FAX

MEGASTAR ARIES and *MEGASTAR TAURUS:* (formerly *Aurora II* and *I*); entered service 1991; 3,264 G.R.T.; 82.2 meters x 14 meters; 72-passenger capacity; 36 cabins; Scandinavian officers, international crew; cruises in Far East for private charters. (**Category A/B—Not Rated**)

MEGASTAR ASIA: (formerly *Europa*); entered service 1982; 33,819 G.R.T.; 658' x 95'; 600-passenger capacity; 316 cabins; Scandinavian officers, international crew. (**Category A/B—Not Rated**)

STAR AQUARIUS: (formerly *Athena*); 40,000 G.R.T.; 176 meters x 30 meters; 1,900-passenger capacity; 728 cabins; Scandinavian officers, international crew; two-, three-, and four-night cruises from Singapore to Malaysian ports. (**Category D—Not Rated**)

STAR PISCES: (formerly *Kalypso*); 40,000 G.R.T.; 176 meters x 30 meters; 2,192-passenger capacity; 746 cabins; Scandinavian officers, international crew; two-night cruises from Hong Kong to Xiamen and Haikou in China. (**Category D—Not Rated**)

SUPERSTAR CAPRICORN: (formerly *Royal Viking Sky* and *Golden Princess*); entered service 1971; 28,078 G.R.T.; 205 meters x 25 meters; 1,375-passenger capacity; 430 cabins; Scandinavian officers, international crew; cruises throughout Southeast Asia. (**Category B/C—Not Rated**)

SUPERSTAR GEMINI: (formerly *Crown Jewel* and *Cunard Crown Jewel*); entered service 1992; 20,000 G.R.T.; 164 meters x 23 meters; 900-passenger capacity; 400 cabins; Scandinavian officers, international crew; two- and five-night cruises from Singapore to Malaysian and Thai ports. (**Category C—Not Rated**)

SUPERSTAR LEO and *SUPERSTAR VIRGO* entered service 1998 and 1999, respectively; 75,000+ G.R.T.; 268 meters x 32 meters; 2,800-passenger capacity; 982 cabins; Scandinavian officers, international crew; cruises throughout Southeast Asia. (**Category B—Not Rated**)

SUPERSTAR SAGITTARIUS: (formerly *Sun Viking*); entered service 1972; 18,556 G.R.T.; 563' x 80'; 882-passenger capacity; 380 cabins; Scandinavian officers, international crew. (**Category B/C—Not Rated**)

(Medical Facilities: Information not provided.)

Formed in 1993 by Tan Sri Liu Goh Tong, Star Cruises is the first major cruise line concentrating on meeting the needs and satisfying the tastes of the Asian cruise market. Although the top ship officers are Scandinavian and the crew is from all over the world, the passenger mix is 70 percent Asian. Languages spoken on board are English and Mandarin.

The line offers three categories of cruise experiences. The *Star Aquarius* and *Star Pisces,* converted ferry liners, are designed to appeal to the Asian mass market of first-time cruisers, vacationing families, and the young at heart seeking a less-expensive cruise on a no-frills ship with an abundance of activities and facilities.

MegaStar Aries and *MegaStar Taurus* are generally booked by private charter groups (up to 72 passengers) seeking a more elegant, yacht-like cruise experience.

SuperStars Gemini, Capricorn, Sagittarius, Leo, and *Virgo* are geared to the more traditional, seasoned traveler seeking a more typical cruise experience on longer voyages to multiple destinations, with international standards for food, service, facilities, etc. *Gemini* is the former *Cunard Crown Jewel,* acquired by Star Cruises in 1995. *Capricorn* was added to the fleet in 1997, having had prior lives as *Royal Viking Sky* and *Golden Princess. Sagittarius,* formerly *Sun Viking* of Royal Caribbean Cruise Line, commenced sailing for Star Cruises in January 1998. *Leo* and *Virgo* are newly constructed 75,000+-ton ships that will enter service in 1998 and 1999, respectively; and *Megastar Asia,* formerly Hapag-Lloyd's 600-passenger *Europa,* begins sailing in 1999.

The *Star Aquarius* and *Star Pisces* are similar vessels, converted from ferry service. The *Aquarius,* based in Singapore, offers two- and three-night cruises to Malaysian ports, including Penang, Kuala Lumpur, and Langkawi. Home for *Star Pisces* is Hong Kong, with itineraries to Xiamen and Haikou in China.

Prices range from $100 per person per night in a very basic, small inside cabin with two to four berths, up to $290 per person for a far more comfortable junior suite. An average room costs about $150 per person per night. All cabins have private bathrooms, TVs, and telephones. The 20 junior and executive suites have additional facilities and amenities and would be my recommendation for those requiring more space and comfort.

Passengers are given meal vouchers that can be used in a variety of ethnic restaurants. Most passengers and families opt for the buffet-style international, Malay, and Chinese dining rooms. The more upscale Italian and Japanese restaurants are à la carte, and passengers can turn in their vouchers for a partial credit. The Chinese restaurants also offer à la carte selections at a surcharge.

Public facilities on both vessels include cinemas; show lounges that convert to discos, several smaller lounges, and bars; Karaoke lounges; indoor pools, small gyms, and health spas; numerous shops; food courts; sun decks; jogging tracks; video arcades; and a child-care center.

SuperStar Gemini, the former *Cunard Crown Jewel,* was acquired in 1995 and is the first of the line's more upscale vessels. It alternates itineraries from Singapore with two-night cruises to Malacca or Tioman departing Fridays and five-night cruises to Kuala Lumpur (Port Klang), Langkawi, and Phuket departing Sundays. Fares range from $150 per person per night to $165 for a deluxe cabin or small suite, $230 for a junior suite, and $350 for an executive suite that includes an outside patio.

The cabin size, amenities, and public areas have not changed since the days the ship sailed for Cunard, where it was marketed as a more understated, popular-priced alternative to the Cunard deluxe market ships.

Cabin size and inside and outside public areas are about average for ships in the 20,000 gross-ton range. Located on the top three decks are the pool, fitness center, children's area, video arcade, cardroom, library, disco and karaoke lounge, the buffet restaurant, and the more expensive cabins and suites. The less expensive cabins are on the bottom three decks, with the show lounge, shops, reception room, bars, and lounges in the middle and the main dining room, Ocean Palace, one deck below.

SuperStar Capricorn is the Star Cruise identity given to the former *Golden Princess* (originally the *Royal Viking Sky*). It is scheduled to offer diverse Asian itineraries.

MegaStar Aries and *MegaStar Taurus* are the former *Aurora II* and *I* of Classical Cruises. These small, yacht-like vessels—which feature more traditional, rather than nautical, décor—are used for groups and business charters or special events and do not offer regular itineraries.

The first of the line's new-builts, *SuperStar Leo,* debuted in the fall of 1998, followed by *SuperStar Virgo* in the summer of 1999. These ships weigh in at 74,500 G.R.T. and can accommodate a maximum of 2,800 passengers in 982 cabins, 608 of which have ocean views and 391 boast balconies. Initially *Leo* offered two- and three-night sailings from Singapore. Present plans will deploy her to Hong Kong when *Virgo* comes on line. There are 6 luxury-theme suites on Deck 10 with private balconies, living areas, separate bedrooms, master bathrooms with whirlpool and separate shower, guest powder rooms, four interactive color televisions (including one above the whirlpool), and fax machines. All of the 370 inside cabins have four berths.

Public areas include an atrium spanning six decks; multiple dining venues composed of the 632-seat, three-meal-a-day Windows Restaurant, the 268-seat, Chinese family-style Garden Room, the 568-seat Raffles Buffet Terrace, offering Malay, Japanese, Thai, Chinese, and Western buffets, the 102-seat Chinese Thai Pan Restaurant, the 52-seat, gourmet Maxim's, the 130-seat Japanese Shogun with Teppanyaki, Sushi, and Tatami rooms, the 50-seat, casual 24-hour Blue Lagoon Café, and the Bavarian-style Beer Gardens; the two-story Moulin Rouge gambling casino, the 957-seat Show Lounge, the 432-seat Gala of the Stars observation lounge and disco; an English-style pub with darts and billiards; Karaoke rooms; young children's and teen facilities that rival the new Disney ships; a Roman-style spa and fitness center; and a Romanesque lido-deck area with pools and Jacuzzis.

Presently the ships are marketed mainly in Singapore, Hong Kong, Malaysia, and Thailand. With the addition of new vessels and more amenities and facilities, a greater number of North Americans and Europeans may be testing the waters.

Strong Points:

Star Cruises offers a variety of cruising styles that are gauged to appeal to international cruisers.

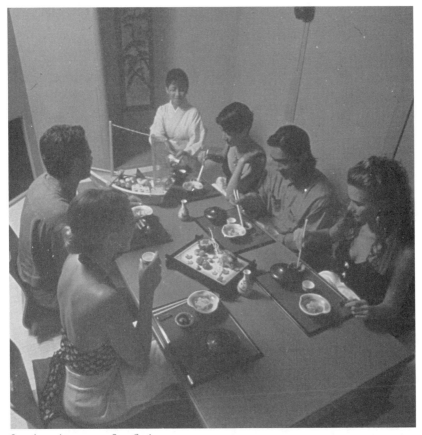

Star Aquarius, *courtesy Star Cruises*

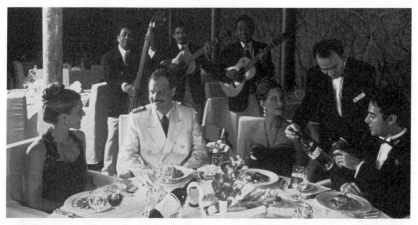

Star Aquarius, *courtesy Star Cruises*

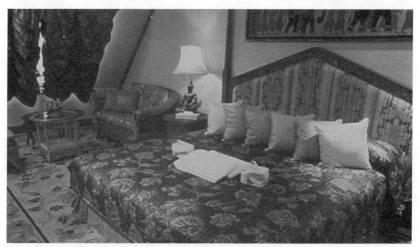

Star Aquarius, *courtesy Star Cruises*

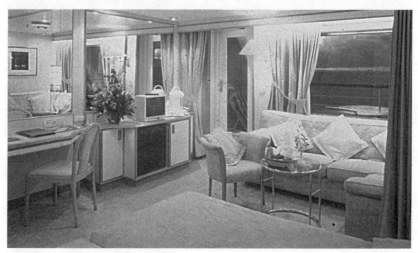

SuperStar Gemini, *courtesy Star Cruises*

DINNER

Appetiser

Symphony of Seafood
Baby scallops, prawns, shrimps and crab meat
on crisp greens, choice of dressings
or
Baked Escargots
in onion, herb and garlic butter

Soup

Gratinated Onion Soup
with bread Swiss cheese crouton
or
Cream of Fresh Broccoli with Almonds

Salad

Crisp Caesar Salad
Sliced romaine lettuce with garlic, parmesan,
anchovies, vinegar dressing and croutons

Main Course

Broiled Fillet of Fresh Fish from Phuket
Lemon grass ginger sauce
stirfried vegetables
or
Stirfried Chilli Prawns
on bell pepper rice and pak choy
or
Deep Fried Escalope Viennose
Breaded and fried veal scaloppine
roast potatoes and sauteed vegetables
or
Roast Rack of New Zealand Lamb
Fresh herb and Dijon mustard marinated lamb
mint gravy, ratatouille, pomme dauphinoise
or
Stirfried Porkloin slices in Satay Sauce
Chinese vegetables, steamed rice

Vegetarian

Vegetables Chop Suey
on laksa noodle

Cheese

Selection of Fine Cheeses
Walnut onion bread and wheat crackers

Dessert

Baked Alaska
a tradition of its own, served with strawberry sauce
or
Black Forest Cake
Sour cherries and whipped cream in a chocolate sponge cake,
flavoured with kirsch wasser

Sherbet

Orange

Coffee or Tea

Courtesy Star Cruises

STAR CRUISES

WHEN	WHAT	WHERE
8.00 am	**TUMMY TONING CLASS** Join Francisca for a class that is designed to tighten & tone the abdominal area	Fitness Centre Deck 8
9.00 am	**STROLL A MILE** Did you know that 5 times around deck 5 equals 1 mile? Please meet Lauren on the starboard(right) outside Deck near Reception	Reception Deck 5
9.30 am	**POOL DECK RING TOSS** Your chance to win great prizes	Pool Deck
10.00 am- 12:00 mn	**THE KARAOKE LOUNGE IS OPEN!** Join the DJ & sing your favourite songs!!!!	Starship Karaoke Deck 7
10.00 am	Get zany at the Pool Deck for **SHUFFLEBOARD**	Pool Deck
10.00 am	**PRE-DINNER WINE PURCHASE** Choose your wine for the Gala Dinner tonight. Great selection on display...	Bar Gemini Deck 5
10.30 am- 11.30 am	**MORNING TEA IS SERVED**	Bar Gemini Deck 5
10.45 am	**GREAT MUSIC FROM THE SUPERSTAR ENSEMBLE**	The Atrium Deck 4
11.00 am	**M/V SUPERSTAR GEMINI ARRIVES IN PULAU LANGKAWI**	
2.30 pm	**TRIVIA QUIZ** Can you beat the Quiz Master?	Gemini Bar Deck 5
WHEN	WHAT	WHERE
3.00 pm	**GOLF PUTTING COMPETITION** Show off those putting skills	Pool Deck
3.30 pm	**PRE-DINNER WINE PURCHASE** Choose your wine for your dinner tonight	Mariners Restaurant Deck 6
3.30 pm- 4.30 pm	**AFTERNOON TEA IS SERVED**	Mariners Restaurant Deck 6
4.00 pm	**KARAOKE JAMMING** Join the DJ and the Cruise Staff & Name That Tune to win a prize	Starship Karaoke Deck 7
6.00 pm & 8.15 pm	**CAPTAIN'S APPRECIATION COCKTAIL PARTY** Captain Kjell Holms cordially invites you for cocktails in the Galaxy of the Stars lounge	Galaxy of the Stars Deck 5
7.00 pm	**M/V SUPERSTAR GEMINI DEPARTS FOR PHUKET**	
7.30 pm	**MUSICAL CHARADES** For all teenagers and teenagers at heart, come & join this fun event and have a chance to meet new friends....	Starship Karaoke Deck 7
9.05 pm & 10.55 pm	Star Cruises & The SuperStar Gemini proudly present SHOWTIME **THE JULIO IGLESIUS SHOW** starring **CLAUDIO PARENTE** with your Cruise Director **GERRY KEATING**	Galaxy of the Stars Deck 5
10.15 pm	**DANCE DATE WITH THE GEMINI BIG BAND**	Galaxy of the Stars Deck 5
11.30 pm	**MUSIC WITH MR PIANO MAN RAUL**	Bar Gemini Deck 5
12.00 mn- 1.00 am	**50's & 60's DANCE DATE** Come and dance to some of the great hits of yesteryears	Starship Disco Deck 7
12.00 mn	MIDNIGHT MOVIE FEATURING **"EYE FOR AN EYE"** starring Sally Field	Galaxy of the Stars Deck 5
1.00 am- 3.00 am	**DANCE THE NIGHT AWAY** Joseph will spin your favourites	Starship Disco Deck 7

Courtesy Star Cruises

WINDJAMMER BAREFOOT CRUISES
1759 Bay Road
Miami Beach, Florida 33139-1413
(305) 672-6543

AMAZING GRACE: entered service 1955; renovated 1985; 1,585 G.R.T.; 257' x 40'; 96-passenger capacity; 48 cabins; international officers, West Indian and Central American crew; 13- and 26-day cruises to the Bahamas and Caribbean year-round. (**Category D—Not Rated**)

FANTOME: entered service 1927; renovated 1969 and 1992; 676 G.R.T.; 282' x 40'; four masts 170' high; 11 sails and 2 engines; 128-passenger capacity; 64 cabins; international officers, West Indian and Central American crew; 6-day cruises to Antigua. (**Category D—Not Rated**)

FLYING CLOUD: entered service 1935; renovated 1968; 400 G.R.T.; 208' x 32'; three masts 140' high; 11 sails and 1 engine; 66-passenger capacity; 33 cabins; international officers, West Indian and Central American crew; 6-day cruises to the British Virgin Islands year-round. (**Category D—Not Rated**)

LEGACY: entered service 1959; renovated 1997; 1,740 G.R.T.; 294' x 40'; four masts 180' high; 11 sails and 3 engines; 122-passenger capacity, 61 cabins; international officers, West Indian and Central American crew; 6-day cruises to the Virgin Islands year-round. (**Category D—Not Rated**)

MANDALAY: entered service 1923; renovated 1982-1984; 420 G.R.T.; 236' x 33'; three masts 140' high; 11 sails and 1 engine; 72-passenger capacity; 36 cabins; international officers, West Indian and Central American crew; 13-day cruises to the Windward and Leeward Islands year-round; 6-day itineraries through the Grenadine Passage year-round. (**Category D—Not Rated**)

POLYNESIA: entered service 1938; renovated 1975; 430 G.R.T.; 249' x 36'; four masts 170' high; 11 sails and 1 engine; 126-passenger capacity; 57 cabins; international officers, West Indian and Central American crew; 6-day itineraries to the Leeward and Windward Islands year-round. (**Category D—Not Rated**)

YANKEE CLIPPER: entered service 1927; renovated 1965 and 1987; 327 G.R.T.; 197' x 30'; three masts 140' high; 9 sails and 1 engine; 64-passenger capacity; 32 cabins; international officers, West Indian and Central American crew; 6-day cruises to the Grenadine and Spice Islands year-round. (**Category D—Not Rated**)

(Medical Facilities: No information supplied by cruise line.)

Windjammer Barefoot Cruises is the largest operator of "tall ships" in the world. Founded in 1947 by Captain Mike Burke, a passionate seaman, the seven-ship fleet of authentic tall ships ranges in size from 327 to 1,740 tons and includes: *Amazing Grace, Fantome, Flying Cloud, Mandalay, Polynesia, Yankee Clipper,* and *Legacy,* the most recent addition to the fleet.

The cruise line, which is still a family business, originated from Captain Mike's vision of creating an intimate, adventurous, and casual sailing environment for travelers seeking a true "wind-in-the-hair" cruise vacation. Steeped in natural heritage and pioneering spirit, Windjammer enables passengers to return to an era when excitement and adventure prevailed on the high seas.

Each Windjammer tall ship boasts a distinctive and unique heritage. Prior to joining the Windjammer fleet, the ships often served as private yachts for the world's most legendary financial moguls, from the Vanderbilts and the Guinnesses to E. F. Hutton and Aristotle Onassis. Over the years, the cruise line has invested millions of dollars to restore these magnificent seafaring vessels to their original grandeur, providing today's passengers with an authentic sailing experience. The accommodations and public areas are more rustic than found on the more upscale sailing vessels, and the atmosphere is more casual.

Visiting more than 60 ports of call throughout the Bahamas, U.S. and British Virgin Islands, West Indies, Belize, and the Bay Islands, Windjammer's ships reach remote, exotic, and eco-rich islands such as Carriacou, Iles Des Saintes, St. Lucia, Utila, Roatan, and Guanaja—the type of locales that often are inaccessible to the larger cruise ships. Having been a major presence in the Caribbean for more than 50 years, the fleet sails year-round throughout the region, offering affordable 6- and 13-day cruises. "Stowaway" nights provide passengers with the opportunity to board their Windjammer vessel the evening prior to sailing for an extra night of relaxation and fun.

The Windjammer philosophy allows its passengers to do as much or as little as they wish during their cruise. Passengers, or "shipmates," may learn the art of seamanship by assisting with the maneuvering and sailing of the "tall ships" and participating in informal, hands-on sailing classes that teach such skills as how to tie a bowline, hoist a sail, or steer a ship. In keeping with the casual atmosphere, Captain Story Time allows for an informal gathering with the shipmaster as he shares the upcoming island's history and culture and references interesting tales, sights, and activities. In the evenings passengers can enjoy live music, join in the fun of costume parties and limbo contests, or simply gaze at the stars under the warm Caribbean sky.

Breakfast, served between 6:30 and 8:30 a.m., includes fresh produce, freshly baked breads, and hot and cold entrees. On-board lunch is buffet style or consists of an impromptu beach barbecue held on a picturesque beach. Windjammer offers two seatings for dinner, 6:30 and 7:45 p.m. The cruise lines tries to accommodate special meal requests, offering vegetarian dishes as well as a children's menu that feature kids' favorites such as pizza, chicken nuggets, and macaroni and cheese, among others.

With an emphasis on beaches, water sports, and the natural surroundings, Windjammer offers some unique and adventurous shore excursions. Thrill seekers can climb the breathtaking mountains and tropical rain forest in Saba, hike the rugged last settlement of the Carib Indians and visit a roaring waterfall on Dominica, or discover a bird and an egg-laying site for the endangered green turtle on Conception Island. Water lovers may scuba-dive in a natural reef and in the Blue Hole, a lagoon with an underwater shaft filled with stalactite-studded caverns on Lighthouse Reef, Belize; snorkel in a protected cove of Gorda Cay; or deep-sea fish off Glover's Reef, Belize.

Windjammer's Dive Vacations call at remote sites that appeal to the most seasoned scuba diver while offering resort courses for beginners. Some of Windjammer's more popular offerings are the singles' cruises. Hosted aboard the *Polynesia,* the singles' cruises sail the Leeward Islands and British Virgin Islands.

With the recent introduction of the Junior Jammers Kids Club, Windjammer has created an organized, fully chaperoned program of fun and wholesome activities that allow children to learn about nature and the environment during a carefree, relaxed barefoot cruise. Available aboard *Legacy* during the summer months, the Junior Jammers program caters to children of all ages. (The minimum age for children to sail aboard Windjammer's tall ships is 6 years old.) Imaginatively designed daily activities for the younger children include participating in pirate hunts, competing in athletic contests, and playing beach games. Teenagers may take sailing lessons, go fishing, or snorkel the tropical Caribbean waters. Babysitting is also available during the events from 7:00 P.M. to midnight for a fee of $5.00 per hour.

Cruise fares range from an average of $129 per day per person for a standard cabin (fleetwide) during off-season to an average of $162 per day per person for a standard cabin in peak season. Special discount values are available on various cruises throughout the year.

Strong Points:

Casual, friendly atmosphere; unique Caribbean itineraries designed for beach and water lovers, as well as excellent scuba-diving expeditions and popular singles' cruises.

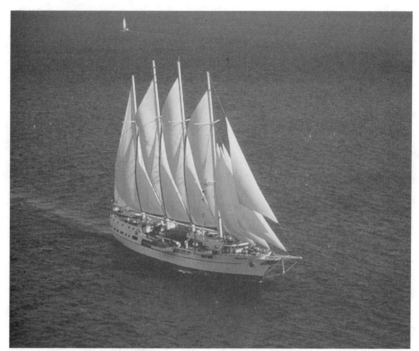

Courtesy Windjammer Barefoot Cruises

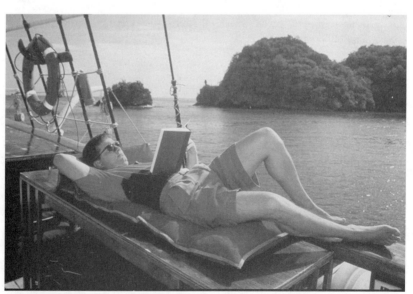

Courtesy Windjammer Barefoot Cruises

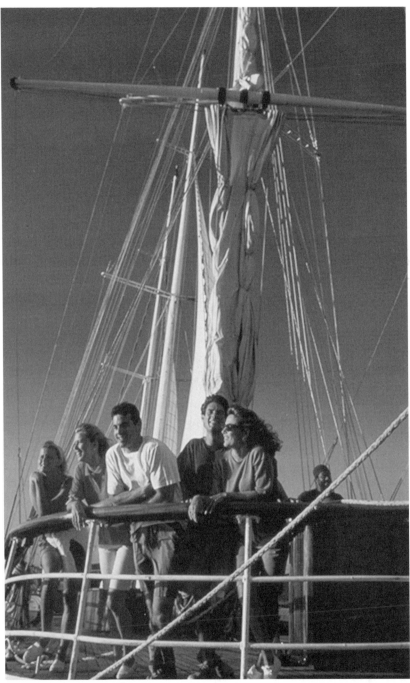

Courtesy Windjammer Barefoot Cruises

WINDSTAR CRUISES
300 Elliott Avenue West
Seattle, Washington 98119
(206) 281-3535

WIND SONG: entered service 1987; 5,350 G.R.T.; 440' x 52'; four masts 204'
high; six sails and three engines; 148-passenger capacity; 74 cabins; European
officers, Indonesian and Filipino crew; seven-day cruises from Costa Rica in the
winter and from Rome in the warmer months.

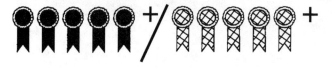

WIND SPIRIT: entered service 1988; 5,350 G.R.T.; 440' x 52'; four masts 204'
high; six sails and three engines; 148-passenger capacity; 74 cabins; European
officers, Indonesian and Filipino crew; seven-day cruises in the Mediterranean
in the summer and in the Virgin Islands the remainder of the year.

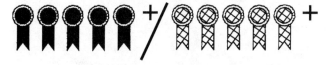

WIND STAR: entered service 1986; 5,350 G.R.T.; 440' x 52'; four masts 204'
high; six sails and three engines; 148-passenger capacity; 74 cabins; European
officers, Indonesian and Filipino crew; seven-day cruises in the Caribbean in
the summer and to Costa Rica in the fall; and will sail the eastern Mexican
Riviera and Central America in the winter and spring of 2000.

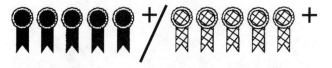

WIND SURF: (formerly *Club Med I*); entered service 1990; 14,745 G.R.T.; 617' x 66';
312-passenger capacity; 156 cabins; European officers, Indonesian and Filipino
crew; seven-day cruises in the Mediterranean in summer and in the Caribbean
the remainder of the year.

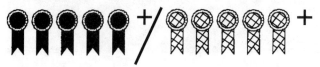

(Medical Facilities: C-0; P-1; EM, CLS, MS; CM; PD; EKG; TC; PO; EPC; OX; WC; OR; ICU; LJ—This is for all ships except *Wind Surf,* which also carries a nurse.)

Windstar Cruises was founded in 1984 by Finnish-born Karl Andren, who put the uniquely designed *Wind Star* into Caribbean service in 1986. Thereafter, *Wind Star* was joined by her two identical sister ships, *Wind Song,* in July 1987 and *Wind Spirit,* in 1988. In 1997 Windstar purchased *Club Med I* from Club Med Cruises, renamed the ship *Wind Surf,* and conducted extensive renovations, including the addition of 31 new suites, a 10,000-square-foot spa, and a bistro-style restaurant. *Wind Surf* commenced service for its new owners in the Mediterranean in the spring of 1998.

Windstar Cruises was purchased by Holland America Line in 1988, and Holland America was subsequently purchased by Carnival Cruise Line. However, a Windstar Cruise bears no resemblance to cruises on the ships of its owners, and remains a uniquely casual yet elegant experience thoroughly enjoyed by those who have been fortunate enough to sail on one of its four sleek vessels. The unique feature of these vessels is the computer-monitored and directed sailing systems with diesel-electric back-up propulsion. However, the ships do not sail the entire time.

All of the cabins on the three original ships are outside, identical, and located on the lower two decks. They are 185 square feet in area and are designed in a modern interpretation of the nautical tradition, with mixed woods and rich fabrics. Each includes a color TV; videocassette player; safe; three-channel radio; CD player; fully stocked refrigerator; mini-bar; terry-cloth robes; direct-dial ship-to-shore telephone; two twin beds that convert to queen size; and a bathroom with separate toilet compartment, sink, shower, generous cabinet space, and hair dryer. Room service is available around the clock. Eleven cabins offer a third bed.

The public areas are located on the top two decks, but the sauna, fitness room, sports shops, watersports platform, and Sillingers are on the third deck down from the top (designated Deck 2). The public areas include a sun deck with a small pool, a casino, an intimate yet elegant dining room, a lounge, a hair stylist, boutique, infirmary, and library. Breakfast and a buffet lunch are served in the glass-enclosed veranda lounge that is lit up at night and converts to a disco. Dinner takes place in the romantic main dining room from 7:30 to 9:30 P.M. without pre-assigned seating. The line describes its cuisine as a combination of French, European, and New American. Menus and recipes have been recently designed by award-winning Chef Joachim Splichal, owner of Patina and Pinot Bistro in Los Angeles. Tipping is accepted, but not solicited.

In the evening there is dance music, local native shows, and a gala deck barbecue under the stars. A large selection of videocassette tapes and CDs can be rented in the library and aired in individual cabins. There is also a small casino with two blackjack tables and 13 slot machines.

The itineraries for the *Wind Star* and *Wind Spirit* include some of the more picturesque islands in the central Caribbean during the fall, winter, and spring; and the ships sail to a number of French, Italian, Greek, and other Mediterranean islands and ports during the summer. The unique ability of these vessels to navigate shallow waters and tender passengers to beaches and harbors permits these ships to call on more unusual destinations that the larger cruise ships cannot negotiate.

The *Wind Song* ceased its Polynesia itinerary in late 1997 in order to initiate cruises from Costa Rica to Isla de Cano, Bahia Drake, Quepos, Tortuga Island, Playa Flamingo, and Isla Coiba in Panama in the winter and cruises from Rome to Mediterranean islands and ports during the warmer months.

The emphasis of all four vessels is on beaches, watersports, small, quaint ports, and making the most of the beauty of the natural surroundings. Each ship is equipped with Zodiac-type inflatable motor launches for water-skiing and transportation to shallow beaches, water skis, scuba and snorkel equipment, windsurfing boards, and small sailboats. A water-sport platform extends from Deck 2 (second deck from the bottom of the ship).

The most enjoyable features of cruises on this line are the impressive comfort, special features, and storage space in all cabins; the intimate dining experience that permits passengers to dine alone or with other passengers of their choice and alfresco for breakfast and lunch (with waiters rather than cafeteria style); the option to dress casually and comfortably; the relaxed and unregimented program; and the ability to visit numerous exotic ports seldom offered by other cruise lines. The Indonesian, Filipino, and European service staff are most attentive and friendly.

The line offers attractive air-sea packages. Cruise fares are the same for every cabin, ranging from about $350 per day per person during intermediate season to $450 per day in peak season. Special discount values are available on various cruises throughout the year.

Following her extensive renovations, *Wind Surf* now boasts thirty-one 376-square-foot suites, twice the size of the 125 deluxe, 188-square-foot cabins. All accommodations are outside with queen beds that convert to twins, color televisions with video cassette players, CDs, safes, mini-bar/refrigerators, international direct-dial telephones, hair dryers, and terry-cloth robes. The suites are really double cabins where one has been converted to a parlor while retaining its storage space and bathroom, affording exceptional space and comfort for its occupants.

The new 10,000-square-foot spa features treatment rooms for body wraps, facials, and massages, as well as steam and sauna. A well-stocked, glassed-in fitness center sits atop ship, permitting those exercising to enjoy interesting panoramas. In addition to the romantic, single-seating main dining room, there is a 90-seat alternative dining bistro featuring rotisserie dining, pastas, wines, and additional tables for two. Meeting facilities can accommodate up to 160 people with special audiovisual equipment and a galley for snacks and refreshments. Complimentary water sports are available off the marina deck, and the ship has two outdoor swimming pools, two Jacuzzis, and a nice lido/lounge/bar area. Other public facilities include a large main lounge, a signature boutique, a library stocked with CDs and videos as well as books, a casino, and infirmary. *Wind Surf,* being almost three times the size of the other three vessels, offers more indoor public areas and far more generous outdoor deck space. Although she retains the sleek appearance of a sailing vessel, the cruise experience is more similar to that on other cruise ships of her size and is less intimate than on the other Windstar ships.

Wind Surf features special spa packages that cost from $259 to $699, and "cruise only" brochure fares start at $400 per person per day in the Caribbean and $600 per day in the Mediterranean, escalating to $775 to $995 per day for the suites. *Wind Surf* will offer seven-day cruises from Nice, Rome, and Venice in the summer, and Caribbean cruises the remainder of the year.

Strong Points:

Unique, beautiful design; comfortable, functional staterooms; great water-sports; casual, yet elegant atmosphere; a more intimate dining experience; and super itineraries for beach lovers wishing to travel in comfort and luxury. The new *Wind Surf* offers an attractive suite option for the more affluent traveler and greater indoor and outdoor public areas, as well as impressive spa facilities.

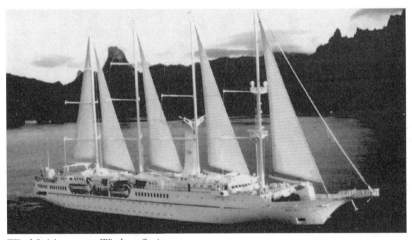

Wind Spirit, *courtesy Windstar Cruises*

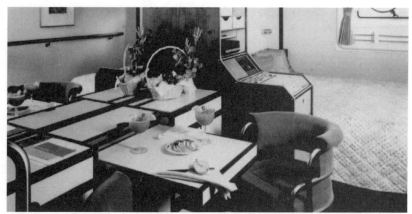

Wind Spirit, *courtesy Windstar Cruises*

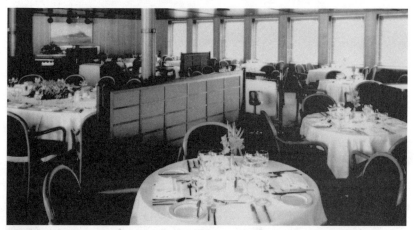

Wind Spirit, *courtesy Windstar Cruises*

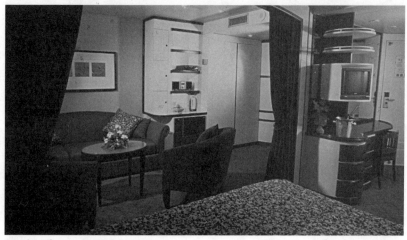

Wind Surf, *courtesy Windstar Cruises*

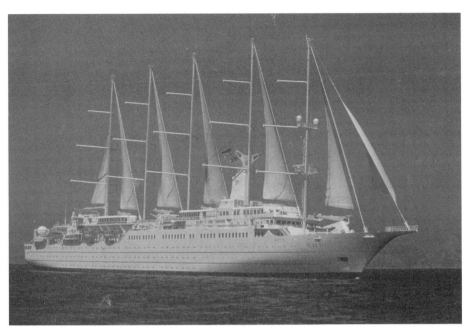

Wind Surf, *courtesy Windstar Cruises*

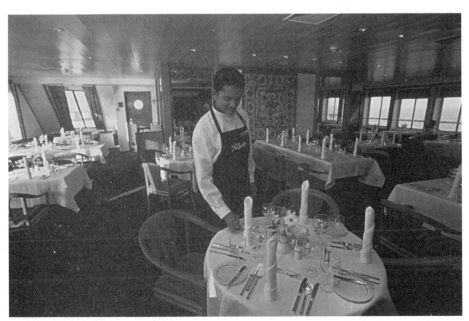

Wind Surf, *courtesy Windstar Cruises*

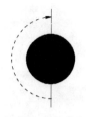

$\mathscr{A}$PPETIZERS

Italian Antipasta

Crispy Risotto Cake a la Putanesca: Capers, Sun Dried Tomatoes,
Grilled Fennel and Anchovy

Array of Tropical Fruit and Fresh Mint

$\mathscr{S}$OUPS

Classic French Pistou Soup

Chilled Cream of Berry with Fresh Mint

$\mathscr{S}$ALADS

Fresh Spinach with Hot Apple Smoked Bacon Dressing

Wind Star Housse Salad with Asparagus, Basil Dressing

or with your choice of:
French, Italian, Thousand Islands, Blue Cheese, Hot Honey Mustard

$\mathscr{E}$NTREES

Poached Orange Roughy with Fresh Dill Beurre Blanc

Steamed Crab Legs with Drawn Butter

Grilled Beef Rib Eye Steak with Bearnaise

Braised Osso Buco a la Milanaise

Sauteed Penne Pasta with Shrimps, Vegetables and Tomato Sauce

Also available upon request Baked Potato and Vegetables of the Day

*Special thanks to Chef Joachim Splichal of Patina and Pinot of Los Angeles
for taking us in new culinary directions, "180° From Ordinary".*

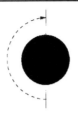

$\mathscr{C}$HEF $\mathscr{M}$ICHAEL'S
$\mathscr{R}$ECOMMENDATIONS

Crispy Risotto Cake a la Putanesca: Capers, Sun Dried Tomatoes, Grilled Fennel and Anchovy

Classic French Pistou Soup

Fresh Spinach with Hot Apple Smoked Bacon Dressing

Grilled Beef Rib Eye Steak with Bearnaise

French Profiteroles with Hot Fudge Sauce

$\mathscr{L}$IGHT AND HEALTHY ENTREE

Grilled Tuna with Tropical Fruit Salsa
Kcal: 305 Fat: 6.00

$\mathscr{V}$EGETARIAN ENTREE

Vegetable Stir Fry
(Prepared without Dairy Products)

$\mathscr{W}$INES BY THE GLASS

White Wine	Red Wine
Chardonnay Haywood, Sonoma, California 4.25	Cabernet Sauvignon R. Amberhill, California 4.25
Chardonnay Chateau Woltner, Napa Valley, California 4.25	Mouton Cadet Rothschild, Bordeaux 4.25
Champagne Maison Deutz, Santa Barbara 5.50	Dessert Wine Quady Essencia, California 4.75

$\mathscr{D}$ESSERTS

French Profiteroles with Hot
Fudge Sauce

Napoleon Cake

Banana Pie with Raspberry Sauce

Assorted French Pastries

International Fromage

COUPE WIND STAR
Peach Melba

ICE CREAM
Mocha

Chocolate

SHERBET
Wild Berries

BEVERAGES
Espresso, Cappuccino, Cafe au Lait,

Chocomilk, Chocolate, Espressochoc,

Tea and Herbal Teas,

Regular or Decaffeinated Coffee

$\mathscr{C}$ORDIALS AND LIQUEURS

Remy Martin Louis XIII 75.00
Martell Cordon Bleu 8.75
Remy Martin X.O 8.75
Remy Martin V.S.O.P. 6.75
Grand Marnier 4.50
Tia Maria 4.50
Cointreau 4.50
Drambuie 4.50
Sambuca 4.50

$\mathscr{C}$OFFEE DRINKS

Coffee Specialties 6.00

Captain's Coffee
with Grand Marnier and Tia Maria

Irish Coffee
with Irish Whiskey

French Coffee
with Cognac

Italian Coffee
with Sambuca

Mexican Coffee
with Kahlua

Almond Dream
with Amaretto and Bailey's

French Chocolate
with Hot Chocolate and Cognac

Tropical
with Hot Chocolate, Kahlua and Rum

WINDSTAR CRUISES

Sunrise: 6:03 am
Sunset: 9:06 pm

Wednesday
July 8th, 1998
Monte Carlo, Monaco

The principality of Monaco covers just 473 acres and would fit comfortably inside New York's Central Park or a family farm in Iowa. Its 5,000 citizens would fill only small fraction of the seats in Yankee Sadium. The country is so tiny that residents have to go to another country to play golf. Passports are required for entrance to most casinos and in the evening men are required to wear a coat and tie to enter the Private Saloon of the Grand Casino. On occasion people have managed to enter without a tie, but most of the time the casino is strict with the rule. (There is also an admission fee of 50ff). Official minimum age for entrance to casinos is 21.

SHORE EXCURSIONS
1:30 pm   " Scenic French Riviera Tour" Please meet at 1:20 pm in the Lounge.

TODAY'S ACTIVITIES
7:30 am - 9:30 am   Breakfast is served in the Veranda.
8:00 am - 10:00 pm   The Wind Surf Spa is open on deck # 2.
8:00 am   Wind Surf arrives in Monte Carlo, Monaco. After the ship has been cleared by the local authorities, local tenders depart the ship on the hour and half hour and depart shore at quarter to and quarter after the hour. Please note there are no tenders going ashore at 8:30 pm and no returning tender at 8:15 pm and 8:45 pm. Please take your ID card.
9:00 am - 11:00 am   The Host & Hostess desk opens for port information & shore excursion sign-ups.
12:30 pm - 2:00 pm   Lunch is served in the Veranda.
4:00 pm - 5:00 pm   Tea is served in the Compass Rose.
5:00 pm - 7:30 pm   The Photo Gallery opens on Main Deck.
6:30 pm - 12:00 pm   Enjoy the music of the "Jordan Heppner Trio" in the Wind Surf Lounge.

7:15 pm   Your Hosts, Walt and Cheri will be in the Lounge for a briefing on your day tomorrow in Cannes, France.

7:30 pm - 9:15 pm   Dinner is served in the Restaurant.
7:45 pm - 9:30 pm   Dinner is served in the Bistro, Star deck forward.
9:30 pm - 1:00 am   Enjoy the sounds of "The Lucky Bridge Trio" in the Compass Rose on Bridge Deck.
9:30 pm - 10:30 pm   The Host & Hostess desk opens for port information & shore excursion sign-ups.
2:00 am (Thurs.)   The last tender returns from shore.

WATERSPORTS
10:00 am - 12:00 noon The Marina opens for watersports activities. Windsurfing, sailing, water-skiing, kayaking and boat rides. Sign-ups are taken on a first come first serve basis. (Access from deck # 3)
1:30 pm - 5:00 pm   The Marina opens for watersports activities. (Access from deck # 3)

Restaurant Hours *(Please, no shorts, jeans or tennis shoes in the Restaurant)*

Continental Breakfast is served in the Compass Rose	6:00 am - 10:00 am
Breakfast is served in the Veranda	7:30 am - 9:30 am
Lunch is served in the Veranda	12:30 pm - 2:00 pm
Tea is served in the Compass Rose	4:00 pm - 5:00 pm
Dinner is served in the Restaurant	7:30 pm - 9:15 pm
Dinner is served in the Bistro **(Reservations only for the Bistro, please)**	7:45 pm - 9:30 pm

Cabin Service Dial # 3450　6:00 am - midnight

If the answer machine is activated please leave a message at the sound of the tone.

Host & Hostess Desk

Receive Port Information & Sign-up for Shore Excursions

9:00 am - 11:00 am	9:30 pm - 10:30 pm

Lounge

Pool Bar	9:30 am - 6:00 pm
Compass Rose (Dial # 3453)	**10:00 am - Closing**
Wind Surf Lounge (Dial # 3553)	6:00 pm - Closing

Reception Dial # 0　Open 24 hours

Casino Dial # 3441 *(Please, no one under 18 years of age and no photos)*

Slot Machines	Closed
Gaming Tables	Closed

Due to Customs regulations, the Casino will be closed while in port.

Shops Onboard Dial # 3701or2

Signature Shop - Kiosk	Closed

Due to Customs regulations, the Shops will be closed while in port.

Photo Center Dial # 3700　5:00 pm - 7:30 pm

Come and see how we have captured your cruise memories. Photographs on display 5 pm to 7:30 pm.

Spa Dial # 3253

Spa & Salon	8:00 am - 10:00 pm
Sauna	8:00 am - 10:00 pm
Fitness Center　**Please see your daily fitness program for scheduled classes.**	6:00 am - 10:00 pm

Infirmary Hours Dial # 3152

For Medical Emergencies outside infirmary hours, please call	8:00 am - 9:30 am
Reception #. 0 (Consultation fee will be charged)	4:30 pm - 6:00 pm

Television Information　*To improve your reception of In-House-Channels, please turn off your VCR*

Channel 0:　THIS CHANNEL RESERVED FOR PLAYING VIDEO TAPES (From the Library)
Channel 1,2,3 SATELLITE TELEVISION (when available)
Channel 4:　DOCUMENTARY - TORVILL & DEAN　3:00 pm until 5:00 pm

SPECIAL FEATURE

Channel 4: "AS GOOD AS IT GETS"　7:00 pm, 10:00 pm, 1:00 am
Channel 5: "FOR RICHER OR POORER" 8:00 am, 11:00 am, 2:00 pm, 5:00 pm, 8:00 pm
　　　　　　　　　　　　　　　　　　　11:00 pm, 2:00 am
Channel 6: "PEACEMAKER"　8:30 am, 11:00 am, 1:30 pm, 4:00 pm, 6:30 pm
　　　　　　　　　　　　　　　9:00 pm, 11:30 pm, 2:00 am, 4:30 am
Channel 7: "WASHINGTON SQUARE"　9:00 am, 11:30 am, 2:00 pm, 4:30 pm, 7:00 pm,
　　　　　　　　　　　　　　　　　　　9:30 pm, 12:00 am, 2:30 am, 5:00 am
Channel 8:　OCEAN SAT. NEWS

WORLD EXPLORER CRUISES

555 Montgomery Street

San Francisco, California 94111-2544

(800) 854-3835

(800) 325-2732

UNIVERSE EXPLORER: (formerly *Brazil, Monarch Sun, Volendam,* S.S. *Canada Star, Liberte, Queen of Bermuda,* and *Enchanted Seas*); entered service 1958; refurbished 1972, 1985, 1990, and 1998; 23,500 G.R.T.; 617' x 84'; 731-passenger capacity; 367 cabins; mixed crew and officers; cruises to Alaska, western Caribbean, Mexico, and South and Central America. (**Category D—Not Rated**)

(Medical Facilities: C-10; P-1; CLS, MS; CM; PD; BC; EKG; TC; PO; EPC; OX; WC; ICU; M.)

World Explorer Cruises offers educational-adventure cruises in Alaska that depart from Vancouver and sail the Inside Passage to Ketchikan, Sitka, Seward, Valdez, Victoria, Hubbard Glacier, Skagway, Glacier Bay, Juneau, and Wrangell.

For years the itinerary was offered on the 550-passenger *Universe.* In late 1995 World Explorer entered into an agreement with Commodore Cruise Line to charter the *Enchanted Seas* (renaming her *Universe Explorer*), which is a faster vessel with larger cabins and more public areas than the *Universe* and can accommodate an additional 200 passengers.

The ship's public areas include a main dining room, casual grill, five lounges, a cardroom, 16,000-volume library, youth center, 150-seat theater, boutique, beauty salon, fitness center, and computer lab.

Entertainment ranges from classical pianists and folk groups to string quartets and vocalists. Shore excursions include white-water rafting and flights to glaciers. Rates for seven-day cruises range from $1,354 to $2,295 and for 14-day cruises from $2,095 to $3,695 per person. Passengers can also opt for biking tours while in port.

Strong Points:

In-depth itineraries with a diverse range of shore excursions offering a more educational experience than most cruise lines and at reasonable prices.

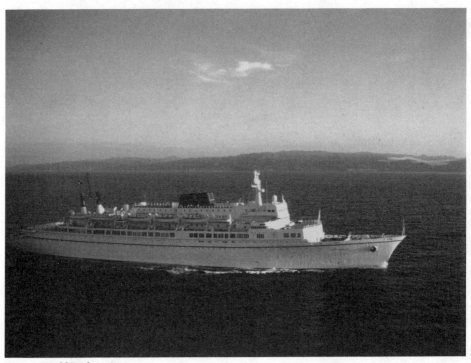

Courtesy World Explorer Cruises

APPETIZERS

Shrimp Cocktail   Prosciutto and Melon

Iced Orange Juice   Chilled Crudities

SOUPS

Beef Consomme   Manhattan Style Fish Soup

SALADS

Spinach with sunflower seeds and
poppyseed dressing

Classic Caesar

Garden Greens with choice of
Thousand Island, Italian, French, Roquefort or Ranch Style Dressing

BEVERAGES

Coffee Black Tea   Herbal Tea   Decaffeinated Coffee

Skim Milk   Low Fat Milk   Milk

Wine List, Sparkling Water, Imported and Domestic Beers and Sodas
are available from the Wine Steward

ENTREES
Served with vegetable du jour

Roast Leg of Lamb served with rosemary sauce and potato du jour

Egg Foo Young with shrimp and fried noodles

↵ Grilled Veal Chop with Dijon mustard sauce on the side
served with roasted potatoes

Ribeye Pepper Steak finished with a brandy sauce

VEGETARIAN ENTREE

Quiche with Fresh Vegetables

DESSERTS

Chocolate Sundae   Fresh Fruit in Season

Strawberry Shortcake with Whipped Cream   International Cheese Board

Black Forest Cake

Executive Chef, Douglas Myhre

↵ Denotes menu items prepared with low fat and low salt content

Courtesy World Explorer Cruises

Sunrise 5:05am

Sunset 9:44pm

THE
DAY AT SEA
DAILY
EXPLORER

6:00-6:30am	Early Riser's Coffee and Tea available-Promenade Deck, Starboard
6:30-9:15am	Continental Breakfast is offered-Promenade Deck, Starboard Side
7:00-9:00am	Breakfast is served (Open Seating)-Marine Dining Room, Main Deck
7:30-8:00am	"WALK-A-MILE" - 12 times around the Promenade Deck. Meet our Fitness Instructor, Karen in the Mandarin Lounge, Promenade Deck.
8:00am	STRETCHERSIZE with Karen, our Fitness Instructor. Join her in the Fitness Room, Sun Deck, Aft.
8:00am	QUIZ TIME! Stop by the Mandarin Lounge for a copy of today's quiz. Spend an hour with it, and you'll find out where the term "Brain-Strain" originated!
8:30am	AEROBICS with Karen in the Fitness Center, Sun Deck, Aft.
8:30-9:20am	HISTORY LECTURE with Dr.Gary Ferngren :EARLY AMERICAN ALASKA & THE GOLD RUSH - Commodore Lounge, Promenade Deck
9:00-10:30am	TOURS OF THE SHIP'S BRIDGE - Please meet in the Mandarin Lounge, Promenade Deck. Passengers will be given tickets on a first come - first serve basis. Groups of twenty guests will depart every twenty minutes with the last tour departing at 10:30am. Additional tours will be given next week.
9:30am	SHORE EXCURSION SALES PRESENTATION for the ports of SEWARD, SITKA, KETCHIKAN & VICTORIA - Tour requests will be accepted immediately following this briefing. Commodore Lounge, Prom Deck
10:00am	BRIDGE LECTURE by Earl Vibbard in the John Muir Room, Boat Deck
10:00-11:40pm	MORNING MOVIE: LITTLE MAN TATE - Starring Jodie Foster. Presented in the Theater on Coral Deck (99 minutes)
11:00am	Friends of Bill W. will meet in the North Star Room, Boat Deck
11:00-11:50pm	SNOWBALL JACKPOT BINGO!!! Come up for fun! The jackpot begins to build! Commodore Lounge, Promenade Deck
11:15-11:45am	EDUCATIONAL VIDEO: PIPELINE AND PERMAFROST - Presented in the Alyeska and Denali Lounges, Promenade Deck
12:00pm	Luncheon is served (1st Seating) - Marine Dining Room, Main Deck
12:10-1:00pm	BIOLOGY LECTURE with Dr. James Gessaman : SEA EAGLES OF ALASKA - Commodore Lounge, Prom Deck - (Repeat at 1:30pm)
1:30pm	Luncheon is served (2nd Seating) - Marine Dining Room, Main Deck
1:30-2:20pm	BIOLOGY LECTURE with Dr. James Gessaman: Repeat of the 12:10 lecture - Commodore Lounge, Promenade Deck
2:00-3:00pm	ARTIST'S WORKSHOP: Join our Artist-in-Residence, John Waldin Space is limited (1st Seating Passengers) Promenade Deck, Aft
2:30pm	Come and see the library's collection of pressed Alaskan flowers and plants Library, Sun Deck, Aft
2:30pm	BRIDGE PLAYERS: Meet with Earl Vibbard for a Bridge get-together in the Mandarin Lounge, Prom Deck.
3:00pm	SPECIAL AFTERNOON CONCERT with our Harpist, Mary-jean Lucchetti Commodore Lounge, Promenade Deck
3:00-4:00pm	ARTIST'S WORKSHOP with Guest Artist - John Waldin - repeat of 2:00pm workshop (2nd Seating Passengers) Promenade Deck, Aft
3:30-5:10pm	AFTERNOON MOVIE: LITTLE MAN TATE - Starring Jodie Foster. Presented in the Theater, Coral Deck

Courtesy World Explorer Cruises

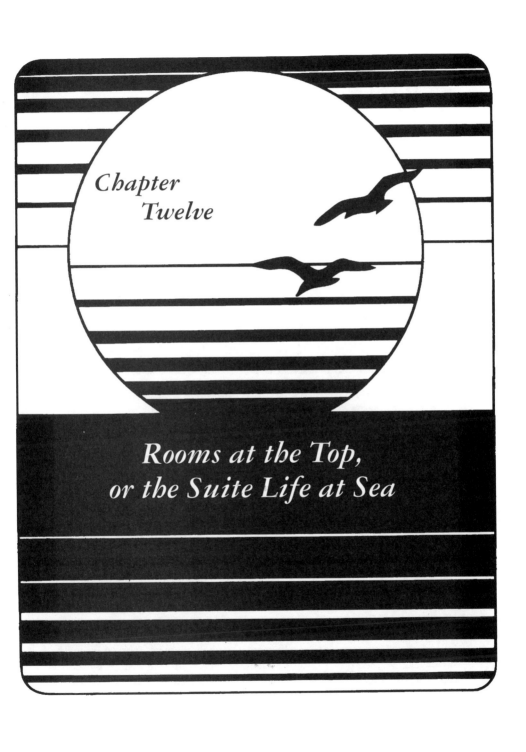

Chapter Twelve

Rooms at the Top, or the Suite Life at Sea

Most fine hotels around the world provide at least one presidential or ultragrand suite or villa where visiting dignitaries, wealthy clientele, or special VIPs can be accommodated with facilities that can house a small entourage, entertain guests, and provide extra services and amenities. In my research for *Stern's Guide to the Greatest Resorts of the World*, I have encountered many awesome accommodations, some measuring up to 5,000 square feet and with price tags as high as $6,000 per night.

Therefore, it is not surprising that "fine hotels at sea" would offer similar luxury accommodations. Historically, the existence of ultragrand suites on ships has undergone a metamorphosis. During the era of the legendary superliners such as the *Titanic, Normandie,* and *Queen Mary,* offering extremely large, ultradeluxe accommodations was de rigueur. However, during the period from 1970 to 1985, when cruising gained popularity with the mass market of vacationers, expensive suites were not a priority, and cruise lines considered a 400- to 600-square-foot stateroom more than sufficient for important clientele.

The final decade of the twentieth century was a period of unprecedented growth for the cruise industry, during which small companies were gobbled up by the major leaguers, who raised funds to acquire and/or build new ships by selling shares of stock to the public. Millions of dollars were spent annually on advertising and publicity in an attempt to stay afloat with the competition and to create the image of having the most prestigious vessels. Savvy cruise operators—seeking top ratings among ship reviewers as well as wishing to appeal to high-profile personalities and a wealthy clientele who could afford and demand the very best—wisely included at least one or two special ultradeluxe suites in the 800- to 1400-square-foot range on their new vessels, at fares ranging from $750 to $1,200 per person per night (for those who pay the published rate).

It is not uncommon for these grand suites at sea to include a master bath with a separate glassed-in shower stall; a large Jacuzzi tub; double vanities; toilet and bidet compartments; a second guest bathroom; an entryway; a large, elegantly furnished living room with a dining area; several giant televisions with VCR and CD attachments; a full-facility, fully stocked pantry where a chef can prepare meals; and one or more large verandas for alfresco entertaining or relaxing. Of course, rooms at the top vary from ship to ship, and some are neither "at the top" (of the ship) nor much more inviting than the deluxe category of suites otherwise available on the ship.

In order to provide my readers with information on options for the "suite life," the following charts and photos may prove helpful.

Top Luxury Suite on Ship				
Name of Cruise Line	Carnival Cruises	Carnival Cruises	Celebrity	Crystal
Name of Ship(s)	Carnival Destiny	Fantasy Class Ships	Century, Galaxy, & Mercury	I. Symphony II. Harmony
Name or Number of Suite	N/A	N/A	Penthouse Suites	Crystal Suite
Square Footage of Suite Without Veranda	345	350	1,101	I. 982 II. 948
Square Footage of Veranda	85	71	118	Not available
Average Published Price per Person per Night	$323	$219-$273	$890	I. $1,791 II. $1,506
Special Facilities (Per Code)	D, F, H	F, H	B, C, D, E, F, G, H, I, J, K	D, F, G, H, I, J, K
Special Amenities (Per Code)			A	A, B, & C Pressing only

CODE TO SPECIAL FACILITIES

A. Second connecting bedroom at no additional charge.
B. Second connecting bedroom option at additional charge.
C. Guest bathroom.
D. Large walk-in closet.
E. Kitchen or pantry where meals can be prepared.
F. Large-screen television.
G. CD player.
H. Jacuzzi in bathroom.
I. Jacuzzi on patio.
J. Dining room or separate dining area.
K. Separate shower stall and separate bathtub.

CODE TO SPECIAL AMENITIES

A. Private butler service.
B. Complimentary soft drinks, liquors, and wines.
C. Free laundry, dry cleaning, and pressing.
D. Complimentary shore excursions.
E. Automatic invitation to Captain's table.

Top Luxury Suite on Ship				
Name of Cruise Line	Cunard	Cunard	Cunard/ Seabourn Cruise Line	Cunard/ Seabourn Cruise Line
Name of Ship(s)	Caronia	QE2	Pride, Spirit, & Legend	Sun
Name or Number of Suite	Penthouse 1 & 2	Queen Elizabeth & Queen Mary	N/A	Owner's Suite
Square Footage of Suite without Veranda	642	831	527	724
Square Footage of Veranda	80' lower level 271 upper level	189	48	160
Average Published Price per Person per Night	Not Available	Not Available	$1,500	Not Available
Special Facilities (Per Code)	B, C, D, E, F, G, H, I, J, K	B, D, E, F	C, D, J	C, D, F, G, H, J, K
Special Amenities (Per Code)	B	A, B	B	B (initial setup only)

CODE TO SPECIAL FACILITIES

A. Second connecting bedroom at no additional charge.
B. Second connecting bedroom option at additional charge.
C. Guest bathroom.
D. Large walk-in closet.
E. Kitchen or pantry where meals can be prepared.
F. Large-screen television.
G. CD player.
H. Jacuzzi in bathroom.
I. Jacuzzi on patio.
J. Dining room or separate dining area.
K. Separate shower stall and separate bathtub.

CODE TO SPECIAL AMENITIES

A. Private butler service.
B. Complimentary soft drinks, liquors, and wines.
C. Free laundry, dry cleaning, and pressing.
D. Complimentary shore excursions.
E. Automatic invitation to Captain's table.

Top Luxury Suite on Ship				
Name of Cruise Line	Disney	Holland America Line	Orient Cruise Line	Premier
Name of Ship(s)	Magic, Wonder	Rotterdam VI	Marco Polo	Oceanic (Big Red Boat)
Name or Number of Suite	Walt Disney & Roy Disney Suites	Penthouse Suite	Dynasty Suite & Explorer Suite	(8) Penthouse
Square Footage of Suite without Verandah	1,023	946	484	Not Available
Square Footage of Verandah	184	180	Not Available	Not Available
Average Published Price per Person per Night	$929	Not Available	$380	$336
Special Facilities (Per Code)	A, C, D, E, F, G, H, J, K	C, D, E, F, G, H, J, K	D	C
Special Amenities (Per Code)	A (Piano)	A, C, E	B	D

CODE TO SPECIAL FACILITIES

A. Second connecting bedroom at no additional charge.
B. Second connecting bedroom option at additional charge.
C. Guest bathroom.
D. Large walk-in closet.
E. Kitchen or pantry where meals can be prepared.
F. Large-screen television.
G. CD player.
H. Jacuzzi in bathroom.
I. Jacuzzi on patio.
J. Dining room or separate dining area.
K. Separate shower stall and separate bath-tub.

CODE TO SPECIAL AMENITIES

A. Private butler service.
B. Complimentary soft drinks, liquors, and wines.
C. Free laundry, dry cleaning, and pressing.
D. Complimentary shore excursions.
E. Automatic invitation to Captain's table.

Top Luxury Suite on Ship				
Name of Cruise Line	Princess	Princess	Radisson Seven Seas Cruises	Renaissance
Name of Ship(s)	Grand Princess	Sun, Dawn, Crown, & Regal	Paul Gauguin	R-1, R-2, R-3, R-4
Name or Number of Suite	N/A	N/A	Grand Suite 801 & 802	Owner's Suites
Square Footage of Suite without Veranda	685	538-695 (includes veranda)	332	598
Square Footage of Veranda	115	See above	197	364
Average Published Price per Person per Night	$898	$450-$550	$765	$600
Special Facilities (Per Code)	D, F, H, I, J, K	D, K	N/A	C, D, F, G, H, J
Special Amenities (Per Code)	A, B (initial stock)	A	None	None

CODE TO SPECIAL FACILITIES

A. Second connecting bedroom at no additional charge.
B. Second connecting bedroom option at additional charge.
C. Guest bathroom.
D. Large walk-in closet.
E. Kitchen or pantry where meals can be prepared.
F. Large-screen television.
G. CD player.
H. Jacuzzi in bathroom.
I. Jacuzzi on patio.
J. Dining room or separate dining area.
K. Separate shower stall and separate bathtub.

CODE TO SPECIAL AMENITIES

A. Private butler service.
B. Complimentary soft drinks, liquors, and wines.
C. Free laundry, dry cleaning, and pressing.
D. Complimentary shore excursions.
E. Automatic invitation to Captain's table.

Top Luxury Suite on Ship		
Name of Cruise Line	Royal Caribbean	Silversea Cruises
Name of Ship(s)	I. Sovereign, Monarch, & Majesty II. Legend & Splendour III. Grandeur & Enchantment IV. Rhapsody & Vision	Silver Cloud Silver Wind
Name or Number of Suite	Royal Suite	Owner's Suite
Square Footage of Suite without Veranda	I. 670 II. 1,020 III. 1,119 IV. 1,326	492-1 Bedroom 7 32-2 Bedroom
Square Footage of Veranda	I. 132 II. 155 III. 148 IV. 132	95
Average Published Price per Person per Night	I. $628 II. $764-$916 III. $642 IV. $640-$964	$1,500
Special Facilities (Per Code)	B, C, D, F, G, H, J, K	B, C, D, F, G, H, J
Special Amenities (Per Code)	A (Piano)	B

CODE TO SPECIAL FACILITIES

A. Second connecting bedroom at no additional charge.
B. Second connecting bedroom option at additional charge.
C. Guest bathroom.
D. Large walk-in closet.
E. Kitchen or pantry where meals can be prepared.
F. Large-screen television.
G. CD player.
H. Jacuzzi in bathroom.
I. Jacuzzi on patio.
J. Dining room or separate dining area.
K. Separate shower stall and separate bathtub.

CODE TO SPECIAL AMENITIES

A. Private butler service.
B. Complimentary soft drinks, liquors, and wines.
C. Free laundry, dry cleaning, and pressing.
D. Complimentary shore excursions.
E. Automatic invitation to Captain's table.

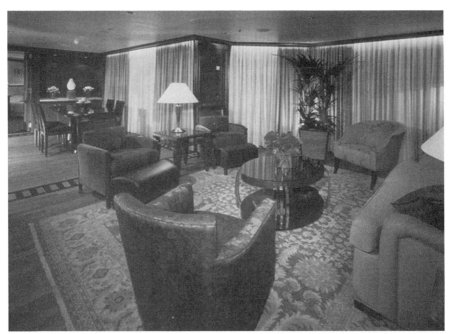

Mercury, *courtesy Celebrity Cruises*

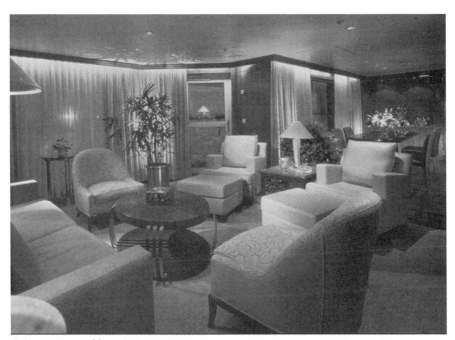

Galaxy, *courtesy Celebrity Cruises*

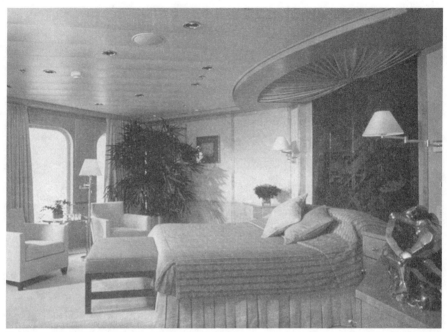

Century, *courtesy Celebrity Cruises*

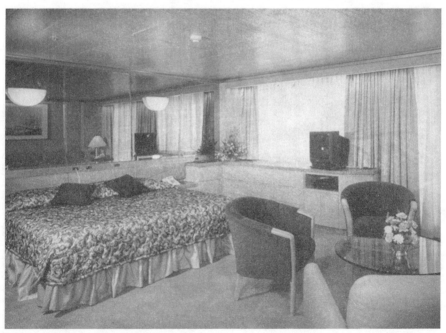

Rotterdam VI, *courtesy Holland America Line*

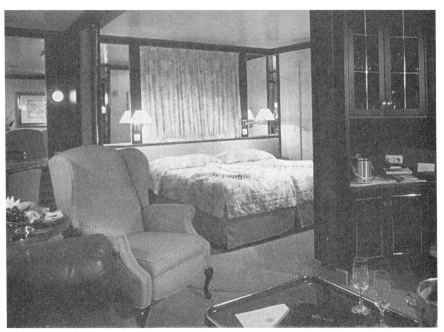

Seabourn Sun, *courtesy Cunard Cruise Line*

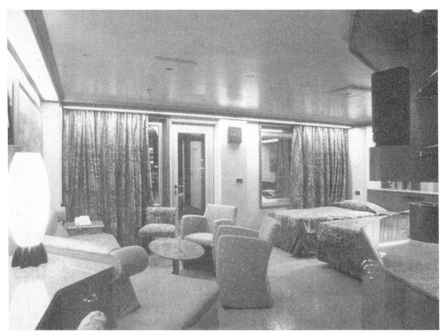

Carnival Destiny, *courtesy Carnival Cruises*

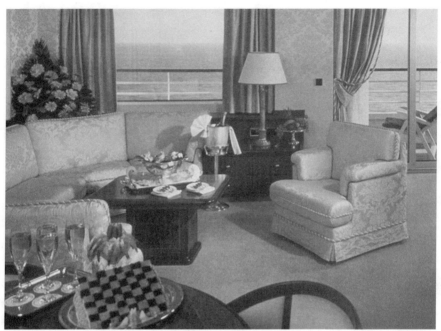

Crystal Symphony, *courtesy Crystal Cruise Line*

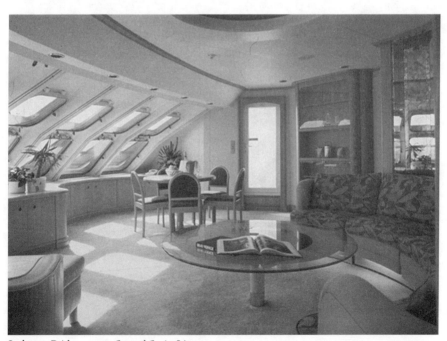

Seabourn Pride, *courtesy Cunard Cruise Line*

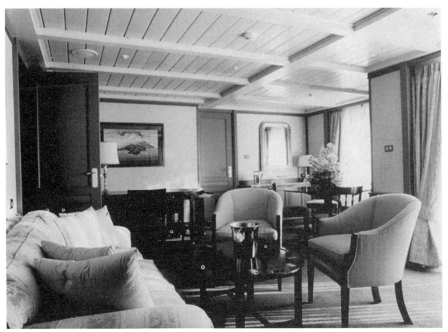

Zenith, *courtesy Celebrity Cruises*

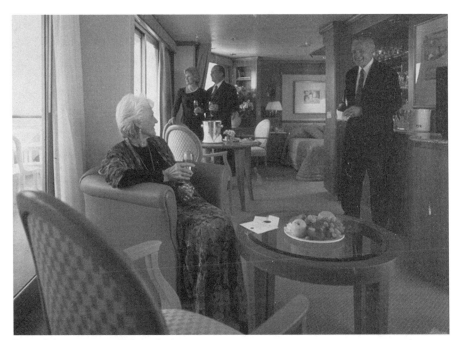

Dawn Princess, *courtesy Princess Cruises*

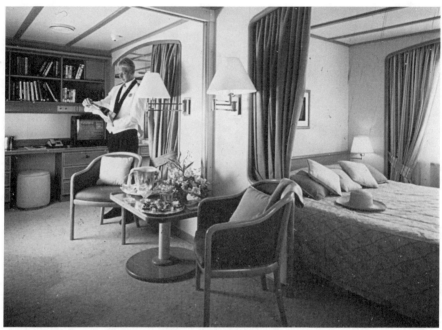

Seabourn Goddess I, *couresty Cunard Cruise Line*

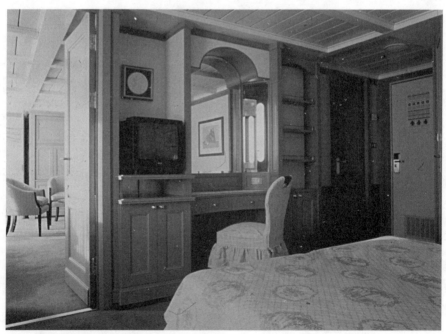

Silver Wind, *courtesy Silversea Cruises*

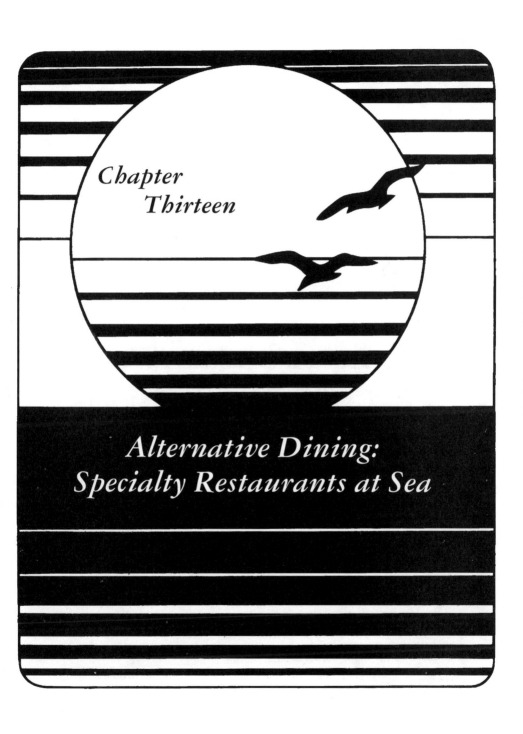

Chapter
Thirteen

Alternative Dining:
Specialty Restaurants at Sea

Passengers on cruise ships generally do not have the option of leaving the ship for dinner as they do when vacationing ashore at a hotel or resort. Therefore, the challenge for cruise operators has been keeping the dining experience sufficiently interesting and diverse to prevent guests from becoming bored or dissatisfied.

The various lines attempt to vary the menus each day of the cruise and to provide theme nights in an effort to make each dinner seem special. However, discerning cruisers soon realize that the environs, the style of preparation, and one's table companions (except on open-seating vessels) are the same and often feel that a change would be welcome.

The existence of an alternate dining venue with a new decor, separate kitchen, different style of cuisine, and an option for a dining companion or companions of your choice becomes a welcome plus, enhancing the cruise experience.

Although Costa, Sitmar, and (later) Princess cruises introduced separate pizza parlors back in the late seventies, Crystal was the first of today's major cruise lines to provide elegant specialty dinner restaurants at no extra charge to their passengers. The concept did not go unnoticed by the other cruise lines, and today many vessels offer alternative dining experiences.

A further development was the recognition of some passengers' preference not to dress for or partake in a multicourse dinner and/or the desire to dine away from their assigned tables. In an attempt to satisfy such preferences, several of the major cruise lines kept their more casual breakfast and lunchtime buffet restaurants open for dinner.

Since more and more cruise lines are experimenting with alternative specialty restaurants, as well as keeping their buffet restaurants open for dinner, those readers who find these features important would be well advised to check with the cruise line at the time of booking.

The following charts, photos, and menus are offered to afford my readers a rough idea of the alternative dining possibilities as they exist at the time of publication on cruise ships that feature these options:

Alternative Dining Restaurants				
Name of Cruise Line	Carnival Cruises	Carnival Cruises	Celebrity Cruises	Crystal Cruises
Name of Ship(s)	Destiny	Fantasy Class Ships	Horizon Zenith	(H) Harmony (S) Symphony
Name of Restaurant	Sun & Sea	Bar & Grill Restaurants	Lido Restaurant	(H) Prego/Kyoto (S) Prego/Jade Garden
A. General Style of Restaurant	C	C	C	E
B. Dress Code	C	C	C	S
C. Type of Cuisine	B, P, I, A	B, P, I	Eclectic P, I, B	Prego I Jade Garden A Kyoto Japanese
D. Additional Charge (if any)	N	N	N	N
E. Seating Capacity	1,252	722	Varies	(H) 55/60 (S) 75/85
F. Availability Throughout Cruise to Passengers	N	N	N	R

Code:

A. Casual - C
   Elegant - E

B. Casual - C
   Same as in dining room - S

C. Buffet - Eclectic - B
   Pizza - P
   Italian - I

Asian - A
Gourmet - Continental - GC
French - F

D. Surcharge - S
   No Charge - N

F. Nightly - N
   Once Per Cruise - O
   Reservation Basis - R

Alternative Dining Restaurants			
Name of Cruise Line	Cunard	Cunard	Cunard/ Seabourn Cruise Line	Cunard/ Seabourn Cruise Line
Name of Ship(s)	Caronia	QE2	Legend Pride Spirit	Sun
Name of Restaurant	Tivoli	Lido	Veranda Café	Venezia
A. General Style of Restaurant	E	C	C	E
B. Dress Code	S	C	C	S
C. Type of Cuisine	I	B, I, A, F	B, I, P, GC	I
D. Additional Charge (if any)	N	N	N	N
E. Seating Capacity	40	200	96	60
F. Availability Throughout Cruise to Passengers	O	N	N	O

Code:

A. Casual - C
   Elegant - E

B. Casual - C
   Same as in dining room - S

C. Buffet - Eclectic - B
   Pizza - P
   Italian - I

Asian - A
Gourmet - Continental - GC
French - F

D. Surcharge - S
   No Charge - N

F. Nightly - N
   Once Per Cruise - O
   Reservation Basis - R

Alternative Dining Restaurants				
Name of Cruise Line	Disney	Holland America Line	Orient Lines	Princess Cruises
Name of Ship(s)	Magic Wonder	Rotterdam	Marco Polo	Grand Princess
Name of Restaurant	Palo	Odyssey	Raffles	(TS) Trattoria Sabatini (PD) The Painted Desert
A. General Style of Restaurant	C	E	C	C
B. Dress Code	C	S	C	C
C. Type of Cuisine	I	I & GC	B (with theme)	(TS) I (PD) SW U.S.
D. Additional Charge (if any)	$5 Gratuity	N	N	N
E. Seating Capacity	148	88	194	(TS) 90 (PD) 92
F. Availability Throughout Cruise to Passengers	N	R	R	R

Code:

A. Casual - C
   Elegant - E

B. Casual - C
   Same as in dining room - S

C. Buffet - Eclectic - B
   Pizza - P
   Italian - I

Asian - A
Gourmet - Continental - GC
French - F

D. Surcharge - S
   No Charge - N

F. Nightly - N
   Once Per Cruise - O
   Reservation Basis - R

Alternative Dining Restaurants

Name of Cruise Line	Princess Cruises	Radisson Seven Seas Cruises	Radisson Seven Seas Cruises	Renaissance
Name of Ship(s)	Crown Princess Regal Princess Royal Princess Sun Princess Dawn Princess Grand Princess	Paul Gauguin	Radisson Diamond	R-1, R-2, R-3, R-4
Name of Restaurant	24-hour café	La Veranda	Don Vito's (The Grill)	1) The Grill 2) The Italian Restaurant
A. General Style of Restaurant	C	C	C	E
B. Dress Code	C	C	C	S
C. Type of Cuisine	B	I, F, & GC	I	1) English/ American Grill - Steakhouse 2) I
D. Additional Charge (if any)	N	N	N	N
E. Seating Capacity	Grand Princess 600 Others 200-300	80	Varies	1) 98 2) 96
F. Availability Throughout Cruise to Passengers	N	R	N	R

Code:

A. Casual - C
  Elegant - E

B. Casual - C
  Same as in dining room - S

C. Buffet - Eclectic - B
  Pizza - P
  Italian - I

Asian - A
Gourmet - Continental - GC
French - F

D. Surcharge - S
  No Charge - N

F. Nightly - N
  Once Per Cruise - O
  Reservation Basis - R

Alternative Dining Restaurants				
Name of Cruise Line	Royal Caribbean	Silversea	Star Cruises	Windstar Cruises
Name of Ship(s)	All Ships	Silver Cloud Silver Wind	Star Aquarius Star Pisces	Wind Surf
Name of Restaurant	Windjammer Cafe	Terrace Cafe	1) Umigawa 2) Marco Polo	The Bistro
A. General Style of Restaurant	C	C	C	C
B. Dress Code	C	S	C	C
C. Type of Cuisine	B	I	1) A 2) GC	I/GC
D. Additional Charge (if any)	N	N	1) $80 2) $60	N
E. Seating Capacity	Varies	148 indoors 30 outdoors	N	90
F. Availability Throughout Cruise to Passengers	N	R	N	O

Code:

A. Casual - C
   Elegant - E

B. Casual - C
   Same as in dining room - S

C. Buffet - Eclectic - B
   Pizza - P
   Italian - I

Asian - A
Gourmet - Continental - GC
French - F

D. Surcharge - S
   No Charge - N

F. Nightly - N
   Once Per Cruise - O
   Reservation Basis - R

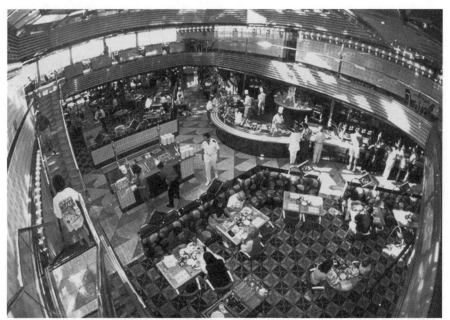

Sun & Sea Restaurant, courtesy Carnival Cruises

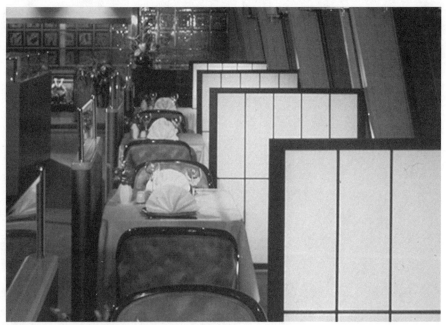

Kyoto, courtesy Crystal Cruises

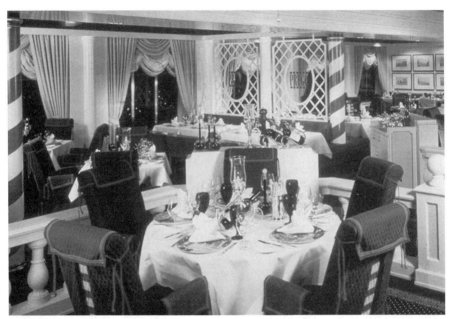

Prego, courtesy Crystal Cruises

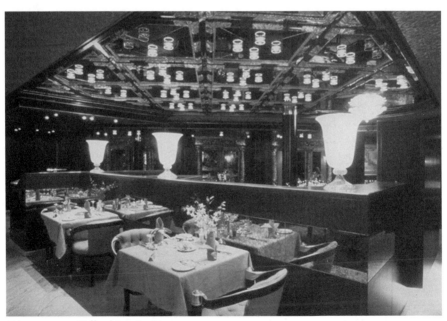

Odyssey, courtesy Holland America Line

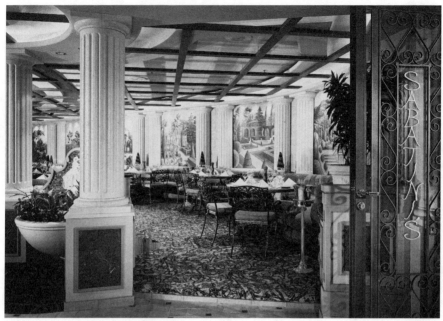

Trattoria Sabatini, courtesy Princess Cruises

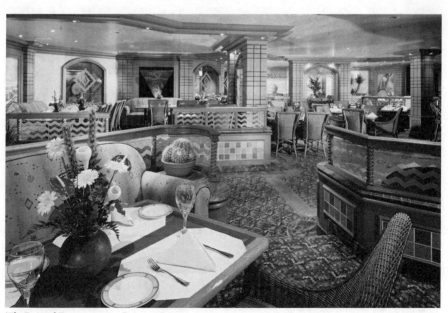

The Painted Desert, courtesy Princess Cruises

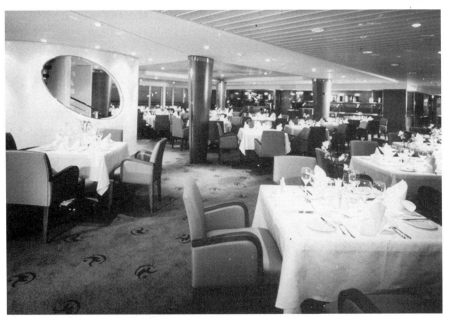

La Veranda, courtesy Radisson Seven Seas Cruises

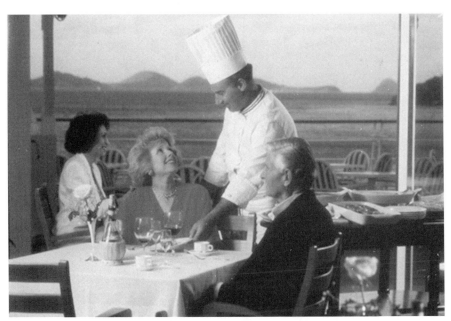

Don Vito's (The Grill), courtesy Radisson Seven Seas Cruises

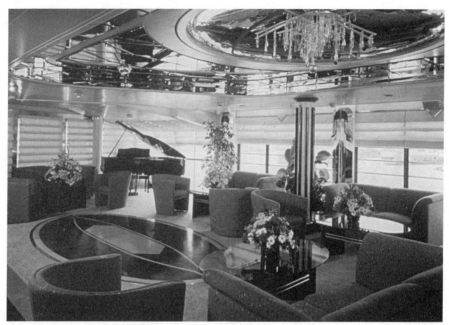

Venezia Restaurant, Seabourn Sun, *courtesy Cunard Line*

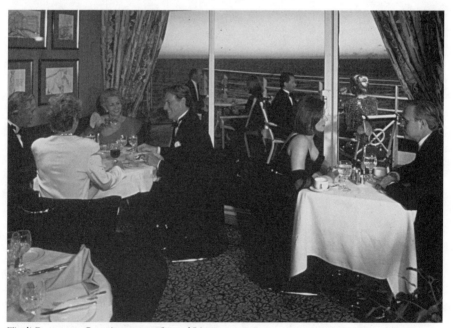

Tivoli Restaurant, Caronia, *courtesy Cunard Line*

LA VERANDA

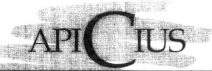

APICIUS

ABOARD M/S PAUL GAUGUIN

~ AT SEA ~ MARCH 29TH, 1998

Chef Jean-Pierre Vigato was born in Paris to an Italian family whose life was built, as is often the case, around food and restaurants. His Father, Mother and Grandmother were all cooks. He had no particular interest in studies and from the age of 14 on, his choice was clear. "I want to be a Chef," he told his parents, who had the intelligence not to disagree with his chosen vocation.

ORIGINS OF APICIUS
The moment came for Jean-Pierre to open his first restaurant. It was called "Grandgousier" and opened in the Pigalle district. In 1982, he earned his first star from Michelin. In 1984, he opened "APICIUS" and quickly was met with an avalanche of favorable reviews that made him well known in France and abroad. In 1984, came the two stars Michelin and soon "APICIUS" was inducted into the prestigious "Relais et Chateaux" group.

BOULANGERIE

BAGUETTE ET PETITS PAINS FRAIS
Fresh baguette and rolls

ENTRÉE FROIDE

CHARLOTTE DE POMMES DE TERRE AU CAVIAR,
SAUCE CRESSONNETTE AU CITRON
Sevruga Caviar resting on a charlotte of potatoes, cressonnette sauce

ENTRÉE CHAUDE

GROS RAVIOLE DE HOMARD EN "DIM SUM",
JUS DE CRUSTACÉS AU BASILIC
Lobster Ravioli in "Dim Sum"
with shellfish gravy and basil

POISSON & VIANDE

BAR AU GRILL ET JUS AUX ÉPICES
Grilled fillet of Seabass with aromatic herbs

FILET DE BOEUF SAUTÉ MINUTE,
BEURRE CRU AUX HERBES FRAÎCHES
ET PARMENTIER DE POMMES DE TERRE
Grilled fillet of Beef with fresh herb butter
and potatoes purée parmentier

DESSERT

CRÈME BRÛLÉE À LA VANILLE TAHITIENNE
Crème Brûlée with Tahitian Vanilla
PETITS FOURS

White : Muscadet 1996
Domaine de la Jousseliniere
"Muscadet", Valle de la Loire, France

Red: Château Ducla 1995
"Cabernet Franc, Merlot & Malbec"
Bordeaux, France

MENU CREATED BY JEAN-PIERRE VIGATO

RADISSON SEVEN SEAS
CRUISES

Courtesy Radisson Seven Seas Cruises

PREGO

Welcome to Prego where we offer our Guests an alternative choice of dining. Our Prego chef prepares your Italian meals individually upon request. This "a la minute" style cooking may require a slightly longer preparation, but allow us to provide our Guests with the freshest and finest Italian cuisine.
Buon Appetito!

PIEDMONTE

In this lushly wooded countryside at the foot of the Alps are the great delicacies of the region's cuisine: pheasant and hare, tiny sweet strawberries and delicately flavored snowy white truffles. The result is elegant, flavorful and beautifully presented. The vine-covered hillsides produce robust full-bodied Barolo, gentler Barbaresco, and Barbera.

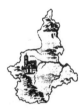

TRE VENEZIE

Risotto, hearty soups and cool seafood salads accented by fresh lemon may be found on tables in this fertile region crisscrossed by rivers. Wine glasses hold pale white wines with overtones of ripe pear. The region also cultivates red wines of French transplants such as rich Cabernet, velvety Merlot and the lighter Malbec.

EMILIA-ROMAGNA

Parma. Simply uttering the name of the culinary capital of this region brings to mind the region's nickname, la grassa—the "fat one". Highlights of the sumptuous cuisine feature tangy Parmesan cheese, creamy fresh mozzarella, fragrant basalmic vinegar and prosciutto di Parma, the satiny, rose-pink ham celebrated worldwide.

ANTIPASTI

ANTIPASTO MISTO
Italian Appetizer Plate with Marinated Seafood, Prosciutto Ham, Marinated Vegetables, Mozzarella-Tomato, Olives, Anchovies, and Grilled Scampi

CARPACCIO DI MANZO
Thinly Sliced Raw Beef Tenderloin with Mustard Sauce and Capers
FROM PIEMONTE

PROSCIUTTO E MELONE
Sweet Melon Slices with Italian Prosciutto
FROM PERUGIA

TORRE DI VEGETALI ALLA GRIGLIA CON FETTE DI ARAGOSTA, GAMBERONI E CAPOSANTE SALTATI
Tower of Grilled, Marinated Vegetables with Slices of Lobster, Sautéed Prawns and Scallops in Truffle Vinaigrette
FROM SICILY

ASSAGGI DI PASTA A VOSTRA SCELTA
All Pasta Dishes are Available as Appetizers

INSALATA

INSALATA MISTA
Chopped Seasonal Salad with Olive Oil and Balsamic Vinaigrette

INSALATA "CESARE"
Caesar Salad Prepared by Your Head Waiter

INSALATA CAPRESE
Sliced Roma Tomatoes and Mozzarella Cheese, Topped with Mesclun of Greens, Tossed in Basil Vinaigrette

ZUPPE

CREMA DI FUNGHI SERVITA NEL PANE ALL'ORIGANO
Cream of Selected Italian Mushrooms: Porcini, Morel, and Champignons, Served in an Oregano Bread Cup
FROM CALABRIA

ZUPPA DI LENTICCHIE CON PETTO D'ANATRA
Country Style Lentil Soup with Duck
FROM VENETO

ZUPPA DI POMODORO CON TORTELLINI RIPIENI DI PATATE
Light Cream of Tomato, Served with Potato Tortellini
FROM LIGURIA AND LOMBARDIA

PIATTO VEGETARIANO

RISOTTO PRIMAVERA
Traditional Italian Vegetable Risotto

PIATTI PRINCIPALE

LASAGNE ALLA CASALINGA
Layers of Pasta with Ground Beef, Porcini Mushrooms, Tomato,
Béchamel, and Mozzarella Cheese
FROM EMILIA ROMAGNA

RAVIOLI AL CARCIOFI' FATTI IN CASA CON BURRO ALLE ERBE E PESTO DI RUCOLA
Homemade Artichoke Ravioli, Tossed in a Light Herb Butter Sauce,
Sprinkled with Arrugula Pesto
FROM LAZIO

SPAGHETTINI AI FRUTTI DI MARE AL VERDE DI PREZZEMOLO
Freshly Cooked Spaghetti with Assorted Seafood,
Garlic, Red Chili, Parsley, and White Wine
FROM PUGLIA

PASTA INTEGRALE CON VERDURA E ERBE ALL' OLIO D'OLIVA
Whole Wheat Linguine with Seasonal Vegetables,
Extra Virgin Olive Oil, and Herbs
FROM LAZIO-TOSCANA

SPAGHETTI O PENNE RIGATE A PIACERE
Spaghetti or Penne Rigate with Your choice of Bolognese, Puttanesca,
Arrabiata, or Tomato-Basil Sauce

GAMBERONI MARINATI ALLA GRIGLIA CON CAPPELLINI SALTATI CON VERDURA MISTA E SALSA AL POMODORO E LIMONE
Grilled Marinated Tiger Prawns, Served on Capellini, Tossed in
Eggplant, Zucchini, Artichoke, and Lemon Flavored Tomato Sauce
FROM CAMPAGNA

SALMONE "DOLCE E FORTE"
Broiled Fresh Salmon Fillet on a Carmalized Green Peppercorn Sauce,
Served with New Potatoes and Grilled Vegetables
FROM PUGLIA

SCALOPPINE DI VITELLO CON CAPELLI D'ANGELO
Sautéed Veal Scaloppine with a Light Lemon Sauce, or Mushroom
Sauce, Served with Angel Hair Pasta and Summer Vegetables
FROM LOMBARDIA

FILETTO DI MANZO AL "BAROLO"
Grilled Filet Mignon of Black Angus Beef, Served with
Barolo Red Wine Sauce, Grilled Polenta, and Seasonal Vegetables
FROM TOSCANA

COTOLETTE D'AGNELLO ARROSTO ALL'AGLIO E ERBE. SERVITE CON PURE DI PATATE ALL'AGLIO E ZUCCHINE ALLA GRIGLIA
Roasted Rack of Baby Lamb with a Herb Crust,
Served with Garlic Mashed Potatoes and Grilled Zucchini
FROM MOLISE-MARCHE-ABRUZZO

TOSCANA

Raise a glass of Chianti to this home of Italy's world-renowned wine. Its blend of four grapes from vineyards rolling over the hills from Florence to Siena dates back to the nineteenth century. Enjoy it with food that is rustically simple and full of flavor: veal and pasta accented by silky Tuscan olive oil and herbs, fresh vegetables and golden-crusted breads.

UMBRIA

The treasure of Umbria's mountain villages is the black truffle. Its big, dense flavor make it a luxurious addition to simply roasted meats and fish, or as the jewel crowning a dish of buttery fettucine. The perfect accompaniments to Umbria's hearty fare are the bold reds and dry whites.

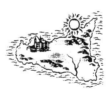

SICILIA

Ripe, red Sicilian tomatoes are enjoyed year round, either fresh and plump or dried in the bright sun that warms the island. This is Italy's produce basket—mellow artichokes, crisp endive, fragrant fennel, olives and figs are plentiful. The region is famous for intense white wines and especially for its dessert wines, Moscato and the famous Marsala.

WINE SUGGESTIONS

VINO BIANCO

Pinot Grigio, Santa Margherita 1997	$7.00 per glass
Orvieto Classico, Villa Antinori, Umbria 1996	$6.00 per glass

VINO ROSSO

Centine, Rosso di Montalcino, Castello Banfi, Toscano 1996	$5.50 per glass
Chianti Classico Riserva, Villa Antinori, Toscano 1994	$6.50 per glass
Brunello di Montalcino, Villa Banfi, Toscano 1992	$11.50 per glass

DESSERT
SPECIALITIES

MOUSSE DI LIMONE E
MASCARPONE CON MERENGA

Lemon Mascarpone Mousse with Meringue

ASSAGGINI DI DOLCI TIPICI

*Dessert Sampler – Flourless Chocolate Nut Cake, Italian
Tiramisu and Panna Cotta with Passion Fruit Sauce
and Berries*

TIRAMISU

*Espresso Flavored Lady Fingers, Layered with Light
Mascarpone Cheese, Lightly Dusted with Cacao*

GELATO ALL'ITALIANA DI VANIGLA,
CIOCCOLATO, FRAGOLE

*Vanilla, Chocolate, Spumoni, Strawberry Ice Cream,
or Sherbet of the Day*

*Espresso, Cappuccino, Coffee, Decaffeinated Coffee,
International Teas, or Café Latte*

AFTER-DINNER DRINKS

As a Digestif, we would like to recommend:

Grappa Marchese de Gresy – $4.50

Sambuca Romana – $3.95

Frangelico – $3.95

Amaretto di Saronno – $3.95

*or your favorite classic after-dinner liqueur,
available from our wine waiter*

TOSCANA

*Raise a glass of Chianti to this
home of Italy's world-renowned
wine. Its blend of four grapes
from vineyards rolling over the
hills from Florence to Siena dates
back to the nineteenth century.
Enjoy it with food that is rustically simple and full of flavor:
veal and pasta accented by silky
Tuscan olive oil and herbs, fresh
vegetables and golden-crusted
breads.*

UMBRIA

*The treasure of Umbria's moun-
tain villages is the black truffle.
Its big, dense flavor make it a
luxurious addition to simply
roasted meats and fish, or as the
jewel crowning a dish of buttery
fettucine. The perfect accompaniments to Umbria's hearty fare
are the bold reds and dry whites.*

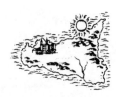

SICILIA

*Ripe, red Sicilian tomatoes are
enjoyed year round, either fresh
and plump or dried in the bright
sun that warms the island. This
is Italy's produce basket—mellow
artichokes, crisp endive, fragrant
fennel, olives and figs are plentiful. The region is famous for
intense white wines and especially
for its dessert wines. Moscato and
the famous Marsala.*

6/98

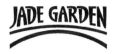

A P P E T I Z E R S

Tempura Shrimp with Dipping Sauce

Vegetable Spring Roll with Mariposa Plum Sauce

Peking Duck in Mandarin Pancakes

Traditional Japanese Sushi and California Roll

Grilled Chicken Satay with Indonesian Peanut Butter Sauce

S O U P S

Chicken Velvet Corn Soup

Tom Yam Goong
Spicy Thai Shrimp Soup Flavored with Lime Leaves and Lemongrass

Clear Broth with Spinach and Tofu

B E V E R A G E   S U G G E S T I O N S

WHITE WINE

Columbia Winery, Riesling, Washington State 1996	$4.50 per glass
Cuvaison Chardonnay, Napa Valley 1996	$7.50 per glass
Gewürztraminer, F.E. Trimbach, Alsace 1994	$6.00 per glass

RED WINE

Acacia Pinor Noir, Carneros 1996	$8.00 per glass
Château Souverain Cabernet Sauvignon, Alexander Valley 1994	$6.50 per glass

BEER

Tsingtao Beer, China	$3.00 per bottle
Asahi Beer, Japan	$3.00 per bottle
Kirin Beer, Japan	$3.00 per bottle

SAKE

Hot Sake, Sho Chiku Bai	$3.50 per carafe
Cold Sake, Hakutsuru	$3.50 per glass
Horin Gekkeikan	$75.00 per Bottle

May we suggest a $6.00 gratuity per guest for your waiter.

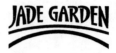

ENTREES

CANTONESE LOBSTER
TENDER LOBSTER MEAT STIR FRIED WITH ORIENTAL VEGETABLES,
ON BLACK BEAN-TRUFFLE SAUCE

KAFIR LIME BEEF
GRILLED, SLICED FILET MIGNON WITH KAFIR LIME-SOY-SHALLOT SAUCE

SESAME SHRIMP
FRESH GULF SHRIMP WITH JULIENNE OF VEGETABLES ON GOLDEN SESAME SAUCE

MANDARIN LEMON-TANGERINE CHICKEN
LIGHTLY FRIED BATTERED BREAST OF CHICKEN
ON FRESH LEMON-TANGERINE SAUCE

SINGAPORE NOODLES
WOK-TOSSED SOFT NOODLES WITH
SEASONAL FRESH VEGETABLES IN A LIGHT OYSTER SAUCE

CATCH OF THE DAY
ASIAN CRUSH HERB MARINATED FRESH FILLET OF FISH,
PAN GRILLED WITH MISO FLAVORED BOK CHOY,
SERVED ON BURMESE RED GINGER SAUCE

ALL DISHES ARE SERVED WITH YOUR CHOICE OF EITHER
STEAMED RICE OR VEGETABLE FRIED RICE

DESSERTS

SAMPLER
ORANGE CREME BRÛLÉE, GINGER CHOCOLATE CAKE, GREEN TEA ICE CREAM,
LYCHEE AND JACK FRUIT

GINGER CRÈME BRÛLÉE WITH CRISP FILO

TAPIOCA PUDDING
TAPIOCA PUDDING IN ORANGE SOUP WITH MANGOS AND BERRIES

GREEN TEA ICE CREAM • MANGO SHERBET

JASMIN TEA, GREEN TEA, GINSENG TEA, ROASTED JAPANESE TEA,
ESPRESSO, CAPPUCCINO, COFFEE, OR DECAFFEINATED COFFEE

4/98

TRATTORIA SABATINI

PIZZA

NORDIC
Topped with Wild Smoked Salmon, Fresh Tomato, Olive Oil and Garlic Sprinkled with Capers and Spring Onions

COSTA SMERALDA
A Seafood Feast of Bay Shrimps, Mussels, Crab Meat, Mozzarella Cheese with Tomato and Pesto Sauce

KING KAMEHAMEHA
*A Tropical Paradise Display of Cooked Ham and Hawaiian Pineapple, Mozzarella Cheese
and Fresh Tomato Slices*

SABATINI'S SPECIALITY
Topped with Cured Parma Ham, Buffalo Mozzarella Cheese, Fresh Tomato Sauce and Sweet Basil

VEGETABLE
*A Combination of Mozzarella and Cheddar Cheese with Tomato Sauce, Bell Pepper, Avocado,
Zucchini, Mushrooms and Chopped Spring Onions*

CALZONE
*Rolled Pizza Dough Filled with Tomato Sauce, Mozzarella and Ricotta Cheeses, Mushrooms,
Sautéed Red Bermuda Onions and BBQ Breast of Chicken*

CARPACCIO DI BRESAOLA
*Lean Thin Slices of Air-Cured Beef with Extra Virgin Olive Oil and Shaved Parmesan Cheese
on a Bed of Celery and Arugula Salad*

MOZZARELLA IN CARROZZA
*Cheese Mozzarella between Slices of White Bread, Batter Dipped
and Deep-Fried and Served with Spicy Fresh Tomato Marinara Sauce*

DELIZIE DEL MEDITERRANEO
A Delicious Warm Seafood Composition Combined with the Famous Florentine White Beans al Fiasco

---

SOUP AND SALAD
Fresh Homemade Soup and Salad of the Day Recommended by Our Chef

PENNE ALL'ARRABBIATA
Pasta Quills Simmered in a Fresh Spicy Garlic-Tomato Sauce

RAVIOLI DI SALMONE IN SALSA VELLUTATA
Homemade Filled Pasta with Salmon Mousse Served in a Fresh Tomato Velvet Cream Sauce

FUSILLI ALLE VERDURE ESTIVE
Corkscrew-Shaped Pasta Simmered with Fresh Seasonal Vegetables and Topped with Parmesan Cheese

PETTO DI POLLO ALLA VALDOSTANA
*Breaded Breast of Chicken Gently Sautéed, Topped with Ham, Mushrooms and Fontina Cheese.
Served with Our Chef's Selection of Premium Fresh Vegetables and Fried Potatoes*

MILK-FED VEAL CHOP WITH A NATURAL SAUCE
*Enhanced by a Marsala Wine. Served with Wild Mushroom Ragout,
Château Potatoes and Wedge of Artichoke*

BRANZINO DEL ADRIATICO AL SALMORIGLIO
*Adriatic Sea Bass Fillet Sautéed with Marinated Fresh Vegetables in Olive Oil.
Served with Parsley Potatoes and Summer Vegetables*

All main entrees are freshly prepared and cooked to order

SWEETS AND SAVORIES

PANNA COTTA
Custard Cream in a Swath of Caramel Sauce Topped with Whipped Cream Curls

TIRAMISU
Homemade Ladyfingers Soaked in Espresso Coffee and Layered with Mascarpone Cream

CROSTATA GENOVESE
A Typical Italian Sweet Crust Filled with Apricot Preserves

SELECTION OF ITALIAN CHEESES AND CRACKERS

SEASONAL FRESH FRUIT PLATE

BUON APPETITO!

PRINCESS CRUISES   GRAND PRINCESS

THE PAINTED DESERT RESTAURANT

APPETIZERS

JALISCO GUACAMOLE
A Mexican Favorite, Homemade Guacamole Dip
Prepared by Your Waiter Table-Side According to Your Request

RAINBOW QUESADILLA
Monterey Jack and Cheddar Cheese Quesadilla Topped with Spicy Colored Pepper Strips

THE SUPREME TARTLET
A Spicy Mixture of Beef and Cheese, Served with a Tomatilla Salsa

SAVORY TORTILLAS
Brie Filled Tortillas, Presented on a Papaya-Poblano Salsa

THE EL PASO ROLL UP
A Mixture of Lean Pork Meat Chili, Tomatoes, Cream Cheese and Nopalitos,
Topped with Sour Cream Served with Guacamole

SOUP
Rancho Santa Fe Tortilla Soup

SALAD

SOUTH OF THE BORDER CAESAR SALAD
Served with El Cliente Dressing and Topped with Polenta Croutons

TACO SALAD
Served with Shredded Beef, Refried Beans, Lettuce and Tomato. Topped with Salsa Fresca

NOGALES SALAD
A Combination of Shredded Lettuce and Vegetables Served in a Flour Tortilla Shell
Topped with Spicy Chicken Breast. Served with a Lime-Cilantro Vinaigrette

VEGETARIAN

VEGETARIAN CHILI
A Spicy Combination of Beans, Tomato, Mushrooms. Served with Corn Tortillas

TOFU TACOS
A Saute of Tofu, Cilantro, Yellow Peppers and Tomato. Garnished with Chopped Walnuts

ENTRÉES

SHRIMP QUESADILLAS
Flour Tortillas Filled with Marinated Shrimp and Mango-Jalapeño Salsa

HACIENDA CHOPPED SIRLOIN
A Mixture of Chopped Sirloin with Garlic and Poblano Chili.
Served with Avocado and Salsa Fresca

SWORDFISH PADRE ISLAND
Grilled Swordfish Steak Served with a Curry-Pepper Chili Sauce

TRADITIONAL CHICKEN FAJITAS
Tender Strips of Free Range Chicken Complemented by a Mosaic of Bell Pepper, Red Bermuda
Onions and Tomatoes in the Old Fashion Style (Served on a Traditional Fajita Plate)

DESSERT

SPICY PUMPKIN CHEESECAKE
Served with a Blueberry Coulis

SANTA FE MARGUERITA
Topped with Fresh Fruit

SOUTHWESTERN DELIGHT
Lime Flan Complemented with Honey Tortilla Strips

APPLE TORTILLAS
Served with a Vanilla Sauce

Courtesy Princess Cruises

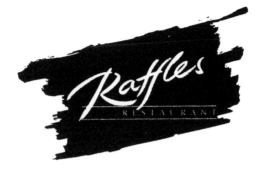

A Taste of Asia

Appetizer   A Selection of Szechuan Appetizers
Lo Han Shrimp - Anise Pork Bites - Crispy Fried Wonton - Sweet Sour Cucumber

Soups   Mandarin Style Chicken and Mushroom

Shrimp and Pea

Seafood   Indonesian Rempah
Chilli Fried Seafood Fritter with Black Bean Ginger Sauce

Entrees   Kung Pao Pork
Cooked Tableside - Red Chillies, Mixed Nuts, Bok Choy, Nonya-Style Sauce

Raffles Duck
Braised Duckling Foukien Style served with Five Spices and Crispy Noodles

Rice   Garlic Fried Rice

Desserts   Tapioca Custard
Mango Nectar

Cream of Fruit Sallis-Style Leche Prita
with Coconut

Kalamay with Maize

Cover and service charge $15.00 per person includes complimentary wines

MARCO POLO

Courtesy Orient Cruise Line

Aboard the

M/v Silver Wind

En Route to Malé, Maldives
Thursday, December 10, 1998

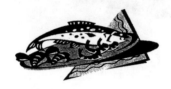

SPECIALITÀ DELLA CUCINA ITALIANA
in the Terrace Cafe

DAL NOSTRO PANETTIERE
Crispy Focaccia and Homemade Grissini

INSALATA MISTA
Assorted Mixed Lettuces with Tomatoes, Cucumbers and Balsamic Vinaigrette
(On Request)

PARMIGIANO REGGIANO
Parmesan Reggiano
(On Request)

GELATI AND FRUTTA FRESCA
Handmade Vanilla Ice Cream and Fresh Fruits

WINES
White Wine: Pinot Bianco, Colli Euganei, D.O.C., Azienda Agricola Vignalta, Italy, 1997
Red Wine: Vino Nobile di Montepulciano, D.O.C.G., Tenuta Lodala Nuova, Tuscany, Italy, 1995

Brian O'Brien   Antonio Amato   Donato Ventura

MENU

ANTIPASTO

**TIMBALLO DI MELANZANE, POLENTA ALLA BRACE GRATINATA
AL FORMAGGIO, PEPERONI ALLA MEDITERRANEA**
Eggplant Terrine, Grilled Polenta Gratinated with Cheese, Marinated Bell Peppers

*****

PASTE

RAVIOLI DI MAGRO AL BURRO FUSO E SALVIA
Handmade Spinach and Cheese Ravioli with Drawn Butter and Sage Sauce

FETTUCCINE ALLA BOSCAIOLA
Fresh Fettuccine Pasta with Fresh Tomato and Mushrooms Sauce

*****

SECONDI PIATTI

PESCE SPADA IN CASSERUOLA
Sword Fish in a Light Tomato, Capers and Olives Sauce

OR

COSTOLETTE DI AGNELLO AL ROSMARINO CON PATATE ARROSTO
Broiled Lamb Chops with Rosemary and Roasted Potatoes

*****

I DOLCI

'TIRAMISU'

*Espresso, Cappucino
Grappa and Limoncello*

Terrace Café, *courtesy Silversea Cruises*

Aboard the

M/V SILVER WIND

En Route to Phuket, Thailand
Tuesday, December 15, 1998

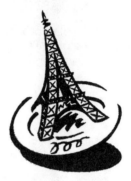

"Tour de France"
in the Terrace Café

In both reality and the popular imagination no other country has approached France in terms of elevating its cuisine to a high art form. In spite of new trends and dietary habits tradition still plays the major role in the French Kitchen. Contemporary French chefs while relying on tradition place at least as much importance today on the quality and flavor of the ingredients. Tonight our Chef de Cuisine, Franck Garanger and Chef, Antonio Amato will echo these themes and they invite you to join them on a grand gastronomic *Tour de France* Our chefs have created tonight's menu not merely to explore the culinary highways and byways of France but to provide you with an extraordinary dining experience that captures the very essence of the country. In perhaps no other country in the world do wine and food complement each other as fittingly as they do in France. This symbiotic relationship between the culinary and oenological arts is no mere accident. As wine styles evolved in areas like Champagne, Burgundy, Bordeaux and the Valley of the Loire regional cuisine evolved to match them. As our chefs take you on a grand culinary tour of the best of contemporary French cuisine you will have an opportunity to try the wines that make such a harmonious match with tonight's dishes.

Brillat-Savarin once said that a day without wine is like a day without sunshine - who would dispute him?

Brian O'Brien	**Antonio Amato**	**Donato Ventura**
Head Sommelier	Chef	Head Waiter

MENU

Assiette d'amuses bouches
Hot Hors d'Oeuvres

Tian de Saint Jacques Tiède sur lit de Ratatouille
Warm Scallops on a Bed of Ratatouille with Assorted Greens
Served with Virgin Sauce

Croustillant de Barbue de Mer et Homard au Beurre blanc
Crispy Fresh John Dorry or Brill o Fillet with Sauce Beurre Blanc
Served on a Bed of Carrot Mousseline with Lobster and "Croquant" Sweet Potatoes

Granité au Champagne et Orange
Refreshing Champagne-Orange Sorbet

Filet de Boeuf roti aux truffes du Perigord
"Recette de ma Grand Mère"
Grandmothers' Recipe for Roast Beef Tenderloin withTruffle Sauce
Served with Garden Fresh Vegetables and Pommes Salardaises
Garnished with Baby Onions, Forest Mushrooms and Strips of Bacon

DESSERT
Tour Eiffel au chocolat et framboises
Chocolate "Eiffel Tower" with Raspberries

Petits Fours et Friandises

Café

VINS FRANÇAIS
Vin Blanc: Clos de Chateau, Chardonnay, Domaine de Chateau de Meursault,
Burgundy, 1993.
Vin Rouge: Château Fombrauge, Grand Crû, St. Emilion, France, 1996

Terrace Café, *courtesy Silversea Cruises*

PALO

Pane Casalingo

Warm Bread from our own Bakery

Pizza

Prepared in our "on-stage" Pizza Oven

Pizza Lucana
Herb-grilled Chicken, Calamata Olives
and Spinach

Pizza del Levante
Funghi Selvaggi e Pesto
Pizza with Roasted Peppers, Wild Mushrooms
and Pesto Sauce

Pizza Palo Chef
Our Chef's Specialty Pizza of the day

Antipasti

Melanzane alla Griglia
Grilled Eggplant with
Triple Tomato Balsamic Relish
and Goat Cheese

Insalata di Rucola alla Palo
Salad Greens with Balsamic Dressing
and shaved Parmesan

Carpaccio alla Cavour
Beef Tenderloin Carpaccio
with stone-ground Mustard Sauce
and a Relish of Tomato,
Red Onion and Citronette

Insalata delle Isole
Fresh Mozzarella and Tomatoes
with extra virgin Olive Oil,
Cracked Black Pepper and
Balsamico di Modena

Calamari alla Veneziana
Lightly-fried Squid with savory
Sauces of Tomato and Garlic

Portobello della Valtellina
Grilled Portobello Mushroom and
Polenta with Shallot Sauce
and shaved Parmesan

Insalata Savoia
Warm Shrimp Salad with
Asparagus and Lemon Dressing

Le Zuppe

Minestrone alla Genovese
A hearty Vegetable Soup

Zuppa ai Frutti di Mare
Traditional Italian Fish Soup
flavored with Basil Leaves

Primi Piatti

Tortelloni alla Granseola
Freshly-made Tortelloni, stuffed
with Crabmeat and Eggplant

Orecchiette alle Verdure
Fire-roasted Vegetables, Garlic,
Basil and shaved Parmesan

Penne del Golfo
Penne Pasta with Pancetta, Onion,
Garlic and spicy Tomato

Ravioli delli Alpi
Homemade Ravioli with Artichoke,
Ricotta Cheese and Oven Dried Tomato

Risotto ai Funghi Selvatici
Risotto with Wild Mushrooms

Secondi Piatti

Pollo Farcito alle Ruspoli
Chicken Breast stuffed with
Vegetables and served with
Roasted Potato and Asparagus

Costolette d' Agnello al Chianti
Rack of Lamb with Chianti Wine Sauce
and Baby Vegetables

Filetto di Vitello alla Bixio
Pan-seared Loin of Veal, served with
Wild Mushroom Sauce

Pesce dello Chef
Pan-sautéed Chef's catch on Risotto
with Olive Tapenade

Dolci

Tiramisú dei Dogi

Soufflé Romantico
Warm Chocolate and Hazelnut Soufflé
with Vanilla Bean Sauce

Panna Cotta della Nonna
A sweet creamy Custard

Cassata alla Siciliana
Honey Citrus-flavored Frozen Custard
with Pistachio Cream

Gelato all' Italiana

Caffè

Cappuccino $2.00
1/3 Espresso, 1/3 Steamed Milk, 1/3 Froth

Espresso $1.50

Caffè Mocha $2.00
1/3 Espresso and Chocolate, 2/3 Steamed Milk,
topped with Whipped Cream

Latte $2.00
1/3 Espresso, 2/3 Steamed Milk

Caffellatte $2.00
1/2 Coffee, 1/2 Steamed Milk

Caffè Melange $2.00
Coffee with Whipped Cream

100% Colombian Coffee

All the above are available decaffeinated

Gran finale

Sambuca Black
Opal Nero $3.95
Italian Anis Liqueur

Amaretto d' Sarenno $3.95
Almond-flavored Italian Liqueur

Grappa $6.95
An old Italian tradition "vinacce"
(distilled from fresh Grape Pomace)

Sorbetto $3.95
Refreshing combination of Vodka,
Champagne and freshly-made
Citron Ice

THE GRILL

APPETIZERS

Cold Gulf Shrimp and Scallops in our own spicy homemade Cocktail Sauce

Refried-Beans and Hot Pepper, Cheese Quesadillas with Pickled Onions

Potato Skins served crispy under melted Cheese, Sour Cream dip

Deep fried Mozzarella, fresh Marinara Sauce

Fire-Roasted Peppers and Marinated Mushrooms with Bitter Green

SOUPS

Boston Clam Chowder

Baked Onion, Three Cheese Croûtons

Bowl of Chili

SALADS

Freshly Torn Romaine Salad with Parmesan and Home-Made Dressing

Sliced Beef Steak Tomato, Red Onion Rings and Scallions

Mixed baby Field Greens

MAIN COURSES

Boneless Breast of Chicken
Grilled with a spicy Southwester Barbecue Sauce

New York Strip Steak
Charbroiled just the way you like it with Baked Potato

Grilled Pork Chop
Rosemary and Lemon marinated, Cranberry-Pear Relish and Garlic Sauce

Broiled Norwegian Salmon
Medley of Vegetables

CHEF'S SPECIAL OF THE DAY
Ask your Waiter about today's selection

Chef's Palette of Vegetables

DESSERTS

Mango Passion Fruit, Cheesecake with Macadamia Nut-Crust

Warm Tarte-Tatin, Caramel Sauce

Crème Brûlée

Joconde Sponge Cake, Hazelnut Mousse, Raspberry and Chocolate

Courtesy Renaissance Cruises

ITALIAN RESTAURANT

ANTIPASTI

Savory layers of Beef-Steak Tomato, Prosciutto and Mozzarella,
crowned with oven-roasted Wild Mushrooms

Paper-thin slices of raw Tenderloin with Olive Oil, Lemon,
shaved Parmesan and Foccacia Crostini

Roasted Eggplant Cakes, mixed Greens, Lemon and Thyme Aïoli

Oven-baked Cheese wrapped in Basil and Parma Ham
on a bed of Baby Leaf Salad and Roast Peppers drizzled with Balsamic Vinaigrette

ZUPPA

ZUPPA DELLO CHEF
See your Waiter for Today's Selection

INSALATE

Caesar Salad with Grated Parmesan, Mustard, marinated Tomato and Foccacia Crôutons

Tender Lettuce Leaves, Roasted Peppers, Olives, toasted Hazelnuts
and charred Herbed Tomato Vinaigrette

PIATTA DEL GIORNO

Spaghetti tossed in a rustic Tomato Sauce and shaved Parmesan

Baked large Green and White Noodles interleaved with
Meat Bolognese, Prosciutto, Porcini and fresh Peas

Tagliatelle with Broccoli, Sugar Snap Peas, Teardrop Tomatoes, Garlic and Extra-Virgin Olive Oil

Fusilli with grilled Chicken, Broccoli, roasted Pine Nuts, Balsamic roasted Chicken Broth,
sundried Tomato and Montrachet Cheese

Mustard and herbed seasoned grilled Salmon, Citrus Vinaigrette,
Sauteed Risotto Cake and Green Beans

Sage Veal Medallions, Prosciutto curls, Grilled Vegetable Polenta on Marsala Wine Sauce

Breast of Chicken, Onion confit, steamed Vegetables,
fresh Garlic and Oregano White Wine

Pan-seared Shrimp and Fettuccine with Tomato, grilled Peppers,
Garlic, Parsley and Extra-Virgin Olive Oil

Grilled Marinated Loin of Beef
Sliced to order, covered with Aged Balsamic Vinegar, Virgin Olive Oil,
Rock Salt, Crushed Pepper, Shallots and Parmesan Chips

DOLCI

Panna Cotta Vanilla Bavaroise with Red Fruits, Caramel Sauce	Cassata Siciliana A Frozen Pistacchio Mousse with Maraschino Liquor
Tiramisu A Classic Italian Dessert with the flavors of Coffee and Chocolate	Chaud-Froid of Pear Poached in Red Chianti and Blueberries

Lemon Mascarpone Brûlée Tart
with a nutty pecan flavor

Courtesy Renaissance Cruises

FaxGram
800.341.4770

CUNARD

FaxGram
Document #111

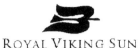

ROYAL VIKING SUN

SAMPLE DINNER MENU

VENEZIA

ANTIPASTI MISTI DAL BUFFET
Selection of Typical Appetizers from the Buffet

ANTIPASTI FREDDI
COLD APPETIZERS

Carpaccio con scaglie di Parmigiano
*Seared Sirloin of Beef sliced thin with shaved parmigiano
reggiano and virgin olive oil caper dressing*

Insalata di mare
*Shrimp, scallops and calamari marinated in wine vinegar
olive oil and lemon juice*

Prosciutto di Parma e melone
*Air-dried cured ham, aged to old Italian
tradition, served with seasonal melon*

ANTIPASTI CALDI
HOT APPETIZERS

Risotto con funghi porcini e crema di tartufo
Cèpes risotto with truffle oil

Pomodori alla Siciliana
*Stuffed tomatoes with olives, sardines, capers, onion,
and garlic bread stuffing, gratinated with parmesan cheese*

Melanzane alla Parmigiana
*layers of aubergines, plum tomatoes, mozzarella cheese
gratinated with parmesan Parma style*

Subject to change without notice.

CUNARD

ROYAL VIKING SUN

SAMPLE DINNER MENU
VENEZIA

PIATTI PRINCIPALI
MAIN COURSE

Costoletta di vitello alla Milanese
Breaded and sautéed veal chop served with saffron risotto

Petto di pollo al rosmarino
Grilled chicken breast served with rosemary potatoes

Filetto di manzo con cipolline glassate
*Grilled tenderloin of beef with glazed red wine onions,
grapes served with polenta*

Fritto di gamberoni al profumo di mare
Jumbo shrimp deep-fried with white wine herb sauce

Fegato alla Veneziana
Calf's liver Venetian style served with Risi-Bisi

Scaloppine al Marsala
Veal scaloppine with marsala wine served with mixed vegetables

Pesce del giorno
Chef's fish choice

CONTORNI E VERDURE - SIDE ORDERS
Risotto alla Milanese
Saffron risotto

Spaghetti, Penne, Fettuccine
Spaghetti, penne, and fettuccine pasta

Polenta alla griglia
Grilled polenta

Verdure primavera
Assorted vegetables

Insalata Mista
Mixed salad

Patate al forno con rosmarino
Rosemary oven-baked potatoes

CUNARD

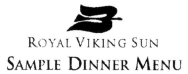

ROYAL VIKING SUN
SAMPLE DINNER MENU

DOLCI
DESSERTS

Tiramisu
Venetian Mascarpone cream

Cassata Siciliana
Vanilla, chocolate, and ricotta iced parfait

Torta di mele e Zabaglione
Warm apple tart with Sabayone

Frutti di bosco con gelato alla crema
Hot mix berries served over vanilla ice cream

Sorbetto al limone e all'arancio
Lemon and orange sorbet served in almond tulip

Scelta di formaggi assortiti
Choice of Italian cheeses

CAFFÉ
COFFEE
Espresso
Cappuccino
American Coffee with or without caffeine

Subject to change without notice.

Courtesy Cunard Line

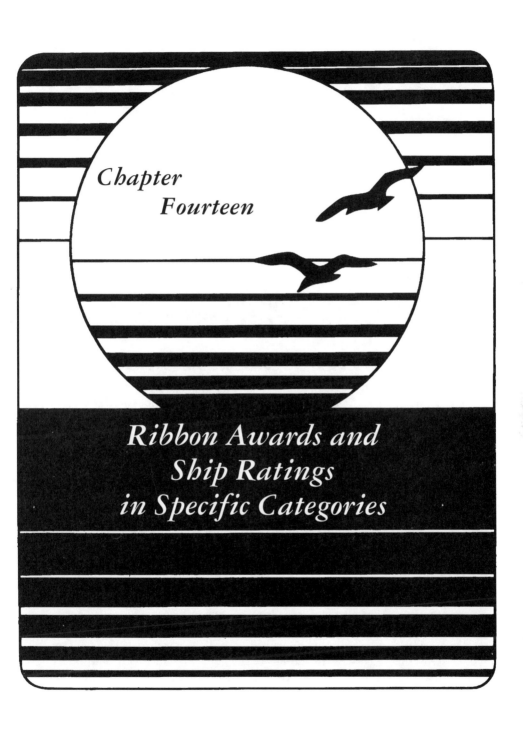

Chapter
  Fourteen

Ribbon Awards and
Ship Ratings
in Specific Categories

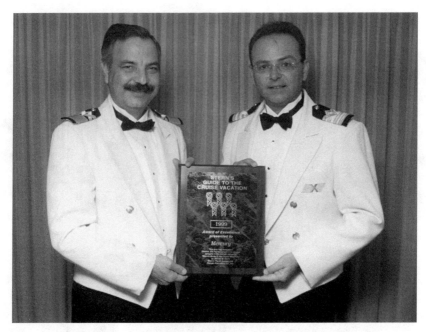

Courtesy Celebrity Cruises

Because the quality of food, service, and entertainment, as well as the general physical condition of ships, is constantly changing, it is risky to attempt to compare or rate cruise ships. Any such attempt must reflect a great deal of personal preference and may be somewhat undependable inasmuch as quality can vary from cruise to cruise on the same ship due to a change in chefs, staff, or company policy. In fact, the quality can even change between the date of this writing and the time you are reading this book.

However, travel agents, potential cruisers, and the cruise industry in general have come to rely upon travel writers' ratings and personal opinions. Having a profound desire to make this guide the most helpful and most valuable cruise guide available, I have succumbed to peer pressure and attempted to rate the ships as definitively as possible.

A system of "Ribbon Awards" (overall ratings) will be found below and after each ship listed previously in chapter 11. In addition, ratings in eleven specific categories will be found for at least one ship from each major cruise line. Again, I must emphasize that these are my personal, subjective opinions, and you may disagree with them after you have cruised on the ships being rated. An intelligent traveler should not take the ratings of any guide as gospel. Obviously, every reviewer has his personal preferences and prejudices that may or may not coincide with your own.

Explanation of Ribbon Awards _____

(overall ratings):

Since all ships are not competing for the same potential passengers, it would be unfair to make overall comparisons of ships with vastly different price structures. Obviously, a ship charging $600 to $1,000 per day per person for an average cabin can afford to give its affluent customers more than one charging $150. Therefore, the various vessels have been divided into four major market categories. As was pointed out in chapter 2, pricing policies of cruise lines are confusing, if not deceptive. Therefore, my division into major market categories is not only based upon published fares, but also upon on-board costs, air-sea packages, the economic passenger market the line seeks to attract, and the market it actually does attract.

CATEGORY A—DELUXE:

"Black ribbon awards" are given to ships competing for business at the top of the market for the affluent, mature traveler whose prime consideration is not cost: minimum cabin in excess of $400 per person per day; average cabin about $500 to $700 per person per day; and top suites may go from $750 to $1,500 per person per day.

CATEGORY B—PREMIUM:

"Crisscrossed ribbon awards" are given to ships competing for business between the middle- and top-priced cruise markets for the upper-middle-class segment: minimum cabin in excess of $300 per person per day; average cabin about $350 to $450 per person per day; and suites may go from $450 to $750 per person per day.

CATEGORY C—STANDARD/MASS MARKET:

"Diagonal ribbon awards" are given to ships competing for business in the middle-priced cruise markets for travelers looking for bargains without sacrificing the total cruise experience: minimum cabin in excess of $175 per person per day; average cabin about $200 to $275 per person per day; and suites may go from $350 to $600 per person per day.

CATEGORY D—ECONOMY:

"White ribbon awards" are given to ships competing for business in the economy cruise market for singles, younger cruisers, and bargain hunters wishing to experience a good time on a cruise but willing to sacrifice comfort, food, and service for price savings: minimum cabin about $100 per person per day; average cabin about $150 to $200 per person per day.

Note: Rates referred to above are based on published prices. In reality, almost every cruise line offers an array of discounted fares that may average considerably less than the official published fare.

Note: Some ships and cruise lines overlap categories and therefore have been assigned "split designations." An "A/B" (black ribbon/crisscross ribbon) category reflects a ship that provides a product geared to travelers who prefer a luxury vessel at a lower price without some of the amenities or bells and whistles as are included on the pure luxury vessels. A "B/C" (crisscross ribbon/diagonal ribbon) category is reserved for ships that cannot quite be described as premium because of condition, age, décor, or facilities, yet provides passengers a higher-level cruise experience than those in the mass-market division.

An award of six ribbons in any given market category—A, B, C, or D—represents overall excellence in dining, service, accommodations, entertainment, facilities, itineraries, condition of the ship, and creature comfort relative to the particular market category. We have given a rating of six-plus ribbons to a limited number of luxury ships where the attention to passenger comfort and satisfaction is so extraordinary as to entitle these vessels to special recognition. Five ribbons represent that the vessel is very good in most areas, although it may be excellent or average in some. Three to four ribbons denote a ship that is average to mediocre in most areas. Two ribbons are reserved for those ships that are well below average in most areas, and one ribbon suggests readers should have second thoughts before booking passage.

Because the ships have first been divided into market categories based on price and clientele, it would not be accurate to compare ratings for ships in different market categories. A five-ribbon award given a ship in Category A does not necessarily mean that that ship offers less overall than a six-ribbon award given vessels in Categories B, C, or D. Be certain you compare apples with apples.

A deluxe-category ship is expected to perform at a higher level than a premium or mass-market category vessel; therefore, the standard of excellence required to receive high ratings for the latter category is less stringent. Be careful not to compare our ratings with those in other cruise guides. Some authors have chosen to utilize anywhere from three to ten stars, ribbons, anchors, etc., or opt for a hundred-point evaluation system. The reader must be aware of the range of categories utilized by each reviewer in order to make a valid comparison. (Be advised that most of the smaller riverboats and barges that do not offer a full cruise program have not been rated in this chapter; some ships that have recently changed ownership or that are not marketed in the United States also have not been rated.)

Alphabetical listing of cruise ships with tonnage, market category, and ratings:

Name of Ship	Cruise Line	Tonnage (G.R.T.)	Market Category	Ratings
Adriana	Odessa America	4,600	N/R	N/R
Agean I	Dolphin Hellas	11,563	D	N/R
Aida	Arkona Touristik	38,600	B	4+
Amadeus I and II	Rivers of Europe/Danube Cruises Austria	N/A	N/R	N/R
Amazing Grace	Windjammer Barefoot Cruises	1,585	D	N/R
Ambassador I	Odessa America	2,573	N/R	N/R
American Queen	The Delta Queen Steamboat Company	3,707	B/C	5
Anni	Sheraton Nile Cruises	N/A	N/R	N/R
Apollo	Royal Olympic	28,570	D	2
Arcadia	P & O	63,524	B	N/R
Arkona	Arkona Touristik/Deutsche Seereederei GmbH	18,519	N/R	N/R
Arlene	Aqua Viva Cruise Line	1,375	N/R	N/R
Astor	TransOcean Tours	20,570	N/R	N/R
Astra II	Hapag-Lloyd	10,563	D	4
Asuka	NYK Cruises	28,717	B	N/R
Aton	Sheraton Nile Cruises	N/A	N/R	N/R
Ausonia	Euro Cruises	12,800	D	N/R
Austria	K D River Cruises of Europe	N/A	N/R	N/R
Awani Dream 2	Awani Cruises	17,593	D	N/R

Ship	Cruise Line			
Azur	First European Cruises	15,000	N/R	N/R
Bali Sea Dancer	Classical Cruises	4,000	N/R	N/R
Belorussiya	Odessa America	17,000	N/R	N/R
Berlin	Peter Deilmann EuropAmerica Cruises	9,570	B	N/R
Big Red Boat	Premier Cruise Line	38,772	D	4
Black Prince	Fred Olsen Lines	11,209	N/R	N/R
Black Watch	Fred Olsen Lines	28,000	N/R	N/R
Blue Danube I and II	Europe Cruise Line	N/A	N/R	N/R
Bolero	Euro Cruises	16,107	N/R	N/R
Bremen	Hapag-Lloyd	6,752	B	N/R
Britannia	K D River Cruises of Europe	N/A	N/R	N/R
Caledonian Star	Special Expeditions	3,095	N/R	N/R
Calypso	TransOcean Tours	11,160	N/R	N/R
Carnival Destiny	Carnival Cruise Lines	101,353	B/C	5
Carousel	Airtours/Sun Cruises	23,200	N/R	N/R
Celebration	Carnival Cruise Lines	47,262	C	4
Century	Celebrity Cruises	70,606	B	6
Cezanne I	Rivers of Europe/Danube Cruises Austria	N/A	N/R	N/R
Cezanne II	Rivers of Europe/Danube Cruises Austria	2,500	N/R	N/R
Cinderella	Euro Cruises (Viking Line)	46,398	D	N/R
Clara Schumann	K D River Cruises of Europe	N/A	N/R	N/R
Clelia II	Golden Sea Cruises	4,077	B	N/R
Clipper Adventurer	Clipper Cruise Line	N/A	C	N/R
Club Med II	Club Med Cruises	14,000	B	4+
Columbus	Hapag-Lloyd	14,903	C	N/R

Costa Allegra	Costa Cruise Lines	30,000	B/C	4
Costa Classica	Costa Cruise Lines	54,000	B/C	4+
Costa Marina	Costa Cruise Lines	25,000	C	4
Costa Riviera	Costa Cruise Lines	31,500	C	4
Costa Romantica	Costa Cruise Lines	54,000	B/C	4+
Costa Victoria	Costa Cruise Lines	76,000	B/C	4+
Crown Princess	Princess Cruises	70,000	B	5
Crystal Harmony	Crystal Cruises	49,400	A	6+
Crystal Symphony	Crystal Cruises	50,200	A	6+
Danube Princess	Peter Deilmann EuropAmerica Cruises	N/A	N/R	N/R
Dawn Princess	Princess Cruises	77,000	B	5+
Delta Queen	The Delta Queen Steamboat Company	3,360	C	4
Deltastar	Rivers of Europe/Danube Cruises Austria	1,550	N/R	N/R
Deutschland	K D River Cruises of Europe	1,180	N/R	N/R
Deutschland	Peter Deilmann EuropAmerica Cruises	22,400	A/B	N/R
Discovery Sun	Discovery Cruises	9,903	N/R	N/R
Disney Magic	Disney Cruise Line	83,000	B/C	5-
Disney Wonder	Disney Cruise Line	83,000	B/C	5-
Dolphin IV	Cape Canaveral Cruise Lines	13,000	D	2
Dresden	Peter Deilmann EuropAmerica Cruises	N/A	N/R	N/R
Ecstasy	Carnival Cruise Lines	70,367	C	4+
Edinburgh Castle	Castle Shipping	32,753	D	N/R
Elation	Carnival Cruise Lines	70,367	B/C	5
Enchanted Capri	Black Sea Shipping/Commodore Cruise Line	15,410	D	3
Enchanted Isle	Commodore Cruise Line	23,395	D	3+

Ship	Cruise Line			
Enchantment of the Seas	Royal Caribbean Cruise Line	74,000	B	5+
Europa	Hapag-Lloyd	28,600	A/B	N/R
Esprit	French Country Waterways, Ltd.	N/A	N/R	N/R
Explorer	Abercrombie & Kent	2,398	N/R	N/R
Fair Princess	P & O Holidays	24,724	D	2
Fantasy	Carnival Cruise Lines	70,367	C	4+
Fantome	Windjammer Barefoot Cruises	676	D	N/R
Fascination	Carnival Cruise Lines	70,367	B/C	5
Fedor Dostoyevsky	TransOcean Lines	21,000	D	N/R
Flamenco	Festival Cruises/Euro Cruises	17,270	N/R	N/R
Flying Cloud	Windjammer Barefoot Cruises	400	D	N/R
Fuji Maru	Mitsui OSK	23,340	N/R	N/R
Galapagos Explorer	Galapagos Cruises	3,990	C	N/R
Galaxy	Celebrity Cruises	77,713	B	6
Grand Princess	Princess Cruises	109,000	B	5+
Grande Caribe	American Canadian Caribbean Line	98	D	N/R
Grande Mariner	American Canadian Caribbean Line	98	D	N/R
Grandeur of the Seas	Royal Caribbean Cruise Line	74,000	B	5+
Gripsholm	TransOcean Tours	24,474	N/R	N/R
Hanseatic	Radisson Seven Seas Cruises	9,000	B	N/R
Heinrich Heine	K D River Cruises of Europe	N/A	N/R	N/R
Helvetia	K D River Cruises of Europe	N/A	N/R	N/R
Holiday	Carnival Cruise Lines	46,052	C	4
Horizon	Celebrity Cruises	46,811	B	6
Horizon II	French Country Waterways, Ltd.	N/A	N/R	N/R

Ship	Line			
Hotp	Sheraton Nile Cruises	N/A	N/R	N/R
Illicb	Euro Cruises	8,000	D	N/R
Imagination	Carnival Cruise Lines	70,367	B/C	5
Independence	American Hawaii Cruises	30,090	C	3+
Inspiration	Carnival Cruise Lines	70,367	B/C	5
Isabela II	Metropolitan Touring's Galapagos Cruises	1,083	N/R	N/R
Islandbreeze	Premier Cruise Line	38,175	D	3+
Italia	K D River Cruises of Europe	N/A	N/R	N/R
Jason	Royal Olympic Cruises	5,250	D	2+
Jubilee	Carnival Cruise Lines	47,262	C	4
Kalypso	Euro Cruises/Viking Line	40,000	D	N/R
Konigstein	Sea Air Holidays, Ltd.	N/A	N/R	N/R
La Palma	Intercruise, Ltd.	11,600	C/D	N/R
Le Levant	Ponant Company	3,500	B	N/R
Le Ponant	Ponant Company/Classical Cruises	850	B	N/R
Leeward	Norwegian Cruise Line	25,000	C	N/R
Legacy	Windjammer Barefoot Cruises	1,740	D	N/R
Legend of the Seas	Royal Caribbean Cruise Line	69,130	B	5+
Leisure World	New Century Tours	16,254	D	N/R
Liberte	French Country Waterways, Ltd.	N/A	N/R	N/R
Lili Marleen	Peter Deilmann EuropAmerica Cruises	750	B	N/R
Maasdam	Holland America Line	55,451	B	5+
Majesty of the Seas	Royal Caribbean Cruise Line	73,941	B	5
Mandalay	Windjammer Barefoot Cruises	420	D	N/R
Marco Polo	Orient Lines	22,080	C	5

Ship	Cruise Line	Tonnage		
Mariella	Euro Cruises/Viking Line	37,799	D	N/R
Maxim Gorki	Black Sea Shipping	25,000	D	N/R
Mayan Prince	American Canadian Caribbean Line	98	D	N/R
MegaStar Aries	Star Cruises	3,264	B	5
MegaStar Asia	Star Cruises	33,819	A/B	N/R
MegaStar Taurus	Star Cruises	3,264	B	5
Melanesian Discoverer	Melanesian Tourist Service	630	N/R	N/R
Melody	Mediterranean Shipping Cruises	36,500	C	N/R
Mercury	Celebrity Cruises	77,713	B	6
Mermoz	Paquet Cruises	13,691	D	N/R
Minerva	Swan Hellenic	12,500	N/R	N/R
Mississippi Queen	The Delta Queen Steamboat Company	3,364	C	4
Mistral	First European Cruises	47,900	N/R	N/R
Monarch of the Seas	Royal Caribbean Cruise Line	73,941	B	5
Monterey	Mediterranean Shipping Cruises	21,051	D	N/R
Mozart	Peter Deilmann EuropAmerica Cruises	2,680	B	5+
Nantucket Clipper	Clipper Cruise Line	95	C	N/R
Nenuphar	French Country Waterways, Ltd.	N/A	N/R	N/R
Neptune	Royal Olympic Cruises	4,000	D	2
Niagara Prince	American Canadian Caribbean Line	99	D	N/R
Nieuw Amsterdam	Holland America Line	33,930	B	4+
Nile Goddess	Sonesta Hotels and Nile Cruises	N/A	N/R	N/R
Noordam	Holland America Line	33,930	B	4+
Nordic Empress	Royal Caribbean Cruise Line	48,563	B	4+
Normandie	Aqua Viva Cruise Lines	1,375	N/R	N/R

Ship	Cruise Line	Tonnage	Rating	Ribbon
Norway	Norwegian Cruise Line	76,044	B/C	N/R
Norwegian Capricorn	Norwegian Capricorn Line	28,078	N/R	N/R
Norwegian Crown	Norwegian Cruise Line	40,000	C	N/R
Norwegian Dream	Norwegian Cruise Line	50,760	C	N/R
Norwegian Dynasty	Norwegian Cruise Line	20,000	C	N/R
Norwegian Majesty	Norwegian Cruise Line	32,400	C	N/R
Norwegian Sea	Norwegian Cruise Line	42,000	C	N/R
Norwegian Sky	Norwegian Cruise Line	76,000	B/C	N/R
Norwegian Wind	Norwegian Cruise Line	50,760	C	N/R
Ocean Majesty	Majestic International Cruises	10,417	D	N/R
Ocean Princess	Princess Cruises	77,000	B	5+
Oceanbreeze	Premier Cruise Line	21,486	D	3+
Oceanic (Big Red Boat)	Premier Cruise Line	38,772	D	4
Oceanic Odyssey	Spice Island Cruises	5,218	B	N/R
Odessa	TransOcean Cruises	13,757	D	N/R
Odysseus	Royal Olympic Cruises	12,000	D	2+
Olympic Countess	Royal Olympic Cruises	17,593	D	3
Oriana	P & O Cruises	69,153	B	N/R
Orient Venus	Venus Cruises	21,884	N/R	N/R
Orpheus	Royal Olympic Cruises	5,092	D	2+
Pacific Princess	Princess Cruises	20,000	B	4+
Pacific Venus	Venus Cruises	26,518	N/R	N/R
Panorama I	Classical Cruises	599	N/R	N/R
Paradise	Carnival Cruise Lines	70,367	B/C	5
Paul Gauguin	Radisson Seven Seas Cruises	18,800	A	6

Pegasus	Royal Olympic Cruises	14,000	D	N/R
Polynesia	Windjammer Barefoot Cruises	430	D	N/R
Princess	French Country Waterways, Ltd.	N/A	N/R	N/R
Princess Danae	Classic International Cruises	17,074	D	N/R
Princess de Provence	Peter Deilmann EuropAmerica Cruises	N/A	N/R	N/R
Prussian Princess	Peter Deilmann EuropAmerica Cruises	N/A	N/R	N/R
Queen Elizabeth 2	Cunard Line	70,327	N/R	N/R
(Grill Rooms)			A	6
(Caronia)			A	5+
(Mauretania)			B/C	5
Queen of Holland	Sea Air Holidays, Ltd.	N/A	N/R	N/R
R-1	Renaissance Cruises, Inc.	30,200	A/B	5
R-2	Renaissance Cruises, Inc.	30,200	A/B	5
R-3	Renaissance Cruises, Inc.	30,200	A/B	5
R-4	Renaissance Cruises, Inc.	30,200	A/B	5
Radisson Diamond	Radisson Seven Seas Cruises	20,000	A	6
Reef Endeavor	Captain Cook Cruises	3,500	N/R	N/R
Regal Empress	Regal Cruises	23,000	D	N/R
Regal Princess	Princess Cruises	70,000	B	5
Rembrandt	Premier Cruise Line	38,645	C	4
Renaissance VII-VIII	Renaissance Cruises, Inc.	4,500	A/B	5
Rhapsody	Mediterranean Shipping Company	17,495	C	N/R
Rhapsody of the Seas	Royal Caribbean Cruise Line	78,941	B	5+
Rhine Princess	Europe Cruise Line	N/A	N/R	N/R
River Cloud	Abercrombie & Kent/	N/A	N/R	N/R

Ship	Line			
Rotterdam VI	Holland America Line	60,000	B	5+
Rousse	Rivers of Europe/Danube Cruises Austria	1,295	N/R	N/R
Royal Clipper	Star Clipper Cruises	5,000	B	N/R
Royal Princess	Princess Cruises	44,348	B	5
Royal Star	Star Lines/Sea Air Holidays	5,360	D	N/R
Ryndam	Holland America Line	55,451	B	5+
Saga Rose	Saga Holidays	25,147	C	N/R
Santa Cruz	Metropolitan Touring's Galapagos Cruises	1,500	C	N/R
Sapphire	Thompson Cruises	12,183	D	N/R
Sea Bird	Special Expeditions	100	D	N/R
Sea Cloud	Special Expeditions	2,323	A	N/R
Seabourn Legend	Cunard/Seabourn Line	10,000	A	6+
Seabourn Pride	Cunard/Seabourn Line	10,000	A	6+
Seabourn Goddess I and II	Cunard/Seabourn Line	4,250	A	6+
Seabourn Spirit	Cunard/Seabourn Line	10,000	A	6+
Seabourn Sun	Cunard/Seabourn Line	37,845	A	6+
Seabreeze 1	Premier Cruise Line	21,000	D	3+
Seawind Crown	Premier Cruise Line	23,306	D	3+
Seawing	Airtours/Sun Cruises	16,607	D	N/R
Sensation	Carnival Cruise Lines	70,367	B/C	5
Silja Europa	Silja Line	59,914	D	N/R
Silja Festival	Silja Line	34,419	D	N/R
Silja Finnjet	Silja Line	25,900	D	N/R
Silja Serenade	Silja Line	58,376	D	N/R

Ship	Cruise Line	Tonnage		
Silja Symphony	Silja Line	58,376	D	N/R
Silver Cloud	Silversea Cruises, Ltd.	16,700	A	6+
Silver Wind	Silversea Cruises, Ltd.	16,700	A	6+
Sky Princess	Princess Cruises	46,314	B	4+
Song of America	Airtours/Sun Cruises	37,584	C	N/R
Song of Flower	Radisson Seven Seas Cruises	8,282	A	6
Southern Cross	Odessa America	17,270	N/R	N/R
Sovereign of the Seas	Royal Caribbean Cruise Line	73,192	B	5
Spirit of Alaska	Alaska Sightseeing Tours	97	N/R	N/R
Spirit of Columbia	Alaska Sightseeing Tours	89	N/R	N/R
Spirit of Discovery	Alaska Sightseeing Tours	94	N/R	N/R
Spirit of Glacier Bay	Alaska Sightseeing Tours	97	N/R	N/R
Splendour of the Seas	Royal Caribbean Cruise Line	69,130	B	5+
Star Aquarius	Star Cruises	40,000	D	N/R
Star Pisces	Star Cruises	40,000	D	N/R
Star Clipper	Star Clippers, Inc.	3,025	C	4+
Star Flyer	Star Clippers, Inc.	3,025	C	4+
Statendam	Holland America Line	55,451	B	5+
Stella Maris	Royal Olympic Cruises	3,500	C	2+
Stella Oceanis	Royal Olympic Cruises	5,500	C	2+
Stella Solaris	Royal Olympic Cruises	18,000	C	3
Sun Dream	Airtours/Sun Cruises	22,945	D	N/R
Sun Goddess	Sonesta Hotels and Nile Cruises	N/A	N/R	N/R
Sun Princess	Princess Cruises	77,000	B	5+
Sun Vista	Sun Cruises	30,440	C	N/R

Ship	Cruise Line	Tonnage		
SuperStar Capricorn	Star Cruises	28,078	B/C	N/R
SuperStar Gemini	Star Cruises	20,000	C	N/R
SuperStar Leo	Star Cruises	75,000+	B/C	N/R
SuperStar Sagittarius	Star Cruise	18,556	B/C	N/R
SuperStar Virgo	Star Cruises	75,000+	B/C	N/R
Switzerland	Leisure Cruises	15,739	D	N/R
Symphony	Mediterranean Shipping Company	16,500	D	N/R
Terra Australis	Odessa America	1,899	N/R	N/R
Theodor Fontane	K D River Cruises of Europe	N/A	N/R	N/R
Topaz	Thompson Cruises	31,500	D	2+
Triton	Royal Olympic Cruises	14,100	D	4
Tropicale	Carnival Cruise Lines	36,674	C	N/R
Tut	Sheraton Nile Cruises	N/A	N/R	N/R
Universe Explorer	World Explorer Cruises	23,500	D	5+
Veendam	Holland America Line	55,451	B	N/R
Victoria	P & O Cruises	27,670	C	N/R
Viking Princess	Palm Beach Cruise Line	6,422	N/R	4
Viking Serenade	Royal Caribbean Cruise Line	40,132	B	5+
Vision of the Seas	Royal Caribbean Cruise Line	78,491	B	5+
Vistafjord	Cunard Line	24,492	A	5+
Volendam	Holland America Line	63,000	B	N/R
Volga	Rivers of Europe/Danube Cruises Austria	2,125	N/R	N/R
Wasa Queen	Silja Line	16,500	D	N/R
Westerdam	Holland America Line	53,872	B	5
Wilhelm Tell	K D River Cruises of Europe	N/A	N/R	N/R

Ship	Cruise Line			
Wind Song	Windstar Cruises	5,350	A/B	5+
Wind Spirit	Windstar Cruises	5,350	A/B	5+
Wind Star	Windstar Cruises	5,350	A/B	5+
Wind Surf	Windstar Cruises	14,745	A/B	5+
World Discover	Society Expeditions	3,153	N/R	N/R
World Renaissance	Royal Olympic Cruises	11,724	D	2+
Yankee Clipper	Windjammer Barefoot Cruises	327	D	N/R
Yangtze Angel	Europe Cruise Line	N/A	B	N/R
Yorktown Clipper	Clipper Cruise Line	97	C	N/R
Zenith	Celebrity Cruises	47,225	B	6

Note: "N/R" indicates that ship was not rated due to changes that have occurred since most recent investigation of ship or author has not recently sailed on ship.

Explanation of Ship Ratings _____

All ships are not excellent, good, or bad across the board; and some excel in one area and fall short in others. For example, there are several Category A—Deluxe Ships that are known for impeccable food and service and fine accommodations, yet offer little entertainment and activities and could be poor choices for younger singles or children. On the other hand, some Category D—Economy Ships have only passable food and service, numerous small or inadequate cabins, yet provide so much fun and entertainment that less demanding, budget-minded, younger cruisers would have a more rewarding experience.

For the purpose of these more detailed ratings, I chose ships from each major cruise line upon which I most recently cruised. The vessel rated is not necessarily the best in the line, and its ratings may not be identical to those of the cruise company's other ships.

I have used a simple five-point system:

*****	excellent	(the best available at sea)
****	very good	(one notch below the best, but better than most)
***	good	(average)
**	fair	(below average)
*	poor	(a rose by any other name)

Explanation of Categories _____

The following thirty ships are ranked according to how they measure up in the following eleven categories:

Food—variety, quantity, and wholesomeness

Gourmet Dining—gourmet quality of food, preparation, presentation, caliber of wines, tableside preparations, and availability of special orders

Service in Dining Rooms

Service in Cabins

Activities and Entertainment—quantity and quality

Average Cabin—spaciousness, decor, and facilities included

Outside Deck Area—spaciousness for passenger capacity, condition, decor, and facilities available

Inside Public Area—spaciousness for passenger capacity, condition, decor, and facilities available

Physical Condition of Ship, Public Areas, and Cabins

Special Activities and Facilities for Children

Good Ship for Singles

	Food	Gourmet Dining	Service in Dining Rooms	Service in Cabins
American Hawaii Cruises *Independence*	★★★★	★★★+	★★★	★★★
Carnival Cruise Lines *Destiny*	★★★★★	NR	NR	NR
Carnival Cruise Lines *Elation Imagination Inspiration Fascination Paradise Sensation*	★★★★+	★★★★	★★★★	★★★★+
Celebrity Cruises *Century Galaxy Mercury*	★★★★★	★★★★★ (dining room)/ ★★★★+ (other)	★★★★★	★★★★+
Celebrity Cruises, Inc. *Horizon Zenith*	★★★★★	★★★★★ (dining room)/ ★★★★+ (other)	★★★★★	★★★★★
Club Med Cruises *Club Med II*	★★★★+	★★★★	★★★+	★★★+
Costa Cruise Lines *Costa Victoria*	★★★★+	★★★+	★★★+	★★★+
Crystal Cruises *Crystal Harmony Crystal Symphony*	★★★★★	★★★★+ (dining room)/ ★★★★★ (specialty restaurants)	★★★★★	★★★★★

Activities and Entertainment	Average Cabin	Outside Deck Area	Inside Public Area	Physical Condition of Ship, Public Areas, and Cabins	Special Activities and Facilities for Children	Good Ship for Singles
***	***	**	**	*	***	*** (young) **** (mature, over 60)
*****	*****	*****	*****	*****	*****	*****
****+	****+	*****	*****	*****	****	***** (young) *** (mature, over 60)
****+	*****	*****	*****+	*****	****	****
****+	****+	****+	*****	*****	****	****
**	****+	****	***	****	**	****
****	****	****	****	****+	****+	****
*****	*****	*****	*****	*****	**	** (young) **** (mature, over 60

	Food	*Gourmet Dining*	*Service in Dining Rooms*	*Service in Cabins*
Cunard Line *Coronia* (Formerly *Vistafjord*)	*****	***** (grill rooms) **** (other rooms)	***** (grill rooms) ****+ (other rooms)	****+
Cunard Line *Queen Elizabeth II*	****+	****+	****+	****+
Cunard/Seabourn Line *Seabourn Goddess I* *Seabourn Goddess II*	*****+	*****+	*****+	*****
Cunard/Seabourn Line *Seabourn Legend* *Seabourn Pride* *Seabourn Spirit*	*****	*****	*****+	*****
Cunard/Seabourn Line *Seabourn Sun*	*****	*****	*****	*****
Peter Deilmann EuropAmerica Cruises *Mozart*	*****	****+	****	****+
The Delta Queen Steamboat Company *American Queen*	*****	****	***+	***+
Disney Cruise Line *Disney Magic* *Disney Wonder*	*****	**** (dining rooms) *****+ (Palo)	****	****

Activities and Entertainment	Average Cabin	Outside Deck Area	Inside Public Area	Physical Condition of Ship, Public Areas, and Cabins	Special Activities and Facilities for Children	Good Ship for Singles
****+	****	****	****+	****	****	****
****	****+	***+	****	***+	*	* (young) ***** (mature, over 60)
**	****+	****	****	*****	*	*
****	*****	****+	*****	*****	*	***
****+	****+	****	*****	*****	*	** (young) **** (mature, over 60)
***	****+	**+	****	*****	**	**
****+	****+	***	*****	*****	**	** (young) **** (mature, over 60)
****	*****	*****	*****	*****	*****+	**

	Food	*Gourmet Dining*	*Service in Dining Rooms*	*Service in Cabins*
Holland America Line *Maasdam* *Rotterdam VI* *Ryndam* *Statendam* *Veendam*	*****	****	****+	****+
Holland America Line *Westerdam*	*****	****+ (dining room) **** (other)	****+	****+
K D River Cruises of Europe *Deutschland*	****	****	****+	***+
K D River Cruises of Europe *Austria* *Britannia* *Italia*	***	***+	****	***+
Orient Lines *Marco Polo*	*****	****+ (dining room) ***+ (other)	****+	****+
Premier Cruise Line *Oceanic*	****+	**** (dining room) *** (cafe)	****	****
Princess Cruises *Dawn Princess* *Sea Princess* *Sun Princess* *Grand Princess*	*****	****	****+	****+
Radisson Seven Seas Cruises *Radisson Diamond*	*****	*****	*****	*****

Activities and Entertainment	Average Cabin	Outside Deck Area	Inside Public Area	Physical Condition of Ship, Public Areas, and Cabins	Special Activities and Facilities for Children	Good Ship for Singles
****+	****	*****	*****	*****	***+	** (young) ***** (mature, over 60)
*****	****	****	****	****	****	*****
*	**+	**	**	*****	*	*
*	**	**	**	****	*	*
****	***+	***	****	****+	**	**
****	***+ (some) **** (some)	***	***	***	*****	**** (young) ** (mature)
****+	****	*****	*****+	*****	*****	****
***	*****	*****	*****	*****	**	**

	Food	Gourmet Dining	Service in Dining Rooms	Service in Cabins
Radisson Seven Seas Cruises *Paul Gauguin*	*****	*****	*****	****+
Radisson Seven Seas Cruises *Song of Flower*	*****	*****	*****+	*****
Renaissance Cruises, Inc. *Renaissance VII-VIII*	*****	****+	*****	*****
Renaissance Cruises, Inc. *R-1* *R-2* *R-3* *R-4*	*****	****+	*****	*****
Royal Caribbean *Enchantment of the Seas* *Grandeur of the Seas* *Legend of the Seas* *Rhapsody of the Seas* *Splendour of the Seas* *Vision of the Seas*	*****	****	****	*****
Royal Olympic Cruises *Stella Solaris*	****	***+	****	****
Silversea Cruises, Ltd. *Silver Cloud* *Silver Wind*	*****	*****	*****	*****
Star Clippers, Inc. *Star Clipper* *Star Flyer*	****	***	****+	***
Windstar Cruises *Wind Song* *Wind Spirit* *Wind Star*	*****	****+	****	****+
Windstar Cruises *Wind Surf*	*****	****+	****	****+

Activities and Entertainment	*Average Cabin*	*Outside Deck Area*	*Inside Public Area*	*Physical Condition of Ship, Public Areas, and Cabins*	*Special Activities and Facilities for Children*	*Good Ship for Singles*
***+	*****	***+	*****	*****	**	**
****	****	****	*****	*****	**	**
**	*****+	**+	*****	*****	*	**
****	****	*****	*****+	*****+	**	**
*****	****+	*****	*****	*****	****+	****
***	***	**	**	**	**	***
****	*****+	*****	*****	*****	*	**
*	***	**	**	***	**	**
**	****+	***	***	*****	**	**
**	****+	****+	****+	*****	**	**

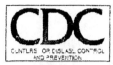

CDC

CENTERS OF DISEASE CONTROL AND PREVENTION

SUMMARY OF SANITATION INSPECTIONS ON INTERNATIONAL CRUISE SHIPS (Green Sheet)

-Summary of the Week ending April 30, 1999 (Updated Every 2 Weeks)
*Indicates inspections during the previous 2 weeks (See notes on page 2)

NAME OF VESSEL	DATE OF INSPECTION	SCORE	NAME OF VESSEL	DATE OF INSPECTION	SCORE
AMERICANA	06/27/98	75	INSPIRATION	12/14/98	91
ARCADIA	01/29/99	90	*ISLAND ADVENTURE	04/17/99	90
ARKONA	03/14/98	89	ISLANDBREEZE	02/07/99	91
ASTOR	01/15/99	91	ISLAND DAWN	09/28/98	86
ASUKA	07/05/98	88	ISLAND PRINCESS	09/02/98	88
BOLERO	03/20/98	94	*JUBILEE	04/28/99	80
C. COLUMBUS	09/23/98	92	LEEWARD	03/22/99	93
CARNIVAL DESTINY	02/21/99	94	LEGACY	01/30/99	90
CELEBRATION	01/10/99	95	LEGEND OF THE SEAS	01/23/99	95
*CENTURY	04/24/99	95	MAASDAM	03/08/99	87
CLIPPER ADVENTURER	09/30/98	93	MAJESTY OF THE SEAS	01/24/99	94
CLUB MED 2	03/04/99	96	MAYAN PRINCE	02/10/98	94
CONTESSA I	12/03/98	87	MAXIM GORKIY	01/16/99	92
COSTA ROMANTICA	03/14/99	91	MELODY	02/17/99	89
COSTA VICTORIA	03/21/99	94	MERCURY	10/18/98	97
CROWN PRINCESS	02/04/99	93	MONARCH OF THE SEAS	04/11/99	98
*CRYSTAL HARMONY	04/25/99	92	NANTUCKET CLIPPER	03/20/99	90
CRYSTAL SYMPHONY	12/22/98	88	NIAGRA PRINCE	09/24/98	63
DAWN PRINCESS	01/30/99	98	NIEUW AMSTERDAM	05/04/98	80
DELPHIN	02/01/99	92	NIPPON MARU	07/04/98	86
DEUTSCHLAND	01/06/99	79	NOORDAM	04/08/99	93
DISNEY MAGIC	01/29/99	88	NORDIC EMPRESS	03/02/99	96
DISCOVERY SUN	12/03/98	94	NORWAY	03/20/99	92
DOLPHIN IV	01/27/99	59	NORWEGIAN CROWN	03/28/99	94
ECSTASY	02/08/99	87	NORWEGIAN DREAM	04/10/99	99
EDINBURGH CASTLE	03/09/98	86	NORWEGIAN DYNASTY	10/09/98	95
ELATION	03/28/99	96	NORWEGIAN MAJESTY	09/20/98	91
EMERALD	02/27/99	89	NORWEGIAN SEA	03/07/99	89
ENCHANTED CAPRI	01/08/99	95	NORWEGIAN WIND	11/15/98	95
ENCHANTED ISLE	01/09/99	96	*OCEANBREEZE	04/23/99	89
ENCHANTMENT OF			OCEANIC	03/29/99	95
THE SEAS	10/25/98	97	ORIANA	03/14/99	93
EUROPA	03/20/98	88	PALM BEACH PRINCESS	11/11/98	88
FANTASY	01/28/99	87	PARADISE	12/06/98	95
FASCINATION	02/28/99	99	PAUL GAUGUIN	12/27/98	86
FLAMENCO	04/10/99	94	QUEEN ELIZABETH 2	01/13/99	87
GALAXY	11/20/98	97	RADISSON DIAMOND	04/12/99	95
GRAND PRINCESS	11/08/98	94	*REGAL EMPRESS	04/27/99	94
*GRANDE CARIBE	04/24/99	92	REGAL PRINCESS	03/08/99	97
GRANDE MARINER	01/15/99	92	REMBRANDT	11/28/98	78
GRANDEUR OF THE SEAS	12/15/98	98	REGAL VOYAGER	10/26/98	88
HANSEATIC	10/05/98	92	*RHAPSODY OF THE SEAS	04/26/99	95
HOLIDAY	03/15/99	89	*ROTTERDAM VI	04/26/99	97
HORIZON	01/08/99	94	ROYAL PRINCESS	02/24/99	94
IMAGINATION	12/05/98	91	*ROYAL VIKING SUN	04/24/99	87

NAME OF VESSEL	DATE OF INSPECTION	SCORE	NAME OF VESSEL	DATE OF INSPECTION	SCORE
RYNDAM	02/02/99	95	TOPAZ	10/17/98	92
SEA BIRD	10/29/98	89	TROPICALE	03/22/99	88
SEA GODDESS I	04/15/99	95	UNIVERSE EXPLORER	06/20/98	95
SEA LION	05/15/98	97	VEENDAM	03/07/99	87
SEA PRINCESS	02/20/99	94	VICTORIA	03/08/99	92
SEABOURN LEGEND	04/09/99	91	VIKING SERENADE	02/05/99	88
SEABOURN PRIDE	04/16/99	95	VISION OF THE SEAS	03/02/99	87
*SEABREEZE I	04/18/99	87	VISTAFJORD	03/30/99	96
SENSATION	03/07/99	93	WESTERDAM	12/12/98	92
SILVER CLOUD	12/28/98	91	WIND SPIRIT	11/22/98	93
SILVER WIND	03/27/99	96	WORLD DISCOVERER	08/21/98	89
*SKY PRINCESS	04/27/99	89	YORKTOWN CLIPPER	05/24/98	91
SONG OF AMERICA	01/17/99	94	ZENITH	01/18/99	93
SOVEREIGN OF THE SEAS	01/11/99	87			
SPIRIT OF COLUMBIA	09/03/98	89			
SPLENDOUR OF THE SEAS	01/06/99	94			
STATENDAM	02/11/99	93			
STELLA SOLARIS	04/14/99	93			
SUN PRINCESS	02/16/99	93			
SUPERSTAR CAPRICORN	04/03/98	70			

Legend: All passenger cruise ships arriving at U.S. Ports are subject to unannounced inspection under the voluntary cooperative inspection program. The purpose of these inspections is to achieve levels of sanitation that will minimize the potential for gastrointestinal disease outbreaks on these ships. Such outbreaks are infrequent, but may be serious when they do occur. Ships are rated on the following items to determine if they meet CDC sanitation standards, **1. Water; 2. Food preparation and holding; 3. Potential contamination of food; 4. General cleanliness, storage and repair.**

Note: Every vessel that has a foreign itinerary and that carries 13 or more passengers is subject to twice-yearly inspections and, when necessary, to reinspection by the Centers for Disease Control and Prevention (CDC). To ensure a clean and healthful environment, cruise ships must meet the criteria established by CDC. The score a ship receives after inspection is published every 2 weeks in the Summary of Sanitation Inspections of International Cruise Ships, commonly referred to as the Green Sheet. The ship's level of sanitation is acceptable to CDC if its score on the inspection is 86% or higher. For further information, contact:

Vessel Sanitation Program
National Center for Environmental Health
Centers for Disease Control and Prevention
1850 Eller Drive, Suite 101
Ft. Lauderdale, FL 33316

Telephone: (954) 356-6650
Fax: (954) 356-6671

Scoring Criteria: In the past, a score of 86 or higher was reported as Satisfactory and a score of 85 and below was reported as Not Satisfactory. Ships unable to achieve at least 86 on a routine periodic inspection will receive a reinspection within a reasonable time frame depending on ship schedules and receipt of the "Statement of Corrective Action" from the ship management.

A score of 86 or higher at the time of inspection indicated that the ship is providing and accepted standard of sanitation. In general, the score, the lower the level of sanitation; however, a low score does not necessarily imply and imminent risk to an outbreak of gastrointestinal disease. CDC reserves the right to recommend that a ship not sail when circumstances so dictate (such as, but not restricted to, contamination of the potable water supply of inadequate treatment of the potable water supply).

Index

CRUISE LINES

CRUISE SHIPS

PORTS OF CALL